Public Health in a Nuclear Disaster
Message from Fukushima

Edited by Seiji Yasumura 1) and Kenji Kamiya 2)

1) Professor, Department of Public Health, Fukushima Medical University School of Medicine, Member, Radiation Medical Science Center for the Fukushima Health Management Survey, Fukushima Medical University

2) Vice President (Reconstruction Support/Radiation Disaster Medicine), Program Director, Phoenix Leader Education Program (Hiroshima Initiative) for Renaissance from Radiation Disaster, Hiroshima University/Vice President, Fukushima Medical University

Authors (in order of writing)

Makoto Akashi	Executive Director, National Institute of Radiological Sciences
Misao Hachiya	Chief, Planning and Promotion Section, Radiation Emergency Medical Assistance Team (REMAT), National Institute of Radiological Sciences
Akira Ohtsuru	Professor, Department of Radiation Health Management, Fukushima Medical University School of Medicine
Kotaro Ozasa	Chief, Department of Epidemiology, Radiation Effects Research Foundation
Yasumasa Fukushima	Councillor, Minister's Secretariat, Ministry of Agriculture, Forestry and Fisheries (MAFF)
Nobuhiro Nakamura	Manager, Health Promotion Division, Public Health and Welfare Department, Fukushima Prefecture
Kenji Sasahara	Director, Fukushima Institute of Public Health
Toshikatsu Shinka	Director, Iwaki City Public Health Centre
Ryoko Miyata	Head/Deputy Director, Kennan Public Health and Welfare Office, Fukushima Prefecture
Ayako Furuyama	Children and Families Division, Public Health and Welfare Department, Fukushima Prefecture
Yukio Endo	Executive Director, Ken-poku Public Health and Welfare, Fukushima Prefecture
Koichi Abe	Director, Koriyama City Public Health Center
Keiko Saito	Chief, Public Health Nurses, Midwives and Nurses Support Section, General Affairs Division, Koriyama City Public Health Center
Yukie Takahashi	Public Health and Welfare Division, Health and Welfare Department, Aizu Public Health and Welfare Office, Fukushima Prefecture
Tomoko Yuda	Chief, Minamiaizu Public Health and Welfare Office, Fukushima Prefecture
Yumiko Toshima	Minamiaizu Public Health and Welfare Office, Fukushima Prefecture
Keiko Abe	Deputy Director/Chief, Tomioka Town
Yuko Owada	Tomioka Town
Maimi Kato	Tomioka Town
Sachiko Inoi	Chief, Health Promotion Section, Health and Welfare Division, Futaba Town
Yumiko Sawada	Chief, Public Health Center, Okuma Town
Keiko Ikari	Chief, Public Health Section, Public Health Division, Kawauchi Village
Yukie Tamane	Residents Welfare Division, Naraha Town
Ryoko Yoshida	Deputy Manager/Head of Radiation Health Management Section, Health and Insurance Division, Namie Town
Kimie Yoshida	Head, Health Promotion Section, Health and Insurance Division, Namie Town
Mihoko Suzuki	Chief, Health Promotion Section, Health and Insurance Division, Namie Town
Chikako Kai	Chief, Health Promotion Section, Health and Insurance Division, Namie Town
Takayo Nemoto	Chief, Nursing Care Insurance Section, Nursing Care and Welfare Division, Namie Town
Tomoko Matsumoto	Head/Chief, Health and Welfare Section, Residents and Living Division, Katsurao Village
Shigeru Nemoto	Head, Public Health Division, Hirono Town
Kazuma Komatsu	Leader, Public Health Division, Hirono Town
Marie Monma	Director, Health Center, Public Health Division, Hirono Town
Keiko Sakuma	Chief, Public Health Division, Hirono Town
Kumiko Matsuda	Technical Chief/Head, Health Promotion Section, Health and Welfare Division, Iitate Village
Mariko Oishi	Health Planning Section, Health Promotion Division, Health and Welfare Department, Minamisoma City
Hitomi Shigihara	Chief, Health Planning Section, Health Promotion Division, Health and Welfare Department, Minamisoma City
Chiharu Okazaki	Chief, Nutritional Management Division, Medical Technology Department, Minamisoma City General Hospital
Yukiko Sugimoto	Chief, Health Promotion Section, Health Promotion Division, Health and Welfare Department, Minamisoma City

Yukiko Iga	Chief, Health Promotion Section, Health Promotion Division, Health and Welfare Department, Minamisoma City
Ikuko Watabe	Manager/Health Guidance Section Chief, Public Health Division, Tamura City
Hiroko Saito	Director, Kawamata Town Health Center
Seiko Kanno	Chief, Maternal and Child Health Section, Health Promotion Division, Health and Welfare Department, Date City
Kayoko Ito	Chief, Health Promotion Section, Health Promotion Division, Health and Welfare Department, Date City
Kanae Hata	Chief, Public Health Section, Health Promotion Division, Health and Welfare Department, Date City
Yoko Watanabe	Deputy Manager, Health Promotion Division, Health and Welfare Department, Date City
Nobutaka Taniguchi	Chief, Health Planning Section, Health Promotion Division, Health and Welfare Department, Date City
Junko Okubo	Chief, Regional Public Health Section, Health Promotion Division, Fukushima City
Yoko Abe	Manager, Health Promotion Division, Civic Affairs Department, Nihonmatsu City
Yoshino Muroi	Health Promotion Division, Aizuwakamatsu City
Koichi Kida	Director, Kida Clinic/Vice President, Fukushima Medical Association
Joji Ikeyama	Director, Arai Dental Clinic/Director, Fukushima Dental Association
Yutaka Tanaka	Managing Director, Fukushima Dental Association
Masahiro Ando	Former Managing Director, Fukushima Dental Association
Osamu Kaneko	President, Fukushima Dental Association
Midori Suzuki	Senior Director, Fukushima Nursing Association
Yasuo Saito	President, Fukushima Association of Radiological Technologists
Hideo Sakurai	Kenkou Yakkyoku Pharmacy/President, Fukushima Pharmaceutical Association
Kazuyuki Yamaguchi	President, Fukushima Physical Therapy Association
Hidenori Oriuchi	Rehabilitation Center, Southern Tohoku Research Institute for Neuroscience
Keiichi Hasegawa	Department of Rehabilitation, Takeda General Hospital/President, Fukushima Association of Occupational Therapists
Keiko Nakamura	President, Fukushima Dietetic Association
Kanae Narui	President, Shirakawa Koriyama Mental Support/Director, Great East Japan Earthquake Reconstruction Project, Fukushima Society of Certified Clinical Psychologists
Seiichi Watanabe	Deputy Manager, Regional Welfare Division, Fukushima Ward Council on Social Welfare
Yohei Imaizumi	Director, Fukushima Acupuncture and Moxibustion Association
Junko Okawara	Former President, Fukushima Association of Medical Social Workers
Aya Goto	Associate Professor, Department of Public Health, Fukushima Medical University School of Medicine
Kenji Kamiya	Vice President (Reconstruction Support/Radiation Disaster Medicine), Program Director, Phoenix Leader Education Program (Hiroshima Initiative) for Renaissance from Radiation Disaster, Hiroshima University/Vice President, Fukushima Medical University
Seiji Yasumura	Professor, Department of Public Health, Fukushima Medical University School of Medicine/Vice Director, Radiation Medical Science Center for the Fukushima Health Management Survey, Fukushima Medical University
Makoto Miyazaki	Assistant Professor, Department of Radiation Health Management, Fukushima Medical University School of Medicine

English Proofreading

Dion Clingwall	Associate Professor, Graduate School of Biomedical and Health Sciences, Hiroshima University

To People Involved in Public Health throughout Japan
— The disaster is still continuing —

The Great East Japan Earthquake occurred on March 11, 2011.

In Fukushima Prefecture, all residents were not only affected by the earthquake and tsunami, but also were forced to face radiation issues caused by the nuclear power station accident. In particular, roughly more than two hundred thousand, who were forced to be evacuated, experienced great distress and are still forced to live inconvenient lives. Other residents, who were not evacuated, also had a highly painful and severe experience. It will take a good amount of time to heal the emotional wounds inflicted by their unhappy experience. Meanwhile, there are concerns that people's memories might fade with time, and that even the tragedy caused by the disaster might be gradually forgotten, although accidents, such as a leakage of contaminated water, may remind people that the nuclear power station accident has not been settled yet.

I planned to write this book for the following three reasons.

1. Fukushima Prefectural Government/Public Health Centers, municipalities and diverse professional organizations also had had various bad experiences due to aspects of the unexpected nuclear power station accident. However, I do not think that their experiences have been fully conveyed to the national government, nor to all prefectures, municipalities and various professional organizations throughout Japan. What is described in this book is part of the public health activities, which were conducted in Fukushima Prefecture in response to the nuclear disaster. Unfortunately, these activities are relatively unknown throughout Japan.

2. Public health activities conducted in Iwate and Miyagi Prefectures at the time of the Great East Japan Earthquake are considerably well known throughout Japan. Their efforts are compiled in the book "*Public Health in Case of Disaster – What We Can Do*" (editor: Osamu Kunii, Nanzando Co., Ltd., 2012). However, "nuclear disaster," "radioactivity/radiation," and "Fukushima Prefecture" are not mentioned in the book. In addition, there had been no books available that focus on public health in cases of nuclear disaster.

3. The most important reason why I planned to write this book is that those involved in public health in Fukushima Prefecture did not have enough time and energy left to communicate the information, because they were caught up in a large amount of disaster-related work that was newly assigned to them in addition to their routine work. Since they had no experience in disaster-related work and had no appropriate manuals for it, they even had to study how to cope with nuclear disaster. Moreover, their work load was extraordinarily high in terms of both the quality of the services required and the quantity. Nevertheless, public health nurses in Fukushima Prefecture had a belief that those involved in public health in Fukushima Prefecture should have the responsibility to preserve peoples' memories of the accident and make use of the experience gained during the accident to prepare for similar disasters in the future.

In this book, only the minimum information is offered so that contributors do not find it a heavy burden to write a manuscript for this book under difficult circumstances in the aftermath of the earthquake. In any examples, what is described in this book might be less than a tenth of the actual activities. If you require additional information, I recommend you come to see the actual situation in Fukushima Prefecture and collect further information.

The planning of this book was carried out through discussions with the following members of a voluntary study group, which mainly comprises public health nurses: Ms. Ikuko Watabe, Ms. Kiyoko Ono, Ms. Yuko Kuroda, Ms. Megumi Hanazumi, Ms. Yoko Abe, Ms. Ayako Furuyama, Ms. Eiko Inage and Ms. Mari Hashimoto.

Lastly, I would like to extend my heartfelt gratitude to Ms. Mayumi Nakao and Ms. Yumiko Kanai for their cooperation in preparing the publication of this book. If this book contributes to the restoration and reconstruction from the disaster, I shall be extremely happy.

January 2014

Seiji Yasumura

Contents

Chapter 1　What Nuclear Disaster Means　　　1

1　Tokyo Electric Power Company Fukushima Daiichi Nuclear Power Station Accident　　　3

A　Radiation Accident and Nuclear Disaster 3
B　Fukushima Daiichi Nuclear Station Accident and Complex Disaster 4
C　Change in the Screening Level for Contamination 6
D　Effects of Radiation and Radiation Dose 7
E　Exposed Dose of Residents 7
F　Report of the World Health Organization (WHO) 8
G　What are Required for Medical Staff 10

2　Medical Actions Taken to Deal with the Tokyo Electric Power Company Fukushima Daiichi Nuclear Power Station Accident　　　12

A　How the Nuclear Station Accident Occurred 12
B　Initial Actions Following the Nuclear Station Accident 12
C　Actions Taken to Deal with the Disaster by Medical Institutions around the Evacuation Area 14
D　Situation of Radioactive Substances in the Environment and Health Risk 15
E　Long-term Support in Cooperation with Local Community 16

3　Health Effects of Radiation　　　18

A　What Radiation Exposure Means 18
B　Atomic Bomb Radiation 18
C　Follow-up survey Study of Atomic Bomb Survivors 19
　　1　Cancer 20
　　2　Disease other than cancer 21
　　3　Atomic bomb survivors exposed in utero 22
D　Genetic Effects 22
E　Summary of Health Effects 23

Chapter 2　Initiatives of Public Administrations　　25

4　Measures Taken by the Japanese Government　　　27

A　Measures Taken to Deal with the Natural Disaster and Radiation Exposure of Residents 27
　　1　Measures taken in response to the large-scale natural disaster 27
　　2　Measures taken specifically to deal with the Fukushima Daiichi Nuclear Station accident 27
B　Measures Taken for Medium- to Long-term Health Management and to Deal with Anxiety 30
　　1　Measures taken for long-term health management 30
　　2　Measures taken to deal with anxiety of residents and the people of Japan ... 31
C　Points to be Improved in Light of the Measures Taken for this Accident 31
　　1　Measures to be taken during the evacuation of resident "people who need support (vulnerable people) in a disaster" 31
　　2　Development of the mechanism to clarify (estimate) the initial exposed dose 32
　　3　Education of health workers 32

4 Provision of information on various health effects of radiation to people on a routine basis 32

5 Measures Taken by Fukushima Prefecture   34

A Measures Taken to Support the Health of Affected People 34

  1 Coordination to secure regional healthcare experts to be engaged in activities to support the health of evacuees 34

  2 Coordination to dispatch and accept healthcare teams 34

  3 Main activities of the dispatched healthcare teams 38

  4 Issues in requesting the dispatch of healthcare teams 39

  5 Securing experts after the coordination for dispatch ended 39

B Nutritional Management for People Living in Shelters, Temporary Houses, and Other Places 40

C Measures to Deal with Infectious Diseases in Shelters, Temporary Houses, and Other Places 41

D Mental Healthcare for Affected People 41

E Supply of Pharmaceuticals and Other Items 42

F Health Management of the Residents of Fukushima Prefecture Associated with the Nuclear Disaster 42

  1 Performing emergency exposure screening 42

  2 Conducting a survey of radioactive substances contained in food and drinking water 43

  3 Conducting the Fukushima Health Management Survey 43

  4 Distribution of personal dose meters and internal exposure inspection 44

6 Measures Taken by the Soso Public Health and Welfare Office   45

A Measures Taken for Hospitals Immediately after the Occurrence of the Disaster 46

B Measures Taken to Deal with the Nuclear Plant Accident and for the Emergency Exposure Screening 46

C Measures to Deal with Medical Care Weakened Due to the Designation of the Emergency Evacuation-Ready Zonefor the Original Indoor Evacuation Zone 49

D Measures to Deal with the Collapse of Psychiatric Care 54

E Necessity of Disaster Simulation 56

7 Measures Taken by the Iwaki City Public Health Center   57

A Outline of Iwaki City and the Iwaki City Public Health Center 58

B March 11 to April 30, 2011 (up to one month) 58

  1 Situation in the city 58

  2 Situation of the medical institutions in the city 59

  3 Activities at shelters 59

  4 Mental healthcare 60

  5 Radiation screening (emergency exposure screening) 60

  6 Distribution of stable iodine tablets 61

C May 1 to September 30, 2011 (two to seven months) 62

  1 Situation in the city 62

  2 Health management and mental healthcare in shelters 62

  3 Support to the affected areas in the city 63

  4 Measures taken for pets 63

D October 1, 2011 to March 31, 2012 (seven months to one year) 64

  1 Situation in the city 64

  2 Measures taken for radiation health management 64

  3 Measures taken for affected people in the city and evacuees from other municipalities 64

E April 1, 2012 to March 31, 2013 (one year and one month to two years) 66

1   Situation in the city 66
2   Influence of the inflow of population from other areas, such as where the nuclear plant is located, on residents' life 66
F   Important matters required in taking measures to control a disaster 67

8   Measures Taken by the Ken-poku Public Health and Welfare Office   68

A   March 11 to April 30, 2011 (up to one month) 69
   1   Situation 69
   2   Main activities 69
   3   Summary and measures to be taken in the future 69
B   May 1 to September 30, 2011 (two to seven months) 70
   1   Situation 70
   2   Main activities 70
   3   Summary and measures to be taken in the future 70
C   October 1, 2011 to March 31, 2012 (seven months to one year) 71
   1   Situation 71
   2   Main activities 71
   3   Summary and measures to be taken in the future 71
D   April 1, 2012 to March 31, 2013 (one year and one month to two years) 72
   1   Situation 72
   2   Main activities 72
   3   Summary and measures to be taken in the future 73

9   Measures Taken by the Ken-chu Public Health and Welfare Office   74

A   March 11 to April 30, 2011 (up to one month) 75
   1   Situation 75
   2   Main activities 75
   3   Summary and measures to be taken in the future 76
B   May 1 to September 30, 2011 (two to seven months) 77
   1   Situation 77
   2   Main activities 77
   3   Summary and measures to be taken in the future 77
C   October 1, 2011 to March 31, 2012 (seven months to one year) 78
   1   Situation 78
   2   Main activities 78
   3   Summary and measures to be taken in the future 78

10   Measures Taken by the Ken-nan Public Health and Welfare Office   79

A   March 11 to April 30, 2011 (up to one month) 80
   1   Situation of the areas under our jurisdiction and main activities 80
   2   Summary and measures to be taken in the future 82
B   May 1 to September 30, 2011 (two to six months) 82
   1   Situation of the areas under our jurisdiction and main activities 82
   2   Summary and measures to be taken in the future 83
C   October 1, 2011 to March 31, 2012 (seven months to one year) 83
   1   Situation of the areas under our jurisdiction and main activities 83
   2   Summary and measures to be taken in the future 83
D   April 1, 2012 to March 31, 2013 (one year and one month to two years) 84
   1   Main activities 84
   2   Summary and measures to be taken in the future 84

11 Measures Taken by the Koriyama City Public Health Center 88

A March 11 to April 30, 2011 (up to one month) 89
  1 Situation 89
  2 Main activities 89
  3 Summary and measures to be taken in the future 91
B May 1 to September 30, 2011 (two to six months) 91
  1 Situation 91
  2 Main activities 92
  3 Summary and measures to be taken in the future 92
C October 1, 2011 to March 31, 2012 (seven months to one year) 92
  1 Situation 92
  2 Main activities 92
  3 Summary and measures to be taken in the future 93
D April 1, 2012 to March 31, 2013 (one year and one month to about two years) 93
  1 Situation 93
  2 Main activities 94
  3 Summary and measures to be taken in the future 94

12 Measures Taken by the Aizu Public Health and Welfare Office 95

A March 11 to April 30, 2011 (up to one month) 96
  1 Situation 96
  2 Main activities 96
  3 Summary and measures to be taken in the future 98
B May 1 to September 30, 2011 (two to six months) 99
  1 Situation 99
  2 Main activities 99
  3 Summary and measures to be taken in the future 101
C October 1, 2011 to March 31, 2012 (seven months to one year) 101
  1 Situation 101
  2 Main activities 101
  3 Summary and measures to be taken in the future 102
D April 1, 2012 to March 31, 2013 (one year and one month to two years) 102
  1 Situation 102
  2 Main activities 103
  3 Summary and measures to be taken in the future 103

13 Measures Taken by the Minami-Aizu Public Health and Welfare Office 104

A March 11 to April 30, 2011 (up to one month) 105
  1 Situation 105
  2 Main activities 105
  3 Summary and measures to be taken in the future 105
B May 1 to September 30, 2011 (two to six months) 106
  1 Situation 106
  2 Main activities 106
  3 Summary and measures to be taken in the future 106
C October 1, 2011 to March 31, 2012 (seven months to one year) 106
  1 Situation 106
  2 Main activities 107
  3 Summary and measures to be taken in the future 107
D April 1, 2012 to March 31, 2013 (one year and one month to two years) 107
  1 Situation 107
  2 Main activities 107
  3 Summary and measures to be taken in the future 107

Chapter 3   Situation of and Countermeasures by Each Individual Municipality   109

14   Efforts of Tomioka Town   111

A   Residents 114
  1   Nutrition (meals/water) 114
  2   Exercise (environmental improvement) 115
  3   Rest (mind, anxiety, suicide, etc.) 117
  4   Others 118
B   Expectant/nursing mothers and children 119
  1   Nutrition (meals/water) 119
  2   Exercise (environmental improvement) 119
  3   Rest (mind, anxiety, suicide, etc.) 120
  4   Others 121
C   People requiring assistance during a disaster (vulnerable peoplein case of a disaster) 121
  1   Nutrition (meals/water) 121
  2   Exercise (environmental improvement) 122
  3   Rest (mind, anxiety, suicide, etc.) 122
  4   Others 123

15   Efforts of Futaba Town   124

A   Residents 127
  1   Nutrition (meals/water) 127
  2   Exercise (environmental improvement) 128
  3   Rest (mind, anxiety, suicide, etc.) 129
  4   Others 130
B   Expectant/nursing mothers and children 132
  1   Nutrition (meals/water) 132
  2   Exercise (environmental improvement) 133
  3   Rest (mind, anxiety, suicide, etc.) 133
  4   Others 134
C   People requiring assistance during a disaster (vulnerable people in case of a disaster) ... 135
  1   Nutrition (meals/water) 135
  2   Exercise (environmental improvement) 136
  3   Rest (mind, anxiety, suicide, etc.) 136

16   Efforts of Okuma Town   137

A   Residents 140
  1   Nutrition (meals/water) 140
  2   Exercise (environmental improvement) 140
  3   Rest (mind, anxiety, suicide, etc.) 141
  4   Others 142
B   Expectant/nursing mothers and children 145
  1   Nutrition (meals/water) 145
  2   Exercise (environmental improvement) 145
  3   Rest (mind, anxiety, suicide, etc.) 146
C   People requiring assistance during a disaster (vulnerable people in case of a disaster) ... 147
  1   Nutrition (meals/water) 147
  2   Exercise (environmental improvement) 147
  3   Rest (mind, anxiety, suicide, etc.) 148

17 Efforts of Kawauchi Village 149

A Residents 152
   1 Nutrition (meals/water) 152
   2 Exercise (environmental improvement) 152
   3 Rest (mind, anxiety, suicide, etc.) 153
B Expectant/nursing mothers and children 153
   1 Nutrition (meals/water) 153
   2 Exercise (environmental improvement) 154
   3 Rest (mind, anxiety, suicide, etc.) 154
C People requiring assistance during a disaster (vulnerable people in case of a disaster) ... 155
   1 Nutrition (meals/water) 155
   2 Exercise (environmental improvement) 155
   3 Rest (mind, anxiety, suicide, etc.) 156
D Others 157

18 Efforts of Naraha Town 158

A Residents 162
   1 Nutrition (meals/water) 162
   2 Exercise (environmental improvement) 162
   3 Rest (mind, anxiety, suicide, etc.) 163
B Expectant/nursing mothers and children 165
   1 Nutrition (meals/water) 165
   2 Exercise (environmental improvement) 166
   3 Rest (mind, anxiety, suicide, etc.) 166
C People requiring assistance during a disaster (vulnerable people in case of a disaster) ... 168
   1 Nutrition (meals/water) 168
   2 Exercise (environmental improvement) 168
   3 Rest (mind, anxiety, suicide, etc.) 170
D Others 170

19 Efforts of Namie Town 173

A Residents 176
   1 Nutrition (meals/water) 176
   2 Exercise (Environmental improvement) 176
   3 Rest (mind, anxiety, suicide, etc.) 177
   4 Others 178
B Expectant/nursing mothers and children 179
   1 Nutrition (meals/water) 179
   2 Exercise (Environmental improvement) 180
   3 Rest (mind, anxiety, suicide, etc.) 181
   4 Others 181
C People requiring assistance during a disaster (vulnerable people in case of a disaster) ... 182
   1 Nutrition (meals/water) 182
   2 Exercise (Environmental improvement) 182
   3 Rest (mind, anxiety, suicide, etc.) 183
   4 Others 183

20 Efforts of Katsurao Village 185

A Residents 188
   1 Nutrition (meals/water) 188
   2 Exercise (Environmental improvement) 189
   3 Rest (mind, anxiety, suicide, etc.) 190
B Expectant/nursing mothers and children 192

	1	Nutrition (meals/water)	192
	2	Exercise (Environmental improvement)	193
	3	Rest (mind, anxiety, suicide, etc.)	194
C	People requiring assistance during a disaster (vulnerable people in case of a disaster)		195
	1	Nutrition (meals/water)	195
	2	Exercise (Environmental improvement)	196
	3	Rest (mind, anxiety, suicide, etc.)	197

21 Efforts of Hirono Town 199

A	Residents		202
	1	Nutrition (meals/water)	202
	2	Exercise (Environmental improvement)	203
	3	Rest (mind, anxiety, suicide, etc.)	203
	4	Others	204
B	Expectant/nursing mothers and children		206
	1	Nutrition (meals/water)	206
	2	Exercise (Environmental improvement)	206
	3	Rest (mind, anxiety, suicide, etc.)	207
	4	Others	207
C	People requiring assistance during a disaster (vulnerable people in case of a disaster)		209
	1	Nutrition (meals/water)	209
	2	Exercise (Environmental improvement)	209
	3	Rest (mind, anxiety, suicide, etc.)	209
	4	Others	210

22 Efforts of Iitate Village 213

A	Residents		216
	1	Nutrition (meals/water)	216
	2	Exercise (Environmental improvement)	216
	3	Rest (mind, anxiety, suicide, etc.)	217
B	Expectant and nursing mothers & children		217
	1	Nutrition (meals/water)	217
	2	Exercise (Environmental improvement)	218
	3	Rest (mind, anxiety, suicide, etc.)	218
C	People requiring assistance during a disaster (vulnerable people in case of a disaster)		219
	1	Nutrition (meals/water)	219
	2	Exercise (Environmental improvement)	219
	3	Rest (mind, anxiety, suicide, etc.)	220
D	Others		221

23 Efforts of Minamisoma City 222

A	Residents		225
	1	Nutrition (meals/water)	225
	2	Exercise (Environmental improvement)	225
	3	Rest (mind, anxiety, suicide, etc.)	226
B	Expectant and nursing mothers & children		227
	1	Nutrition (meals/water)	227
	2	Exercise (Environmental improvement)	227
	3	Rest (mind, anxiety, suicide, etc.)	228
C	People requiring assistance during a disaster (vulnerable people in case of a disaster)		229
	1	Nutrition (meals/water)	229
	2	Exercise (Environmental improvement)	229
	3	Rest (mind, anxiety, suicide, etc.)	230

D   Others 231

24 Efforts of Tamura City   232

A   Residents 235
   1   Nutrition (meals/water) 235
   2   Exercise (Environmental improvement) 235
   3   Rest (mind, anxiety, suicide, etc.) 236
   4   Others 238
B   Expectant/nursing mothers and children 239
   1   Nutrition (meals/water) 239
   2   Exercise (Environmental improvement) 239
   3   Rest (mind, anxiety, suicide, etc.) 240
   4   Others 241
C   People requiring assistance during a disaster (vulnerable people in case of a disaster) ... 242
   1   Nutrition (meals/water) 242
   2   Exercise (Environmental improvement) 242
   3   Rest (mind, anxiety, suicide, etc.) 242
   4   Others 243

25 Efforts of Kawamata Town   244

A   Residents 247
   1   Nutrition (meals/water) 247
   2   Exercise (Environmental improvement) 247
   3   Rest (mind, anxiety, suicide, etc.) 247
   4   Others 248
B   Expectant/nursing mothers and children 248
   1   Nutrition (meals/water) 248
   2   Exercise (Environmental improvement) 249
   3   Rest (mind, anxiety, suicide, etc.) 249
   4   Others 250
C   People requiring assistance during a disaster (vulnerable people in case of a disaster) ... 250
   1   Nutrition (meals/water) 250
   2   Exercise (Environmental improvement) 251
   3   Rest (mind, anxiety, suicide, etc.) 251
   4   Others 252

26 Efforts of Date City   253

A   Residents 256
   1   Nutrition (meals/water) 256
   2   Exercise (Environmental improvement) 256
   3   Rest (mind, anxiety, suicide, etc.) 257
B   Expectant/nursing mothers and children 257
   1   Nutrition (meals/water) 257
   2   Exercise (Environmental improvement) 258
   3   Rest (mind, anxiety, suicide, etc.) 259
C   People requiring assistance during a disaster (vulnerable people in case of a disaster) ... 260
   1   Nutrition (meals/water) 260
   2   Exercise (Environmental improvement) 260
   3   Rest (mind, anxiety, suicide, etc.) 261
D   Others 261

27 Efforts of Fukushima City 263

A Residents 268
   1 Nutrition (meals/water) 268
   2 Exercise (Environmental improvement) 269
   3 Rest (mind, anxiety, suicide, etc.) 270
B Expectant/nursing mothers and children 272
   1 Nutrition (meals/water) 272
   2 Exercise (Environmental improvement) 274
   3 Rest (mind, anxiety, suicide, etc.) 275
C People requiring assistance during a disaster (vulnerable people in case of a disaster) ... 277
   1 Nutrition (meals/water) 277
   2 Exercise (Environmental improvement) 278
   3 Rest (mind, anxiety, suicide, etc.) 279
   4 Summary/measures in the future 280
D Others 281

28 Efforts of Nihonmatsu City 284

A Expectant/nursing mothers and children 288
   1 Nutrition (meals/water) 288
   2 Exercise (Environmental improvement) 289
   3 Rest (mind, anxiety, suicide, etc.) 290
   4 Others 291

29 Efforts of Aizu-Wakamatsu City 294

A Residents 297
   1 Nutrition (meals/water) 297
   2 Exercise (Environmental improvement) 297
   3 Rest (mind, anxiety, suicide, etc.) 297
B Expectant/nursing mothers and children 298
   1 Nutrition (meals/water) 298
   2 Exercise (Environmental improvement) 298
   3 Rest (mind, anxiety, suicide, etc.) 299
C Public health activities at evacuation centers 299

Chapter 4 Activities of Various Professional Organizations 301

30 Fukushima Medical Association 303

A Activities after the occurrence of the earthquake 303
   1 Establishment of a disaster response headquarters and its initial activities 303
   2 Establishment of JMATs and their activities in Fukushima Prefecture 304
   3 Activity situation of county and city medical associations after the occurrence of the earthquake 305
B Issues related to nuclear disaster responses 307
   1 Participation in disaster administration of Fukushima Prefecture 307
   2 Countermeasures against exposure to radiation 307
   3 Suggestions related to recovery and reconstruction from nuclear disaster 308

31 Fukushima Dental Association 309

A Report about dental health support activities 309

1 Survey method 309
2 Frequency of going out for relief activities 309
3 Number of people engaged in support activities 309
4 Number of targets for relief activities 310
5 Contents of support activities 311
B Consideration of dental health support activities 311
1 Situation at the time of support activities 311
2 Survey method and dental health support activities 312
3 Results of the survey 313
C Dental care support activities in the future 314

32 Fukushima Nursing Association — 315

A Outline of the Fukushima Nursing Association 315
B Contents and progress of support activities related to the earthquake 315
1 Survey of the damage situation 315
2 Request for the dispatch of disaster relief nurses 316
3 Situation of the dispatch of disaster relief nurses 316
C Disaster support activities conducted as a general operation by the Fukushima Nursing Association 318
D Outsourcing business from Fukushima Prefecture to promote measures to secure nursing staff 319
E Health assistance projects in municipalities using health-care professionals 319
F Future issues 320

33 Fukushimaken Association of Radiological Technologist — 322

A Initial response of the Fukushimaken Association of Radiological Technologist 322
B Screening activities for emergency radiation exposure 323
C Screening before a postmortem examination of bodies 326
D Future activities and expected roles 327

34 Fukushima Pharmacists Association — 329

A Summary of the nuclear power station accident 329
B Initial responses at the occurrence of the earthquake 329
C Radiation pharmacists 331
D Stock and distribution of stable iodine preparations 332
1 Medication of stable iodine preparations 332
2 Storing of stable iodine preparations 333
3 Prescription records 333

35 Fukushima Physical Therapy Association — 335

A Disaster support activities immediately after the earthquake 335
B Disaster support activities at the intermediate stage 335
C Disaster support activities at the later stage 335
D Rehabilitation continuing into the future 336

36 Fukushima Association of Occupational Therapists — 337

A Initial responses (confirmation of the safety of members) 337
B A period when members took action not as an organization but as an individual 337
C A period when the Fukushima Association of Occupational Therapists commenced activities as an organization 338
D Support activities of the Aizu branch commenced 338
E Activities of the Fukushima Counseling and Support Professional Team 339

F   Support activities in temporary housing 340
G   People become healthy through activities 340
H   Support activities in Minamisoma City 341
I   Support activities in the future 341

37 Fukushima Dietetic Association 342

A   Overall activities of the Fukushima Dietetic Association at the time of the earth-
quake 342
B   Outline of major support activities in collaboration with administrative bodies and
relevant institutions/organizations 343
C   Concrete support activities 343
  1   Providing relief supplies more promptly to those who cannot eat ordinary food 343
  2   Improving a dietary environment in evacuation centers 343
  3   Activities for supporting the health preservation and promotion and independence of disaster victims by request from Fukushima Prefecture and affected
municipalities 346
D   Issues and future activities 346
  1   Present situation and issues 346
  2   Future activities 346

38 Fukushima Society of Certified Clinical Psychologists 347

A   Psychosocial situation of residents in Fukushima Prefecture 347
  1   Psychologically traumatic experience 347
  2   A vague sense of anxiety 347
  3   A vague sense of loss 347
  4   Self-determination 347
  5   Prolonged living as evacuees with no promise of the future 348
  6   Compensation issues 348
  7   Restrictions on topics of daily conversation 348
  8   An extremely large number of disaster-related deaths 349
B   Devising ways to provide support 349
  1   Parent-and-child Play and Parent Meeting 349
  2   Fukushima version of Class Meeting 352
C   Summary of support activities 354
D   Toward the future 354

39 Fukushima Ward Council on Social Welfare 356

A   Issues in support 356
B   Activities of disaster volunteer centers 356
C   Activities of welfare counselors 357
D   Importance of support activities 358

40 Fukushima Acupuncture and Moxibustion Association 359

A   Acupuncture and moxibustion 359
B   Support activities 359
C   Issues 361
D   To contribute to support activities with acupuncture and moxibustion therapies in case
of a disaster 361

41 Fukushima Association of Medical Social Workers 363

A   Immediately after the disaster (activitiesas hospital personnel) 363
B   What was learned through support activities for special nursing care facilities for the

elderly 365
   C   Activities of the Fukushima Professional Team for Counseling and Support 365
   D   Toward the reconstruction of lives 366

42 Universities and other educational research institutions (1) —Guidelines for childcare support in areas around evacuation zones   368

   A   Changes in lives 368
   B   Collaboration between a university and a local government 369
   C   Short-term measures 369
   D   Long-term prospects 371
   E   Residents and scientists 372
   F   Conclusion 373

43 Universities and other educational research institutions (2) —Overview of the Fukushima Health Management Survey   374

   A   Major activities of universities in Fukushima Prefecture 374
     1   University of Aizu 374
     2   Iwaki Meisei University and Higashi Nippon International University 375
     3   Ohu University 375
     4   College of Engineering, Nihon University 375
     5   Fukushima University 375
     6   Fukushima Medical University 375
   B   Efforts of Fukushima Medical University (Fukushima Health Management Survey) ... 376
     1   Roles of the university 376
     2   Overview of the Fukushima Health Management Survey 376

44 Expectations for public health from medical perspectives   381

   A   Health consultationYorozu 381
   B   What was learned through the health consultation Yorozu 382
     1   Aging of the population 382
     2   Decentralization of population 382
     3   Changes in lifestyles 383
     4   Collapse of communities 384
   C   How can medical professionals work together? 384
     1   Time-oriented collaboration between public health nurses and medical profession-als 384
     2   Listening to residents, arranging personnel serving as a liaison and identifying on-site needs 384
     3   Toward the establishment of a sustainable medical care system 385
   D   How to respond to the appearance of structural vulnerability 385

Chapter 5 Measures taken by Hiroshima University   389

45 Recovery Support and Carrying out Radiation Emergency Medicine at the Main Site —As a Tertiary Radiation Medical Institution—   391

   A   Radiation Emergency Medical Assistance 392

B   Support services at Fukushima Medical University 393
C   Risk Communication 394
D   Monitoring Environmental Radiation 394

46   Initiation of Measures for Human Resource Development —Establishment of the Phoenix Leader Education Program (Hiroshima Initiative) for Renaissance from Radiation Disaster—   396

Chapter 6   Suggestions —Toward the Future—   399

47   Measures to be Taken   401

A   Features of the nuclear disaster (its position in disasters) 401
B   Attitudes of the national government, prefectures and municipalities toward responses in public health in case of a nuclear disaster 402
   1   Responses of the national government 402
   2   Responses of prefectures (Fukushima Prefecture) and public health and welfare offices 403
   3   Responses of municipalities 404
C   Major issues in public health at the time of a nuclear disaster 405
   1   Radioactive contamination & screening 405
   2   Preventive medication of stable iodine preparations 406
   3   Support for people requiring assistance during a disaster 406
   4   Handling of dead bodies contaminated by radioactive materials 408
   5   Preparations during ordinary times 408
D   Aiming to provide appropriate information (Toward better risk communication) 410
E   Importance of accumulating experience and transmitting information 411

Materials 413

Index 427

Prefatory Materials

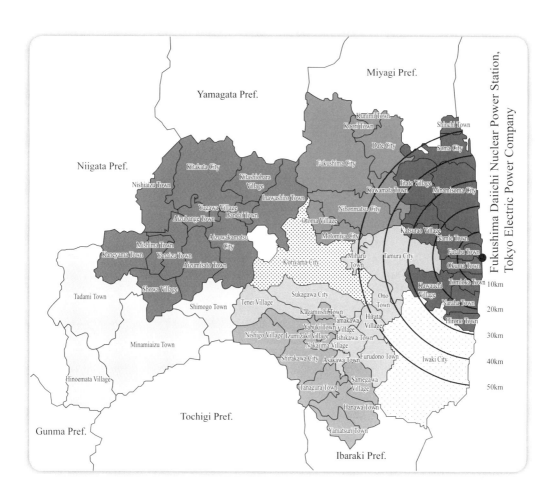

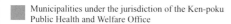 Municipalities under the jurisdiction of the Ken-poku Public Health and Welfare Office
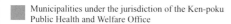 Municipalities under the jurisdiction of the Ken-chu Public Health and Welfare Office
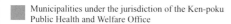 Municipalities under the jurisdiction of the Ken-nan Public Health and Welfare Office
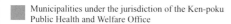 Municipalities under the jurisdiction of the Soso Public Health and Welfare Office
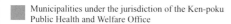 Municipalities under the jurisdiction of the Aizu Public Health and Welfare Office
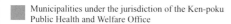 Municipalities under the jurisdiction of the Minamiaizu Public Health and Welfare Office
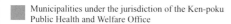 Municipalities under the jurisdiction of the Koriyama City Public Health Center
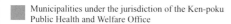 Municipalities under the jurisdiction of the Iwaki City Public Health Center

Calendar of Major Events in Individual Regions

Date	Common	Aizu Region
3/11 (Fri)	• At 14:46, the earthquake occurred. • At 19:03, an emergency situation was declared. (Fukushima Daiichi Nuclear Power Station, Tokyo Electric Power Company) ("Fukushima Daiichi Station") • At 21:23, an evacuation order was issued for the 3-km radius area, and an indoor evacuation order for the 10-km radius area. (Fukushima Daiichi Station)	• JR conventional lines were blocked. • Aizu Railway lines were blocked.
3/12 (Sat)	• At 5:44, an evacuation order was issued for the 10-km radius area. (Fukushima Daiichi Station) • At 7:45, an evacuation order was issued for the 3-km radius area, and an indoor evacuation order for the 10-km radius area. (Fukushima Daini Nuclear Power Station, Tokyo Electric Power Company) ("Fukushima Daini Station") • At 15:36, a hydrogen explosion occurred at Unit 1 of the Fukushima Daiichi Station. • At 17:36, an evacuation order was issued for the 10-km area. (Fukushima Daini Station) • At 18:25, an evacuation order was issued for the 20-km area. (Fukushima Daiichi Station)	• The operation of Aizu Railway lines was resumed.
3/13 (Sun)		• Water supply was fully restored in Aizuwakamatsu City. • The operation of express buses was resumed between Wakamatsu and Niigata, and Wakamatsu and Nozawa (Aizu Bus/Niigata Kotsu).
3/14 (Mon)	• At 11:01, a hydrogen explosion occurred at Unit 3 of the Fukushima Daiichi Station.	
3/15 (Tue)	• At 6:10, an explosion sound was heard at Unit 2 of the Fukushima Daiichi Station. (There was a doubt that a pressure suppression chamber might have been damaged.) • At 6:14, it was confirmed that the outer wall of Unit 4 of the Fukushima Daiichi Station was damaged. • At 9:38, a fire occurred at Unit 4 of the Fukushima Daiichi Station. (The fire was brought under control at 11:00.) • At 11:00, an indoor evacuation order was issued for the 20- to 23-km radius area. (Fukushima Daiichi Station)	
3/16 (Wed)	• At 8:30, white smoke arose from Unit 3 of the Fukushima Daiichi Station.	• Prefectural high schools and special needs schools announced successful applicants, who were selected through the second stage examination and the first stage examination, respectively. • Water supply was fully restored in Inawashiro Town.
3/17 (Thu)	• In the morning, seawater was dropped into Unit 3 by helicopters of the Self-Defense Forces. (a total of four times)	• The operation of express buses was resumed between Wakamatsu and Koriyama (Aizu Bus/Fukushima Transportation).
3/18 (Fri)		• A graduation ceremony was held at Hinoemata Village Hinoemata Elementary School.
3/19 (Sat)	• Water was sprayed onto Unit 3 of the Fukushima Daiichi Station. (Hyper Rescue Team of the Tokyo Fire Department) • Approximately 700 residents in Iitate Village began to be evacuated to Tochigi Prefecture.	
3/20 (Sun)		
3/21 (Mon)	• White smoke was discharged from Units 2 and 3 of the Fukushima Daiichi Station. • The shipment of raw milk, spinach and *kakina* (green leafy vegetable) was blocked.	
3/22 (Tue)	• White smoke was discharged from Units 2 and 3 of the Fukushima Daiichi Station.	• The operation of express buses was resumed between Wakamatsu and Shinjuku (Aizu Bus/JR Bus Kanto).
3/23 (Wed)	• White smoke was discharged from Units 2 and 3 of the Fukushima Daiichi Station. • The shipment of head leafy vegetables, cruciferous flower buds, turnips and non-head leafy vegetables (other than those announced on March 21) was blocked. • Japan Post's domestic parcel delivery service was resumed in Fukushima Prefecture. • The 83rd National Invitational High-School Baseball Tournament opened.	• Graduation ceremonies were held at municipal elementary schools in Aizuwakamatsu City, Kitakata City, Kitashiobara Village, Nishiaizu Town, Bandai Town, Inawashiro Town, Aizubange Town, Yugawa Village, Yanaizu Town, MishimaTown, Kaneyama Town, Showa Village, Shimogo Town, Tadami Town and Minamiaizu Town.
3/24 (Thu)	• Foot contamination was detected in two workers at Unit 3. • After being taken to Fukushima Medical University, they were transferred to the National Institute of Radiological Sciences on the following day.	• The operation of express buses was resumed between Wakamatsu and Sendai (Aizu Bus).
3/25 (Fri)	• A voluntary evacuation request was issued for the 20- to 30-km radium area. (Fukushima Daiichi Station)	• The operation of express buses was resumed between Wakamatsu and Fukushima (Aizu Bus/Fukushima Transportation).
3/26 (Sat)		• The operation of the Ban-etsu West Line was resumed.

Central Region	Coastal Region
• The Tohoku Expressway was closed. • The Tohoku Shinkansen Line was all blocked. • JR conventional lines were all blocked. • The Iizaka Line was all blocked. • The Abukuma Kyuko Line was all blocked. • The Ban-etsu Expressway was closed. • The Abukuma Kogen Road was closed.	• The Joban Expressway was closed. • JR conventional lines were all blocked. • The Ban-etsu Expressway was closed.
• Water supply was fully restored in Otama Village.	• At 9:00, residents in Futaba Town began to be evacuated to Kawamata Town by microbuses. • At 19:30, approximately 1,800 residents living within the 10-km radius in Namie Town moved to the Tsushima District.
• The operation of the Iizaka Line was resumed. • Water supply was fully restored in Kawamata Town and Yamatsuri Town.	
• The operation of express buses was resumed between Fukushima and Koriyama (Fukushima Transportation), Fukushima and Sendai (Fukushima Transportation/Miyagi Transportation/JR Bus Tohoku). • The closure of the Abukuma Kogen Road was lifted. • Water supply was fully restored in Tanagura Town.	• Water supply became partly available in Iwaki City (Taira/Uchigo/Nakoso).
• The operation of the Tohoku Shinkansen Line was resumed between Tokyo and Nasushiobara Stations.	• Nihonmatsu City expressed its intention to receive evacuees from the Tsushima District in Namie Town.
• Prefectural high schools and special needs schools announced successful applicants, who were selected through the second stage examination and the first stage examination, respectively.	
• The operation of express buses was resumed between Koriyama and Wakamatsu (Fukushima Transportation/Aizu Bus). • Water supply was fully restored in Motomiya City, Koori Town and Nakajima Village.	• Approximately 250 residents out of the disaster victims in Tomioka Town and Kawauchi Village moved to Sugito Town, Saitama Prefecture.
• The operation of express buses was resumed between Fukushima and Shinjuku (Fukushima Transportation/JR Bus Tohoku/JR Bus Kanto). • The operation of express buses was resumed between Koriyama and Shin-Koshigaya (Fukushima Transportation/Tobu Bus Central). • Water supply was fully restored in Miharu Town and Ono Town.	• Residents in Minamisoma City began to be evacuated to Niigata Prefecture and Gunma Prefecture, when they wanted to be evacuated. • Futaba Town announced that its administrative operations would be conducted in Saitama Prefecture. • The operation of express buses was resumed between Iwaki and Tokyo (Shin Joban Kotsu/JR Bus Kanto/Tobu Bus Central).
• The operation of express buses was resumed between Koriyama and Niigata (Fukushima Transportation/Niigata Kotsu). • Water supply was fully restored in Tamura City.	• Approximately 700 residents began to be evacuated from Iitate Village to Tochigi Prefecture. • The administrative operations of Futaba Town began to be conducted at the Saitama Super Arena in Saitama City. • The Soma Port was partly restored.
• Fukushima University announced successful applicants, who were selected through the second stage entrance examination. • Fukushima Medical University announced successful applicants, who were selected through the second stage entrance examination. • Water supply was fully restored in Date City. • The operation of express buses was resumed between Koriyama and Iwaki (Fukushima Transportation/Shin Joban Kotsu).	• The operation of express buses was resumed between Iwaki and Koriyama (Shin Joban Kotsu/ Fukushima Transportation).
• Private water-supply systems were restored in some areas (Dake, Towa and Obama) in Nihonmatsu City.	• The closure of the Joban Expressway to unauthorized vehicles was lifted between Iwaki-Chuo IC and Mito IC.
• Fukushima Medical University partly resumed outpatient care (for only patients with appointments). • Water supply was fully restored in Fukushima City. • A graduation ceremony was held at Sakurano Seibo Gakuin Elementary School.	• Prefectural high schools and special needs schools announced successful applicants, who were selected through the second stage examination and the first stage examination, respectively.
• Water supply was fully restored in Kunimi Town. • Graduation ceremonies were held at municipal elementary schools in Date City, Otama Village, Nishigo Village, Izumizaki Village, Tanagura Town, Yamatsuri Town and Hanawa Town.	• The earthquake with an intensity of upper 5 on the Japanese seismic scale occurred in Iwaki City (at around 7:12, 7:36 and 18:55).
• The Tohoku Expressway became open to unauthorized vehicles. • The Ban-etsu Expressway became open to unauthorized vehicles. • The Abukuma Kogen Road became open to unauthorized vehicles. • Water supply was fully restored in Tenei Village, Nihonmatsu City and Izumizaki Village.	
• The operation of express buses was resumed between Fukushima/Koriyama and Narita (Fukushima Transportation/Chibakotsu). • The operation of express buses was resumed between Fukushima and Wakamatsu (Fukushima Transportation/Aizu Bus).	
• The operation of the Banetsu West Line was resumed.	

(Fukushima Health Management Survey)

Chapter 1

What Nuclear Disaster Means

1 Tokyo Electric Power Company Fukushima Daiichi Nuclear Power Station Accident

Radiation and radioactive substances exist in nature. Radiation is emitted from space and radioactive substances exist in soil, rocks, and the air, causing us to be exposed daily to radiation, albeit in extremely small amounts. We are also exposed to the rays from the sun. Ultraviolet rays and infrared rays, as well as radiation (γ-rays and x-rays), and included in the sunlight are also certain types of electromagnetic waves, which can be classified into radio waves (electromagnetic waves as are emitted from, for example, mobile phones), infrared rays, visible rays (visible to human eyes), ultraviolet rays, and ionized radiation. In most cases, people do not notice their exposure to radiation even if they are exposed to high radiation because radiation has no color, odor, or taste; meaning that people can detect nothing about what is happening even if they are at a nuclear accident site. Even in the event of the exposure to a dose that requires medical treatment, people do not immediately know of their exposure because it takes time for the symptoms to appear. The explanation of radiation and its effects is by no means easily comprehensible, even for medical personnel. For example, there are various units used to describe radiation, such as counts per minute (cpm), becquerel (Bq), gray (Gy), and sievert (Sv), and, furthermore, the dose expressed in Sv includes the effective dose, equivalent dose, and committed effective dose.

The Tohoku Earthquake, which occurred off the Pacific Coast at 2:46 pm on March 11, 2011, and the subsequent tsunami hit the Tokyo Electric Power Company Fukushima Daiichi Nuclear Power Station (hereinafter referred to as the "Fukushima Daiichi Nuclear Station"). This caused the release of a large amount of radioactive substances into the environment, leading to an unprecedented large-scale and long-term nuclear accident. This accident is a complex disaster with the earthquake, tsunami, and the nuclear power plant accident that released radioactive substances, and countermeasures are still being taken even though two years have passed since the occurrence of the accident. This paragraph describes what happened during the accident and how the effects of radiation were evaluated, as well as the basic knowledge of radiation and radiation exposure required for health workers.

A Radiation Accident and Nuclear Disaster

The radiation exposure in aircraft is several tens of times greater than that on the ground while it varies to some extent depending on the altitude and geomagnetic latitude. People are exposed to radiation in some cases in a hospital for diagnosis or treatment; however, radiation exposure within the controlled range is not regarded as an accident even if side-effects appear. A radiation exposure accident refers to unexpected and unintended radiation exposure, which eventually, or potentially, leads to the emergence of its effects. Accordingly, a nuclear disaster means a radiation accident attributable to nuclear facilities or equipment. The malicious practice of radiation exposure is not an accident but a crime. A radiation exposure accident is characterized by causing not only physical effects but also mental discomfort and having a significant influence on society. Roentgen published a research paper on x-rays in November 1895 and it is generally said that Becquerel discovered uranium ore two months later in 1896. Already reported in that year were hair loss, pain, and water blisters caused by x-rays as well as skin reddening caused by radioactive substances. It was reported that a hazardous phenomenon occurred due to radiation only one year after the discovery of x-rays, although many prominent scholars denied such a fact. It took four years before the fact was accepted that frequent exposure to x-rays caused heat burn-like symptoms on the skin. As indicated in these cases, the fact that radiation cannot be sensed by the five senses and no symptoms develop immediately after radiation exposure is one of the reasons that make it difficult to clarify the effects of radiation. There were many examples in past accidents in which it took a long time to find that the accidents had actually occurred, including an accident that was found to have occurred only after symptoms had developed, even though the radiation exposure was at such a level that it required medical treatment. The following is another example of an accident: In 1982 in Taiwan, the disposed source of ^{60}Co (cobalt) radiation were mixed into iron scraps and used for the reinforced concrete for school and apartment buildings. Stable cobalt is an important alloy for industrial use, and radioactive cobalt has the same property as non-radioactive metal. This contamination was found in 1992, which revealed an accident in which 10,000 residents and students had been exposed to radiation[1]. The investigation from 1983 to 2005 found some people with a total dose of more than 2 Sv[2].

B : Fukushima Daiichi Nuclear Station Accident and Complex Disaster

The earthquake that occurred off the Sanriku coast (at 38°06.2'N, 142°51.6'E at a depth of 24 km) on March 11, 2011 had a moment magnitude of 9.0 and a maximum seismic intensity of 7 (Kurihara City, Miyagi Prefecture). This earthquake was named the 2011 off the Pacific coast of Tohoku Earthquake[3], and the subsequent tsunami caused a serious accident at the Fukushima Daiichi Nuclear Station. After the earthquake, the nuclear power generation reactors automatically shut down immediately. Since the fuel continued to generate very high heat even after the reactors had shut down, it was essential to cool the nuclear reactors; however, the functions of the emergency power supply and equipment necessary to cool the reactors were lost due to the earthquake and tsunami. Subsequently, the fuel temperature increased and the fuel reacted with water to generate hydrogen, resulting in hydrogen explosions at reactors Nos. 1, 3, and 4, which released radioactive substances into the environment (Table 1-1)[4].

The main nuclides released were ^{133}Xe (xenon), ^{131}I (iodine), ^{132}Te (tellurium), ^{134}Cs (cesium), and ^{137}Cs. The nuclide ^{133}Xe is a gas with a short half-life of 5.2 days and used for lung examination. The nuclide ^{131}I (γ-rays and β-rays) with a half-life of 8.04 days is accumulated specifically in the thyroid gland if taken into the body. The nuclides ^{134}Cs (γ-rays and β-rays) and ^{137}Cs with half-lives of about 2 years and 30.17 years, respectively, behave similarly to K (potassium) in the body. In addition, other nuclides, such as ^{89}Sr (strontium, β-rays) and ^{239}Pu (plutonium, α-rays) were released, although the amount released was extremely low compared to the other nuclides. Since ^{132}Te and ^{131}I have a short half-life, the problem that remains is ^{134}Cs and ^{137}Cs in the environment on the ground and underground as well as in plants and trees, causing a high dose in the air in the environment.

In the event of a nuclear disaster, it is necessary for all the personnel concerned in the government, prefectures, and municipalities to meet together and for the Nuclear Emergency Response Headquarters of the government and the Emergency Response Headquarters of the local governments to share information and cooperate with each other to smoothly promote activities to take measures to control the nuclear disaster. As the local base for this purpose, an off-site center (OFC) is in place as base facilities for emergency response measures. In Fukushima Prefecture, the OFC was at Aza-Ono, Oaza-Shimonogami, Okuma Town, located about five kilometers from the Fukushima Daiichi Nuclear Station. After this earthquake, there was trouble with communication and radiation measurement equipment that occurred due to the complex disaster with the earthquake and tsunami. This significantly restricted the activities at the OFC and also caused significant difficulties in emergency medical treatment for radiation exposure. The emergency medical treatment system for radiation exposure in the case of a nuclear accident was established only in the municipality where the nuclear facilities are located, while in the neighboring municipalities there was only a limited

Table 1-1 Radioactive substances released from reactors Nos. 1, 2, and 3 in the Fukushima Daiichi Nuclear Station accident and their respective amounts (Unit: Bq)

Nuclide	Half-life	Reactor No. 1	Reactor No. 2	Reactor No. 3	Total
^{133}Xe	5.2 days	3.4×10^{18}	3.5×10^{18}	4.4×10^{18}	1.1×10^{19}
^{134}Cs	2.1 years	7.1×10^{14}	1.6×10^{16}	8.2×10^{14}	1.8×10^{16}
^{137}Cs	30.0 years	5.9×10^{14}	1.4×10^{16}	7.1×10^{14}	1.5×10^{16}
^{89}Sr	50.5 days	8.2×10^{13}	6.8×10^{14}	1.2×10^{15}	2.0×10^{15}
^{90}Sr	29.1 years	6.1×10^{12}	4.8×10^{13}	8.5×10^{13}	1.4×10^{14}
^{140}Ba	12.7 days	1.3×10^{14}	1.1×10^{15}	1.9×10^{15}	3.2×10^{15}
^{127m}Te	109.0 days	2.5×10^{14}	7.7×10^{14}	6.9×10^{13}	1.1×10^{15}
^{129m}Te	33.6 days	7.2×10^{14}	2.4×10^{15}	2.1×10^{14}	3.3×10^{15}
^{131m}Te	30.0 hours	2.2×10^{15}	2.3×10^{15}	4.5×10^{14}	5.0×10^{15}
^{132}Te	78.2 hours	2.5×10^{16}	5.7×10^{16}	6.4×10^{15}	8.8×10^{16}
^{103}Ru	39.3 days	2.5×10^{09}	1.8×10^{09}	3.2×10^{09}	7.5×10^{09}
^{106}Ru	368.2 days	7.4×10^{08}	5.1×10^{08}	8.9×10^{08}	2.1×10^{09}
^{95}Zr	64.0 days	4.6×10^{11}	1.6×10^{13}	2.2×10^{11}	1.7×10^{13}
^{141}Ce	32.5 days	4.6×10^{11}	1.7×10^{13}	2.2×10^{11}	1.8×10^{13}
^{144}Ce	284.3 days	3.1×10^{11}	1.1×10^{13}	1.4×10^{11}	1.1×10^{13}
^{239}Np	2.4 days	3.7×10^{12}	7.1×10^{13}	1.4×10^{12}	7.6×10^{13}
^{238}Pu	87.7 days	5.8×10^{08}	1.8×10^{10}	2.5×10^{08}	1.9×10^{10}
^{239}Pu	24065 years	8.6×10^{07}	3.1×10^{09}	4.0×10^{07}	3.2×10^{09}
^{240}Pu	6537 years	8.8×10^{07}	3.0×10^{09}	4.0×10^{07}	3.2×10^{09}
^{241}Pu	14.4 years	3.5×10^{10}	1.2×10^{12}	1.6×10^{10}	1.2×10^{12}
^{91}Y	58.5 days	3.1×10^{11}	2.7×10^{12}	4.4×10^{11}	3.4×10^{12}
^{143}Pr	13.6 days	3.6×10^{11}	3.2×10^{12}	5.2×10^{11}	4.1×10^{12}
^{147}Nd	11.0 days	1.5×10^{11}	1.3×10^{12}	2.2×10^{11}	1.6×10^{12}
^{242}Cm	162.8 days	1.1×10^{10}	7.7×10^{10}	1.4×10^{10}	1.0×10^{11}
^{131}I	8.0 days	1.2×10^{16}	1.4×10^{17}	7.0×10^{15}	1.6×10^{17}
^{132}I	2.3 hours	1.3×10^{13}	6.7×10^{06}	3.7×10^{10}	1.3×10^{13}
^{133}I	20.8 hours	1.2×10^{16}	2.6×10^{16}	4.2×10^{15}	4.2×10^{16}
^{135}I	6.6 hours	2.0×10^{15}	7.4×10^{13}	1.9×10^{14}	2.3×10^{15}
^{127}Sb	3.9 days	1.7×10^{15}	4.2×10^{15}	4.5×10^{14}	6.4×10^{15}
^{129}Sb	4.3 hours	1.4×10^{14}	5.6×10^{10}	2.3×10^{12}	1.4×10^{14}
^{99}Mo	66.0 hours	2.6×10^{09}	1.2×10^{09}	2.9×10^{09}	6.7×10^{09}

number of medical personnel engaged in treatment for radiation exposure.

As the central organization of the emergency medical treatment system for radiation exposure as well as the tertiary radiation emergency hospital at a nationwide level, the National Institute of Radiological Sciences (hereinafter referred to as the "NIRS") dispatched the first team for emergency medical treatment for radiation exposure, consisting of doctors, nurses, and health physics experts, to the OFC at Okuma Town using Self-Defense Force aircraft about 17 hours after the occurrence of the earthquake[5]. However, due to the destruction of the infrastructure caused by the earthquake, such as the Internet and the mobile phone and fixed phone communications, not only did the OFC not function but also the team had to be fully involved in the contamination monitoring for disaster control personnel and residents on the site.

Chapter 1 — What Nuclear Disaster Means

C: Change in the Screening Level for Contamination

Prior to this accident, the screening level set by Fukushima Prefecture for contamination caused by radioactive substances was 40 Bq/cm^2 for γ and β nuclides. At this level, with an assumption that the contamination is caused by ^{131}I (iodine), about 10,000 to 13,000 cpm can be detected by a standard (GM counter-type) survey meter available in the market. After this accident, there were many residents with contamination exceeding this level at, for example, their head hairs and shoes. At the shelters, however, the decontamination work could not be performed due to water outage, no clean clothes were available to change into, and people could not undress due to low air temperature. Since a significant problem might potentially result under such situations if nothing was done, some measures had to be taken. According to the EPR-First Responders 2006 Manual for First Responders to Radiological Emergency[6] of the International Atomic Energy Agency (IAEA), from the viewpoint of first responders, the contamination level of the skin and clothes that was determined to require decontamination is set to 1 μSv/h or more when measured at a distance of 10 cm. With an assumption that a contaminated person is completely undressed and ^{131}I contamination remains only at the head and neck and their area is 500 cm^2, 100,000 cpm is equivalent to about 1 μSv/h, as indicated in the Manual for First Responders to Radiological Emergency of the IAEA[7]. If the contamination by ^{131}I is 100,000 cpm and this dose rate continues without attenuation for the half-life period (8.02 days), the accumulated skin dose is about 90 mSv based on the skin dose calculation according to the ICRU Report 56[8]. Considering that there is actually a half-life and decontamination progresses naturally through metabolism, the effects on the skin are sufficiently insignificant. Accordingly, the screening level had to be changed to 100,000 cpm but it was not the level to influence health. However, where contaminated patients were found at the Fukushima Daiichi Nuclear Station early after the event, there were for various reasons scarcely any medical institutions in Fukushima Prefecture that could accept such patients. This revealed the fact that the principle of medical care to give "higher priority to saving life over decontamination" had not penetrated well into the education for radiation exposure medical care to be pro-

Table 1-2 Request for health consultation concerning radiation issued by the Ministry of Health, Labour and Welfare

Office Memo
March 21, 2011

Attention:
Local health responsible division of each prefectural/city establishing public health centers/special ward

Office of Community Health, General Affairs Division, Health Service Bureau,
Ministry of Health, Labour and Welfare

Health consultation concerning the effects of radiation (Request) (Partial revision and addition)

In light of the Fukushima Nuclear Station accident, for the health consultation concerning the effects of radiation, we have requested you to take appropriate measures, such as the development of a system that meets the situation of consultation from residents at the respective public health centers, etc., based on the office memo "Health consultation concerning the effects of radiation (Request)" dated March 18, 2011.

The example of the flow of measures to be taken for residents shown in the exhibit of the Office Memo indicated that the level that required decontamination was 13,000 cpm where a survey was conducted using a survey meter. In response to the change in the screening level for contamination to 100,000 cpm indicated by the Nuclear Safety Commission (see the attached sheet), the level that requires decontamination indicated in Exhibit 1 of the said Office Memo shall be changed from 13,000 cpm to 100,000 cpm.

Some people among those who want to receive health consultations, etc. may want the issuance of a certificate, etc. of having taken the survey using a survey meter. However, since we do not think it desirable to issue such a certificate, etc. because doing so does not match the purpose of health consultation and imposes an excessive load on the survey facilities, you are requested to deal with this matter accordingly.

Note: The above memo indicates the change in the screening level for decontamination and requests that the issuance of the certificate of the completion of contamination inspection shall not be requested at a health consultation.

vided for health workers. Both disaster control personnel and medical personnel were also the residents in the affected area in many cases and they were also subject to evacuation. At the time of the accident, what was not supposed to happen actually happened, such as the denial of transportation of contaminated patients by transportation personnel and the denial of acceptance of contaminated patients by medical institutions. In addition, it was reported that some of those who had evacuated to outside of Fukushima Prefecture were requested to submit their certificate of completion of screening or even suffered discrimination when they visited a medical institution[9]. (Table 1-2.)

In the emergency medical treatment for radiation exposure, the situation where a risk more significant than the radiation exposure risk cannot be avoided must be avoided.

D Effects of Radiation and Radiation Dose

The symptom that appears at the lowest dose induced by one-time radiation exposure is the temporary decrease in the number of sperm and said to appear for 1% of men who have received a radiation exposure of 100 mSv[10]. It is only in the case of external radiation exposure of 1 to 2 Sv or more to the whole body at a high dose rate that symptoms appear within several hours after radiation exposure and this level of radiation exposure represents the lowest dose that is subject to medical care. Considering that the exposed dose from the CT scan of the upper abdomen is 10 to 20 mSv, the above is obviously a very high dose. In terms of the period until symptoms appear, for example, even in the case of local exposure of only the hand exceeding 10 Sv by γ-rays, it is at least a week to 10 days until skin problems appear. According to the experience of past contamination accidents, there were no cases where the medical staff who engaged in transportation or medical care of contaminated patients received radiation exposure at the level affecting their health. Furthermore, no cases are found where any person who suffered radiation exposure but had no other complication died soon. For the genetic influence of radiation, the survey result of the children of atomic bomb survivors (second-generation survey with a median exposed dose of their parents of about 140 mSv) is available[11]; however, no genetic influence on humans was observed in the epidemiological surveys for humans to date. Even though this kind of knowledge is necessary for medical personnel, the effects of radiation and the radiation dose are very frequently misunderstood.

E Exposed Dose of Residents

The NIRS has conducted the "Basic Survey (Estimation of External Exposed Dose)" for the health management survey of Fukushima Prefecture residents. While this paragraph omits the details, the NIRS developed the system whereby the whole prefecture was divided into a grid of 2 km × 2 km areas. The dose rate (μSv/h) of each area was calculated on a time-series basis from March 12 to July 11, 2011, based on the results of the System for Prediction of Environmental Emergency Dose Information (SPEEDI) to calculate the external exposed dose of individuals according to the behavior records of the residents (place, outdoors/indoors, duration of stay, building structure of the place in which residents stayed, traveling time)[12]. Information was used to estimate the external exposed dose of the residents.

The results up to a recent date are shown in Tables 1-3 and Figure 1-1)[13]. The maximum value among 451,364 residents (excluding those engaged in radiation work) was 25 mSv and there were 11 people whose maximum value exceeded 15 mSv. All of these 11 people were residents of the Soso Area (Soma City, Minamisoma City, Hirono Town, Naraha Town, Tomioka Town, Kawauchi Village, Okuma Town, Futaba

Chapter 1 — What Nuclear Disaster Means

Table 1-3 Estimation of external exposed dose of the residents (Unit: person; % indicates the ratio in each area) as of September 30, 2013.

Effective dose (mSv)	Ken-poku	Ken-chu	Ken-nan	Aizu	Minamiaizu	Soso	Iwaki	Cumulative total
Less than 1	40,602 (31.7%)	65,167 (59.0%)	23,076 (90.7%)	36,971 (99.4%)	3,732 (99.4%)	59,689 (77.9%)	69,095 (99.2%)	298,332
1 to less than 2	74,887 (58.4%)	38,989 (35.3%)	2,364 (9.3%)	217 (0.6%)	23 (0.6%)	12,782 (16.7%)	555 (0.8%)	129,817
2 to less than 3	12,136 (9.5%)	6,057 (5.5%)	12 (0.0%)	8 (0.0%)	0 —	1,908 (2.5%)	20 (0.0%)	20,141
3 to less than 4	439 (0.3%)	290 (0.3%)	0 —	1 (0.0%)	0 —	699 (0.9%)	3 (0.0%)	1,432
4 to less than 5	44 (0.0%)	6 (0.0%)	0 —	0 —	0 —	524 (0.7%)	2 (0.0%)	576
5 to less than 6	25 (0.0%)	2 (0.0%)	0 —	0 —	0 —	405 (0.5%)	0 —	432
6 to less than 7	8 (0.0%)	0 —	0 —	0 —	0 —	245 (0.3%)	0 —	253
7 to less than 8	1 (0.0%)	0 —	0 —	0 —	0 —	126 (0.2%)	0 —	127
8 to less than 9	0 —	0 —	0 —	0 —	0 —	82 (0.1%)	0 —	82
9 to less than 10	0 —	0 —	0 —	0 —	0 —	46 (0.1%)	0 —	46
10 to less than 11	0 —	0 —	0 —	0 —	0 —	45 (0.1%)	0 —	45
11 to less than 12	1 (0.0%)	0 —	0 —	0 —	0 —	31 (0.0%)	0 —	32
12 to less than 13	0 —	0 —	0 —	0 —	0 —	14 (0.0%)	0 —	14
13 to less than 14	0 —	0 —	0 —	0 —	0 —	13 (0.0%)	0 —	13
14 to less than 15	0 —	0 —	0 —	0 —	0 —	11 (0.0%)	0 —	11
15 or more	0 —	0 —	0 —	0 —	0 —	11 (0.0%)	0 —	11
Total	128,143	110,511	25,452	37,197	3,755	76,631	69,675	451,364 (100%)

Town, Namie Town, Katsurao Village, Shinchi Town, Iitate Village), where the dose was determined to be higher than that in other areas. However, of a total of 76,631 residents in the Soso Area, residents with less than 1 mSv accounted for 77.9% and those with less than 10 mSv accounted for 99.9%. Also shown are the results of the inspection of the internal exposed dose from cesium using a whole-body counter; conducted mainly by the Japan Atomic Energy Agency (JAEA) and partially by the NIRS and other organizations (Tables 1-4)[14]. Of a total of 156,858 people, the maximum value was 3 mSv for two people.

 Report of the World Health Organization (WHO)

Since the exposed dose due to an accident has obscure factors, unlike a planned exposure, an excessively high dose, which can be by no means exceeded, is often computed as obscure factors and are often expressed using the terms, "safe side" or "conservative side." A modification is made, needless to say, if details are clarified. Specific examples are as follows: If it is unknown what is the percentage of contaminated food eaten by a certain person, everything eaten by the person is assumed to be contaminated food. If

Tokyo Electric Power Company Fukushima Daiichi Nuclear Power Station Accident

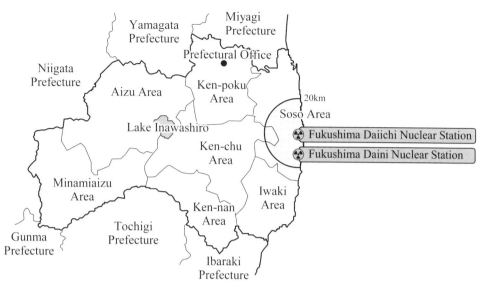

Fukushima Prefecture divides its municipalities into seven areas.
Ken-poku Area: Fukushima City, Date City, Koori Town, Kunimi Town, Kawamata Town, Nihonmatsu City, Motomiya City, Otama Village
Ken-chu Area: Koriyama City, Sukagawa City, Tamura City, Kagami-ishi Town, Tenei Village, Ishikawa Town, Tamakawa Village, Hirata Village, Asakawa Town, Furudono Town, Miharu Town, Ono Town
Ken-nan Area: Shirakawa City, Nishigo Village, Izumizaki Village, Nakajima Village, Yabuki Town, Tanagura Town, Yamatsuri Town, Hanawa Town, Samegawa Village
Aizu Area: Aizuwakamatsu City, Kitakata City, Kitashiobara Village, Nishiaizu Town, Bandai Town, Inawashiro Town, Aizubange Town, Yugawa Village, Yanaizu Town, Mishima Town, Kaneyama Town, Showa Village, Aizumisato Town
Minamiaizu Area: Shimogo Town, Hinoemata Village, Tadami Town, Minamiaizu Town
Soso Area: Soma City, Minamisoma City, Hirono Town, Naraha Town, Tomioka Town, Kawauchi Village, Okuma Town, Futaba Town, Namie Town, Katsurao Village, Shinchi Town, Iitate Village
Iwaki Area: Iwaki City

Figure 1-1 Names of the areas in Fukushima Prefecture

Table 1-4 Results of the internal exposed dose inspection conducted using a whole-body counter (June 27, 2011 to September 30, 2013)

(Unit: person)

Area	Committed effective dose				Total
	Less than 1 mSv	1 mSv	2 mSv	3 mSv	
Ken-poku	38,572	2	1	0	38,575
Ken-chu	33,197	0	0	0	33,197
Ken-nan	23,471	0	0	0	23,471
Aizu	18,902	0	0	0	18,902
Minamiaizu	2,880	0	0	0	2,880
Soso	21,338	12	9	2	21,361
Iwaki	18,472	0	0	0	18,472
Cumulative total	156,832	14	10	2	156,858

it is unknown how long a certain person has stayed at the place where the person may be exposed to radiation, the maximum possible duration is taken into consideration. On February 28, 2013, the World Health Organization (WHO) released "Health risk assessment from the nuclear accident after the 2011 Great East Japan earthquake and tsunami based on preliminary dose estimation"[15]. This report assessed the effects of

Chapter 1 | What Nuclear Disaster Means

radiation from the perspective of the dose. This report was primarily based on the results of "Preliminary dose estimation from the nuclear accident after the 2011 Great East Japan Earthquake and Tsunami[16]" that was released by the WHO in May 2012 and assessed the dose using the data up to September 2011. The report on health effects assessed the risk according to the dose based on the assumption that "people did not evacuate during the four months after the accident," "residents in Fukushima ate only food produced in Fukushima Prefecture," and "no restrictions were placed on food," resulting in an overestimation with applicable people perhaps not existing. The report states that this is intended to minimize the possibility to underestimate the health effects. Even though the above assumption is referred to in the text, the figures alone concerning the dose and risk will bring about significant misunderstanding. For example, the WHO determined the effective exposed dose during one year after the accident to be 10 to 50 mSv, including the contamination from food, in the area with the highest dose in Fukushima Prefecture (i.e., Soso Area) and 1 to 10 mSv in the other areas in the prefecture. According to the external exposed dose evaluation by Fukushima Prefecture, however, residents with less than 1 mSv account for 77.9% in the Soso Area, a significantly lower dose, even including internal exposure, than in the WHO report. This is not an exception, but is one of the examples of overestimation resulting from a small sample size of data.

G: What are Required for Medical Staff

What surprised us in the actions taken after this accident was a lack of correct knowledge about radiation and its exposure that was possessed by the medical staff closely engaged in handling radiation on a daily basis. Included in what needs to be considered in a nuclear or radiation disaster are the medical/biological influence, environmental influence, psychological influence, and socioeconomic influence. All of these significantly relate to the understanding of health effects, and particularly the psychological influence and socioeconomic influence can potentially be reduced depending on the actions taken after the accident.

> "To conclude this paragraph, the authors would like to express a deep gratitude to Aki Yamamoto, the secretary, who devoted herself to the difficult office work that was necessary."

(Makoto Akashi, Misao Hachiya)

References

1) Chang WP, Chan CC, Wang JD: 60Co contamination in recycled steel resulting in elevated civilian radiation doses: causes and challenges. Health Phys, 73: 465–72, 1997.

2) Hwang SL, Hwang JS, Yang YT, Hsieh WA, Chang TC, Guo HR, Tsai MH, Tang JL, Lin IF, Chang WP: Estimates of Relative Risks for Cancers in a Population after Prolonged Low-Dose-Rate Radiation Exposure: A Follow-up Assessment from 1983 to 2005. Radiation Research, 170: 143–148, 2008.

3) Japan Meteorological Agency, Great East Japan Earthquake — The 2011 off the Pacific coast of Tohoku Earthquake — related portal site: http://www.jma.go.jp/jma/menu/jishin-portal.html

4) Nuclear and Industrial Safety Agency, Partial error in the data of the amount of radioactive substances released (October 20, 2011): http://www.meti.go.jp/press/2011/10/20111020001/20111020001.pdf

5) Tominaga T, Hachiya M, Akashi M: Lessons learned from response to the accident at the TEPCO Fukushima Dai-ichi Nuclear Power Plant: from the viewpoint of radiation emergency medicine and combined disaster. Radiation Emergency Medicine, 1: 56–61, 2012.

6) IAEA, EPR-First Responders 2006 Manual for First Responders to a Radiological Emergency, Vienna, Austria, 2006 October.

7) Ogino H, Ichiji T, Hattori T: Verification of screening level for decontamination implemented after Fukushima nuclear accident. Radiat Prot Dosimetry, 51: 36–42, 2012.

8) ICRU, Dosimetry of External Beta Rays for Radiation Protection. International Commission on Radiation Units

and Measurements (ICRU) Report 56, 1997.

9) Office of Community Health, General Affairs Division, Health Service Bureau, Ministry of Health, Labour and Welfare: Health consultation concerning the influence of radiation (Provision of information) (March 23, 2011): http://www.mhlw.go.jp/stf/houdou/2r98520000015rt9-img/2r98520000016399.pdf

10) ICRP J. Valentin (Edt): The 2007 Recommendations of the International Commission on Radiological Protection. ICRP Publication 103 Annals of the ICRP, vol 37: Nos. 2–4, 2007.

11) Nakamura N: Genetic effects of radiation in atomic-bomb survivors and their children: Past, Present and Future. Journal of Radiation Research, vol. 47 (Suppl): B67–73, 2006.

12) Akahane K, Yonai S, Fukuda S, Miyahara N, Yasuda H, Iwaoka K, Matsumoto M, Fukumura A, Akashi M: NIRS external dose estimation system for Fukushima residents after the Fukushima Dai-ichi NPP accident., National Institute of Radiological Sciences, 2013.

13) Fukushima Prefecture homepage: http://www.pref.fukushima.jp/imu/kenkoukanri/251112siryoul.pdf

14) Fukushima Prefecture homepage: http://www.pref.fukushima.jp/imu/wbc/20131101wbc_joukyou.pdf

15) World Health Organization (WHO) 2013 Health risk assessment from the nuclear accident after the 2011 Great East Japan earthquake and tsunami based on preliminary dose estimation WHO Press, Geneva, Switzerland

16) World Health Organization (WHO) 2012 Preliminary dose estimation from the nuclear accident after the 2011 Great East Japan Earthquake and Tsunami, WHO Press, Geneva, Switzerland

2. Medical Actions Taken to Deal with the Tokyo Electric Power Company Fukushima Daiichi Nuclear Power Station Accident

A. How the Nuclear Station Accident Occurred

The Great East Japan earthquake, which occurred on March 11, 2011, was the world's fourth largest earthquake since 1900. Due to the subsequent tsunami that reached the Pacific coast of the Tohoku district, the nuclear power stations in four locations in Miyagi, Fukushima, and Ibaraki Prefectures faced a crisis of station blackout attributable to the loss-of-offsite-power despite the success of the emergency reactor shutdown at all of the 11 nuclear reactors in operation.

In Fukushima Prefecture, an unprecedented complex disaster occurred due to the earthquake, tsunami, and nuclear plant accident. On the first day of the earthquake, the government issued a nuclear emergency situation declaration shortly after 7 pm and issued an evacuation order shortly after 9 pm for the area within 3 km from the Tokyo Electric Power Company Fukushima Daiichi Nuclear Power Station (hereinafter referred to as the "Fukushima Daiichi Nuclear Station") and issued an evacuation order for the area within 10 km on the early morning of the following day, the 12th. Due to the hydrogen explosion of the reactor No. 1 that occurred shortly after 3 pm on the 12th and to other situations, an evacuation order was issued on the evening of the 12th for the area within 20 km from the Fukushima Daiichi Nuclear Station and within 10 km from the Fukushima Daini Nuclear Station (included the area within 20 km from the Fukushima Daiichi Nuclear Station). The reactor cores were able to be cooled in the nuclear plants other than the Fukushima Daiichi Nuclear Station. At the Fukushima Daiichi Nuclear Station, however, since all of the AC power supplies, including emergency batteries were lost, the reactor cores could not be cooled and they melted. Explosions associated with the hydrogen generation occurred and a large amount of radioactive substances, which must be confined inside, spread to vast areas outside the reactor. The level of radioactive substances released is estimated to be one sixth to one tenth of that of the Chernobyl Nuclear Plant accident and this situation developed into a nuclear plant accident of level 7 on the International Nuclear Event Scale (INES), the same level as that of the Chernobyl Nuclear Plant accident.

A large amount of radioactive substances spread to the Pacific Ocean side due to the weather conditions and the amount deposited in soil is estimated to be lower than the amount released. However, there are areas with a high concentration of radioactive cesium contamination of the soil, mainly to the northwest of the nuclear plant, and the air dose rate is approximately proportional to the concentration. The off-site center (OFC) originally located at Okuma Town in Fukushima Prefecture, which had been prepared as a place where actions are taken to deal with the accident in the event of a nuclear disaster, had to be relocated to an alternative location in Fukushima City due to the power and water outage caused by the earthquake as well as the expansion of the evacuation zone.

B. Initial Actions Following the Nuclear Station Accident

Apart from the initial actions common to complex disasters, important matters for the initial actions particular to a nuclear disaster include; indoor evacuation when a radioactive plume (radioactive cloud) passes to prevent internal exposure through inhalation, and use of stable iodine tablets and evacuation from the area the radioactive plume passes when thyroid exposure is predicted to exceed 100 mSv. Since radioactive substances may adhere during evacuation, screening must be performed at the shelter. If the screening level is exceeded, shoes and clothes must be changed and if skin contamination is found, the relevant region must be decontaminated. However, in the case of this accident, since radiation protection measures in a disaster, such as evacuation guidance using the System for Prediction of Environmental Emergency Dose Information (SPEEDI) did not function, evacuation was initially instructed in accordance with the distance from the nuclear plant. Even though stable iodine tablets to prevent internal thyroid exposure were supposed to be taken by those who needed them (based on the instructions of the Nuclear Emergency Response Headquarters) such measures were not always applied due to confusing information. Stable iodine tablets were taken in some locations and not taken in other locations depending on the discretion of the different people at the different sites. At the initial stage, the criterion for the screening level was not clear either. As a result of discussions in, for example, the Nuclear Emergency Response Headquarters, to comprehensively minimize the damage with various factors taken into consideration (such as the weather condition at the time of the accident, the water and power outage condition, and the fact that screening was necessary for many people), 100,000 cpm by a GM counter-type survey meter is said to have been determined as the criterion for decontamination and 13,000 cpm as the criterion for simplified wiping of the contaminated area. Screening following the initial evacuation was performed for more than 200,000 people, and 110 people are reported to have been undressed and decontaminated because of counts exceeding 100,000 cpm.

What made it difficult to make decisions about the initial actions during this nuclear accident was not only that the accident was beyond the scope of the assumption about the necessary measures in the regional nuclear disaster prevention plan, but also that it was a complex disaster, involving the earthquake and tsunami, in broad areas with various types of infrastructure interruptions. Utmost efforts were made under conditions of significant confusion for; the transportation and medical treatment of many people, securing the destinations and means of transportation for patients and inmates for their evacuation from hospitals and care facilities in the evacuation zone, determination of the range and route of residents' evacuation and establishment of their information system, preparation of new shelters and securing evacuation means, searching for missing people, and postmortem examinations. For the emergency medical treatment of injured and sick people exposed to radiation during the restoration work of the nuclear plant where the accident has occurred, five institutes for initial health care and one institute for secondary health care (Fukushima Medical University Hospital) were designated in Fukushima Prefecture prior to the accident. However, since three of these hospitals were in the evacuation zone and the other two were affected by the earthquake and tsunami and busy with the treatment of injured and sick people, it was only Fukushima Medical University Hospital that could accept people with radiation exposure.

The initial actions for the nuclear accident were taken not only in the evacuation area, but also at the shelters and the surrounding areas of the evacuation zone. A system to inspect drinking water and food was established and based on inspection information and the provisional regulation values for radioactivity in food the shipment and safety of food were promptly regulated.

As of March 15 to 16, when the nuclear disaster situation was deteriorating and likely to linger, the range of not only hospital patients but also people who needed support (vulnerable people) in the disaster area was further expanded. There were many matters which required consideration even for healthy victims, such as sanitation and nourishment, mental healthcare, measures against infectious diseases, and measures against cold. In the evacuation area, a total of more than 2,000 people were in hospitals and long-term care facilities. As of March 13, when the evacuation of general affected people was completed, the transportation of 840 patients was not yet completed. Utmost efforts were made to transport patients with the corporation of the Emergency Response Headquarters of Fukushima Prefecture, the Disaster Medical Assistance Team

Chapter 1 | What Nuclear Disaster Means

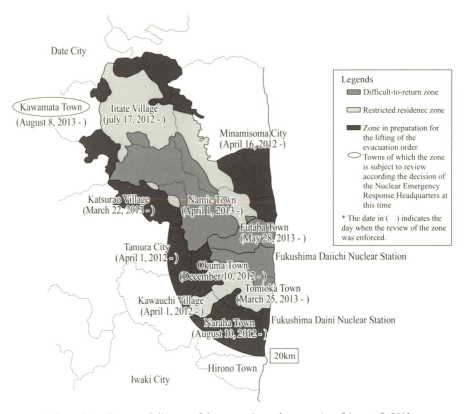

Figure 2-1 Conceptual diagram of the evacuation order zones (as of August 7, 2013)

(DMAT), the Self-Defense Forces, and other organizations. However, it was reported that 12 patients died during transportation and another 50 patients immediately after transportation[1]. The disaster-related death toll during the year until March 2012 compiled by the Reconstruction Agency was 761 in Fukushima Prefecture, the largest among the affected prefectures. Physical and mental fatigue at shelters accounted for most of the deaths, followed by physical and mental fatigue during the transportation to shelters. It was also reported that the mortality rate of evacuees at long-term care facilities in Fukushima Prefecture during the several months after the earthquake was three times higher than during ordinary years[2].

About 120,000 people lived in this evacuation area, including those in the planned evacuation zone. However, a total of about 210,000 people in the relevant municipalities had to evacuate, including those in the emergency evacuation-ready zone. The schematic map showing the change in evacuation order zones and warning zones in 2011 and at present is shown abase (Figure 2-1).

C : Actions Taken to Deal with the Disaster by Medical Institutions around the Evacuation Area

Medical institutions in Fukushima Prefecture, mainly advanced critical care and emergency medical institutions on the initial three days after the earthquake, accepted emergency patients from the earthquake and tsunami and provided them with medical treatment with support from the parties inside and outside the prefecture, such as the DMAT. These medical institutions also functioned as intermediate base hospitals to transport hospital patients and inmates from the hospitals and care facilities in the Hamadori area on the Pacific coast to the hospitals and care facilities in other areas. In addition, many hospitals performed screening for the patients who visited the hospitals from the evacuation area and their attending family members. Furthermore, since it was necessary to provide emergency treatment to and decontamination of radioactive substances at the same time for injured or sick people from the explosion and other events at the Fukushima Daiichi Nuclear Station because of their potential contamination by various types of nuclides, Fukushima Medical University Hospital was engaged in medical care of 12 patients who had an onset of disorder at the initial stage of the accident. Since life sustaining medical care was totally suspended, various patients, such as those under artificial dialysis who needed water, those in an unstable condition, and those who required special curative drugs, were transported to remote areas. In addition, not only general hospitals but also long-term care hospitals and facilities in the Nakadori Area and Aizu Area of Fukushima Prefecture also accepted affected people in the hospitals from the Hamadori Area on the Pacific coast of Fukushima Prefecture[3].

D : Situation of Radioactive Substances in the Environment and Health Risk

It was reported that after the Chernobyl Nuclear Plant accident, which occurred on April 26, 1986, the incidence of thyroid cancer increased in proportion to the internal exposed dose[4]. In addition to the fact that Chernobyl was a region with a lack of iodine from the beginning, the measurement of and regulation of the allowable radiation dose of food, artificial milk (powder milk), drinking water, etc., was extremely insufficient. According to the reports of the International Commission on Radiological Protection (ICRP) and the United Nations Scientific Committee on the Effects of Atomic Radiation (UNSCEAR) and other reports, due to the intake of, for example, raw milk contaminated by radioactive iodine (^{131}I), the average thyroid equivalent dose for children six years old or younger due to internal exposure by radioactive iodine was 1,800 mSv for those who had been evacuated from within 30 km from the Chernobyl Nuclear Plant, 610 mSv for those in the whole Gomel region, and 150 mSv in the whole of Belarus[5].

In Fukushima Prefecture, even though the SPEEDI could not be fully utilized for the evacuation or for the use of stable iodine tablets, an evacuation or indoor evacuation order was issued early and the measurement of radioactive substances in drinking water and food was made with the consequent restrictions on their shipment and intake imposed at an early stage through the efforts of many people concerned. In addition, since a high level of iodine is contained in food in Japan, the amount of radioactive iodine taken into the thyroid gland is predicted to be less when compared to regions with a lack of iodine in the food. However, according to the results of the estimation by the SPEEDI, there were some areas where the internal exposed dose of radioactive iodine might potentially exceed 100 mSv. This was based on the conservative estimation whereby a one-year-old infant was kept outdoors. According to the simplified thyroid screening performed in late March 2011 for about 1,000 children living in the area, the highest thyroid equivalent dose was about 35 mSv, estimated based on a continuous dosage scenario since March 12 and the children with their dose not exceeding the detection limit accounted for 55%. It was also reported in the estimation combined with the atmospheric dispersion simulation (with 90% accuracy) that the highest thyroid equivalent dose would be about 30 mSv[6]. Also, according to the data of direct measurement with a thyroid monitor done by Hirosaki University, radioactive iodine was detected in 74% of 54 adults among the residents who had evacuated to the area where the air dose rate increased during the initial stage, with a maximum value of 33 mSv and a median value of 3.6 mSv. Radioactive iodine was detected in six children among eight, with a maximum value of 23 mSv and a median value of 4.2 mSv[7]. Using the whole-body counters available within one month after the nuclear plant accident, 173 temporary evacuees were inspected to support the residents in the evacuation zone and radioactive iodine could be detected in about

Chapter 1 | What Nuclear Disaster Means

32% of them. The highest thyroid equivalent dose was 20 mSv[8]. Radioactive cesium ^{134}Cs or ^{137}Cs was detected in fewer than 40% of people, with the highest dose not exceeding 0.12 mSv. From the perspective of only comparing these results of the initial internal exposed dose estimation, the risk of thyroid cancer is considered low; however, the dose is expected to be more accurately estimated in the future.

Radioactive cesium in the environment is considered to be the most significant element that contributes to the external exposed dose. The basic survey for the Fukushima Health Management Survey included an initial external exposed dose that was estimated through computer analysis of the external exposed effective dose during the initial four months based on the behavior records in the interview sheet, together with the data of the air dose rate and others factor that have now become clarified. According to the announcement in November 2013, the analysis of about 460,000 residents of Fukushima Prefecture was completed and, consequently, the estimated effective dose during the four months from March 11 to July 11, 2011 was 1 mSv or less for 66.1%, 2 mSv or less for 94.9%, and 5 mSv or less for 99.8%. The highest effective dose was 25 mSv. The subsequent chronic external exposed dose has been measured using a personal dose meter (glass badge in most cases). According to the announcement of Koriyama City, it was reported that the result as of November 2012 converted to an annual dose was 0.59 mSv/year on the average for more than a score of thousands of children of junior high school age or under.

The environmental behavior of nuclides other than radioactive iodine and radioactive cesium (shown above) was researched (i.e., strontium and plutonium) and their ratio was generally extremely low as compared to iodine and cesium, even when compared with the environmental data from Japan at the time of past nuclear experiments and the Chernobyl Nuclear Plant accident data. Consequently, being careful about radioactive cesium will lead to almost complete measures to deal with internal exposure in the chronic phase caused by long half-life nuclides associated with oral intake.

E   Long-term Support in Cooperation with Local Community

As a result of the nuclear power plant accident, higher background (low dose exposure) areas than before the accident emerged, making it necessary to acknowledge radiation as one of the risks that may potentially affect health. It has become necessary to make consistent efforts to reduce external exposure from the environment and from internal exposure due to, for example the food chain. Since the initial stage after the accident it has been becoming a general practice to monitor food, soil, and the environment not only at the distribution level but also the daily life exposure. The comprehensive monitoring requires the efforts of many people. Taking an example of a meal, it is considered necessary not merely to be careful about internal exposure caused by intake of radioactive substances but also to coordinate with the dietary education and the culture with consideration given to various factors, such as the nutrition balance and the limitation of salt intake[9]. Consequently, it is considered important to establish a long-term interactive support system for individual people in cooperation with local public health and medical services. In the Fukushima health management survey being conducted with Fukushima Medical University Hospital as a core organization, an analysis is made by area on the health checkup and individual detailed survey results to utilize the information for health activities of each area. Furthermore, doctors and nurses of the university visit the place where, for example, the health checkup is conducted to directly provide health consultations in cooperation with public health nurses of the area. This can lead to the primary and secondary prevention of disease.

In the future, in addition to providing emergency medical care for exposure during the long-term decommissioning of the nuclear reactors where the accident occurred, it is important to establish efficient and effective preventive measures with multifaceted determination of health risks attributable to chronic low dose (low dose rate) radiation exposure. Accumulating scientific evidences will provide valuable information to the residents of Fukushima Prefecture, people in Japan, and the world for determining individual health risk.

> The author sincerely hopes that efforts made by local communities, including people involved in public health, can be a help to individual residents to lead a healthy life and meaningful life.
> The author would like to express deep gratitude for the heartfelt support to Fukushima Prefecture from the whole country and world.

(Akira Ohtsuru)

References

1) Tanigawa K, Hosoi Y. Hirohashi N, et al: Loss of Life after evacuation: lessons learned from the Fukushima accident. Lancet, 379: 889–891, 2012.

2) Yasumura S, Goto A, Yamazaki S, Reich MR. Excess mortality among relocated institutionalized elderly after the Fukushima nuclear disaster. Public Health, 127: 186–188, 2013.

3) Hasegawa A: Facing a Radiation Disaster, Chapter 1: 10–61. Life Science Publishing Co., Ltd., Tokyo, 2013.

4) Brenner AV, Tronko MD, Hatch M, et a1: I-131 dose response for incident thyroid cancers in Ukraine related to the Chernobyl accident. Enviorn Health Perspect, 119: 933–939, 2011.

5) Cardis E, Hatch M. The Chernobyl accident- an epidemiological perspective. Clin Oncol CR Coll Radiol, 23: 251–260, 2011.

6) Kurihara, 0, Kim, E, Suh S, et al: Reconstruction of early internal dose in the TEPCO Fukushima NPS accident. The 2nd NIRS Symposium on Reconstruction of Early Internal Dose in the TEPCO Fukushima Daiichi Nuclear Power Station Accident: 140–163, 27 Jan 2013, Tokyo.

7) Tokonami S, Hosoda M, Akiba S, et al: Thyroid dose for evacuees from the Fukushima nuclear accident. Scientific Reports, 2: 507, 2012.

8) Matsuda N, Kumagai A, Ohtsuru A, et al: Assessment of internal exposure doses in Fukushima by a whole body counter within one month after the nuclear power plant accident. Radiat Res, 179 (6) : 663–668, 2013.

9) Ohtsuru A, Miyazaki M: Situation in Fukushima Prefecture after the Tokyo Electric Power Company Fukushima Daiichi Nuclear Power Station accident and the present initiatives <Review>. Journal of the National Institute of Public Health 62 (2): 132–137, 2013.

10) Kondo H, Shimada J, Tase C, et al: Screening of Residents Following the Tokyo Electric Fukushima Daiichi Nuclear Power Plant Accident. Health Physics, 105: 11–20, 2013.

11) Yasumura S, Hosoya M, Yamashita S. et al: Study protocol for the fukushima health management survey. J Epidemiol, 22: 375–383, 2012.

3 Health Effects of Radiation

A What Radiation Exposure Means

If cells are exposed to radiation, the cells will die or suffer a functional disorder if exposed to a high dose. Hence, if there are a large number of such cells, the relevant tissue or organ will suffer a functional disorder. This is the deterministic effect (tissue reaction) and generally there is a threshold value showing the exposed dose up to which no functional disorder occurs and over which the degree of the disorder increases with an increase in the exposed dose. In most cases, a deterministic effect leads to the appearance of acute radiation symptoms soon after radiation exposure, and it will be critical if, for example, the bone marrow suppression or the disorder of the epithelium of digestive organs becomes severe. Among health effects that emerge long after radiation exposure, a health disorder other than cancer, such as cataracts and circulatory disorder, can also occur based on this mechanism.

On the other hand, in the case of low dose exposure, the death or functional disorder of cells will not appear but abnormalities such as damage to DNA in cells occurs. These kinds of abnormalities can constantly arise due to various influences other than radiation and those are normally repaired in living organisms; however, abnormalities that cannot be repaired eventually remain and the number of abnormalities remaining can increase with an increase in the exposed dose. The occurrence of cancer and the influence of genetic effects based on this kind of mechanism are called probabilistic effects. Even though the risk of occurrence of cancer increases with an increase in exposed dose, the degree of severity of the cancer that has occurred is not considered to depend on the exposed dose level. In terms of radiation protection, it is not assumed that there is any threshold value of the exposed dose in the risk of occurrence of probabilistic effects, and the concept that the risk increases with an increase in the exposed dose is called the linear non-threshold (LNT) hypothesis [1, 2].

Even if the total exposed dose is the same, the effects of radiation on living organisms differ depending on the radiation exposure for a short time (high-dose-rate exposure) or a long time (low-dose-rate exposure). The effects of low-dose-rate exposure on living organisms are generally considered less significant than those of high-dose-rate exposure because low-dose-rate exposure is considered to provide more opportunities to restore abnormalities than high-dose-rate exposure [1]. Atomic bomb radiation exposure, particularly exposure to the initial radiation, is typical high-dose-rate exposure, whereas exposure to radioactive substances in the environment is generally low-dose-rate exposure.

B Atomic Bomb Radiation

Atomic bomb radiation can be classified into the radiation emitted by nuclear fission of uranium and plutonium inside the bomb and from their products within about one minute after the explosion (the so-called initial radiation and mainly γ-rays) and the residual radiation. The latter is derived from the induced radioactivity produced in the substances (such as soil and buildings) rendered radioactive by neutron beams included in small amounts in the initial radiation and from the radioactive substances (radioactive fallout) produced as a result of nuclear fission. For the initial radiation emitted from the atomic bomb, since such factors as the air dose by traveling distance and the attenuation by shielding when it passes through buildings and human bodies are not established as a dose system, the exposed dose by organ of individual people is estimated based on the interview survey of the exposure location of the exposed persons, shielding condition, and other factors [3, 4]. Since γ-rays and neutron beams differ in their influence on living organisms, the value obtained by adding ten times (equivalent to the biological effect ratio) the neutron ray dose and the γ-ray dose is described in Gy (gray) as the weighted absorbed dose for the assessment of the health effects of atomic bomb radiation [5]. The estimated doses without shielding at locations 1 km away from the center of explosion are about 7 Gy in Hiroshima and about 10 Gy in Nagasaki, both critical. However, they are reduced to about one tenth, about 0.6 Gy and about 1 Gy, respectively, at locations 1.5 km away, and further reduced to about 80 mGy and about 140 mGy at locations 2 km away and about 13 mGy and about 23 mGy at locations 2.5 km away [3].

For induced radioactivity, the radiation dose with respect to the distance from the center of the explosion and the time after the explosion can be estimated based on the neutron dose emitted from the atomic bomb and the elemental composition of the ground and buildings. However, in order to estimate the exposed dose of individual people, the behavior record showing where and when they were is necessary. The radiation exposure attributable to radioactive fallout is considered to be related not only to the radioactive intensity and geographical distribution of the radioactive fallout but also to the situation of people, such as how they contacted rain or other things containing radioactive fallout. Internal exposure due to inhalation of soil dust containing induced radioactivity and intake of water and food containing radioactive fallout is also possible, which is difficult to evaluate. Accordingly, it is extremely difficult to estimate the exposed dose of an individual person caused by the residual radiation. However, as described later, since the risk assessment of contracting cancer and mortality relies on the fact that the estimated risk value of people exposed to a high dose of 1 to 3 Gy shows a clear dose-response relationship with respect to the exposed dose, the estimated risk value based on the initial radioactivity is not considered significantly affected, if at all, by the influence of the residual radiation.

Consequently, the follow-up study of atomic bomb survivors eventually assessed the late health effects (probabilistic effects and late probabilistic effects) caused by the low to high dose external exposure at a high dose rate due to the initial radiation of the atomic bomb. This kind of exposure is significantly different from the exposure of residents caused by, for example, the nuclear power plant accident. However, the tracking study is regarded as the standard document to assess health effects from various perspectives, such as the high accuracy in estimating the amount of exposure to initial radiation, a large number of people tracked, a long period of follow-up, and the high accuracy in obtaining the result indices of mortality, cause of mortality, number of cases of cancer contracted, and others [6].

C Follow-up survey Study of Atomic Bomb Survivors

A long-term epidemiological follow-up study is essential to clarify the late health effects of radiation [5, 7]. For atomic bomb survivors, a follow-up study (life span study: LSS) of about 120,000 people is being conducted with 1950 as the starting year. In addition, another follow-up study is being conducted for about 3,600 atomic bomb survivors exposed in utero and about 77,000 children of atomic survivors born between 1946 and 1984 whose parents' exposure condition is clarified. The main result indices in these follow-up studies are mortality, cause of mortality, and contracting cancer. Also, for some of the people under the LSS and the group of atomic bomb survivors exposed in utero, the adult health study (AHS) is being conducted, whereby their health condition is checked every other year in the health checkup at the

Chapter 1 What Nuclear Disaster Means

Radiation Effects Research Foundation. Recently, a study of the children of atomic survivors through their health checkup has also started.

1 Cancer

The excessively high rate of onset of leukemia for atomic bomb survivors could be observed starting about two years after exposure and peaked six to eight years after exposure. The increase in the risk of cancer other than leukemia (solid tumors) became obvious about 10 years after exposure and has continued to date[5]. The risk of mortality from all solid tumors caused by radiation, based on the follow-up from 1950 to 2003, is about 42% greater on average for men and women when the person who was exposed to 1 Gy radiation at the age of 30 has reached 70 years old as compared to non-atomic bomb survivors in the same generation[8]. As shown in Figure 3-1, the dose-response relationship between the exposed radiation dose and the risk of all solid tumors is decisive according to the approximate line based on the results in the high dose area, while a significant variability can be observed in the low dose area of less than 0.25 Gy. The estimated straight line for the dose-response relationship crossed the origin and the upper limit of the threshold value in the 95% confidence interval was 0.15 Gy and the risk attributable to radiation was significant for 0.2 Gy or more.

For every 10 years older a person was when exposed to radiation, the risk of mortality from all solid tumors when the person reached 70 years old decreased by about 30%. The younger a person when exposed to radiation, the greater the risk; for example, for a person 70 years old exposed to 1 Gy at the age of 20 the risk is about 60% higher than that for a person with no radiation exposure. This value can be obtained by dividing 0.42 (in the case of radiation exposure at the age of 30) by 0.7. According to the results of the study from 1950 to 1997, the lifetime risk for those exposed to 0.1 Gy at the age of 30 was estimated to

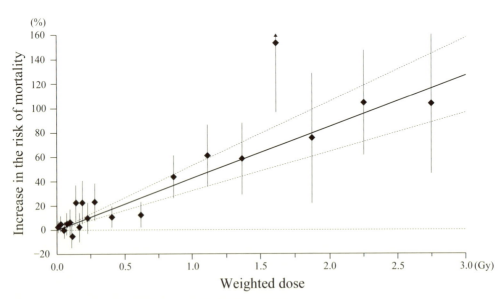

Figure 3-1 Exposed radiation dose and excessive risk of mortality from all solid tumors when an atomic bomb survivor who was exposed at the age of 30 has reached 70 years old
Note: Showing how much the risk of mortality from all solid tumors increases in percentage as compared to a person with no radiation exposure (0 Gy). The risk of mortality increases by about 42% at an exposed dose of 1 Gy.
(Partial revision from Ozasa K, et al.: Studies of the mortality of atomic bomb survivors, Report 14, 1950–2003: An overview of cancer and noncancer diseases. Radiat Res 2012; 177: 229–243 (Errata in April, 2013))

increase by 0.9 percentage points for men and 1.1 percentage points for women from the lifetime risk of mortality from all solid tumors for those in the same generation with no radiation exposure, namely 25% for men and 19% for women. In the case of radiation exposure at the age of 10, the increase in lifetime risk is 2.1 and 2.2 percentage points for men and women, respectively, whereas it is 0.3 and 0.4 percentage points for men and women, respectively, in the case of radiation exposure at the age of 50[9].

The risk of cancer attributable to radiation differs depending on the site and significantly increases at a number of main sites. There is an increase in stomach, lung, liver, colon, breast, gallbladder, esophagus, bladder, ovary, and thyroid gland cancer, whereas no significant increase is observed for pancreas, uterus, prostate gland, or kidney parenchyma, for which the reason is not clear[8-11].

Leukemia is a rare disease that is increased at an early stage after exposure, which makes it difficult to estimate its risk. However, the risk of mortality for people exposed to 1 Gy at the age of 10 from all leukemias is estimated to have increased to several tens of times that of non-atomic bomb survivors at the peak period. The risk of mortality significantly decreased with an increase in age at the time of exposure and it also rapidly decreased even for young people after 10 years after exposure[12]. Since the dose-response relationship for leukemia forms a concave curve instead of a straight line, the risk, for example, after 0.1 Gy exposure is less than one tenth the risk for 1 Gy exposure.

2   Diseases other than cancer

Conventionally, the relationship between radiation exposure and diseases other than cancer has been mainly observed as a deterministic effect at a high dose, such as that of radiation therapy, and its after effect. Also in the case of atomic bomb radiation, radiation cataracts due to posterior subcapsular opacification of the lens relatively soon after exposure has been considered to be a deterministic effect with a threshold value present [13, 14]. In recent years, the increase in the risk of, for example, a cardiovascular disease has been observed for atomic bomb survivors at an exposed dose of 1 to 2 Gy. In the case of a cardiovascular disease with a clear disease type, such as hypertension and cardiac infarction in young atomic survivors, the increase in the morbidity risk is observed at a high dose of 2 Gy or more. In the case of mortality caused by a disease with an unclear disease type, such as a cardiac failure and pneumonia, the risk increases in proportion to the dose. For the latter, it will be also necessary to investigate the possibility of a latent malignant tumor [8, 15, 16]. Since the accuracy of the morbidity investigation of non-cancerous disorders is affected by the diagnostic measures, a standardized method must be used to conduct an investigation; such as a health checkup. In the investigation of the prevalence of thyroid disease from 2000 to 2003, the increase in the risk of a thyroid nodule, benign nodule, and benign tumor (such as thyroid adenoma) was observed in the ultrasonography and the subsequent histological examination[17]. The prevalence of an ophthalmic disease diagnosed from 2000 to 2002 mainly for those who were less than 13 years old when exposed, found dose effects on the cortical cataract in addition to a posterior subcapsular cataract[18]. Since a parathyroid disease is a rare disease there are only a few cases; however, the increase in the prevalence of parathyroid adenoma and parathyroid hypertension were observed in the investigation from 1986 to 1988[19]. While these investigations reported that the risk was higher for those who were exposed when young, it must be noted that, in the prevalence investigation the investigation period and subjects to be investigated are limited in some cases [17-19]. For other disorders, studies are also conducted on their relationship with the atomic bomb radiation exposure[14]. For the relationship between radiation exposure and non-cancerous disorder, studies must be conducted on whether the cause-and-effect relationship is truly indicated through the longitudinal investigation with diagnostic criteria strengthened from the epidemiological perspective, as well as on the mechanism of the clinical condition.

3 Atomic bomb survivors exposed in utero

Atomic bomb survivors exposed in utero are those who were exposed to radiation in their mother's body after conception. The risk of occurrence of microcephaly and mental retardation increased with an increase in the exposed dose. Significant mental retardation occurred, particularly for those who had been exposed eight to 15 weeks after conception, and even although a threshold value is assumed, the occurrence ratio was 0.8% for a exposed dose of less than 5 mGy whereas it was about 25% for a exposed dose of about 0.7 Gy and further increased with an increase in the exposed dose[20]. According to the results of the follow-up study of the risk of cancer for atomic bomb survivors exposed in utero conducted from 1958 to 1998, the risk of developing solid tumors at the age of 50 after exposure to 1 Gy was considered to increase by 42%, which was not, however, necessarily significant compared to the risk of young atomic bomb survivors who had been exposed within six years after birth (170% increase)[21].

D Genetic Effects

Genetic effects are the effects of radiation exposure of the germ cells of the parents before conception, for which there has been a strong concern from the beginning among health effects due to the atomic bomb and of which many investigations have been conducted. Investigations of the children of atomic bomb survivors through, for example, the health checkup that includes birth defects (1948–1954), gender ratio of the children (1948–1962), chromosomal abnormalities of the parents and children (1967–1985), and comparison of DNA abnormalities (1985–present), as well as the investigation of the mutation of blood

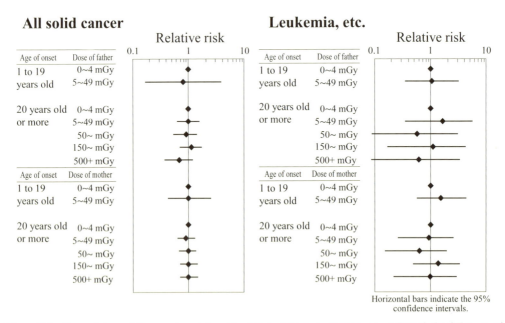

Figure 3-2 Exposed dose of the parents and the risk of their children to develop cancer through the follow-up of the children of atomic bomb survivors (Year of birth between 1946 and 1984, follow-up from 1958 to 1997)
Note: The relative risk by exposed dose of the parents is indicated as the risk of the children, whose parent's respective expose doses were 0 to 4 mGy, to contract all solid tumors or leukemia as the standard (relative risk = 1). Since the 95% confidence interval crosses 1 in all dose ranges, it is determined that no increase can be observed in the risk of the children due to the exposure of their parents. Apart from this, no increase in the risk can be observed in the assessment with the dose as a continuous variable and with 0 Gy as the standard.

proteins (1975–1985), and in any other investigations, observed no increase in the abnormalities in children attributable the radiation exposure of the parents [5, 22]. In the results of the follow-up study from 1957 to 1998, no relationship between the exposed dose of the parents and the risk of the children developing solid tumors or leukemia could be observed (Figure 3-2)[23]. In the prevalence investigation from 2002 to 2006 through health checkups, no increase in lifestyle-related diseases which develop in adulthood, (hypertension, diabetes, hypercholesterolemia, cardiac infarction, angina, or stroke) was found[24]. For these results, follow-up is needed in the future because the people concerned are still young.

E : Summary of Health Effects

Health effects of radiation exposure that were clarified in the studies mainly by following up atomic bomb survivors are considered as follows: (1) The excessive onset of leukemia can be observed soon after the exposure, (2) the excessive onset of other cancers lasts for life in that the number of such cancer cases are added to those developing in ordinary people depending on the exposed dose, and (3) the excessive onset of disorders other than cancer can be observed for specified diseases at a relatively high dose range. For atomic bomb survivors exposed in utero, the effects associated with the development process of organs in fetal life appear in cases of high dose exposure and the risk of cancer after birth increases. For the children of atomic bomb survivors, no genetic effects can be observed to date. Many of the epidemiological surveys on the health effects caused by radiation exposure have been conducted as follow-up studies of those exposed to medical radiation and engaged in radiation work. In recent years, the results of the investigation of, for example, the environmental pollution caused by the Chernobyl Nuclear Plant accident and the nuclear industry in the former Soviet Union are also available. These results are considered roughly consistent with the results of the follow-up study of atomic bomb survivors. The United Nations Scientific Committee on the Effects of Atomic Radiation (UNSCEAR) and the International Commission on Radiological Protection (ICRP) summarize these results to scientifically evaluate the health effects of radiation exposure and establish the criteria for radiological protection[1,6].

The Radiation Effects Research Foundation in Hiroshima and Nagasaki is a public interest corporation funded by the Ministry of Health, Labour and Welfare of Japan and the United States Department of Energy (DOE) (for the latter, partly through the DOE research grant DE-HS0000031 from the National Academy of Sciences). The author's view does not necessarily reflect the views of the governments of either country.

(Kotaro Ozasa)

References

1) ICRP, Publication 103, Recommendations of the ICRP, 2007 (Recommendations of the International Commission on Radiological Protection (ICRP), 2007, The Japan Radioisotope Association (JRIA), 2009)
2) ICRP. Publication 118, ICRP Statement on Tissue Reactions and Early and Late Effects of Radiation in Normal Tissues and Organs. 19–54, 2012.
3) Young RW, Kerr GD, eds. Reassessment of the atomic bomb radiation dosimetry for Hiroshima and Nagasaki—Dosimetry system 2002. Radiation Effects Research Foundation, 2005.
4) Cullings HM, et al: Dose estimation for atomic bomb survivor studies: Its evolution and present status. Radiat Res, 166: 219–254, 2006.
5) Homepage of the Radiation Effects Research Foundation, Directory–2008. http://www.rerf.or.jp/shared/briefdescript/briefdescript.pdf
6) United Nations Scientific Committee on the Effects of Atomic Radiation. Effects of Ionizing Radiation. UNSCEAR 2006 Report, 2008.
7) Ozasa K: Subjects and investigation plan. Effects of atomic bomb radiation on humans, Version 2: 14–19, BUN-KODO Co., Ltd., 2012.

Chapter 1 | What Nuclear Disaster Means

8) Ozasa K, et al: Studies of the mortality of atomic bomb survivors, Report 14, 1950-2003: An overview of cancer and noncancer diseases. Radiat Res 2012: 177: 229–243. (Errata in April, 2013)

9) Preston DL, et al: Studies of mortality of atomic bomb survivors. Report 13: Solid cancer and noncancer disease mortality: 1950-1997. Radiat Res, 160: 381–407, 2003.

10) Preston DL, et al: Solid cancer incidence in atomic bomb survivors: 1958-98. Radiat Res, 168: 1–64, 2007.

11) Furukawa K, et al: Long-term trend of thyroid cancer risk among Japanese atomic-bomb survivors: 60 years after exposure. Int J Cancer, 132: 1222–1226. 2013.

12) Richardson D, et al: Ionizing radiation and leukemia mortality among Japanese Atomic bomb survivors, 1950–2000. Radiat Res, 172: 368–82, 2009.

13) Nefzger MD, et al: Eye findings in atomic bomb survivors of Hiroshima and Nagasaki: 1963–1964. Am. J. Epidemiol, 89: 129–138, 1969.

14) Otake M, et al: Radiation-related posterior lenticular opacities in Hiroshima and Nagasaki atomic bomb survivors based on the DS86 dosimetry system. Radiat Res, 121: 3–13, 1990.

15) Shimizu Y, et al: Radiation exposure and circulatory disease risk: Hiroshima and Nagasaki atomic bomb survivor data, 1950-2003. Br Med J. 2010; 340: b5349: 1–8.

16) Yamada M, et al: Noncancer Disease Incidence in Atomic Bomb Survivors, 1958-1998. Radiat Res, 161: 622–632, 2004.

17) Imaizumi M, et al: Radiation dose-response relationships for thyroid nodules and autoimmune thyroid diseases in Hiroshima and Nagasaki atomic bomb survivors 55–58 years after radiation exposure. JAMA, 295: 1011–1022, 2006.

18) Nakashima E, et al: Comparison of methods for ordinal lens opacity data from atomic-bomb survivors: Univariate worse-eye method and bivariate GEE method using global odds ratio. Ann Inst Stat Math, 60: 465–482, 2008.

19) Fujiwara S, et al: Hyperparathyroidism among atomic bomb survivors in Hiroshima. Radiat Res, 130: 372–378, 1992.

20) Otake M. et al: Radiation-related brain damage and growth retardation among the prenatally exposed atomic bomb survivors. Int J Radiat Biol, 74: 159–171. 1998.

21) Preston DL, et al: Solid cancer incidence in atomic bomb survivors exposed in utero or as young children. J Natl Cancer Inst, 100: 428–36, 2008.

22) Nakamura N, Kodama Y, Asakawa J: Investigation of genetic effects on the birth defects, gender ratio, chromosomal abnormalities, and protein level, and the subsequent investigation on DNA. Effect of atomic bomb radiation on human bodies, Version 2: 319–325, 326–328, 329–333, 334–340, BUNKODO Co., Ltd., 2012.

23) Izumi S, et al: Cancer incidence in children and young adults did not increase relative to parental exposure to atomic bombs. Br J Cancer, 89: 1709–1713, 2003.

24) Fujiwara S, et al: Prevalence of adult-onset multifactorial disease among offspring of atomic bomb survivors. Radiat Res. 170: 451–457, 2008.

Chapter 2

Initiatives of Public Administrations

4 Measures Taken by the Japanese Government

This section overviews the measures taken by the Japanese government in the wake of the accident of the Tokyo Electric Power Company Fukushima Daiichi Nuclear Power Station (hereinafter referred to as the "Fukushima Daiichi Nuclear Station") from the perspective of ensuring the health of the residents of Fukushima Prefecture and the people of Japan, as well as explains various issues to be addressed in the future.

The initial measures taken by the government (Ministry of Health, Labour and Welfare) in the wake of the Fukushima Daiichi Nuclear Plant accident can be roughly classified into; (1) those taken immediately after the occurrence of the accident to deal with the great natural disaster and reduce the radiation exposure of residents and other people to the greatest extent possible, and (2) those for the medium- to long-term health management of the residents and to deal with their anxiety about radiation and radioactivity. While the latter measures (2) must continue to be taken in the future, the measures described in this section are limited to those taken only at the initial stage.

A Measures Taken to Deal with the Natural Disaster and Radiation Exposure of Residents

Of the measures taken by the government from the perspective of ensuring the health of the residents of Fukushima Prefecture and the people of Japan immediately after the occurrence of the Great East Japan Earthquake and the Fukushima Daiichi Nuclear Station accident, those in response to the large-scale natural disaster and those specific to the nuclear plant accident to reduce the exposure of the residents and other people are mainly as follows:

1 Measures taken in response to the large-scale natural disaster

At 14:50 on March 11, 2011, immediately after the occurrence of the earthquake, the Cabinet Response Office was established and the Emergency Meeting Team, consisting of crisis management staff members (bureau director-general class officials) of the related ministries and agencies, was convened. At the same time, the Headquarters for Emergency Disaster Control was established in the Ministry of Health, Labour and Welfare. At 15:04, the Ministry of Health, Labour and Welfare issued an order to stand by to the Disaster Medical Assistance Teams (DMAT) across the country (an order for the dispatch to Fukushima Prefecture was issued at 16:05). At 15:14, the Headquarters for Emergency Disaster Control of the government was established, and the government, under the Disaster Relief Act, cooperated with the municipalities concerned to rescue the affected people, establish shelters, provide meals, secure drinking water, build temporary houses, and provide clothes, bedclothes, and other necessities.

2 Measures taken specifically to deal with the Fukushima Daiichi Nuclear Station accident

At 15:37 on March 11, all of the AC power supplies were lost at the Fukushima Daiichi Nuclear Station, and Tokyo Electric Power Company informed the government and other parties concerned of the situation at 15:42, pursuant to Article 10 of the Act on Special Measures Concerning Nuclear Emergency Preparedness and at 16:45 pursuant to Article 15 of the same Act. In response, a nuclear emergency situation declaration under the same Act was issued at 19:03 and the Nuclear Emergency Response Headquarters of the government was officially established.

Chapter 2 | Initiatives of Public Administrations

a. Evacuation and indoor evacuation of the residents

At 21:23 on March 11, the head of the Nuclear Emergency Response Headquarters of the government (Prime Minister) issued an evacuation order to the residents in the area within 3 km from the Fukushima Daiichi Nuclear Station and issued an evacuation order to the residents in the area within 10 km at 05:44 on the following day, March 12, and to the residents in the area within 20 km at 18:25 on March 12.

The residents subject to these evacuation orders evacuated using their own cars, the busses arranged by their municipalities, or other means, whichever were appropriate. In the area within 20 km, however, there were seven hospitals with a total of about 850 inpatients at that point in time. For the evacuation of the inpatients from these hospitals, the individual hospitals regrettably had to make efforts to secure their evacuation means as well as define the medical institutions accepting these evacuee patients. For their actually evacuation, the Self-Defense Forces, the Fukushima Prefecture Police Department, and other organizations provided transportation in many cases; however, the support was not, and could not be, systematically provided. Furthermore, medical care during the evacuation could not be sufficiently ensured because hospital staff members themselves had also evacuated. Consequently, significant burdens were forced on a large number of patients, resulting in a number of cases of mortality.

On March 15, an indoor evacuation order was issued to the residents in the area of 20 to 30 km. This order was for indoor evacuation but not for evacuation and did not restrict entry to the relevant area. However, the number of people entering the area was extremely reduced, causing difficulties for people in the area to obtain commodities necessary for daily life. On March 25, voluntary evacuation was recommended for the residents in this area.

In this area, there were about 700 inpatients in six hospitals who had to be transported and about 1,000 inmates in 18 care and other facilities. However, since it had become difficult to secure food and other items in medical institutions and other facilities, it was decided to evacuate them in a planned manner. With the experience of the evacuation of people in the area within 20 km as a lesson, the following system was urgently established: The transportation of these patients was provided by the Ministry of Defense (Self-Defense Forces), the Ministry of Land, Infrastructure, Transport and Tourism, and the Japan Coast Guard, as well as the police and fire departments. The coordination with the medical institutions accepting the patients and inmates was made by Fukushima Prefecture (for those within the prefecture) and the Ministry of Health, Labour and Welfare (for those outside the prefecture). Furthermore, the DMAT provided medical support during transportation as necessary. Fukushima Prefecture firstly clarified the requests from individual facilities and subsequently the Ministry of Health, Labour and Welfare coordinated as necessary to receive people in wide areas in response to the request from Fukushima Prefecture. Consequently, mortality during transportation could be avoided.

Subsequently in April, the planned evacuation zones and specific spots recommended for evacuation were determined; however, since the residents in these zones and spots did not have to evacuate all at once, no significant confusion is considered to have occurred for the people who needed support to evacuate.

b. Restriction of the distribution and/or consumption of food

The main forms of exposure due to the radioactive substances released associated with the nuclear plant accident are external exposure (cloud shine) due to the radiation emitted into the atmosphere from radioactive substances, or external exposure (ground shine) due to the radiation emitted from radioactive substances adsorbed to the surface of the ground, and internal exposure due to the inhalation or oral intake of radioactive substances. Among these forms, the basic means to reduce internal exposure through oral intake of water and food contaminated by radioactive substances is to restrict the intake of such water or food.

For the Fukushima Daiichi Nuclear Station accident, the provisional regulation values under the Food Sanitation Act concerning radioactive substances were set on March 17 with the indices concerning the limits on food and drink ingestion in Nuclear Emergency Preparedness and Response Guidelines used for reference. These provisional regulation values were set to a level with the annual committed effective dose equivalent to 5 mSv.

However, it is specified in the Food Sanitation Act that, where food violating the provisional regulation values is found, the relevant prefectural governor, etc. shall order the individual food producers/distributors concerned to prohibit the sale, etc. of the said food (in the same lot). In this case, where distribution and intake of food must be broadly restricted to reduce internal exposure from food from the preventive perspective, measures taken under the Food Sanitation Act were eventually judged as insufficient.

Consequently, in this accident, it was determined to take measures through the order issued by the head of the Nuclear Emergency Response Headquarters (Prime Minister) to prefectural governors as urgent measures under the Act on Special Measures Concerning Nuclear Emergency Preparedness. While food monitoring had already started on March 16, several cases of exceeding the provisional regulation values were reported by March 20 and the government issued an order to restrict the distribution of spinach and kakina (green leafy vegetable of the genus Brassica) in the name of the head of the Nuclear Emergency Response Headquarters on March 21 to the governors of Fukushima Prefecture, Tochigi Prefecture, Ibaraki Prefecture, and Gunma Prefecture (also raw milk for Fukushima Prefecture). Subsequently, every time food exceeding the provisional regulation value was found as a result of monitoring, the range of the items and the areas subject to the restriction were expanded. Furthermore, on April 4, the "concepts of inspection planning and the establishment and cancellation of items and areas to which restriction of distribution and/ or consumption of food concerned applies" were announced. On April 5, the provisional regulation values of radioactive iodine (^{131}I) for fishery products were established.

Starting on April 1, 2012, the provisional regulation values under the Food Sanitation Act were revised so that the committed effective dose from food might be 1 mSv or less per year.

This food monitoring, and the mechanism to establish and cancel the restriction of distribution based on it, have been implemented to date. It has contributed to reducing internal exposure not only at the initial stage after the accident but also from the medium- to long-term perspective.

c. Management of tap water

For tap water, on March 19, 2011, the Ministry of Health, Labour and Welfare established the indices for the restriction of intake of radioactive substances contained in tap water. The actual restriction of intake started on March 21 in Iitate Village (Iitate Small Waterworks; the restriction was cancelled on April 1 for general people, such as adults and children, and on May 10 for infants) followed by other water utilities (municipalities) at which the index value was exceeded. On April 4, the Ministry of Health, Labour and Welfare announced the "concepts of the restriction of tap water intake and the cancellation of the restriction."

d. Others

Medical doctors, public health nurses, and other members were dispatched for the screening and the health management of residents in shelters performed by Fukushima Prefecture.

Chapter 2 | Initiatives of Public Administrations

B: Measures Taken for Medium- to Long-term Health Management and to Deal with Anxiety

1 Measures taken for long-term health management

a. Clarification (estimation) of the exposed dose

Considerable knowledge has already accumulated on the health effects of radiation and the degree of health effects in the future can be predicted by clarifying and estimating the exposed dose associated with the accident. In order to study whether low dose exposure has effects on health, an epidemiology study is needed whereby the relationship between the exposed dose of individuals and long-term health effects are determined (disease registry, cause of death registry, etc.). As basic information for this kind of study, it is very important to clarify and estimate the exposed dose of individual people.

As for the external exposure dose, two methods can be considered; one to directly measure it using an integrating dose meter or a similar device, and the other is to estimate it by using the behavior (traveling) records and the air dose levels by location and time in combination. However, since it is unknown when an accident might occur, instruments for direct measurement were not always available for ready use and such direct measurements could not be made in the accident this time.

For the air dose rate, however, the results of the monitoring performed in several locations and the mobile measurement could be utilized, and consequently it was decided to estimate the exposed dose of individual people by utilizing these data and combining them with the behavior records of individual people. This external exposure dose estimation system was developed by the National Institute of Radiological Sciences (hereinafter referred to as the "NIRS") utilizing subsidies from the Ministry of Education, Culture, Sports, Science and Technology. The behavior survey was conducted as part of the Fukushima Health Management Survey commissioned by Fukushima Prefecture to Fukushima Medical University.

As for the internal exposure dose, a whole-body counter or thyroid monitor was used to estimate the inhaled amount or oral intake amount, based on which the internal exposure dose was estimated as a committed dose.

For the thyroid dose, in order to clarify the effects on children's health based on the estimation on March 23, 2011 by the System for Prediction of Environmental Emergency Dose Information (SPEEDI), the local Nuclear Emergency Response Headquarters performed the thyroid screening (simplified measurement) for 1,149 children 0 to 15 years old from March 24 to 30 at Iwaki City, Kawamata Town, and Iitate Village upon the request (dated March 23) by the emergency advisory group of the Nuclear Safety Commission. It was found that for all of the 1,080 children, excluding 66 for whom the measurement results could not be properly obtained and three whose age was unknown, the value was lower than that equivalent to a thyroid dose of 100 mSv for a one-year old infant established by the Nuclear Safety Commission.

The government did not perform the measurement through thyroid monitor at the early stage after the accident to clarify the overall situation of the thyroid exposure dose attributable to radioactive iodine.

Measurements using a whole-body counter were made by the government and Fukushima Prefecture with the cooperation of the NIRS for 173 residents in the areas (Namie Town, Iitate Village, Yamakiya district of Kawamata Town, etc.) where the internal exposure dose was considered higher than in other

30

areas. The internal exposure attributable to ^{134}CS or ^{137}CS was less than 1 mSv for both of them. Even though measurement using a thyroid monitor was also made at the same time as the measurement using a whole-body counter, radioactive iodine was less than the detection limit because of a short half-life.

According to these results, it was clarified that neither external exposure nor the internal exposure attributable to ^{134}CS or ^{137}CS was at the level posing a significant problem for health according to the current medical knowledge. However, since the estimation of the exposed dose of the thyroid gland was insufficient, it was decided that the government would make further efforts for the estimation.

b. Ensuring the budget for the long-term health management (Health Fund for Childeren and Adults Affected by the Nuclear Incident)

In response to the view announced by the Fukushima Prefecture Governor that the medium- to long-term health management of the residents of Fukushima Prefecture should be performed by Fukushima Prefecture as the responsible organization, the government decided to provide financial and technological support to Fukushima Prefecture. To be specific, the government granted a subsidy of ¥78.2 billion to the "Health Fund for Childeren and Adults Affected by the Nuclear Incident" founded by Fukushima Prefecture and is also providing technical support to the Fukushima Health Management Survey and other projects implemented by Fukushima Prefecture utilizing this fund.

2 Measures taken to deal with anxiety of residents and the people of Japan

Since many disaster victims and people of Japan have significant anxiety about the health effects of radiation due to the accident, measures have been taken, such as establishing a contact for consultation at the NIRS, since immediately after the accident. However, since their anxiety did not seem to have been sufficiently relieved, the government established the "Conference to Coordinate Actions to Deal with the Anxiety about Health of People Affected by the Nuclear Accident," chaired by the Minister of the Environment, on April 20, 2012 and developed an action plan on May 31 in the same year. This conference established uniform actions in taking measures to deal with the anxiety about health.

C Points to be Improved in Light of the Measures Taken for this Accident

While we should never have an accident like the one at the Fukushima Daiichi Nuclear Station again, appropriate measures must be taken anticipating the unlikely occurrence of such an accident. To this end, in light of what we could not do to deal with this accident, we should review manuals, make necessary preparation, and repeatedly conduct drills so that appropriate actions can be taken in the event of an accident.

1 Measures to be taken during the evacuation of resident "people who need support (vulnerable people) in a disaster"

It is necessary to study in advance how and where to transport inpatients and inmates of various facilities, such as medical institutions, care facilities, and welfare facilities, as well as home-care patients and people who need support. It is also necessary to consider how to take measures for patients, such as artificial dialysis patients, whose life will be threatened unless an alternative medical institution can be immediately found. To this end, it is necessary to have sufficient information available on a daily basis as to what kinds of patients are in medical institutions and other facilities within a certain distance from a relevant nuclear plant.

Chapter 2 | Initiatives of Public Administrations

Since an extremely large-scale transportation of inpatients may be needed, depending on the scale of the accident and the location of the nuclear plant, it is also necessary for the prefecture where a nuclear plant is located to have sufficient discussions with neighboring prefectures in advance.

Even though this time the DMAT played a significant role transporting patients from the area 20 to 30 km from the nuclear plant, activities in the event of a nuclear plant accident are not originally within the scope of its activities. It is considered necessary to clarify its role during the process to improve the system to transport patients and provide emergency exposure medical care.

2 Development of the mechanism to clarify (estimate) the initial exposed dose

Included in the issues in dealing with this accident was a lack of and/or deficiency of the detailed monitoring mechanism (of the external dose and the concentration of radioactive substances in the air) that should allow direct clarification of the initial exposed dose or its estimation based on, for example, the behavior survey. Even though it is considered difficult to make direct measurement for all people during the initial confusing period, direct measurement for a certain number of people by gender, by age group, and by evacuation route is extremely important to conduct a study of the people and specific matters subject to subsequent health management. In addition, it is necessary to establish the mechanism in advance that allows the measurement.

3 Education of health workers

With regard to the purpose of screening, it is hard to say that a consensus was formulated in terms of whether it was for screening people who needed emergency exposure medical care, for preventing contamination from being brought out of the evacuation zone (i.e., selecting people who needed decontamination), for selecting people who should take iodine tablets, or for other purposes.

In addition, insufficient information given to medical service workers on radiation/radioactivity and health effects of radiation caused confusion in accepting people at medical institutions.

Accordingly, it is considered necessary to enhance training programs to disseminate information about radiation as a basis for emergency measures, and information about radiation exposure medical care.

4 Provision of information on various health effects of radiation to people on a routine basis

Included in the causes that brought about anxiety about health effects associated with this accident was a lack of basic information on radiation/radioactivity and their health effects. Another cause was the difficulty in understanding the concept of epidemiological cause-and-effect relationship. Furthermore, even the provision of such information after the accident will not lead to relief or elimination of anxiety without a feeling of trust in those providing information.

The dissemination of information about radiation and epidemiology and the study on how to provide reliable information will be issues to be addressed in the future.

4 Measures Taken by the Japanese Government

The relation of facts in this section may not be necessarily accurate due to the diversity of information and your understanding of this matter is appreciated. Also, please note that the views expressed in this section are the private views of the author.

**(Yasumasa Fukushima, Former Director, Health Sciences Division,
Minister's Secretariat, Ministry of Health, Labour and Welfare)**

5 Measures Taken by Fukushima Prefecture

A Measures Taken to Support the Health of Affected People

1 Coordination to secure regional healthcare experts to be engaged in activities to support the health of evacuees

In the case of this disaster, immediately after the Great East Japan Earthquake, the accident of the Tokyo Electric Power Company Fukushima Daiichi Nuclear Power Station (hereinafter referred to as the "Fukushima Daiichi Nuclear Station") occurred, and as the situation of the accident changed, so did the situation of evacuees, with new evacuation orders and other instructions being issued one after another. For example, as the number of evacuees increased a remarkable change occurred in their relocation and dispersion. In the towns/villages around the Fukushima Daiichi Nuclear Station, even the municipal offices had to be evacuated and relocated.

Consequently, evacuation effects were not limited to each municipality but dispersed broadly both the inside and outside of the prefecture. Furthermore, some evacuees had to relocate themselves to two or more shelters overtime, and as of March 16, 2011 (the fifth day after the earthquake), there were primary shelters established at 556 locations in 52 out of a total of 59 municipalities in the prefecture and the number of evacuees in shelters reached 73,608.

Under such circumstances, there were limited human resources engaged in health support activities, such as public health nurses at each public health and welfare office (hereinafter referred to as "public health center"), due a focus being placed on radiation screening of evacuees. To strengthen the system to promote the activities to support the health of evacuees promptly and broadly, the prefecture requested the government on March 12 to dispatch healthcare teams for support (consisting of public health nurses, national registered dietitians, public health doctors, sanitary management personnel, administrative personnel, and other members) from outside of the prefecture.

2 Coordination to dispatch and accept healthcare teams

As shown in Table 5-1, there are roughly three routes to dispatch public health nurses for support; public health nurses are the core members in the dispatched healthcare teams. The Health Promotion Division, Social Health and Welfare Department made arrangements to accept the dispatched teams for support through the Ministry of Health, Labour and Welfare route (Fig. 5-1 shows the flow of the request and coordination to dispatch healthcare teams) and the inter- municipality route. Fukushima Prefecture requested the dispatch of personnel through both routes and accepted them to perform their duties in the affected areas.

Table 5-2 shows how the dispatch of healthcare teams was requested and how they were accepted. The prefecture started accepting healthcare teams under the circumstances where the support of healthcare teams from outside of the prefecture was extremely limited compared to that of other prefectures due to the influence of the nuclear plant accident. In April, the number of evacuees relocating from primary shelters, such as schools and gymnasiums, to secondary shelters, such as private accommodation facilities leased by public administrations, increased. Furthermore, with an increase in the number of locations of

5 Measures Taken by Fukushima Prefecture

Table 5-1 Route to accept public health nurses for support

Route for acceptance	Outline	Division to coordinate the acceptance
Ministry of Health, Labour and Welfare route	- Public health nurses, etc. are dispatched for support through the coordination and mediation of Office of Public Health Guidance, General Coordination Division, Ministry of Health, Labour and Welfare pursuant to Article 30 of the Disaster Countermeasures Basic Act. - The prefecture requests the dispatch of personnel and accepts the dispatched personnel. - The dispatched personnel conduct support activities in the affected areas (affected municipalities, prefectural public health centers, etc.) designated by the prefecture.	Health Promotion Division
Ministry of Internal Affairs and Communications route	- The affected municipalities, etc. request the dispatch and the prefecture puts together the content of the requests and reports it to the Ministry of Internal Affairs and Communications, based on which the Ministry of Internal Affairs and Communications requests the Japan Association of City Mayors and the National Association of Town and Village Mayors for cooperation on the dispatch. - Dispatch is classified into a short-term dispatch and a medium- to long- term dispatch. - The coordination for accepting the dispatch and the content of specific activities, etc. is made between the municipalities concerned (concluding an agreement for the dispatch of personnel).	Local Administration Division of municipalities
Inter-municipality route	- Negotiation is made directly between the municipalities concerned based on a support agreement, proposals, etc. between the municipalities to accept the support personnel.	Health Promotion Division (Only for inter-prefectural coordination)

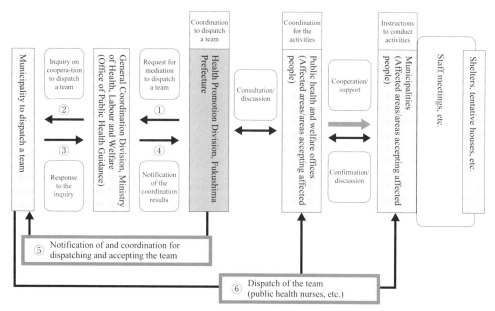

Figure 5-1 Flow of the request and coordination to dispatch healthcare teams through the Ministry of Health, Labour and Welfare route

shelters inside the prefecture, the number of support teams from across the country increased in the middle of April. In the last week of April, 89 people from 26 teams a day were accepted at maximum for support. In the prefecture, the prolonged relocation and dispersion of evacuees as well as the significant change in the administrative functions of the municipalities affected by the nuclear disaster caused the municipalities and human resources inside the prefecture continued difficulties in dealing with the situation, and forced

Chapter 2 | Initiatives of Public Administrations

Table 5-2 How measures have been taken to support the health of affected people

Situation in the prefecture	Main measures taken by the prefecture	Main issues
Within 24 hours after the earthquake (March 11 to 12)		
- Occurrence of the earthquake and tsunami - Establishment of the Emergency Response Headquarters and Regional Chapters of Fukushima Prefecture - Prefectural office building also affected (Difficulty in entering the building) - Lifeline interruption - Public transportation system interruption	- Collecting information on the extent of damage, etc. - Inquiries to municipalities and public health centers on the needs for dispatch of public health nurses, etc. - Request to the Ministry of Health, Labour and Welfare for the mediation to dispatch public health nurses, etc.	- Difficulty in clarifying the extent of damage at each area due to limited communication means, etc. - Difficulty in clarifying the situation, etc. through public health centers - Measures taken only by a limited number of prefectural government personnel
One to three days after the earthquake (March 12 to 14)		
- Intermittent aftershocks - Interruption and limitation of communication means - Hydrogen explosion at the Fukushima Daiichi Nuclear Power Station Unit 1 (Evacuation order for the area within 20 km) - Primary evacuees (52,998 as of March 14) - Increase in the number of evacuees and shelters due to repeated evacuation orders being issued due to the nuclear disaster - Radiation screening started (March 13)	- Coordination to determine the place of activities of dispatched public health nurses, etc. - Inquiry on whether public health nurses in the prefecture (prefecture, municipalities) can be dispatched to affected areas	- Fully involved in clarifying the situation of the whole area in the prefecture due to the rapid increase in and broad dispersion of evacuees and shelters - Difficulty in clarifying the extent of damage and the needs for support due to the continued difficulty in communicating with municipalities because of the start of the relocation of municipality offices, etc.
Three to seven days after the earthquake (March 14 to 17)		
- Intermittent aftershocks - Lifeline interruption - Hydrogen explosion at the Fukushima Daiichi Nuclear Power Station Unit 3 (March 14) and Unit 2 (March 15) (Evacuation order for the indoor evacuation zone in the area of 20 to 30 km)	- Continued coordination to determine the place of activities of dispatched public health nurses, etc. The dispatch of public health nurses for support from the outside of the prefecture was temporarily suspended due to the nuclear plant accident (March 15). - Inquiry and coordination on whether public health nurses in the prefecture (prefecture, municipalities) can be dispatched to affected areas - Public health centers, where possible, started visiting shelters, etc. in line with the timing of radiation screening. - Support for the coordination, etc. on medical care and welfare services for the cases that required emergency measures - Issuance of the notification on "Visits to shelters" to each public health center	- Continued fully involved in clarifying the situation of the whole area in the prefecture due to the rapid increase in and broad dispersion of evacuees and shelters - Shortage of public health nurses, etc. engaged in visiting shelters and conducting activities to support the health of evacuees (Public health nurses of public health centers were involved in radiation screening 24 hours a day and the dispatch of public health nurses from the outside of the prefecture was suspended due to the nuclear plant accident.) - Difficulty in clarifying the extent of evacuees because shelters were built by various organizations and human resources were also insufficient at the same time
Two to three weeks after the earthquake (March 18 to 31)		
- Intermittent aftershocks - Lifeline interruption, shortage of gasoline, food, etc. - Public transportation system interruption - Continued and repeated relocation of evacuees due to the influence of the nuclear plant accident	- Visits to shelters and activities to support health mainly by medical care teams - Visits to shelters, consultations on health, etc. by public health centers - Dispatch of public health nurses in the prefecture to towns and villages in the Coastal Region for support (a total of 100 nurses between March 22 and April 13) - Assisting activities to support health in shelters by public health nurses from the School of Nursing, Fukushima Medical University, Fukushima office of the Japan Health Insurance Association, and the Fukushima Preservative Service Association of Health	- Continued difficulty in clarifying the situation concerning shelters and the health issue of evacuees - Continued shortage of public health nurses, etc. engaged in visiting shelters and conducting activities to support the health of evacuees - Continued difficulty in clarifying the situation of the people who needed support (vulnerable people) in the disaster and supporting them mainly in the municipalities where their office functions were relocated

Situation in the prefecture	Main measures taken by the prefecture	Main issues
One month after the earthquake (April)		
- Shortage of gasoline, food, etc. gradually relieved - After shock of intensity 6 lower in Iwaki City and the Central Region - Relocation started to the secondary shelters (Relocation accelerated since the middle of April) - Number of evacuees (Primary shelters: 14,400, Secondary shelters: 12,422 (April 15)) - Dispatch of healthcare teams from the outside of the prefecture fully in progress	- Continued visits to shelters, consultations on health, coordination on how people who needed health support should be treated, etc. by each public health center - Health condition survey conducted for people living in secondary shelters with the mutual cooperation of healthcare teams in the affected municipalities, the municipalities to which people evacuated, the prefecture (public health centers), outside of the prefecture, etc. (for 13,479 people in 466 facilities in 31 municipalities from the middle of April to the end of June) - Living environment survey in shelters conducted by each public health center	- Difficulty in clarifying the health condition of evacuees and controlling the information about the people who needed support due to the continued relocation of evacuees - Continued issue of the living environment and diet in shelters, etc. and disparity in the quality of shelters, etc. - Continued health issues, such as colds, constipation, and stress symptoms such as sleeplessness as well as functional decline, etc. mainly in elderly people - Continued needs for experts engaged in health support activities with the dispersion of evacuees to broader areas
Two to three months after the earthquake (May to June)		
- Prolonged evacuation life - Residents in the planned evacuation zone starting evacuation - Relocation of and change in the functions of the municipality office in the affected municipalities (Katsurao Village, Iitate Village) - Fukushima Health Management Survey (Basic survey) - Inspection by whole-body counter started	- Measures taken in April continued - Employment of healthcare experts started in the Emergency Job Creation Fund Program for the purpose of developing the system to conduct health support activities of the affected people in each area - Support to create places for the exchange among evacuees and establish and operate the health salons, etc. after the health condition survey	- Worsening of chronic disorders, etc. and progress of functional decline, etc. due to the burden and the change in daily life attributable to prolonged evacuation life - Increase in anxiety, fatigue, stress, etc. associated with life in an unfamiliar area, evacuation life dispersed to broader areas, change in family structure, change in daily life, etc. - Continued shortage of healthcare experts in the affected municipalities, etc.
Four to five months after the earthquake (July to August)		
- Relocation from evacuation facilities to temporary houses and municipally subsidized rental houses fully in progress -Increase in evacuees to the inside of Iwaki City - Dispatch of healthcare teams from the outside of the prefecture diminished - Restart of health services in the affected municipalities	- Support to the health condition survey for the residents in temporary houses in accordance with the intention of the affected municipalities - Continued visits to the people who needed health support and coordination on how they should be treated, etc. by sharing the roles with the affected municipalities, etc. - Provision of health education and consultation at the meeting places, etc. of temporary houses and support to establish and operate the exchange salons, etc. - Support to health services in the affected municipalities by public health centers	- Less active exchange and mutual support among residents with the progress in relocation to temporary houses and municipally subsidized rental houses in progress - Shortage of healthcare experts engaged in health support activities due to the dispersion to temporary houses and municipally subsidized rental houses over broader areas - Securing healthcare experts with the Emergency Job Creation Fund Program not making progress as expected. - Difficulty in developing the medium- to long-term health support plan for residents due to the increased workload in the affected municipalities
Six to 12 months after the earthquake (September to March 2012)		
- Relocation to temporary houses and municipally subsidized rental houses fully in progress - Number of evacuees in Iwaki City from Futaba-Gun exceeding 10,000 - Two public health nurses of the prefecture allocated to the Iwaki Regional Promotions Bureau of the prefecture (Stationing of public health nurses in December, with the organization eventually consisting of three public health nurses of the prefecture, one clerk, and six temporary staff members) - Primary shelters in the prefecture closed (December 2011) - Reduction in the scale of the dispatch of healthcare teams from the outside of the prefecture →Termination of dispatch (March 2012)	- Measures taken in July and August continued - Activities to support affected municipalities with the public health center of the municipalities to which people evacuated as a contact point - Support activities by the healthcare teams from the outside of the prefecture to support the evacuees in Iwaki City with the Promotions Bureau as a base - Start of the health support project for the affected people for the purpose of securing experts in the affected municipalities, etc. (starting in January 2012) - Explanatory meeting of the health support project for the affected people held for FY2012 (for 13 municipalities in the coastal area)	- Increase in the number of people who needed health support due to prolonged evacuation life and a significant change in the living environment, etc. - Continued shortage of healthcare experts in the affected municipalities, etc. (At issue is to conduct and continue the health support activities in other than the areas where the municipality office was located.) - Insufficiency in cooperation, common understanding, etc. among the projects of individual divisions, etc. pertaining to the health support for the affected people both in the prefecture and municipalities.

Situation in the prefecture	Main measures taken by the prefecture	Main issues
Since one year after the earthquake (Since April 2012)		
- Continued situation of prolonged evacuation life with no prospect of returning home - Number of evacuees to Iwaki City still likely to increase even now (including removal and reconstruction of temporary houses, etc.) - Change in the municipality office organization structure of the affected municipalities (Relocation of the functions of the municipality office, new establishment of branches, etc.) - Establishment of the Iwaki branch of the Soso public health center in the Iwaki regional joint government building of the prefecture (June 2012).	- Continued activities to support the health of the affected people and support the healthcare activities, etc. of the affected municipalities with the public health center as a contact point. - Support to secure healthcare experts (public health nurses, nurses, national registered dietitians, etc.) in the affected municipalities, etc. in the projects commissioned to the Fukushima Nursing Association, etc. - Support activities for the nutrition/diet and oral health care of the affected people in the projects commissioned to the Dietetic Association and Dental Hygienists' Association of the prefecture. - Implementation of the projects to grant subsidies for the expenses for the health support projects for the affected people, as well as the expenses for the employment of healthcare experts implemented by the affected municipalities, etc.	- Many people with psychological stress and anxiety due to prolonged evacuation life, a significant change in the living environment, the life with no future prospects, etc. - Insufficiency in clarifying the health condition of and providing support to the residents in municipally subsidized rental houses, who were more broadly dispersed

the prefecture to continue to repeatedly request the Ministry of Health, Labour and Welfare to extend the mediation activities for dispatch. Under such circumstances, the prefecture had a hard time determining until when the dispatched support from outside of the prefecture would be requested. It was difficult to obtain the understanding of the municipalities dispatching the teams concerning the details of the support activities that were needed under the circumstance where no progress could be seen. Eventually, the period of dispatch of healthcare teams for support was about one year from March 15, 2011 to March 2, 2012. Support activities were conducted inside the prefecture by many people; a total of 7,442 people (5,667 public health nurses and other 1,775 people) from 18 prefectures (special wards, government ordinance cities, and municipalities are included in the prefecture where they are located).

(Summarized by Health Promotion Division, Fukushima Prefecture)

3　Main activities of the dispatched healthcare teams

In addition to healthcare teams from municipalities outside the prefecture, support was provided by nurses via the Japanese Nursing Association, the Fukushima Nursing Association, the Japanese Psychiatric Nurses Association, the Hospital Bureau, and other organizations (with the coordination made by the Infection Control and Nursing Care Unit to accept the nurses and determine the places of their activities), as well as by the associations and groups concerned in the prefecture (such as the School of Nursing, Fukushima Medical University, the Fukushima Preservative Service Association of Health, Fukushima office of the Japan Health Insurance Association, and the Fukushima Dietetic Association). The public health nurse teams consisting of the members of the prefecture and the municipalities of the prefecture were also dispatched to the cities and towns in the coastal area. These teams conducted the following or similar activities:

(i) Health /sanitary management in shelters

The dispatched teams were stationed at or paid visits to shelters, depending on the situation of the municipality to which they were dispatched, to conduct various activities such as the health management of the affected people and the sanitary management of the shelters as well as nutrition and diet support.

(ii) Conducting health surveys of various people, such as the residents in secondary shelters, temporary houses, and municipally subsidized rental houses and the evacuees staying at home

The dispatched teams visited evacuation facilities, houses of the affected people, and other places in cooperation with the affected municipality and the public health center to clarify the health conditions and provide health consultations, as well as facilitate coordination, such as turning over the people who were found to need support to a medical care team, mental healthcare team, or other organizations concerned.

(iii) Providing health consultations, health education, and such at, for example, a meeting place of temporary houses

After the completion of the health survey of residents in temporary houses, the dispatched teams planned and supported the management of, for example, health consultations and health education with an eye to promoting exchanges among affected people and preventing lifestyle-related diseases, life function decline, and other problems.

(iv) Cooperation with health services and other related services in the affected municipalities

After routine work resumed, the dispatched teams provided support for, for example, the preparation and management of medical checkups, such as medical checkups for babies and specific medical checkup.

4   Issues in requesting the dispatch of healthcare teams

Coordination is essential to accept support personnel for health support activities for affected people and for cooperation and information sharing with other support teams dispatched, such as medical care teams and mental health care teams. At this time, however, each division of the Social Health and Welfare Department independently requested the dispatch of personnel and coordinated the acceptance of the dispatched personnel. This caused confusion due to insufficient information sharing and insufficient coordination for where the personnel should conduct activities.

In addition, there were two or more routes to request the dispatch of public health nurses and other personnel, as shown in Table 5-1. Such support personnel were dispatched through more than one request routes in some cases, sometimes causing duplication of requests and of assigning support personnel.

Under such circumstances, to allow the dispatched healthcare teams to conduct activities effectively and efficiently in the respective areas, it is necessary for the parties accepting the teams to appropriately provide the support personnel prior to and during their activities with necessary information. For example, necessary information would include the damage situation and health issues in the area of their activities and the prospects of their activities. The parties accepting services also need to prepare a unified form of recording and organizing the flow of information in order to appropriately facilitate clarifying the situation of the support activities.

It is necessary in ordinary times to have the initial response system for health support activities in the event of a disaster organized and clarified and the common understanding thereof formulated through, for example, education and training.

5   Securing experts after the coordination for dispatch ended

Even though the dispatch of healthcare teams from the municipalities outside of the prefecture through the Ministry of Health, Labour and Welfare ended in fiscal 2011, the shortage of healthcare experts

Chapter 2 | Initiatives of Public Administrations

engaged in health support activities for residents, such as public health nurses and nationally registered dietitians, has continued in areas such as the affected municipalities from which residents were evacuated to live inside and outside the prefecture. In order to continue health support activities for affected people by securing expert healthcare human resources, the prefecture implemented an alternative method to the dispatch request to the Ministry of Health, Labour and Welfare; the "Health Support Program for Affected People" utilizing the government's Exceptional Subsidies for Health Support in Affected Areas. Thus, with the cooperation of the Fukushima Nursing Association, the prefecture endeavored to secure experts to conduct activities in the affected municipalities, such as public health nurses. The prefecture allocated public health nurses starting in September 2011 in Iwaki City, where the number of evacuated residents from the affected municipalities had increased (the Iwaki branch of the Soso public health center was established later), and still continues support activities and coordination to secure human resources in response to the request from individual municipalities.

B : Nutritional Management for People Living in Shelters, Temporary Houses, and Other Places

In this earthquake, problems with food supply started immediately after the occurrence of the disaster. The damage to transportation networks, shortage of gasoline, and other problems interrupted the distribution of food and other items and residents living in shelters and at home requested consultation on the shortage of artificial milk (power milk), high density liquid diet, and other items. Thus, food issues occurred in various forms in the time series, staring with "securing water and food to maintain life" and including "taking measures to, for example, prevent under- nutrition and deal with food allergies" and "preventing the increase in severity of chronic disorders such as diabetes and hypertension."

Consequently, the prefecture cooperated with the Fukushima Dietetic Association to endeavor to secure and provide relief supplies for "people unable to eat ordinary meals" and requested the Association to dispatch volunteers and the Fukushima Prefecture Council for Promotion of Diet Improvement to cooperate to provide hot meals for the people living in shelters. The prefecture also made the personnel of the public health centers and national registered dietitians and dieticians of municipalities visit all shelters to conduct a survey on diet in primary shelters (twice in total). Based on the survey results, the requests for improvement were submitted to the Emergency Response Headquarters of Fukushima Prefecture and thus the prefecture endeavored to improve the dietary environment for people living in primary shelters in cooperation with various parties concerned, such as associations and groups, municipalities, and the Self Defense Force.

Furthermore, the prefecture still continues nutrition and diet support activities now with an eye to maintenance and promotion of health and ability to eat independently for the affected people, including the development of the "nutrition and diet leaflet for affected people" and the provision of individual or group nutritional guidance and cooking lessons in temporary houses and other places (Table 5-3).

Table 5-3 Main nutrition and diet support activities for the affected people in Fukushima Prefecture

- Securing and appropriate provision of food and nutrition to support health
- Individual nutrition support for "people unable to eat ordinary meals"
- Support for nutrition assessment and smooth hot meal supply activities and improvement of the dietary environment
- Prevention of the increase in severity of lifestyle-related diseases and support for the ability to eat independently for people living in temporary houses and municipally subsidized rental houses, etc.

C : Measures to Deal with Infectious Diseases in Shelters, Temporary Houses, and Other Places

In prolonged evacuation life, the risk management for infectious diseases is crucial. The prefecture made efforts to promptly identify symptoms of infectious diseases and take various countermeasures to thoroughly prevent the infectious diseases from spreading. These included distribution of disinfectants to shelters and other places, periodic provision of reminders concerning the prevention of infectious diseases (such as shelter wall newspapers, posters, and the distribution of educational literature), visits of medical care teams and healthcare teams to shelters, and surveillance of shelters with the cooperation of the National Institute of Infectious Diseases.

The distribution of disinfectants and the provision of reminders concerning the prevention of infectious diseases started one week after the occurrence of the disaster. However, the epidemic outbreak of infectious diseases, such as infectious gastroenteritis, occurred under the circumstances where it was difficult to ensure the hygienic environment due to various problems in primary shelters; including the density of inmates, ventilation, a source of water, and other factors. The outbreak terminated in about two weeks thanks to various remedial measures, such as the guidance on measures to prevent infection through frequent visits to shelters, the improvement of the hygienic environment such as securing a source of water, and the establishment of observation rooms. However, since there is a concern about, for example, the increase in infectious diseases due to the decrease in immunity and other factors associated with prolonged evacuation life, it is necessary to continue to make efforts to provide prompt and accurate information on infectious diseases to residents, and institutions and other concerned parties.

For the countermeasures to be taken against infectious diseases in temporary housing, a meeting of the people in charge from public health centers and other organizations was held on July 26, 2011 remind everyone concerned about the countermeasures to be taken against infectious diseases in temporary housing.

D : Mental Healthcare for Affected People

Mental healthcare teams visited shelters in the all areas of the prefecture starting on March 19, 2011. Fukushima Medical University, the medical association in each area in the prefecture, the Mental Health and Welfare Centre, and medical care teams dispatched from outside the prefecture, and other members, in cooperation with the medical care teams such as the Japan Medical Association Team (JMAT), provided medical care and pharmaceuticals to the evacuees who needed medical care and conducted consultation activities for them.

Subsequently, since the evacuation was expected to be prolonged and thus the development of a medium-to long-term support system was required for the prefecture, "Guideline for Fukushima Prefecture Mental Healthcare Team Activity" were established in May 2011. The system for visiting evacuees was strengthened through, for example, the increase in the number of public health nurses and experts such as clinical psychotherapists in each public health center utilizing the Emergency Job Creation Fund Program.

On February 1, 2012 the prefecture opened the "Fukushima Center for Disaster Mental Health (base center)," utilizing the Mental Healthcare Human Resource Network established by the government from the appropriation of the third supplementary budget for fiscal 2011. The base center accepted experts from outside of the prefecture for providing medium to long term mental healthcare. On April 13, 2012, six district centers were opened at the Ken-poku, Ken-chu, Ken-nan, Aizu, Soma, and Iwaki Districts.

Additional experts are also stationed in other cities, such as Minamisoma City and Kazo City in Saitama Prefecture.

E   Supply of Pharmaceuticals and Other Items

Starting on the day of occurrence of the disaster, the supply of pharmaeuticals, medical equipment, and other items was requested by municipalities, first-aid stations in shelters, medical institutions and various medical care teams, including the Disaster Medical Assistance Team (DMAT). Measures were taken to respond to the request for pharmaceuticals, medical equipment, and other items based on the "Fukushima Pharmaceuticals Stockpile and Supply System for Disasters" in cooperation with the Fukushima Pharmaceutical Wholesalers Association and the Fukushima Health Industry Distributors Association.

The prefecture also accepted proprietary drugs and ethical pharmaceuticals as well as medical support goods such as hand disinfectants sent from across the country and supplied them to various places and parties concerned, such as secondary stockyards, first-aid stations, and medical care teams.

F   Health Management of the Residents of Fukushima Prefecture Associated with the Nuclear Disaster

1   Performing emergency exposure screening

Immediately after the Fukushima Daiichi Nuclear Station accident, the prefecture started performing emergency exposure screening for evacuees and other people based on the "Fukushima Radiation Emergency Medicine Activities Manual."

At the initial stage, screening was performed mainly by each public health center. However, due to the shortage of manpower, the prefecture requested municipalities, universities, and research institutes across the country to dispatch personnel through the Ministry of Education, Culture, Sports, Science and Technology and the Ministry of Health, Labour and Welfare. Equipment and devices, such as GM counter-type survey meters, were those brought by the support personnel, universities, and research institutes from across the country.

Emergency exposure screening immediately after the accident was performed intensively in March and April 2011. Since the initial stage of the activities, field information has been collected and instructions have been shared by, for example, holding meetings every morning and evening involving experts to take daily improvised measures to meet a situation that was changing by the minute. The subsequent anxiety of local residents about their health could not be eliminated and it was decided to continue the screening.

On April 22, 2011 when the warning zone was designated, temporary visits to the zone started for a public benefit purpose with permission of the head of the relevant municipality and consent of the off-site center (OFC) of the government. There was a rapid increase in the number of visits after the consecutive holidays in May, and screening was also performed at J-Village and other locations.

After the consecutive holidays in May, many residents also started to pay temporary visits to their homes in the area within 20 km, where mainly the medical team members of the OFC of the government lived then, and screening was performed at each transfer station.

Screening is still continuing by the local Nuclear Emergency Response Headquarters of the government, mainly for those paying a temporary visit for public benefit purposes.

2 Conducting a survey of radioactive substances contained in food and drinking water

Since there was a concern about the health effects of food and drinking water contaminated due to the diffusion of radioactive substances associated with the nuclear disaster, the prefecture submitted a written request to the director-general of the local Nuclear Emergency Response Headquarters to perform emergency monitoring inspections of agriculture, forestry and fishery products and drinking water. On March 19, 2011, emergency monitoring inspections of agriculture, forestry and fishery products and drinking water started utilizing private inspection agencies.

In tap water, radioactive iodine (^{131}I) and other substances were detected at the Fukushima City Waterworks on March 16 and at the Iitate Small Waterworks on March 20. For the latter, measures were taken to restrict intake. Furthermore, radioactive iodine exceeding 100 Bq/kg, the maximum dose allowed for babies, was also detected in other tap water and the relevant water utilities were requested to take measures, such as distribution of mineral water in PET bottles. Under such circumstances, the prefecture extended the scope of tap water to be inspected in a phased manner starting on March 17 and started monitoring inspections of radioactive substances in all tap water in the prefecture on March 26.

Since radioactive iodine had a short half-life of about 8 days, the detected value decreased with the passage of days after the accident. However, the inspection of drinking water for radioactive substances had to be continued because there was a concern about long-term effects of radioactive cesium (^{134}Cs, ^{137}Cs) due to its long half-life.

To improve the monitoring inspection system, germanium semiconductor detectors had been deployed starting in October 2011 first to the Fukushima Prefectural Institute of Health, followed by the Meat Hygiene Inspection Office, and subsequently to eight water utilities. Monitoring inspections were started in accordance with the "Fukushima Drinking Water Monitoring Implementation Plan," which specified the frequency of monitoring by zone based on the environmental dose and the distance from the Fukushima Daiichi Nuclear Station.

3 Conducting the Fukushima Health Management Survey

In the light of the radioactive contamination in the prefecture caused by the nuclear disaster, the prefecture is conducting the Fukushima Health Management Survey for the purpose of monitoring the health of the residents of Fukushima Prefecture and promoting their health in the future. For the purpose of obtaining a broad range of advice and opinions from a technical perspective, the prefecture established the Review Committee for the Fukushima Health management Survey on May 19, 2011 to determine how to conduct the survey and to manage the progress of the survey.

The programs being conducted now include the "basic survey," the "detailed surveys," the creation of

Chapter 2 | Initiatives of Public Administrations

the "Fukushima resident health management file," and "Fukushima resident health management program support." The database to register the survey results is also being constructed.

The "basic survey" covers all the residents of Fukushima Prefecture because the external exposure dose during the period when the air dose was highest is estimated and used as the foundation of the health management for the long-term. Included in the "detailed surveys" are "thyroid ultrasound examination", "comprehensive health check", "mental health and lifestyle survey", and "pregnancy and birth survey" (refer to page 341 in Chapter 43).

Furthermore, the "Fukushima resident health management file" has been created so that the residents in Fukushima Prefecture can put together and record and store the survey and inspection results concerning their own health to facilitate their health management. The file is sent to the residents together with, for example, a notification of the basic survey results. In addition, as the "Fukushima resident health management program support," the "radiation and health advisory group" of Fukushima Prefecture are established to provide advice and support to municipalities based on expert knowledge. Training workshops are also held for the personnel of, for example, municipalities and prefectural public health centers, who are providing more familiar health services to the residents of Fukushima prefecture, as well as for educators and other people engaged in the health management of children.

4 Distribution of personal dose meters and internal exposure inspection

With the increasing anxiety of the residents of Fukushima Prefecture about health effects caused by radiation, the prefecture decided to promote the "Urgent Project to Protect Children" in June 2011. As part of the project, in addition to the Fukushima Health Management Survey, the prefecture established a system to support the municipalities distributing, for example, personal dose meters (glass badges) and performed internal exposure inspection using a whole-body counter for the health management of the residents of Fukushima Prefecture. They also held explanatory meetings by radiation experts, thus endeavoring to promote the understanding and eliminate the anxiety of residents.

The costs of the personal dose meters that were used in the "Project to Support the Urgent Preparation of Dose Meters" are subsidized in the case where municipalities distributed the meters to people, such as children, expectant mothers, and prepared (calibrated) survey meters (scintillation type).

As for "internal exposure inspection," starting with the inspection at the National Institute of Radiological Sciences for the residents in the planned evacuation zone in June 2011, the prefecture is promoting visiting inspections inside and outside the prefecture using an in-vehicle whole-body counter. The priority is to be placed on the children 18 years old or younger and expectant mothers in the prefecture. There was also inspection available, mainly for evacuees who were outside the prefecture, at medical institutions or conducted by organizations outside the prefecture owning a whole-body counter.

(Nobuhiro Nakamura)

6 Measures Taken by the Soso Public Health and Welfare Office

1 Outline of the areas under jurisdiction

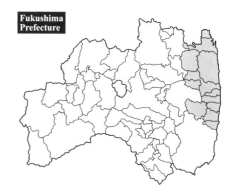

(1) Municipalities under jurisdiction

The following two cities, seven towns, and three villages are under jurisdiction: Soma City, Minamisoma City, Hirono Town, Naraha Town, Tomioka Town, Kawauchi Village, Okuma Town, Futaba Town, Namie Town, and Katsurao Village of Futaba-Gun, and Shinchi Town and Iitate Village of Soma-Gun

(2) Population/population aging rate (as of January 1 each year)

	2011	2013
Population	195,717	181,934
Population aging rate	25.8	27.3

2 Damage situation caused by the earthquake and nuclear disaster in the areas under jurisdiction

(1) Damage situation (as of March 12, 2013)

Physical damage	Completely destroyed	Half destroyed	Partially destroyed
Residential buildings	7,995	3,706	9,968
Public facilities		27	
Others		3,505	

Human damage	Direct deaths	Associated deaths	Missing	Injured
	1,273	1,213	188	81

(2) Evacuation situation (as of March 12, 2013)

	End-March 2011	End-September 2011	End-March 2012	Latest
Installation of shelters	16	2		
No. of evacuees	77,647	46,431	29,953	10,768
No. of evacuees accepted				
No. of residents living in temporary houses for residents and evacuees accepted				11,644

(Emergency Response Headquarters of Fukushima Prefecture: Calculated based on the flash report on the damage situation caused by the 2011 off the Pacific coast of Tohoku Earthquake)

Chapter 2 | Initiatives of Public Administrations

The Soso Public Health and Welfare Office (hereinafter referred to as the "public health center") is the only public health center in Japan that has under its jurisdiction the Tokyo Electric Power Company Fukushima Daiichi Nuclear Power Station (hereinafter referred to as the "Fukushima Daiichi Nuclear Station"), where the accident equivalent to a level 7 on the International Nuclear Event Scale (INES) occurred. The office is responsible for keeping in order the measures taken in response to this accident that will be very important to study measures to be taken in the future. Measures taken during the approximately one year since the occurrence of the disaster until March 2012 are as follows:

A Measures Taken for Hospitals Immediately after the Occurrence of the Disaster

At 2:46 pm on March 11, 2011, an unprecedented large disaster occurred. In the public health center building with a seismic resistance level "C," I waited under the desk until the tremors stopped, for fear that the building might collapse. After the tremors of aftershock settled, the first thing for the public health center personnel to do was to clarify the damage situation of medical institutions and support them. I assigned two public health nurses to have them contact 16 hospitals under our jurisdiction over the phone every two to three hours. Even though phone calls were hard to complete, it was eventually clear that matters of urgency were occurring one after another. It was said that Minamisoma Municipal General Hospital, near the place hit by tsunami, was like a military hospital with many victims, such as drowned persons, being brought in. Triage tags, stocked in the public health center, were immediately provided. Other problems continued to be raised, such as artificial dialysis could not be undergone due to the disrupted water supply and that the fuel for the private power generator being operated to deal with electric power failure would run out in several hours. We were heavily involved in taking measures to deal with these problems. We requested a supply of diesel oil and kerosene for private power generation of the Local Emergency Response Headquarters of the Soso District; however, the response was "not available." As for artificial dialysis, it was determined based on the communication among hospitals to consolidate patients to the unaffected hospitals.

Wasting time with no phone calls getting through left a sense of futility. Electricity of the hospitals interrupted was restored before the following morning. At 10 pm on the following day, the 12th, it was determined that all possible necessary measures for hospitals that could be taken had been taken and I came home. We felt keenly that we needed some means of communication that could be connected to hospitals even in the event of a disaster.

B Measures Taken to Deal with the Nuclear Plant Accident and for the Emergency Exposure Screening

On the 11th, when the TV in the center was kept on, bad news was broadcasted. I do not know at exactly what time it was but the news said, "The seismic tremor was detected and all reactors of the Fukushima Daiichi Nuclear Station stopped. Immediately after that, the emergency power supply to operate the emergency core cooling systems (ECCS) for Unit 1 to 3 broke down and the cooling function was lost. The government issued a declaration of a nuclear emergency situation pursuant to the Act on Special Measures Concerning Nuclear Emergency Preparedness. The water level inside the nuclear reactors decreased and fuel rods inside the nuclear reactors may become exposed." Accordingly, the government issued an evacuation order for the residents in the area within a 3 km radius from the Fukushima Daiichi Nuclear Station and an indoor standby order for those in the area from 3 to 10 km in radius. On the following day, the range of the evacuation order was expanded to a 10 km radius from the Fukushima Daiichi and Daini Nuclear

6 Measures Taken by the Soso Public Health and Welfare Office

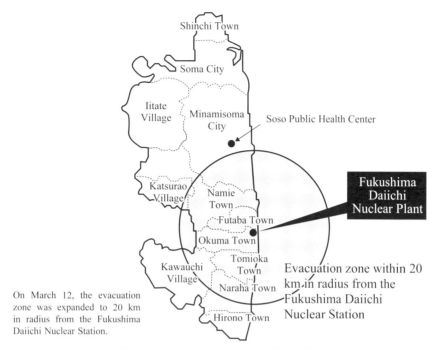

On March 12, the evacuation zone was expanded to 20 km in radius from the Fukushima Daiichi Nuclear Station.

Figure 6-1 Evacuation zone as of March 12

Stations and the evacuation zone around the Fukushima Daiichi Nuclear Station was expanded from a range of 10 km to a 20 km radius (Figure 6-1).

On the 12th, in response to the request of the local Nuclear Emergency Response Headquarters in the off-site center (OFC), several staff members of the public health center were dispatched as the personnel in charge of the medical team. On the same day, a news report told that at about 3:36 pm, a loud explosion occurred together with white smoke generated around the Unit 1 of the Fukushima Daiichi Nuclear Station and the nuclear reactor building was blasted away with only the frame left standing. On that day, I came home at around 10 pm and went to bed. In the middle of the night, however, the doorbell woke me up and I saw the clock indicating that it was half past one in the morning. I saw two staff members of the public health center, who were standing by at night, on the door phone monitor screen. I hurriedly changed clothes and opened the door. Then a staff member of the National Institute of Radiological Sciences (hereinafter referred to as the "NIRS") in a Tyvek suit with a mask started talking fast. In short, he told that he wanted me, the head of the local public health center, to be the leader of the medical team in the OFC and coordinate the study of the future policy on the measures to deal with exposure of residents. Even though I felt very anxious because an explosion had just occurred, I immediately agreed and headed for the public health center by my car. I think that, during the nuclear emergency response drills repeated every year, I had become very familiar with the idea that this kind of situation might happen someday. At the public health center, I changed my clothes to a fully equipped protective suit and headed for the OFC in a vehicle of the Self-Defense Forces. Since I had no idea of what and how to do everything that would be required of me, I ask various questions of the personnel of the NIRS to confirm how to deal with the situation. After arriving at the OFC, I was told that there were many people in health care facilities for the elderly requiring long-term care who had failed to evacuate, and they were supposed to be transported by the Self-Defense Forces.

Chapter 2 | Initiatives of Public Administrations

I was also told that there were many other residents who might have been exposed to radiation because it had taken a long time for them to evacuate. I determined the priority of screening of the people having failed to evacuate promptly and dispatched the medical doctors of the NIRS to the relevant sites.

What I had to do on the night of the 13th was surveillance and decontamination of emergency patients at the OFC; however, the staff of neighboring hospitals had already evacuated. Since even the medical institutions that were capable of accepting patients did not accept patients unless the certificate of non-contamination was obtained as a result of surveillance, a routine was established whereby an ambulance always came to the OFC first and subsequently headed to the relevant medical institution. The NIRS personnel and the author divided the responsibilities, the former conducting surveillance and decontamination and the latter clarifying the whole body condition of the patient. Six patients were accepted between 11 pm and 2 am on the following day and I was out of the center almost all the time during this period.

In the early morning of the 14th, instructions were sent from the Prime Minister's Office to the OFC by facsimile. It was a hand-written list including the names of the facilities, such as health care facilities for elderly requiring long-term care mentioned above, where people were still not evacuated, as well as the number of such people and where they were planned to be transported. The list had an additional statement that these people should first be screened at the Soso public health center and subsequently transported to a shelter. At about 10 am, I returned to the public health center after I had conveyed this matter to the personnel of the public health center who were dispatched as members of the medical team of the OFC from the public health center. According to the list, 840 people had failed to evacuate, and these people arrived at the public health center in buses of the Self-Defense Forces and the police department and screening was performed for them according to instructions and with the cooperation of the medical doctors of Hiroshima University and the personnel that the NIRS dispatched. As taught by the personnel of the NIRS at the OFC, since the people who had been in the same facilities were considered to have been exposed to the same degree of radiation, surveillance of all the people was not needed. The surveillance was conducted on only two people in the front row and two people in the last row in each bus. The above list included many hospital patients and indicated that they should be transported to the shelter at the senior high school in Iwaki City, where no medical facilities were available; however, without having time for more detailed planning, we had to continue to perform the screening operation at the public health center because new patients continued to be transported to the center.

Later, the screening operation peaked with the number of people screened exceeding 2,000 a day when a group of citizens from Minamisoma City evacuated to Niigata Prefecture, and then the number of people requiring screening gradually diminished. About 100 people were screened on a daily basis. The cumulative number of people screened was 58,930 as of December 18, 2011 (Figure 6-2). At the initial stage, almost all of the personnel were involved in the screening operation; however, support from other prefectures as well as a full-scale backup by the Federation of Electric Power Companies of Japan that was begun in April allowed us to engage in primary disaster control operations of the public health center, such as visiting shelters and dealing with health risk management cases.

Media representatives in Japan and from abroad visited us and took photos of screening scenes. I had one thing in mind that I should tell to visiting media persons: That was the issue of unfair discrimination associated with radiation. There were countless examples of discrimination: Some people were rejected at check-in simply because the person had come from Minamisoma City. Some people were asked to wash their car in the town to which he/she had evacuated simply because the car had a Fukushima license plate. In addition, as was reported by the media, when a person found that a child had come from Fukushima

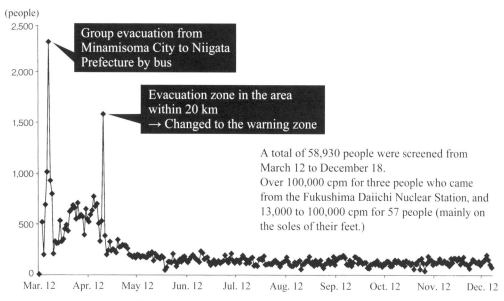

Figure 6-2 Change in the number of people screened

Table 6-1 Proliferation of excessive prejudice and discrimination associated with radiation

It emerged that there were cases where evacuees in the wake of the Fukushima Daiichi Nuclear Station accident could not have a medical examination at medical institutions unless they showed the certificate of "nothing abnormal" from a screening inspection to check the radiation dose. There were also some cases where the screening inspection was obligated when evacuees entered a shelter. An expert points out that this is an excessive reaction based on unscientific prejudice. (snip) Kenji Sasahara, head of the Soso public health center located in the central part of Minamisoma City, shows anger saying, "Inspection has been performed for more than 8,000 people to date.   However, there was no person exceeding the criterion value that requires decontamination. It is ridiculous that Minamisoma is treated as if it were a contaminated area." (Mainichi Newspaper on March 28, 2011)

Prefecture, the person said, "We may be infected by your radioactivity." According to the screening results, there were no residents with radiation exceeding 100,000 cpm, the level that required decontamination, and I kept emphasizing how unreasonably the residents of Fukushima Prefecture had been treated and hurt.

Consequently, these comments were taken up in the articles in the Yomiuri Shimbun Newspaper and Newsweek magazine (http://www.newsweek.com/2011/04/03/inside-the-danger-zone.html) and frequently quoted by, for example, blog sites on the Internet (Table 6-1). However, for something like radiation that cannot be sensed by the five senses, it is a fact of life that knowledge does not necessarily mean understanding, and I am concerned about the deep-rooted issue of discrimination, which may become the root of trouble for the future.

C Measures to Deal with Medical Care Weakened Due to the Designation of the Emergency Evacuation-Ready Zone for the Original Indoor Evacuation Zone

On March 15, the government issued an order of indoor evacuation for the residents in the area 20 to 30 km from the Fukushima Daiichi Nuclear Station (Figure 6-3). The symptoms of problems with medical care had already appeared earlier, immediately after the hydrogen explosion of Unit 1.

Chapter 2 | Initiatives of Public Administrations

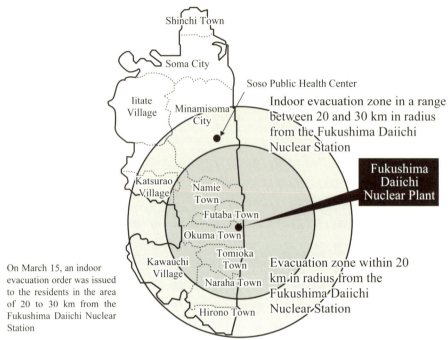

Figure 6-3 Evacuation zone as of March 15

On March 14, when we were heavily involved in the screening operation, an ambulance entered the premises of the public health center with its siren blaring. I wondered what had happened and asked the ambulance personnel and he told us, "In Haramachi-ward of Minamisoma City, the personnel of the hospitals have evacuated causing a shortage of manpower and it takes a long time to identify a place to accept a patient. We are forced to move from one place to another. Manpower should be concentrated in a certain place to allow the place to function as a disaster emergency hospital." However, the difficult situation in Haramachi-ward prevented us from holding an urgent meeting for coordination.

Several days later, the personnel of a certain psychiatric hospital stormed into the public health center in a rage saying, "Give us stable iodine tablets!" We explained that iodine tablets were allowed to be orally taken under the instruction of the government only when the projected dose in the thyroid gland by radioactive iodine (^{131}I) exceeded 100 mSv. The director of the nursing department, who came together with him, told us seriously that adequate medical care could not be provided because the staff members continued to evacuate or to take a leave of absence.

Following the Unit 1 on March 12, hydrogen explosions occurred at the Units 3 and 2 on the 14th and 15th, respectively, and all residents evacuated at once. Only those people who could not evacuate by themselves were left in Minamisoma City within an area of a 20 to 30 km radius from the Fukushima Daiichi Nuclear Station. Staff members of hospitals had also evacuated one after another and the ability to meet medical care demands was lost. Consequently, as a result of discussions between the government and the Emergency Response Headquarters of Fukushima Prefecture, the Ministry of Health, Labour and Welfare decided on March 18 to transport all of the patients in the hospitals within 20 to 30 km to outside of Fukushima Prefecture and requested a total of 11 prefectures, including those in the Kanto-Koshinetsu region and Yamagata Prefecture, to cooperate by accepting the patients.

6 Measures Taken by the Soso
Public Health and Welfare Office

On March 22, the transportation of all of the inpatients was completed. For four hospitals in the indoor evacuation zone, all the hospital admission and outpatient service functions were suspended and all that was left at Minamisoma Municipal General Hospital was the provision of the medicines that a patient was already taking, if a patient brought the "medicine notebook" or something similar with him/her. Consequently, a number of outpatients from Minamisoma City visited two hospitals in Soma City, which was outside the 30 km range from the Fukushima Daiichi Nuclear Station, and the people concerned in Soma City voiced a request for the four hospitals in Minamisoma City to restart outpatient services.

On March 19, it was determined that three volunteer medical doctors from other prefectures would come from the Emergency Response Headquarters of Fukushima Prefecture. We contacted the director of Public Soma General Hospital and it was decided that they would work as the support personnel for outpatient doctors. We felt very grateful.

In addition, on the 22nd, the secretary general of the Soma-gun Medical Association contacted us to ask the procedures under the Medical Care Act for several medical doctors of the Medical Association having their clinic in Minamisoma City to provide outpatient services by rotation at the Medical Association Building and other places. We responded that legal procedures might be considered later on since the situation constituted a disaster. On March 25, outpatient services started as a "provisional clinic of the Soma-gun Medical Association" in a part of the Kashima Kosei Hospital, which was located several kilometers outside the 30 km line from the Fukushima Daiichi Nuclear Station. About 100 patients a day visited the clinic and the inflow of patients from Minamisoma City to Soma City is estimated to have been reduced to a certain extent.

On March 25, it was announced that there was a phone call from the Vice President of Nagasaki University to the vice leader of the rescue team of the Emergency Response Headquarters of Fukushima Prefecture. Nagasaki Prefecture wanted to extend total support to medical care in Fukushima Prefecture starting in April and Fukushima Prefecture wanted to request the visiting medical care for about 140 home-care patients in a radius of 20 to 30 km. The governor of Fukushima Prefecture immediately issued solicitation documents to the governor of Nagasaki Prefecture pursuant to the Disaster Relief Act. Consequently, the personnel of Nagasaki University and the Nagasakiken Medical Association took turns every week to visit home-care patients and shelters together with the teams of the Fukushima Medical University and the Self-Defense Forces for eight weeks in April and May and discovered a total of five people with symptoms of, for example, bedsore and dehydration, and transported them to the hospitals outside the 30 km range. From our public health center, about three members were dispatched to Minamisoma City on consecutive days and an experienced public health nurse (Deputy Director ate Department of Health and Welfare) chaired the conference held every morning and evening and two public health nurses joined the visiting medical care team.

On April 4, outpatient services were restarted at all of the four hospitals in Minamisoma City. However, it was pointed out by the professor of Fukushima Medical University engaged in the visiting medical care that there was no hospital accepting inpatients in Minamisoma City; this report was taken up by the local newspaper on April 18. All beds in the hospitals in Soma City continued to be occupied and it was impossible to fulfill medical care needs only within the Soso District (Figure 6-4).

Back on March 31, the director of Watanabe Hospital located in Minamisoma City visited our public health center. His visit was intended to tell us his proposal as follows: The government did not approve the admission to hospitals in the indoor evacuation zone; however, considering the critical medical

Chapter 2 — Initiatives of Public Administrations

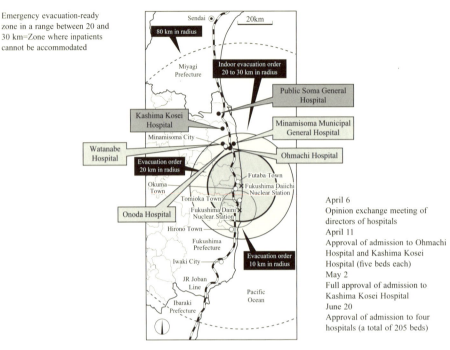

Figure 6-4 Securing inpatient beds

situation, such as some had died of stroke and some elderly persons living alone at home had starved to death, short-term admission to hospitals south of Soma City should be approved. To that end, an opinion exchange meeting should be held with the participation of the directors of the hospitals in Soma City and Minamisoma City and the fire defense headquarters. In response to this proposal, it was decided to hold a meeting on April 6 and we discussed the agenda in advance with the vice leader of the rescue team of the Emergency Response Headquarters of Fukushima Prefecture.

The situations including the following were taken into consideration: Beds must be secured in the zone where the government did not approve the admission to hospital; if an emergency situation occurred at the Fukushima Daiichi Nuclear Station, inpatients must evacuate again; however, there were lives that must be saved. Consequently, it was suggested to establish a policy to secure 10 beds in this area for patients who could be discharged in about three days and find a volunteering hospital for implementation. Since the representative of the Emergency Response Headquarters of Fukushima Prefecture was not available on this day, the Director of Medical and Pharmaceutical Affairs Division of our public health center explained the above suggestion.

The meeting was thrown into confusion by various opinions given on this matter, such as that no hospital could volunteer unless the guidelines of the prefecture showed what the medical care in this district should be. Also, that compensation was needed during a situation where the income was significantly decreased due to the services limited to those for outpatients whereas salaries must be paid to the personnel taking a leave of absence. The meeting was concluded with a comment saying "Anyway, no conclusion can be reached unless a meeting attended by the Vice Governor is held with the directors of hospitals." We reported to the Emergency Response Headquarters of Fukushima Prefecture that the issue was no longer at a level that could be addressed by the public health center, only by one of the agencies. On April 11, the vice

Table 6-2 "Indoor evacuation zone" in the area of 20 to 30 km designated as the "emergency evacuation-ready zone."

Instruction

| Attachment |

April 22, 2011, 09:44

(ii) Emergency evacuation-ready zone

The residents and other people in the following zone shall be always ready to be able to move out or evacuate indoors for emergency evacuation. In this zone, residents continue to be expected to voluntarily evacuate, and especially those people, such as children, expectant mothers, people dependent on care, and inpatients, shall not enter said zone. In addition, in this zone, nursery centers, kindergartens, and elementary, junior high, and senior high schools shall be closed. Even though the entry of people into said zone to perform unavoidable tasks, such as services, is not prevented, such people shall be always ready to independently move out or evacuate indoors even in such cases.

---

leader of the rescue team of the Emergency Response Headquarters of Fukushima Prefecture negotiated individually with hospitals and it was approved to secure five beds in Ohmachi Hospital and also five beds in Kashima Kosei Hospital located outside the 30 km range. The discussion between the government, which had not yet approved the admission to hospitals, and the prefecture made no progress. It is said that the prefecture defined this matter as a "matter implicitly agreed upon" by the government. Furthermore, through the instruction document dated April 22, the government notified that the area of 20 to 30 km was designated as the "emergency evacuation-ready zone" and inpatients must not enter this area (Table 6-2).

At the same time, this means substantially relaxed measures whereby the conventional "indoor evacuation zone" was changed to the zone where residents should be prepared to be able to evacuate or evacuate indoors in case of an emergency. Accordingly, the population of Minamisoma City, once reduced to several thousand people, recovered to about 30,000 in May with a gradual increase in the number of people coming back. Consequently, a significant contradiction developed between the restriction by the government not to approve admission to hospitals and the actual increase in medical care demand with an increase in population.

The medical care issues in the Soso District were often reviewed by mass media. On May 2, all of the 80 beds in Kashima Kosei Hospital became available for inpatients, and on June 20, a total of 205 beds in the four hospitals in the 20 to 30 km range became available for inpatients. The ratio of the emergency patients in Minamisoma City who could be accommodated in the hospitals in the city was 50.7% in April, which recovered to 83.1% in June.

On August 28, Minamisoma City established the "Review Committee on the Medical Care in the Soma City Area" in an attempt to find a breakthrough to improve the situation caused by a lack of medical staff in the city. The appointed members of the Committee included the directors of the five hospitals in the city having beds for general patients and two psychiatric hospitals, the Vice President of the Soma-gun Medical Association, and other people. The author also attended the Committee meetings as a head of the public health center. The personnel concerned in the government and the prefecture also participated in the Committee meetings as observers, which made the meetings full of extraordinary tension. The mayor also attended the first meeting and commented that the government should be responsible for the restoration of medical care in Minamisoma City. The draft medical care restoration program shown in the meeting also included the same content, which was unanimously agreed upon in the meeting. The author commented that, to obtain the support of the government, the needs of the region as well as of the diagnosis and treatment departments and the number of medical doctors required must be clarified.

On September 30, the government declared the removal of the designation of the "emergency evacuation-

Chapter 2 | Initiatives of Public Administrations

ready zone" because the Fukushima Daiichi Nuclear Station was in stable condition. However, residents and medical staff members started to return to the area only very slowly and the local healthcare remained unrestored. Under such circumstances, on October 7, the government opened the "Ministry of Health, Labour and Welfare's Support Center to Secure Health Workers in the Soso District" in the Soso public health center. Two staff members were allocated and they continually worked hard and very effectively collecting information not only from the hospitals in the district but also more widely from, for example, Fukushima Medical University and the Fukushima Medical Association. In three months, they accomplished a great achievement to secure five full-time doctors for Minamisoma City Hospital.

Meetings had been held repeatedly of the "Study Committee on the Medical Care in the Soma City Area" and, since it was tiring for individual hospitals to conduct similar functions with limited manpower, the Study Committee members started to think of role sharing among individual hospitals. Under such circumstances, a member of the secretariat frequently consulted us and we discussed ideas together. The idea of role sharing was approved in a meeting and Yomiuri Shimbun Newspaper on January 17, 2012 posted an article with the headline "Five hospitals to share roles in medical care for their survival."

D : Measures to Deal with the Collapse of Psychiatric Care

Under the jurisdiction of our public health center, there were five hospitals having psychiatric care beds (Hibarigaoka Hospital and Odaka-akasaka Hospital (Minamisoma City), Futaba Kosei Hospital (Futaba Town), Futaba Hospital (Okuma Town), and Takano Hospital (Hirono Town)) and three of them were in the evacuation zone in the area within 20 km and closed by March 13. The other two hospitals were also closed because of their location within the indoor evacuation zone and eventually no beds were available for inpatients in the Soso District (Figure 6-5). Three clinics providing psychiatric services in Minamisoma City could not accept patients either and consequently the patients followed by the outpatient clinics were left behind in the district.

On March 22, the director of Public Soma General Hospital contacted us saying, "Many mental disease patients are coming from south for clinic visits. We are in great trouble because they have no medicine notebooks and our medical doctors have no knowledge about psychiatric medicines. We really want a psychiatrist dispatched to us to work fulltime for the time being if possible, or, otherwise, certain times a week."

We immediately called the director of the Fukushima Mental Health and Welfare Centre and received an answer that a psychiatrist of the Center would be dispatched on the 25th. Subsequently, thanks to the consideration of a professor of Department of Neuropsychiatry, Fukushima Medical University, staff members came from both inside and outside of the prefecture as "Mental Healthcare Teams" and consequently the clinical psychiatry operation functioned as a "provisional clinic." Also in response to the request by the director of the hospital to dispatch other staff members, such as nurses, public health nurses of our public health center were dispatched for the clinic. It was decided that our public health center would receive reservations for clinical examinations. "Mental Healthcare Teams" also visited shelters, with public health nurses of our public health center accompanying. Accordingly, with the cooperation of many medical care staff members outside and inside the prefecture, measures could be taken in various aspects of providing care, including the stress reaction to the disaster, such as sleeplessness and flashback, and the worsening of the integration dysfunction syndrome. On the other hand, even though the system of medical examination for the time being had been established, patients and their family members voiced their anxiety about how long they would be able to have access to medical examinations, as well as the fact that they took medical

6 Measures Taken by the Soso Public Health and Welfare Office

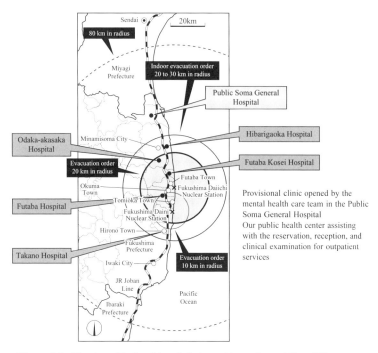

Figure 6-5 Number of beds of the clinical psychiatry changed from 901 to zero.

advice from a different psychiatrist every time.

Three clinics in Minamisoma city started medical examinations in April. Takano Hospital and Hibarigaoka Hospital restarted outpatient services in May and June, respectively, and thus started the reconstruction of psychiatric care by full-time psychiatrists.

Pursuant to Article 34 of the Psychiatric Social Workers Act, many patients were transported after the earthquake and the workload to the personnel of the public health center was increased because, for example, they accompanied the patients for their transportation to hospitals beds for inpatients in such cities as Fukushima City and Koriyama City.

On December 15, 2011, the "Soma Wide Area Mental Health Care Center Nagomi" was commissioned by the prefecture to start the outreach project dealing with the earthquake disaster. This project supported the lives of mentally disordered people through the visits of teams with members having various specialties, including medical care. The teams included of the medical staff, such as psychiatrists and nurses, and the welfare staff, such as psychiatric social workers and clinical psychotherapists. Their visits led to a significant sense of security for people concerned. The staff worked around the clock and the drastic reduction in emergency transportation cases involving the public health center personnel was considered to be substantially attributable to their success.

On January 10, 2012, "Mental Health Clinic Nagomi" was opened in Soma City. The director of the clinic flew from Okinawa every week. This was also considered to have significantly contributed to relieving the anxiety of the local residents caused by the earthquake and the nuclear plant accident and the worsening of mental diseases.

Chapter 2 | Initiatives of Public Administrations

Furthermore, on January 17, 2012, the medical examination of inpatients restarted for 60 beds of Hibarigaoka Hospital, which was achieved because psychiatrists from psychiatric hospitals across the country could be dispatched through the support of the "Ministry of Health, Labour and Welfare's Support Center to Secure Health Workers" established in the public health center in October 2011.

E : Necessity of Disaster Simulation

In the light of this accident, we felt keenly that elaborate simulations should be made in advance to determine how many people cannot evacuate by themselves and fail to escape and where they are and by whom, how, and where they should be transported in the case of the occurrence of the events such as those subject to the declaration of a nuclear emergency situation pursuant to Article 10 or 15 of the Act on Special Measures Concerning Nuclear Emergency Preparedness. We also found many cases where inpatients were left behind in the evacuation zone. Assuming such situations may occur, it is also necessary to develop an advanced plan on, for example, where outside of the evacuation zone, by whom, and how they should be transported and how many of them can be accepted and in which hospitals. Furthermore, of those people with health support needs who were transported by bus from the evacuation zone on March 14, there was no one whose screening level exceeded 100,000 cpm. It will have to be reviewed whether it is necessary to transport people in bad health conditions all the way to the public health center to perform their screening.

Finally, in the wake of this nuclear plant accident that drove more than 160,000 residents from their homes and caused huge damage to various industries, including not only the agricultural and fishery industry but also the medical care industry, it will be necessary to discuss on a nationwide basis whether it is reasonable to continue nuclear power generation in the future. If it is to be continued, we need to take maximum safety measures, fundamentally review the measures to be taken in the case of occurrence of an accident, and thoroughly disclose information.

(Kenji Sasahara, former head of the Soso public health center)

Measures Taken by the Iwaki City Public Health Center

1 Outline of the areas under jurisdiction

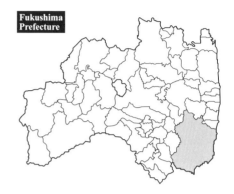
Fukushima Prefecture

(1) Municipalities under jurisdiction

Iwaki City, one of the core cities of Japan, is under its jurisdiction.

(2) Population/population aging rate (as of January 1 each year)

	2011	2013
Population	341,904	329,879
Population aging rate	25	26.3

2 Damage situation caused by the earthquake and nuclear disaster in the areas under jurisdiction

(1) Damage situation (as of March 12, 2013)

Physical damage	Completely destroyed	Half destroyed	Partially destroyed
Residential buildings	7,916	3,706	9,968
Public facilities		27	
Others		3,505	

Human damage	Direct deaths	Associated deaths	Missing	Injured
	293	111	37	4

(2) Evacuation situation (as of March 12, 2013)

	End-March 2011	End-September 2011	End-March 2012	Latest
Installation of shelters	60			
No. of evacuees	3,518			
No. of evacuees accepted				
No. of residents living in temporary houses for residents and evacuees accepted				7,683

(Emergency Response Headquarters of Fukushima Prefecture: Calculated based on the flash report on the damage situation caused by the 2011 off the Pacific coast of Tohoku Earthquake)

Chapter 2 Initiatives of Public Administrations

A year and half have passed since the Great East Japan Earthquake and the accident of the Tokyo Electric Power Company Fukushima Daiichi Nuclear Power Station (hereinafter referred to as the "Fukushima Daiichi Nuclear Station"). Since the occurrence of the unprecedented complex disaster, efforts have been made to restore the affected areas. Particularly in Fukushima Prefecture, however, the restoration work has actually made no significant progress due to the problem of contamination by radioactive substances from the nuclear plant accident, resulting in many people unable to return to their home town. Under such circumstances, mixed feelings, such as irritation, impatience, and resignation, are gradually arising among residents.

Iwaki City is the only core city in Japan that has experienced the earthquake, tsunami, and nuclear plant accident caused by the Great East Japan Earthquake. While Iwaki City is one of the areas significantly affected by the earthquake, it has also now accepted many residents who have evacuated mainly from the area where the nuclear plant is located, thus facing challenges different from those in other areas in Fukushima Prefecture.

A Outline of Iwaki City and the Iwaki City Public Health Center

Iwaki City has a total population of 330,352, consisting of 160,017 males and 170,335 females with 127,614 households (as of September 1, 2012), and an area of 1,231.35 km^2 and it is one of the core cities of Japan with its area the 16th largest among municipalities across the country (as of October 1, 2011). Iwaki City also has a coast line of about 60 km and the sea represents an important tourist resource for the city. Before the earthquake, the fishery industry was flourishing and the beaches were very crowded with sea bathers in summer.

Iwaki City alone forms a secondary medical care area and, with no prefectural public health and welfare office (hereinafter referred to as "public health center"), the only public health center in the city is the Iwaki City Public Health Center.

B March 11 to April 30, 2011 (up to one month)

1 Situation in the city

At 2:46 pm on March 11, the 2011 off the Pacific coast of Tohoku Earthquake occurred with its epicenter off the Sanriku coast (with a seismic intensity of 6 lower in Iwaki City). Due to the influence of the subsequent tsunami and aftershocks (aftershocks with a seismic intensity of 6 lower occurred on April 11 and 12, 2011 with their epicenters near Iwaki City), the city suffered significant damage particularly along the coastal area. As of March 4, 2013, a total of 441 people had been killed: the direct death toll was 293, the disaster-related death toll 111, and missing people certified dead was 37.

On the day of the disaster, information from other areas could be seen on TV and the Internet; however, the public health center had difficulty obtaining local information and the extent of damage in the city gradually became clarified on the following day, the 12th. A number of consultations and inquiries came from residents to the public health center and the roles were shared among the staff members of the public health center to start taking various necessary measures. On the afternoon of the same day, a hydrogen explosion occurred at Unit 1 of the Fukushima Daiichi Nuclear Station, and Iwaki City started accepting many evacuees from Futaba-Gun, where the nuclear plant was located, and other towns and villages. A total of 19,813 people, including Iwaki City residents, were evacuated to 127 shelters in the city at the peak of the evacuation. However, as mentioned before, Iwaki City, which was supposed to accept evacuees, also had significant damage, particularly along the coastal area, and had to accept evacuees in the midst of great confusion in the city with disrupted water and gas services.

Since water services were not available in most areas in the city due to the damage to the water works network, water tank tracks were used to supply water to various areas in the city with support from municipalities across the country and the Self-Defense Forces.

Fortunately, the electricity supply was not interrupted. However, significant damage was caused to much of the infrastructure, such as the water and gas supply, and the restoration took longer than a month.

2 Situation of the medical institutions in the city

At the initial stage, no contact could be made with medical institutions and the personnel of the public health center were directly dispatched to clarify the damage situation of hospitals. To assess the situation of clinics, information was collected with the cooperation of the local medical association utilizing, for example, the SNS (social networking service) of the medical association. The information about the medical institutions in the city was obtained directly from the officers and other staff members of the local medical association.

Life in the city became increasingly difficult due to significant damage to the infrastructure, such as water and gas supply, as well as the interrupted distribution of food, gasoline, and other goods caused by the influence of rumors associated with a series of hydrogen explosions at the nuclear plant. Under such circumstances, health workers also had to consider the evacuation of their children and other family members. Furthermore, various factors, notably including anxiety about the influence of radiation, forced health workers themselves to make a decision as to whether or not they should stay in the city.

The disrupted water supply in most areas in the city caused significant trouble for medical institutions to continue medical care. It was particularly difficult for the medical institutions where artificial dialysis was being conducted to continue the medical care and many artificial dialysis patients in the city had to be transported to other hospitals, mainly in the Kanto region.

Rumors concerning the nuclear plant accident caused a shortage of gasoline and prevented pharmaceutical products from being delivered to medical institutions. The evacuation of health workers outside the city caused medical institutions, pharmacies, and other health related facilities to be unable to function normally.

Thus, a negative chain reaction occurred due to the influence of not only the earthquake but also the nuclear plant accident, leading to increased difficulties for those living in the city.

3 Activities at shelters

The medical care, mainly at shelters, had the support of the Japan Medical Association Team (JMAT) that started on March 12. Since the public health center was simultaneously involved in many activities, such as radiation-related work, consultation from residents, and healthcare work related to shelters, it was impossible to allocate many of its staff members to support medical care at the shelters. While accepting

| Chapter 2 | Initiatives of Public Administrations |

support from the JMAT, following a discussion with the local medical association, it was decided to dispatch public health nurses from the public health center to support the medical association. Together with the medical association, the Local Medical Care Office, and the Health and Social Welfare Department of the city, the dispatched public health nurses coordinated with the JMAT and arranged the visiting schedule. They also played a role in communicating information obtained through the visits of the JMAT to shelters to the public health center.

Many elderly people with chronic diseases evacuated to shelters had their medicines swept away by the tsunami or were unable to take them out of their home. Since many private-practice doctors had joined the JMAT, they provided chronic disease patients with medical care on a daily basis, and their activities met the medical needs at shelters. Through visits of the JMAT, information could be obtained on the health condition of evacuees and on the infectious disease outbreak situation, which allowed the public health center to take necessary measures. Together with the JMAT, the local pharmacist association members and the disaster relief volunteer pharmacists dispatched from across the country conducted activities, including visiting shelters.

Along with medical care activities, various healthcare activities were deployed at shelters. Since there was a concern about the deterioration in the nutritional condition of evacuees, various activities were conducted, such as consultations on nutrition, mainly by dietitians from the public health center, who distributed dietary supplements and provided hot meals. Dental and oral health support by dental hygienists included checking the dental and oral health condition of evacuees. The dental health consultations provided for evacuees included providing necessary dental health materials.

4   Mental healthcare

For mental healthcare, the mental healthcare teams of Fukushima Medical University visited shelters starting on March 19 with the support of many universities and hospitals from across the country. The public health center provided coordination and the teams not only visited shelters but also visited homes and conducted various activities in the citizens' salons and other places in each area of the city.

Various cases were observed from immediately after the earthquake, for which the mental healthcare teams took measures.

(Example of cases for which the mental healthcare teams took measures)
• Cases of mental disorders associated with the experience of the earthquake and tsunami
• Cases of mental disorders associated with the death of close members of the family due to the earthquake and cases where the potential problem in the family surfaced, triggered by the earthquake
• Cases where people could not become independent and were unable to leave the shelter
• Cases of the worsening of the original mental disease

5   Radiation screening (emergency exposure screening)

In response to the accident of the Fukushima Daiichi Nuclear Station on March 12, radiation screening for surface contamination was started on March 13 using survey meters (GM counter- type). The number of examinees screened, which had been 13 a day on March 13, increased to 1,181 a day on March 18 and screening was performed for a total of 36,800 people during half a year. With Fukushima Prefecture, universities across the country, the Disaster Medical Assistance Team (DMAT), and the Federation of Electric

Power Companies of Japan as core members, screening was performed with the cooperation of the Iwaki City Public Health Center. To facilitate whole body decontamination, tents of the Self-Defense Forces were set up beside the General Health and Welfare Center of the city, where the public health center was located. There was no case that exceeded the criterion (100,000 cpm) at that time for whole body decontamination. Many of the residents who wanted to be screened lived outside the evacuation zone or the indoor evacuation zone and screening was actually not needed for these residents according to the notification issued by the government at that time. However, many of the residents who visited the screening site had strong anxiety and eventually it was decided to perform screening for the residents who wanted screening.

6 Distribution of stable iodine tablets

Stable iodine tablets are to be taken to prevent and/or relieve thyroid disorders caused by radioactive iodine (^{131}I). Even though stable iodine tablets were stockpiled in advance in the areas where the nuclear plant was located to deal with a potential nuclear plant accident, they were not stockpiled in the neighboring municipalities because they were not defined as areas that would be affected in the event of a nuclear plant accident. However, Iwaki City stockpiled stable iodine tablets at its own discretion in light of the experience of the JOC criticality accident at Tokai-mura. Immediately after the nuclear plant accident, when Iwaki City residents met evacuees at a shelter who came from the areas where the nuclear plant was located, fear increase in some of the Iwaki City residents after they found that stable iodine tablets had already been distributed to the people from those areas by their respective local municipalities. There was also a concern that some residents might take antiseptics containing iodine by mistake. Consequently, considering all factors, it was decided to distribute stable iodine tablets that had been stockpiled in the city to the residents after this nuclear plant accident. Tablets were distributed to the residents while the city let them know well in advance that the tablets should only be taken when the mayor issued an instruction to take them and should never be taken before the instruction was issued. However, under the circumstances where mail and door-to-door delivery services were suspended and many residents were evacuating to outside the city, which made it difficult to fully utilize the local medical association, tablets had to be distributed to more than 150,000 people (all residents less than 40 years old and pregnant women 40 years old or older) in a short period of time and consequently this became a project to be implemented through the collective efforts of the whole municipal government. In this project, the main force was the public health center and the pharmacists of the public health center played a significant role.

According to the experience in Iwaki City, it is difficult to distribute stable iodine tablets to many residents in the midst of great confusion in the event of a nuclear plant accident. In light of this experience, it is necessary to distribute stable iodine tablets to each household in the areas within a certain range from a nuclear plant before a disaster. As in this case, the area where tablets should be distributed in advance should not be assumed to be limited to a narrow area. If the influence of the nuclear plant accident spreads more than expected, the residents relatively near the evacuation zone will experience great confusion, as was seen during this accident.

According to the manual, stable iodine tablets for children should be prepared as a syrup from powder and this preparation will take a significant amount of time in the event of the actual nuclear plant disaster. It is children on whom the influence of radioactive iodine should be minimized. It is necessary to develop a stable dosage form of iodine preparation for the use by children in the future.

Currently, the Nuclear Regulatory Authority is discussing the distribution and administration of stable iodine tablets, and we hope that the experience with this event can be fully utilized.

Chapter 2 — Initiatives of Public Administrations

C May 1 to September 30, 2011 (two to seven months)

1 Situation in the city

On April 11 and 12, one month after March 11, earthquakes with a seismic intensity of 6 lower occurred and some houses collapsed and mud and rock slides occurred in the city, which significantly affected the city. However, in April when the distribution of goods restarted with the distribution of gasoline fully restored, the situation in the city was remarkably improved. Furthermore, thanks to the support from other municipalities, water services were restored in the middle of April and residents and health workers who had evacuated to outside of the city started returning to the city.

Various lectures and study meetings presented by, for example, academic experts and hosted by various groups and associations were held in various places in the city. However, some of those meetings fomented significant disorder. Also, on the Internet and in other media, many "instant experts" provided a large amount of information that was not fully confirmed, which eventually caused confusion among residents. Any experts must be responsible for what they have done and said, and they must recognize the significance of their responsibility from the perspective of how much anxiety and pain an irresponsible comment can cause to residents struggling with the crisis they faced.

2 Health management and mental healthcare in shelters

During this period, the health management of evacuees as well as the sanitary management and environmental improvement was continued in shelters. One of the important factors that has an influence on the outbreak of infectious diseases in shelters is the density of the people in each shelter and an excessive concentration of evacuees makes it difficult to manage sanitation of common spaces, such as lavatories. In Iwaki City, the overcrowded situation lasted only for a relatively short period of time partly because evacuees started moving into municipally subsidized rental houses relatively early in the middle of April, which was fortunate in terms of taking measures to deal with infectious diseases.

On April 25, Iwaki City started operating the infectious disease surveillance system in shelters that was developed by the Infectious Disease Surveillance Center of the National Institute of Infectious Diseases (hereinafter referred to as the "Surveillance Center of the NIID"). This eventually made it possible to clarify the change over time in, and the total picture of, the outbreak of infectious diseases in typical shelters in the city. It was decided that the information for the input to the infectious disease surveillance system in shelters be collected by the staff members operating the respective shelters (mainly non-medical workers), which enhanced their awareness of preventing the outbreak of infectious diseases in shelters. Furthermore, the infectious disease surveillance feedback files for shelters in Fukushima Prefecture provided by the Surveillance Center of the NIID were used to periodically summarize the infectious disease outbreak trends in shelters in the city.

This facilitated taking efficient countermeasures against infectious diseases based on the risk assessment and proposals made by the Iwaki City Public Health Center. The activities of the JMAT were concluded on May 3 because there was a prospect that evacuees would increasingly move from shelters to temporary houses or temporary municipally subsidized rental houses and the local medical institutions could then adequately deal with the various situations.

Measures Taken by the Iwaki
City Public Health Center

For mental healthcare, care teams continued to pay visits to shelters to provided consultations as requested, prescribe medicine, and give a dose of medicine, as well as take care of babies who needed to be followed up as a result of, for example, baby health checkups and they provided consultations in response to requests from nursery schools and kindergartens.

After all the confusion, it was on August 20, 162 days after the earthquake, when shelters were closed.

3 Support to the affected areas in the city

After the occurrence of the earthquake, we repeatedly requested the prefecture and the government to dispatch public health nurses. However, we continued to have a difficult situation for a while because public health nurses were not immediately dispatched; possibly due to the concern about the influence of the nuclear plant accident. In early April 2011, with the cooperation of public health nurses dispatched from many municipalities and universities across the country, comprehensive home visits were started with a focus on the affected coastal areas. Home visits were fully implemented in late April. Through these visits, public health nurses checked the health condition of evacuees and gave advice, as well as clarified the needs for support and provided the information on mental healthcare and where to contact an appropriate professional for consultations. This facilitated defining the living and health conditions of people in the coastal area and could also provide a sense of security to the residents.

After the earthquake, people's attention was attracted to shelters; however, many elderly people actually continued to live at their homes near the coastal area that had been affected by the tsunami, and during the home visits, many of them voiced their opinion saying "We wanted you to come earlier." It must be kept in mind that, in providing support to affected people the affected people are not only those in shelters.

As residents returned to the area where they had lived, cleanup activities were started for their homes and the surrounding areas. The public health center distributed hydrated lime as needed to the areas that had been inundated by the tsunami or other events.

In the coastal area, marine products, such as fish and shellfish, stored in refrigerators started to spoil due to power failure and complaints were made on associated problems, such as abnormal odors spreading and flies. The staff members of the public health center applied remedial chemicals in an attempt to prevent such problems in some cases.

4 Measures taken for pets

There were some evacuees living in a vehicle with their pet because they did not wish to bother other people in the shelter.

Late April 2011, Iwaki City Animal Rescue Headquarters, consisting of the representatives of the city (public health center), the veterinary medical association of the city, volunteer groups, and other parties concerned, was established to protect affected animals. In addition, since pets were not allowed in many temporary houses and temporary municipally subsidized rental houses, the Iwaki City Pet Protection Center was established to facilitate pet owners to move into these restricted houses. This was intended to provide people who could not live with their pet with a temporary place for the pet to live. The center was established originally for the purpose of protecting the pets of the residents; however, with the passing of time, pets accompanied by the evacuees from the area where the nuclear plant was located were increasingly

Chapter 2 — Initiatives of Public Administrations

accommodated in the center.

It seems that the evacuation of pets was not considered so important before this earthquake. Now that many families have pets, it is necessary for both the pet owners and the public administration to think of measures in advance for how to evacuate pets in the event of a disaster.

D October 1, 2011 to March 31, 2012 (seven months to one year)

1 Situation in the city

The life of residents was gradually returning to normal, and after shelters had been closed, the routine work of the public health center could be gradually resumed.

However, under the circumstances where residents had a strong anxiety about exposure to low dose radiation, decontamination was promoted in areas where the radiation dose was relatively high and for the living spaces for children, such as child-care facilities and educational facilities.

2 Measures taken for radiation health management

In January 2012, the Radiation Health Management Center was newly established in the public health center, consisting of two sections. Namely, the Health Management Section in charge of, for example, distributing personal dose meters (glass badges) and iodine tablets and the Health Inspection Section in charge of radioactivity inspection of food products and other items and internal exposure inspection (Figure 7-1).

Programs implemented by the Radiation Health Management Center of the public health center now include, (i) internal exposure inspection using a whole-body counter, (ii) inspection of well water for drinking water and food products using a germanium semiconductor detector, and (iii) leasing of digital dose meters.

Internal exposure inspection was performed with the cooperation of the prefecture for the children 18 years old or younger and for expectant mothers after the nuclear plant accident occurred (still performed as of March 31, 2013).

3 Measures taken for affected people in the city and evacuees from other municipalities

As a monitoring and health support system for affected people in the whole city, the system shown in Figure 7-2 was established and the support to affected people was started in line with the system.

It was decided to provide evacuees from other municipalities with various services pursuant to the Special Act on Evacuees from Nuclear Accidents. It was also decided that the clerical work concerning protective vaccination as well as health checkups of expectant and nursing mothers should continue to be provided by the evacuees' original municipality utilizing the existing wide area framework in the prefecture.

People even from a single municipality had evacuated diversely to various areas in the prefecture. This caused difficulty for public health nurses and other staff of the evacuees' original municipality to conduct

7 Measures Taken by the Iwaki City Public Health Center

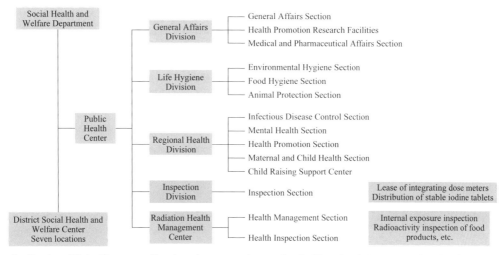

Besides the public health center, radioactive substances are inspected at the Water Supply Department, branch offices, etc.

Figure 7-1 Organization of the Iwaki City Public Health Center (As of March 31, 2013)

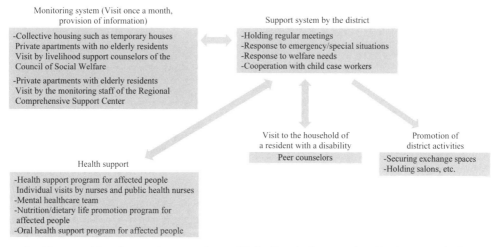

Providing support to various people concerned as a public health center in cooperation with relevant organizations

Figure 7-2 Monitoring and health support system of Iwaki City for affected people

their activities, which led to the disparity in the health services for evacuees depending on the area to which they had evacuated.

To continually provide mental healthcare, the Fukushima Center for Disaster Mental Health (base center) was founded in February 2012 and subsequently district centers were established in six districts in the prefecture in March. In Iwaki City, where there were many evacuees from the areas where the nuclear plant was located, the Iwaki District Center was established and started its activities.

65

Chapter 2 | Initiatives of Public Administrations

E : April 1, 2012 to March 31, 2013 (one year and one month to two years)

1 Situation in the city

Concerning radiation and radioactivity, most of the residents can now accept the current situation in the city in a relatively objective manner. However, more than few residents are concerned about the effects of the initial exposure on the thyroid gland of children. Fukushima Prefecture plans to continually perform thyroid inspection for the residents 18 years old or younger at the time of the nuclear plant accident with the inspection schedule determined in advance. The development of thyroid cancer in children is known as one of the effects of the Chernobyl nuclear plant accident. Even though the Chernobyl nuclear plant accident differs from the Fukushima Daiichi Nuclear Station in various aspects, such as measures taken subsequent to the accident, the inspection results must continue to be carefully monitored into the future.

According to the results of the answers to doctors' questions in the health checkup of babies in the city, some parents do not let their babies go out or play outdoors too often and they are also concerned about low dose exposure of their babies; although the number of such parents have significantly decreased. This restriction on outdoor play has reduced the exercise volume and decreased the physical strength of children. In addition, children are significantly more likely to be obese. Since Iwaki City is the area in Fukushima Prefecture where many people already die of lifestyle-related diseases, measures must be taken to deal with child obesity and child lifestyle- related diseases to prevent their development of future lifestyle-related diseases.

2 Influence of the inflow of population from other areas, such as where the nuclear plant is located, on residents' life

While 7,838 residents of Iwaki City have evacuated to outside of the city (as of February 25, 2013), the number of evacuees into Iwaki City from other areas, such as Futaba-Gun, by far exceeds it, reaching as many as 23,901 people when including only those officially registered (as of March 1, 2013). The number of vacant rental houses in the city continues to be extremely low. In addition, many workers are in the city from across the country to engage in the operations to deal with, for example, the nuclear plant accident, and hotels and Japanese inns are already reserved for many days to come. Some estimates are that the population has increased by more than 30,000 as a whole, meaning that the population in the city has increased by about 10% in only one to two years. The remarkable increase in population during this short period has significantly changed the living environment, such as more severe traffic congestion in the morning and evening and on holidays. Some action needs to be taken to secure a place where evacuees from Futaba-Gun can lead a stable life, the so-called "temporary town," but no definite action has been decided upon.

Even prior to the earthquake there was a lack of medical doctors that has continued in Iwaki City (168 doctors to 100,000 residents as a whole and 82.7 hospital doctors to 100,000 residents according to the Survey of Physicians, Dentists and Pharmacists 2010 by the Ministry of Health, Labour and Welfare), placing a significant load on medical institutions. With an increase in the number of evacuees in the city, a further load is placed on medical institutions. There are some who say that the residents' life is affected due to, for example, the longer waiting time and the difficulty in making reservations at a medical institution.

Considering the influence on medical care in the city in the future, included among the most significant issues is the prevention of diseases for those who have evacuated into the city due to the nuclear plant accident. There is a particular concern for those living in dispersed temporary municipally subsidized rental houses, as it is difficult to monitor them only through healthcare activities. Unless this issue is firmly addressed, the load on the medical institutions in the city will increase in the future. The government, the prefecture, and the municipalities concerned are requested to take firm measures.

In any event, the government, the prefecture, and individual municipalities must make a clear decision in terms of how to deal with the issue of evacuees as soon as possible. Immediate actions must be taken for regional healthcare and medical treatment sites.

F. Important matters required in taking measures to control a disaster

Required at the initial stage in dealing with an earthquake disaster is the "strength of public health sanitation of the region," particularly the comprehensive strength of a public health center. Provided that reporting to, contacting, and consulting with a superior is ensured, it is important to give as much discretion as possible to the personnel in charge at the site to deal with the actual situation. While it is important to develop a disaster management manual and have it in place, individuals' ideas and ability to take action are also absolutely necessary, and it is important to develop before a disaster the personnel capable of creating and executing flexible plans.

Measures to deal with the earthquake disaster have not been completed yet and we will continue to keep an eye on the health of residents on a long-term basis in cooperation with the departments and organizations concerned.

(Toshikatsu Shinka)

8 Measures Taken by the Ken-poku Public Health and Welfare Office

1 Outline of the areas under jurisdiction

(1) Municipalities under jurisdiction

The following four cities, three towns, and one village are under the jurisdiction: Fukushima City, Nihonmatsu City, Date City, Motomiya City, Koori Town, Kunimi Town, and Kawamata Town of Date-Gun, and Otama Village of Adachi-Gun

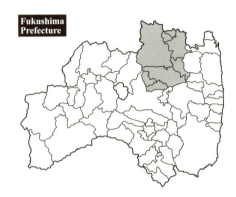

(2) Population/population aging rate (as of January 1 each year)

	2011	2013
Population	496,586	481,140
Population aging rate	25.1	26.6

2 Damage situation caused by the earthquake and nuclear disaster in the areas under jurisdiction

(1) Damage situation (as of March 12, 2013)

Physical damage	Completely destroyed	Half destroyed	Partially destroyed
Residential buildings	532	5,666	26,479
Public facilities	418		
Others	6,586		

Human damage	Direct deaths	Associated deaths	Missing	Injured
	7	9	0	46

(2) Evacuation situation (as of September 26, 2013)

	End-March 2011	End-September 2011	End-March 2012	Latest
Installation of shelters	69			
No. of evacuees	256	1,274	13	1,892
No. of evacuees accepted	8,265			
No. of residents living in temporary houses for residents and evacuees accepted				5,592

(Emergency Response Headquarters of Fukushima Prefecture: Calculated based on the flash report on the damage situation caused by the 2011 off the Pacific coast of Tohoku Earthquake)

8　Measures Taken by the Ken-poku
Public Health and Welfare Office

A : March 11 to April 30, 2011 (up to one month)

1　Situation

- At 2:46 pm on March 11, the 2011 off the Pacific coast of Tohoku Earthquake occurred. The seismic intensity was 6 upper at Kunimi Town and the town office building was completely collapsed. The seismic intensity was 5 lower to 6 lower in other municipalities. Electricity and water supply were disrupted, the transportation system was cut off, and gasoline was in short supply.
- On March 12, an evacuation order was issued for the area within 20 km due to a hydrogen explosion of the Unit 1 of the Tokyo Electric Power Company Fukushima Daiichi Nuclear Power Station (hereinafter referred to as the "Fukushima Daiichi Nuclear Station").
- The Japanese Red Cross Society opened a first-aid station at Azuma gymnasium.
- Hydrogen explosions occurred at Unit 3 and 2 of the Fukushima Daiichi Nuclear Station on the March 14 and 15, respectively (indoor evacuation order issued for the area of 20 to 30 km).
- Medical care meetings were held in the Ken-poku Public Health and Welfare Office (hereinafter referred to as the "public health center") between March 23 and the end of April to coordinate the places to be visited as well as to share information.
- Health support teams came into the district from outside of the prefecture starting on March 30.

2　Main activities

- Starting at night on March 12, inpatients were transferred from the hospitals in the Soso district to the Fukushima Gender Equality Centre (Nihonmatsu City) used as a shelter and screening was performed for all of the team members engaged in transportation and of the transportation vehicles.
- Since hospitals that were expected to accept patients had actually rejected those who could not confirm whether they were contaminated by radioactive substances, certificates showing the completion of screening were issued.
- We checked the damage and evacuation of individual facilities.
- We checked whether patients were safe, including those with intractable disease.
- On March 18, we started confirming the situation in shelters and providing support.
- Starting on March 22, patients who needed a private room could be accommodated in the Training Center for Local Officers at the discretion of the head of the public health center.

3　Summary and measures to be taken in the future

- Radiation screening was the top-priority job of our public health center, which was required to secure the personnel and many equipment items to perform screening.
- Priority was placed on screening and it was one week after the occurrence of the disaster that we could start health consultations for evacuees. Providing early support is necessary to prevent a work overload on public health nurses of municipalities.
- The notices from the government could not be thoroughly communicated due to the power failure and damage to municipality office buildings, causing disparity in measures taken by the municipalities to which residents had evacuated. It is necessary to study how to thoroughly communicate the notification.
- Private rooms that can accommodate evacuees who need them, such as those with new born infants and children with special needs, must be secured at an early stage.

69

Chapter 2 Initiatives of Public Administrations

 May 1 to September 30, 2011 (two to seven months)

1 Situation

- On April 22, the Yamakiya district of Kawamata Town was designated as the planned evacuation zone and 1,234 residents from 469 households were evacuated.
- Starting on June 15, a total of eight staff members (five for nursing or similar jobs and three including psychiatric social workers) were urgently employed.
- On June 30, 104 spots in part of Date City was designated as specific spots recommended for evacuation, and residents of 78 households, who wanted to relocate, out of a total of 103 relevant households were evacuated to, for example, municipal houses.
- On November 25, spots for an additional 15 households were designated as specific spots recommended for evacuation.
- On September 23, primary shelters (in the Azuma Sports Park) were closed, resulting in no primary shelters available in the municipalities under the jurisdiction of the Ken-poku Public Health Center.

2 Main activities

- Staring on March 30, support from outside of the prefecture was provided, and activities were started with our public health center as well as Date City, Otama Village, and Namie Town, which had requested support, as bases of activities.
- Visiting health consultations by public health nurses and other staff was started in Namie Town and Minamisoma City on April 11 and for secondary shelters on April 22.
- Starting on May 12, meetings were periodically held with the municipalities from which people had evacuated to conduct a study on the support for affected people.
- On June 28, visiting health consultations were started for temporary houses along with that for secondary shelters.
- On September 30, the final visit was paid to the secondary shelters in Namie Town (Tsuchiyu Spa).
- Psychiatric social workers and clinical psychotherapists were urgently employed to start conducting visiting health consultations and paying visits to psychiatric hospitals.

3 Summary and measures to be taken in the future

- Health support teams from the outside of the prefecture were effective. However, it took time to communicate with and to coordinate them; for example, introduce lodging places for them. In addition, the support was for a short period of about one week. Consequently, an orientation had to be given almost every day. Some of the support workers did not have a driver's license and we had to provide transportation in some cases. From the perspective of the party that is supported, we want them to assist us for the longest term possible using a system whereby they can support affected people by themselves.
- Since the municipality from which residents have evacuated is fully involved in dealing with issues at hand, the long stay of, for example, public health nurses of the public health center who can work as coordinators in the a municipality, will facilitate cooperation.

C October 1, 2011 to March 31, 2012 (seven months to one year)

1 Situation

- The number of new applications for nursing care insurance payment, which used to be about 16.4 per month at ordinary times, increased to 64.4.

2 Main activities

- While visits to all temporary houses in Namie Town were continued, the health guidance and light exercise classes and the consultation by a clinical psychotherapist at the meeting place of temporary houses started on October 3 (Figures 8-1 and 2).
- On November 11, visits to municipally subsidized rental houses in Iitate Village started (a total of 209 residents 75 years old or older in 14 households). On December 5, visits to municipally subsidized rental houses in Namie Town started (263 households with residents 65 years old or older). On January 19, visits to municipally subsidized rental houses in Futaba Town started (38 residents in 17 households).

3 Summary and measures to be taken in the future

- With evacuation time prolonged, a study must be conducted on measures to be taken for people who have few opportunities to move and whose need of nursing care may be eventually authorized, as well measures taken to address dietary imbalance.
- A study must be conducted on measures to be taken for people who do not show up at the meeting place and other public places.
- Health consultations were held at Iizaka Spa and other places for the residents of municipally subsidized rental houses. However, the means allowing many people to gather should have been studied because there were many elderly people who did not drive, or had difficulty coming to the place where consultations were conducted.

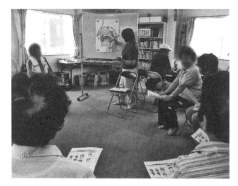

Figure 8-1 Dental health guidance at the meeting place of a temporary house

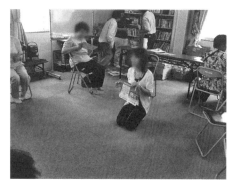

Figure 8-2 Mental healthcare at the meeting place of a temporary house

Chapter 2 | Initiatives of Public Administrations

D April 1, 2012 to March 31, 2013 (one year and one month to two years)

1 Situation

- In order to identify the health condition of affected people who have been forced into a long evacuation in temporary housing or municipally subsidized rental houses, and prevent health conditions from getting worse, to relieve anxiety about health and to promote exchanges among affected people, support is provided through various activities. These group activities and onsite instructions were conducted by people from various occupations; such as public health nurses, nurses, dental hygienists, physical therapists, occupational therapists, Judo therapists, clinical psychotherapists, psychiatric social workers, and dietitians. In addition, exchange meetings with parents and children playing together and also among parents are held to provide mental and emotional support to parents and children based on the meetings with affected municipalities in the "Liaison Conference for Health Support Activities."

2 Main activities

- Various group activities were conducted, including health consultation, health education, and recreation activities such as light exercise and games, using the meeting places of temporary houses and municipally subsidized rental houses in cooperation with the Ken-poku district center of the Fukushima Center for Disaster Mental Health (Figure 8-3).
- Onsite instructions were provided to the people who needed support.
- As a mental healthcare program for children, various events, such as exchange meetings with parents and children playing together and exchange meetings among parents, were held to provide mental support to parents and children.
- Liaison Conference for Health Support Activities: Meetings were held periodically with the affected municipalities that the public health center supported (e.g., scheduling of the health support activities, reporting their results, and exchanging information).
- Since an issue concerning baby health checkups arose in the municipalities from which affected people had evacuated and the municipalities where their health checkups were performed, maternal and child health liaison meetings were held.
- Group meetings with psychiatrists were held mainly for the support workers from the affected municipalities, namely Namie Town, Iitate Village, and Date City.

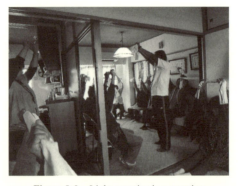

Figure 8-3   Light exercise in a meeting

3 Summary and measures to be taken in the future

- Although the municipalities from which residents have evacuated have regained their equanimity, there are some municipalities that have to support their residents who have evacuated to more than 30 locations, in the most extreme case, even within the prefecture. Affected people must be supported; however, since the public administration providing support is also affected, there will also be an issue as to how to support the support worker.
- As the situations differ depending on the affected municipality, it is also necessary for the local public health center to make proposals resulting from meetings that are held on a periodic basis, as to how to support the affected people.

(Ryoko Miyata, former head of the Ken-poku Public Health and Welfare Office)

9 Measures Taken by the Ken-chu Public Health and Welfare Office

1 Outline of the areas under jurisdiction

(1) Municipalities under jurisdiction

The following two cities, six towns, and three village are under the jurisdiction: Sukagawa City; Tamura City, Kagamiishi Town and Tenei Village of Iwase- Gun, Ishikawa Town, Tamakawa Village, Hirata Village, Asakawa Town, and Furudono Town of Ishikawa-Gun, and Miharu Town and Ono Town of Tamura-Gun

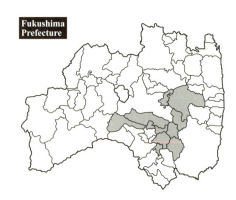

(2) Population/population aging rate (as of January 1 each year)

	2011	2013
Population	212,647	206,851
Population aging rate	25.0	25.9

2 Damage situation caused by the earthquake and nuclear disaster in the areas under jurisdiction

(1) Damage situation (as of March 12, 2013)

Physical damage	Completely destroyed	Half destroyed	Partially destroyed
Residential buildings	1,550	4,967	25,773
Public facilities		389	
Others		7,220	

Human damage	Direct deaths	Associated deaths	Missing	Injured
	9	6	1	23

(2) Evacuation situation (as of March 12, 2013)

	End-March 2011	End-September 2011	End-March 2012	Latest
Installation of shelters	34			
No. of evacuees	3,410	2,539	580	580
No. of evacuees accepted	3,498			
No. of residents living in temporary houses for residents and evacuees accepted				2,747

(Emergency Response Headquarters of Fukushima Prefecture: Calculated based on the flash report on the damage situation caused by the 2011 off the Pacific coast of Tohoku Earthquake)

* In Fukushima Prefecture, Koriyama City is included in the Ken-chu District in terms of the medical care area; however, since Koriyama City is one of the core cities of Japan, it is not under the jurisdiction of the Ken-chu Public Health and Welfare Office.

9 Measures Taken by the Ken-chu Public Health and Welfare Office

A   March 11 to April 30, 2011 (up to one month)

1   Situation

- An earthquake with a seismic intensity of 6 upper (Sukagawa City and Tenei Village) occurred and shelters were set up in the area under their jurisdiction.
- The Miyakoji District of Tamura City, which was under our jurisdiction, was designated as a warning zone and an evacuation order was issued.
- Many houses, mainly in Koriyama City, Sukagawa City, and Kagamiishi Town, completely collapsed.
- The medical institutions where artificial dialysis was performed suspended their services due to the water outage.
- Many evacuees from the municipalities of Futaba-Gun and Iwaki City rushed to the municipalities along National Routes 49 and 398. Shelters were set up in all of the municipalities under our jurisdiction (Figure 9-1).
- On March 16, a medical care team from Tokyo Metropolis entered Tamura City to provide support.
- On March 22, a public health team from Shiga Prefecture started its activities. The activities lasted until the end of August 2011.
- The suspension of the JR line and express way services caused difficulty for our office staff members to make their commute.
- The office function of the towns in Futaba-Gun from which people had evacuated was relocated; Tomioka Town and Kawauchi Village to Koriyama City, Hirono Town to Ono Town, Okuma Town to Tamura City and relocated again to Aizuwakamatsu City on April 3.
- On April 6, support teams from outside of the prefecture started their activities: Including the public health teams from Hokkaido and Wakayama Prefecture and the public health nurse teams from Fukuoka Prefecture and Hiroshima Prefecture.
- Each medical association under our jurisdiction visited shelters to provide medical care.

2   Main activities

- On March 13, our office staff members started visiting shelters under our jurisdiction to perform external exposure screening (Figure 9-2).
- On March 18 and 19, our office worked to clarify the actual situation of the health support activities at

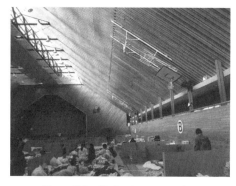

Figure 9-1   Shelter in a gymnasium

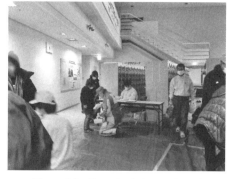

Figure 9-2   Screening being performed

Chapter 2 Initiatives of Public Administrations

the shelters in the municipalities under our jurisdiction.

- On March 20, the public health nurses and dietitians of the Public Health and Welfare Office (hereinafter referred to as the "public health center") started visiting shelters (except those in Koriyama City) to provide consultations.

  The public health center had 15 public health nurses (including one on sick leave) and three dietitians (including one on child-care leave) for these activities.

- We conducted coordination for patients admitted to and discharged from the medical institutions and for artificial dialysis patients in the areas under our jurisdiction.

- We conducted coordination for external support (medical support teams, mental healthcare teams, and health support teams).

- On April 3, the office function of Okuma Town was relocated to Aizuwakamatsu City, and consequently many of the evacuees were also relocated.

- Since evacuees relocated to the Aizu District and support teams from the outside of the prefecture started their activities, the support team system in the public health center was changed. Starting on April 5, the public health nurses of the public health center were stationed in or visited the shelters in the prefectural facilities in Koriyama City to provide health consultations.

- Starting at the end of March, outbreaks of infectious gastroenteritis occurred in some shelters and measures were taken to prevent the spread of infection.

  Measures included distributing antiseptic solution, hand-wash soap and paper towels, providing guidance for evacuees on how to wash hands and dispose of vomited matter, cleaning lavatories, identifying symptomatic people, and providing assistance for medical examinations.

- Many support workers from outside of the prefecture gathered in the shelter at the Big Palette Fukushima convention center in Koriyama City after the Shinkansen and express way services had been restored. At this point in time, the major duty of the public health nurses from the public health center was the coordination of the support workers.

3 Summary and measures to be taken in the future

- For visiting consultations at shelters, teams in charge of the respective municipalities were formed. The formation of teams could support the activities of public health nurses with little experience and allowed the team members to take days off in turn.

- It took time to clarify the actual situation in municipalities. Assigning a person in charge of a specific municipality in advance would have clarified the person who would gather information and help coordinate support.

- Since the timing of the disaster fell at the end of the fiscal year, routine paperwork for, for example, subsidizations and contracts had to be performed together with the tasks associated with the support shelters. Consequently, such paperwork had to be performed at night. The work load of public health nurses who supported shelters should have been reduced if, for example, the office work in the public health center was well coordinated.

- In shelters, outbreaks of infectious diseases, such as infectious gastroenteritis and influenza, occurred. Workers in shelters must be equipped with the basic knowledge and skills to take infection prevention measures.

9 Measures Taken by the Ken-chu Public Health and Welfare Office

B : May 1 to September 30, 2011 (two to seven months)

1 Situation

- The time living as evacuees was prolonged and evacuees relocated from primary shelters to other places, such as secondary shelters that included spring inns and municipally subsidized rental houses.
- Shelters for residents who had evacuated from Futaba-Gun continued to be used for them. As evacuation life was prolonged, evacuees relocated from shelters, such as gymnasiums and community halls, to secondary shelters that included spring inns and municipally subsidized rental houses, such as apartment houses. This allowed shelters to gradually close.
  The shelter at the Big Palette Fukushima convention center, where the number of evacuees had peaked at about 2,300 in late March, was closed at the end of August and all of the shelters in the areas under our jurisdiction were eventually closed.
- In June, evacuees started moving into temporary houses and relocated from shelters.
- In July, Katsurao Village relocated its office function from Mishima Town to Miharu Town, and residents who were mainly living in temporary houses were relocated.
- The dispatch of public health nurses who were supported from outside of the prefecture ended in August. Public health nurses and dietitians were secured as a project of the prefecture and a team was organized together with the public health nurses of the public health center to conduct activities for health support until March 2012.

2 Main activities

- In May, public health nurses started visiting secondary shelters, such as Japanese inns, to provide health consultations.
  In June, with the change in personnel from the prefecture, a new organization was established to implement the health support project.
- For the organization of the public health nurses of the public health center, the system to support municipalities was introduced with public health nurses in charge of the municipality from which evacuees had come, instead of the municipality to which evacuees had relocated.
- To deal with life inactive diseases (disuse syndrome) associated with prolonged evacuation life, health education, such as health classes (classes for diabetics), was provided in shelters.
- A public health nurse accompanied an elderly person who was concerned about life in a temporary house to check the house before the person moved in. They checked the operation of gas appliances and other apparatus and also reviewed whether any auxiliary fixtures should be mounted.
- In June, temporary houses were completed and the health survey was started for those moving into the temporary houses.
- In July, a health salon was started in the meeting room of temporary housing to promote exchanges among residents and prevent residents from being isolated.

3 Summary and measures to be taken in the future

- As the life in shelters was prolonged, the life function of many people, particularly aged people, became remarkably decreased.
  It is necessary to support evacuees with an eye to their life after leaving the shelter. For example by

Chapter 2 Initiatives of Public Administrations

- letting them have a role in activities in the shelter.
- After evacuees have relocated to temporary houses and municipally subsidized rental houses, it is mainly elderly people who stay in the house during daytime, which makes it difficult to contact children and adults to clarify health issues. Cooperation with, for example, schools is necessary.
- There was food poisoning caused by hot meal that had been supplied, and countermeasures were taken in cooperation with the food hygiene department.
- We could visit evacuees living in municipally subsidized rental houses only after visiting temporary houses. There were many cases where evacuees were isolated in the district and support and information from the public administration did not reach them easily. A study is necessary into conducting activities in cooperation with organizations in the district of the municipality to which people have been evacuated.

C October 1, 2011 to March 31, 2012 (seven months to one year)

1 Situation

- Neighborhood community associations were founded for residents in temporary houses and thus the system allowing the residents to conduct regional activities was gradually established.

2 Main activities

- Jointly with life support counselors of the social welfare council, we held health salons at meeting places for evacuees living in temporary houses and we visited municipally subsidized rental houses.
- We mainly visited municipally subsidized rental houses for elderly people and people who needed support, in collaboration with the municipalities from which they had come.
- Roles were shared with the life support counselors from the municipalities from which or to which evacuees had come to conduct support activities. This included support for the counselors in the cases where, for example, they were asked for advice on health issues that were difficult to respond to during their monitoring activities.

3 Summary and measures to be taken in the future

- In our visits to the residents of municipally subsidized rental houses, it was difficult to determine their health condition because they were often out of the house during the daytime.
- The information about the residents of the municipalities whose office function was in the area under our jurisdiction could be shared; however, the information about the residents of the municipalities whose office function was not in the area under our jurisdiction was not available, thus visiting activities were not provided. It is necessary to study how to share information when people have evacuated over a wide area.
- In terms of interactions among residents in temporary houses, it was difficult to establish good neighborly ties. Elderly people and people with disabilities were more likely to be homebound in when municipalities assigned temporary housing for evacuees by a drawing as compared to the municipalities whose residents moved into temporary houses as a group based on their old residential areas. It is important to give advice to people about moving into temporary housing from the perspective of health management.
- With evacuation life was prolonged and no future prospects seen, mental health issues and consultations became diversified and individuated. It was necessary to deal with problems of individuals and the work load of support workers increased. It is necessary to establish a support system for support workers.

(Ayako Furuyama, former staff member of the Ken-chu Public Health and Welfare Office)

10 Measures Taken by the Ken-nan Public Health and Welfare Office

1 Outline of the areas under jurisdiction

(1) Municipalities under jurisdiction

The following one city, four towns, and four villages are under the jurisdiction: Shirakawa City; Nishigo Village, Izumizaki Village, Nakajima Village, and Yabuki Town of Nishishirakawa-Gun; and Tanagura Town, Yamatsuri Town, Hanawa Town, and Samegawa Village of Higashishirakawa-Gun

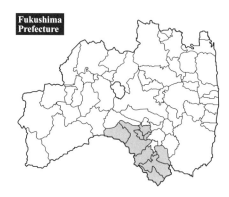

(2) Population/population aging rate (as of January 1 each year)

	2011	2013
Population	149,885	146,847
Population aging rate	23.8	24.6

2 Damage situation caused by the earthquake and nuclear disaster in the areas under jurisdiction

(1) Damage situation (as of March 12, 2013)

Physical damage	Completely destroyed	Half destroyed	Partially destroyed
Residential buildings	677	4,070	12,969
Public facilities		180	
Others		3,365	

Human damage	Direct deaths	Associated deaths	Missing	Injured
	15	0	0	13

(2) Evacuation situation (as of March 12, 2013)

	End-March 2011	End-September 2011	End-March 2012	Latest
Installation of shelters	15			
No. of evacuees	152			
No. of evacuees accepted	724			
No. of residents living in temporary houses for residents and evacuees accepted				559

(Emergency Response Headquarters of Fukushima Prefecture: Calculated based on the flash report on the damage situation caused by the 2011 off the Pacific coast of Tohoku Earthquake)

Chapter 2 | Initiatives of Public Administrations

 March 11 to April 30, 2011 (up to one month)

1 Situation of the areas under our jurisdiction and main activities

- There was only minor damage to the building of our Public Health and Welfare Office (hereinafter referred to as the "public health center"). Water supply and gas supply started to be restored on March 23 and 24, respectively. Electric power was restored by the end of March 11 and phone lines were almost restored on March 18.
- We checked damage to ten hospitals under our jurisdiction on the day of the earthquake and damage to clinics on March 22. In collaboration with medical institutions, we coordinated efforts to secure water tank trucks and provisions for their food services.
- On March 11, it could be confirmed that there was no human injuries and only minor damage to a total of 37 facilities in the areas under our jurisdiction; namely eight facilities accommodating people with disabilities, four facilities accommodating children, 23 welfare and health facilities for elderly people, and two social aid facilities.
- On March 11, we started collecting information on the damage and the current situation of water works facilities and providing consultation and conducting research in response to requests from, for example, water supply installers. The water supply had been disrupted for a total of 32,630 households in seven municipalities, and it was restored by April 18.
- Support for animals at shelters started on March 17. The main items of support and the respective starting dates are as follows:
  - No commission any longer charged to accept disaster-affected animals (from March 18)
  - Setting up facilities (temporary tents) to accommodate disaster-affected animals (from April 4)
  - Starting to bring in animals and managing their rearing (from April 5)
  - Protection activities in the warning zone (from April 28)
- Immediately after the occurrence of the earthquake, we paid visits to primary shelters at gymnasiums, community halls, meeting places, schools, and other facilities (Table 10-1). In order to check various situations, such as the situation of the evacuees who needed immediate medical support, the supply and demand situation of goods, and the situations of water supply, hygiene management, and animal protection management, public health nurses cooperated with people in various occupations. These included environmental health officers, food sanitation inspectors, national registered dietitians, pharmacists, and dental hygienists, as well as with the respective municipalities, and conducted activities from the occurrence of the disaster until around the end of April. To be specific, in coordination with the public health nurses and medical institutions in the respective municipalities their top priority was placed on dealing with emergency situations, they conducted various activities, such as provision of health consultation, provision of stockpiled pharmaceuticals, coordination for facilities to accept people who needed support (vulnerable people) in a disaster, and transportation to medical institutions of the affected people who needed medical treatment.
  Furthermore, while fulfilling the coordination function for the visiting medical care by the Disaster Medical Assistance Team (DMAT), the Japan Medical Association Team (JMAT), and healthcare teams from the outside of the prefecture, and for the visits to shelters by mental healthcare teams of psychiatric medical institutions under our jurisdiction, the public health center continued to keep the records of individuals based on its own visits, provided stockpiled pharmaceuticals, and played a role in providing the visiting staff with the information on the affected people who needed medical support (Figure 10-1).
- We provided and distributed posters and fliers about infectious disease prevention and gave advice on

10 Measures Taken by the Ken-nan Public Health and Welfare Office

Table 10-1 Change in the number of primary/secondary shelters and evacuees (total number of facilities and evacuees)

Date to start accepting refugees in primary shelters: March 13, 2011, Date of closure: August 31, 2011*

Month	March	April	May	June	July	August
Primary shelters	223	302	137	78	62	56
No. of evacuees in primary shelters	18,420	16,402	9,404	6,592	4,992	3,086

Date to start accepting refugees in secondary shelters: April 4, 2011, Date of closure: November 14, 2011**

Month	March	April	May	June	July	August	September	October	November
Secondary shelters		433	822	868	767	413	218	173	37
No. of evacuees in secondary shelters		5,774	14,404	13,148	9,797	4,392	1,352	711	55

* Peak date: March 19, 2011, 1,929 people, 23 shelters
** Peak date: May 19, 2011, 532 people, 26 facilities

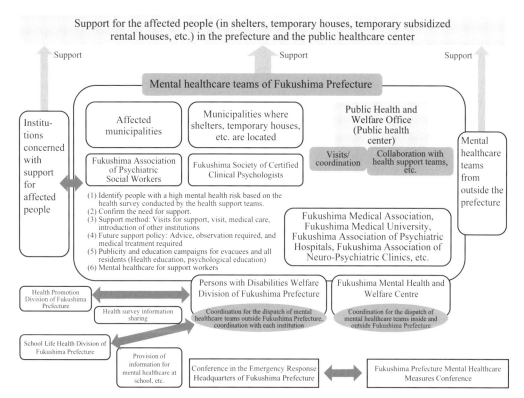

Figure 10-1 Support for affected people and evacuees by mental healthcare teams and the public healthcare center

hygiene management and measures to prevent food poisoning. We also started on March 31 to implement the shelter surveillance program developed by the National Institute of Infectious Diseases to detect infectious disease at an early stage and take measures to prevent the spread of infection.

- In response to a notice from the Ministry of Health, Labour and Welfare, we provided necessary pharmaceuticals free of charge when a medical support team visited shelters.
- In our public health center, emergency exposure screening was started on March 13, which was on a round-the-clock basis at the initial stage, and a certificate of the completion of screening was issued starting on the 14th. For emergency exposure screening, teams were formed with the support of healthcare

teams from the outside of the prefecture, and screening was performed in various areas in the prefecture by paying visits to shelters or establishing a place for screening. We also took necessary measures in response to the restriction of the distribution and intake of food contaminated with radioactive substances.
- Many inquiries were received about the storage of stable iodine tablets; however, stable iodine tablets were not stockpiled and no directions were issued by the Emergency Response Headquarters of Fukushima Prefecture to administer tablets.

2 Summary and measures to be taken in the future

- Immediately after the earthquake, the public health center was required to have a coordinating function to clarify which shelter needed what level of medical support and to match the medical support with such needs. The contact point was centralized within the public health center to share information on the actual situation of the shelters and their needs and establish a system at an early stage to accept healthcare teams. Holding meetings with healthcare teams was effective. It is significant if a network of institutions concerned, such as medical institutions, is established in ordinary times.
- It is necessary to establish systems utilizing cloud computing in the event of a disaster, including the following features: Information sharing by many users, real time information update, backup of medical record information through storage outside the hospital, information referable even when patients are transported, registration and dispatch of various teams. Dispatch of teams in the event of a disaster such as advance health support teams, public health dispatch teams, the Disaster Public health Assistance Team (DPAT), the Disaster Health Emergency Assistance Team (DHEAT), the Radiation Emergency Medical Assistance Team (REMAT), and the Disaster Psychiatric Assistance Team (DPAT). It is also necessary to establish systems for sharing the health management information of affected people, and health support system.
- It is also necessary to continue to conduct a study on how exposure screening should be handled and what should be the consulting system for residents.
- Dosing instructions for stable iodine tablets that prevent thyroid exposure must be clarified in advance.
- It is necessary in the future to strengthen mutual cooperation with the institutions concerned and communication with various parties concerned, including residents, as well as improve risk communication, such as information sharing at ordinary times, and crisis communication, such as information disclosure to minimize damage in case of emergencies.

 # B May 1 to September 30, 2011 (two to six months)

1 Situation of the areas under our jurisdiction and main activities

- From the start of accepting evacuees at primary shelters until their closure (March 13 to August 31, 2011)
- From the start of accepting evacuees at secondary shelters until their closure (April 4 to November 14, 2011): At the same time, various events were held in the secondary shelters, such as recreation classes and dental health consultations.
- Start of accepting evacuees at temporary houses and temporary privately- or municipally- owned subsidized rental houses (May 9, 2011 to date): We could pay visits to temporary houses from the very beginning; however, we could not pay visits to temporary subsidized rental houses because the personal information of their residents was not available. After it had become possible to collect personal information, we could pay visits. Our public healthcare center held the Ken-nan District Evacuees' Health

Support Liaison Conference to strengthen mutual cooperation among the parties concerned, which made it possible to survey the health needs of evacuees and identify people who needed support. Thus we promoted healthy town and new community development.
- In an example of our involvement in cases of acute vomiting and diarrhea at shelters through shelter surveillance, we detected the increase in infectious gastroenteritis cases at an early stage and immediately started our involvement, isolated patients, and thoroughly promoted environmental and hand hygiene, and thus we could ultimately prevent the infection from expanding. In addition, mass outbreaks of acute respiratory tract infection were detected through shelter surveillance and the involvement of the public health center contributed to reducing the number of newly infected patients.
- We held a symposium on the Great East Japan Earthquake and medical care (September 22, 2011).

2 Summary and measures to be taken in the future

- Through the experience of the support for shelters based on shelter surveillance it was clarified that taking measures against infectious disease in the event of a disaster utilizing shelter surveillance was useful.
- The symposium jointly held with the Shirakawa Medical Association provided an opportunity to share information on various matters of medical care, such as the current situation, issues, and measures taken, in the wake of the Great East Japan Earthquake. In addition, the concerted measures taken by the medical institution and public administration were significant in terms of future preparedness of the region for earthquakes.

C October 1, 2011 to March 31, 2012 (seven months to one year)

1 Situation of the areas under our jurisdiction and main activities

- Secondary shelters were closed (November 14, 2011).
- Temporary houses and temporary subsidized rental houses started accepting evacuees on May 9, 2011 and the number of evacuees living there was 3,189 as of March 31, 2012.
- Public health nurses and other members continued to pay visits to temporary houses and temporary privately- or municipally-owned subsidized rental houses and various events, such as recreation classes, were held at the same time.
- Inspection for radioactive substances in processed and other foods was performed. Sampling of specimens and the inspection started on October 13 and 19, 2011, respectively. Radioactive substances exceeding the new standard were detected in, for example, some dried wild grass and accordingly instructions were given to the manufactures to voluntarily reframe from selling.
- Temporary welfare facilities in the areas under our jurisdiction were completed and evacuees started moving into the facilities on March 1, 2012. All of the evacuees from Namie Town who had been dispersed in the areas under our jurisdiction moved into the temporary facilities.
- We reviewed the evacuation route from the welfare facilities in Namie Town to, for example, the public welfare facilities in the areas under our jurisdiction.
- The results of measurements from exposure screening during about one year showed 13,000 cpm or less for all of 6,002 people screened (Table 10-2). Recently, people rarely visit us for measurements.

2 Summary and measures to be taken in the future

- The notice on the scope of the development and improvement of emergency temporary facilities

Chapter 2 — Initiatives of Public Administrations

Table 10-2 Exposure screening situation

By month	No. of people measured in the center (in working hours) (people)	No. of people measured in the center (out of working hours) (people)	No. of people measured in visits (people)	No. of people engaged in screening (people)	Total hours (hours)
March 2011	3,151	698	560	171	2,901
April	850	22	0	74	732
May	350	6	0	83	664
June	184	0	0	64	512
July	77	0	0	51	408
August	50	0	0	31	248
September	18	0	0	20	140
October	19	0	0	20	140
November	7	0	0	20	140
December	8	0	0	19	133
January 2012	0	0	0	19	133
February	0	0	0	21	147
March	2	0	0	21	147
Total	4,716	726	560	614	6,445

Note) Peak date of measurement: 1,165 people on March 15, 2011, Total number of people measured: 6,002 people Support for measurements by other groups: Total of 225 people from March 21 to May 9, 2011

acknowledged by the Minister of Health, Labour and Welfare in "Government subsidies for disaster relief expenditures for social welfare facilities, etc. pertaining to the Great East Japan Earthquake" was issued on August 11, 2011 by the Vice Minister of Health, Labour and Welfare. However, this applied only to social welfare facilities damaged by the earthquake. The cases where people evacuated from, for example, the welfare facilities of Namie Town in the warning zone during this disaster have been included within the scope of the "provision of accommodations (including emergency temporary housing) in Article 23, Paragraph (1), Item (i) of the Disaster Relief Act" for about two years after the nuclear plant accident: Showing that the government has flexibly taking measures in accordance with the purpose of the legal system.

- For those people, such as the residents of the welfare facilities of Namie Town, who may have a problem if they live in a general shelter, it is necessary to have a certain accommodation capacity secured as welfare shelters in the region where they can receive livelihood and other support. This can be accomplished by, for example, concluding an agreement in advance with social welfare facilities with the system in place whereby people who need support (vulnerable people) in a disaster can lead a secure life, including a barrier-free life.

D April 1, 2012 to March 31, 2013 (one year and one month to two years)

1 Main activities

- Table 10-3 shows the outline of measures taken by the public health center in a time series during the two years after the earthquake.

2 Summary and measures to be taken in the future

- When the disaster occurred, a water supply was requested by medical institutions and we passed the

Table 10-3 Measures taken by the Ken-nan public health center in a time series during the two years after the earthquake.

Division / Category	Measures (with dates, 2011–2013)
Events, etc.	Occurrence of the earthquake; Surges of the tsunami
General Affairs Planning Division (Damage in the public health center)	Mobilization of the General Affairs Group of the Ken-nan District Emergency Response Headquarters (March 11 to August 28); Investigation of the damage to the public health center (March 11); Lifeline; * The Ken-nan Public Health and Welfare Office started coordination for the health support activities of Futaba Town. (From September 26); Water supply restored (March 23); Gas supply restored (March 24); Gasoline supply restored (March 31)
(Work system)	24 hours-a-day system (March 11 to April 8); Services on weekends and holidays (April 9 to August 28)
(Coordination for medical support teams)	Activities of the Shirakawa Medical Association (March 16 to April 30); Activities of the healthcare teams from Hokkaido: 5 teams (March 24 to April 8); Activities of other healthcare teams (March 25 to April 14)
Health and Welfare Division (Welfare facilities)	Confirmation of the damage to welfare-related facilities (37 facilities; March 11)
(Mental health)	Visits to shelters for mental healthcare (April 7 to August 9); * The Ken-nan district center of the Fukushima Center for Disaster Mental Health started activities. (From April 9); Visits to the households of evacuees with an immature infant (June 20 to date)
(Maternal and child health)	Visits to the households of evacuees with babies (May 17 to date); Parents and children playing together (December 20 to date) *Twice a month
Social Aid Division	Acceptance of the application for social aid by evacuees started (March 22 to date)
Health Promotion Division (Coordination for health support activities)	Coordination for visits to shelters and health support activities (March 16 to date); Establishment of the Ken-nan District Evacuees' Health Support Liaison Conference (August 24; Meetings held twice a year now)
(Nutrition management)	Investigation of the nutrition condition (April to May)
Medical and Pharmaceutical Affairs Division	Confirmation of the damage to medical-related facilities (March 11 to June 15); Involvement in screening (March 13 to date); Involvement in dealing with pharmaceutical products (March 24 to October 14)
Hygiene Promotion Division	Confirmation of the damage to waterworks (March 11 to April 18); Visits to shelters to take epidemic prevention measures (May 31 to December 5); Confirmation of the damage to waterworks (March 11 to April 18 (Restored)); Provision of consultation on radioactive substances in drinking water, etc. (March 13 to date); Consolidation of tap water samples in our public health center started (October 3 to date); Monitoring inspection of tap water, etc. started (March 17 to date); Confirmation of the damage to crematoriums (March 14 to May 23); Visits to primary shelters for hygiene guidance (March 17 to July 13); Visits to secondary shelters for hygiene guidance (April 23 to July 13); Involvement in dealing with radioactive substances in food (March 16 to date); Involvement in the inspection of radioactive substances in processed food (October 13 to date); Measures to rescue pet animals (March 17 to December 27)
Public health activities (General Affairs Planning Division)	Visits to primary shelters (March 16 to August 16); Visits to secondary shelters (April 26 to September 7)
(Health Promotion Division)	Health/nutrition/dental consultations, health/nutrition/recreation/relaxation classes, etc. (April 26 to September 7); Visits to temporary houses in the areas under our jurisdiction (August 2 to date); Health/nutrition/dental consultations, recreation/relaxation classes, etc. (December 10 to date); Health/nutrition/recreation/relaxation classes, etc. (June 22 to July 22); Visits to the households of evacuees (September 15 to date)
(Health and Welfare Division)	Administrative meeting with the Futaba Town office and other various support groups (October to date, as needed); Visits to temporary houses and municipally subsidized rental houses in Futaba Town started (October 17 to date); Mental healthcare consultation on an individual basis and for group support ("Gathering to chat leisurely and comfortably") in temporary houses and municipally subsidized rental houses in Futaba Town (November 21 to date); "Ippongi Room" in the temporary house in Yabuki Town (May 10 to date)
(Medical and Pharmaceutical Affairs Division)	

Chapter 2 | Initiatives of Public Administrations

requested for support to the parties concerned, such as water utilities, but the number of, for example, water trucks was insufficient. Hence, it is necessary to ensure a sufficient water supply system.

- The number of lavatories in shelters was insufficient. Hence, it is necessary to provide portable toilets.
- Relief goods were distributed to shelters and other facilities from across the country: however, due to the mismatch in distribution, goods were in short supply in some shelters and in excess in other shelters. Hence, it is necessary to develop a nationwide distribution system in the event of a disaster and build a smooth and efficient system that can match the needs in the affected area with relief goods on the support side through the utilization of clouds.
- As a means of communication for the Fukushima Prefectural government, public health centers, medical institutions, municipalities, and residents, as well as for guidance to an evacuation destination in the event of a disaster, it is necessary to develop a secure communication and information system through multiplex communications, including satellite phone systems, priority telephone links in disasters, MCA radio systems, and radios.
- Some medical institutions refused to perform medical examinations on those who had not received radiation exposure screening. Health workers did not fully understand what radiation was. Hence, it is necessary to provide health workers with information on radiation and provide them with education on radiation.
- It is necessary to secure venues and manpower to establish a system to perform emergency exposure screening, secure clean clothing and have facilities for people to take a shower for decontamination following screening. It is also necessary to have a source of information about taking stable iodine tablets, have evacuees file an application for registration, and standardize measurement equipment and methods for radiation screening.
- In addition it is necessary at ordinary times to review the educational curriculum about radiation for children and the risk communication for residents as well as crisis communication, such as information disclosure to minimize damage in case of an emergency.
- Medical institutions and social welfare facilities were damaged and the personal information of patients and inmates was lost. Hence, it is necessary to digitize information, such as medical records, dispensing information, and medical information on nursing care, and establish a large-scale personal healthcare and welfare information system whereby clouds are utilized and data are accumulated in an integrated manner at an earthquake-resistant data center. The necessary data can then be browsed in various facilities, such as shelters, other medical institutions, and welfare facilities via an Internet dedicated line.
- The mutual aid agreement for disaster response is a broad-based aid system. However, the system's quick response and the support for individual and specific measures, such as securing the lifeline requested by the public health center, are needed. Hence, it is necessary to develop an autonomous aid system to promote immediate mutual aid even without a request.
- It is necessary to establish a continual information dissemination system of information from experts to prevent the anxiety of residents concerning radiation damage from being unnecessarily increased by, for example, mass media.
- It is necessary during ordinary times to establish systems to register and dispatch various teams, such as advance health support teams with an autonomous aid system, public health dispatch teams, the Disaster Public health Assistance Team (DPAT) the DHEAT, the REMAT, and the DPAT, and to share the health management information of affected people, and utilize the data of the restoration and recovery support system.
- For nuclear disasters, it is necessary to develop and improve medical institutions for treating radiation exposure and designate base hospitals for heavily exposed patients from across the country, as well as to establish a Nuclear Disaster Medical Assistance Team (NMAT), or a nuclear disaster version of the DMAT.

- There were only a few hospitals that used the Wide-Area Disaster & Emergency Medical Information System (EMIS) of the government among disaster base hospitals in the affected three prefectures. Therefore, it is necessary to develop and improve various systems for public health centers, including the installation of terminals and the support, input, and training for the transmission of information; for example, the establishment of the Joint Conference of Local Disaster Medical Institutions and the development of the Emergency Response Manual for Disaster Medical Institutions.
- It is necessary to establish the system to provide information and health support to evacuees outside Fukushima Prefecture to facilitate them to, for example, respond to the Fukushima Health Management Survey and get health checkups, cancer examinations, and vaccinations.
- The public health center must take prompt action as a regional health crisis management center and also promote new community development through its efforts to visit residents, including shelters and temporary houses, because of the prolonged influence of the Great Earthquake. The center must place full emphasis on software aspects to meet evacuees' needs and to fully utilize the regional potential.
- The public health center must provide health support to, for example, the evacuees from the warning zone and also continually provide mental healthcare, particular to the evacuees having difficulty in visualizing the reconstruction of their future life.
- Public health institutions, such as public health centers, must conduct inspections and provide proper information on food and drinking water to ensure residents' safety and security from contamination by radioactive substances.
- Public health institutions, such as public health centers, must promptly communicate to residents training information during ordinary times and emergency information at the occurrence of a disaster. They must establish an information system to secure the safety of individuals as well as establishing a safety and security system by reviewing the local disaster management plan and taking disaster mitigation measures.
- Public health institutions, such as public health centers, must play an active role by taking opportunities to get involved in the development of various plans, such as the medical care plan of the prefecture, the reconstruction plan and disaster prevention plan of the prefecture or region, the regional public health care and welfare plan, and the regional medical care revival plan.
- Through the support by the government and municipalities, it is necessary to establish a stress care system that can be used by support workers for affected people and evacuees, such as public health nurses.
- It is necessary to develop comprehensive activities, including health, welfare, and nursing care measures for affected people and evacuees, and reconstruct the comprehensive regional care system.
- It is necessary to construct a new healthcare provision system through the integration and collaboration of medical care functions and the promotion of home medical care by taking into consideration the future vision of the community and the town.
- It is necessary to allow municipalities to issue instructions to take stable iodine tablets at their discretion if the information about taking iodine tablets cannot be communicated from the Nuclear Emergency Response Headquarters of the government, and also to distribute stable iodine tablets and information about taking them to each of the households in the areas within a certain range of a nuclear plant before a disaster.

(Yukio Endo, former staff member of the Ken-nan Public Health and Welfare Office)

11 Measures Taken by the Koriyama City Public Health Center

1 Outline of the areas under jurisdiction

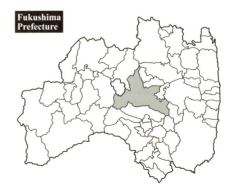

(1) Municipalities under jurisdiction

Koriyama City, one of the core cities of Japan, is under the jurisdiction.

(2) Population/population aging rate (as of January 1 each year)

	2011	2013
Population	339,025	328,210
Population aging rate	20.3	21.9

2 Damage situation caused by the earthquake and nuclear disaster in the areas under jurisdiction

(1) Damage situation (as of March 12, 2013)

Physical damage	Completely destroyed	Half destroyed	Partially destroyed
Residential buildings	2,447	21,615	33,996
Public facilities		69	
Others		6,211	

Human damage	Direct deaths	Associated deaths	Missing	Injured
	1	0	0	4

(2) Evacuation situation (as of March 12, 2013)

	End-March 2011	End-September 2011	End-March 2012	Latest
Installation of shelters	37			
No. of evacuees	642			
No. of evacuees accepted	3,693			
No. of residents living in temporary houses for residents and evacuees accepted				1,875

(Emergency Response Headquarters of Fukushima Prefecture: Calculated based on the flash report on the damage situation caused by the 2011 off the Pacific coast of Tohoku Earthquake)

11 Measures Taken by the Koriyama City Public Health Center

A March 11 to April 30, 2011 (up to one month)

1 Situation

- At 2:46 pm on March 11, an earthquake with a seismic intensity of 6 lower occurred and the Koriyama City Emergency Response Headquarters was immediately established in the conference room of the Kaiseizan Baseball Stadium.
- The main city office building became unusable due to the collapse of the rooftop observation room and the damage to the water storage tank (Figure 11-1).
- About 10,000 residents evacuated to the shelters in a total of 105 locations in the city, including, notably, Kaiseizan Baseball Stadium, which also functions as a shelter.
- On March 22, radioactive iodine (^{131}I) exceeding the level allowed for infants was detected in drinking water in the water purification plant and a restriction was imposed of its intake. The restriction was lifted on the 25th.
- It became an urgent task for medical institutions in the city to secure water for artificial dialysis and procure medical and welfare goods, such as pharmaceutical products, stoma products, various types of catheters, and surgical gowns.
- Residents of Futaba-Gun started evacuation on March 12 and the facilities located in the city under the jurisdiction of the prefecture were used as shelters. There were 13 shelters at the peak period.
- The "post-disaster mental healthcare project for children" was formed.
- In April, water services were completely restored.
- On April 6, an outbreak of infectious gastroenteritis caused by norovirus occurred in the shelter at the Big Palette Fukushima convention center, where there were about 2,000 evacuees.
- The collapse of buildings at two hospitals in the city made it difficult to ensure the medical service provision system.

2 Main activities

a. Activities of public health nurses and other people concerned
- Public health nurses paid visits to shelters to check the health of evacuees and provide them with consultations. Public health nurses and dietitians provided telephone consultation services every day including weekends.
- The staff members of the public health center performed external exposure screening for evacuees from

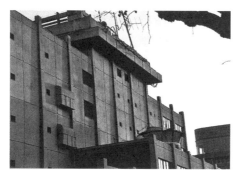

Figure 11-1   Collapsed observation room of the main city office building

the Soso District in the parking lot of the general gymnasium.
- Support was provided from the outside of the city by the sister cities of Koriyama City, namely Tottori City in Tottori Prefecture (March 18) and Kurume City in Fukuoka Prefecture (April 7 to 18).
- As part of the mental healthcare project of Fukushima Prefecture, psychiatrists and psychiatric social workers from Yamagata Prefectural Tsuruoka Hospital were dispatched (March 30 to 31).
- During the period of the outbreak of infectious gastroenteritis caused by norovirus, two medical doctors from the Field Epidemiology Training Program (FETP) of the National Institute of Infectious Diseases also provided support.
- Teams of two, consisting of a member of the public health center and a retired public health nurse, volunteer nurse, temporary nurse, or nurse of the Japan Health Insurance Association, were formed to pay visits to shelters. We requested the Midwives' Association to check the health of expectant mothers and infants in shelters and also requested that the nurses from the hospital wards that were closed due to complete collapse of their buildings perform health checks at shelters on a round-the-clock basis when there were disabled people who needed care.
- In cooperation with exercise instructors working at a private hospital, we paid visits to shelters to have the evacuees to take organized exercise to relieve the lack of normal exercise and stress (Figure 11-2).

b. Activities of dietitians
- In collaboration with the Fukushima Dietetic Association we delivered food to elderly people who had evacuated to the prefectural facilities; we distributed food they can chew, such as rice gruel and nutritional supplements.
- We endeavored to evaluate the food and nutrition conditions at care facilities for elderly people and distributed food.

c. Activities of healthcare teams and medical associations
- In response to the request from Nishinomiya Municipal Central Hospital for the dispatch of a healthcare team, we requested assistance to deal with the dysfunctional emergency medical system. During the period between March 17 and April 5, cooperation was provided by a total of 30 people (10 medical doctors, 10 nurses, and 10 administrative staff members).
- The Koriyama Medical Association paid visits to shelters to provide, for example, health consultation in order to clarify the health condition of evacuees in shelters and provide them with medical care.

d. Activities of pharmacists and pharmaceutical associations
- We managed relief goods, such as pharmaceutical products.
- We prepared and prescribed medicines on a round-the-clock basis at the medical treatment room in the

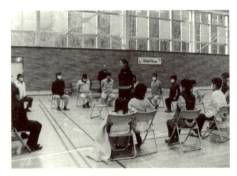

Figure 11-2 Exercises instructed by an exercise instructor from a private hospital

shelter in Kaiseizan Athletic Stadium.

3 Summary and measures to be taken in the future

- Since both the number of shelters where public health nurses can pay visits and the number of people to whom consultation can be provided are limited, it is important for the department of the city that is managing and operating shelters to obtain information in advance on, for example, the number, age group, and the health of the evacuees in shelters to establish a collaborative system that allows public health nurses to effectively respond to the evacuees' needs during their visit to shelters.
- In the wake of the outbreak of infectious gastroenteritis caused by norovirus, it is necessary to establish a system whereby the health of evacuees not only in the shelter where the outbreak has occurred but also in all shelters in the city is reported. This system will allow a small number of staff members to efficiently manage the health condition of evacuees in shelters. Furthermore, when establishing a shelter, it is important to build in a system to prevent the outbreak of infections of, for example, influenza or norovirus and also secure the room and/or space to manage infected patients on an individual basis.
- Due to anxiety about radiation, it was three weeks after the occurrence of the disaster when support teams from other prefectures entered the city. Instead of assuming that support will include support from outside the prefecture, maintaining a social network in the community at ordinary times will lead to prompt measures taken to deal with a disaster.
- The mental health of some of the staff members of the public health was compromised because they blamed themselves that they had not evacuated their children while they heard that some parents had temporarily evacuated their children to remote areas due to the concern about radiation. As specialists, the personnel dealing with a disaster are likely to focus their attention on the health condition of residents; however, it is also important to manage their own health concerns.
- In Koriyama City, public health nurses are allocated to various places and organizations, such as the public health center, Nursing Insurance Division, Child Support Division, and each administration center. This causes a limited number of public health nurses who can pay visits to shelters to provide consultations in the event of a disaster. It is necessary to build a system with an eye to providing efficient support through the integration (centralization) of the chain of command for specialists.
- The staff members of the public health center must learn about the health effects of radiation.
- Since there were many inquiries about the closure of pharmacies, it is necessary not only to clearly describe the respective roles of medical institutions, pharmacies, and the public administration in the relevant manual but also to have collaborative relationships in place before a disaster that function after a disaster.
- Since shortages of supplies in medical institutions and welfare facilities could not be known in advance, relief goods were distributed to the medical institutions and welfare facilities only upon their request. It is necessary to establish a system whereby necessary relief goods can be distributed to medical institutions and welfare facilities by an appropriate allocation method.
- The disaster prevention system of Koriyama City did not assume radiation exposure of residents. It is necessary in the future to establish a system preparing for residents to be exposed to radiation.

B May 1 to September 30, 2011 (two to six months)

1 Situation

- Shelters were gradually closed and the frequency of visits of public health nurses to shelters to provide

consultation also decreased.
- Facilities, such as the main city office building, municipal gymnasiums, and community halls, continued to be unusable as they were completely or half collapsed. This remained as an obstacle to operating or holding various programs and classes even though regular operations were resumed.
- Among the municipalities in Futaba-Gun, temporary municipality offices and temporary houses were constructed in two municipalities (Tomioka Town and Kawauchi Village).

2 Main activities

- Collaborations were made with the operators of shelters to pay a visit to perform health checks when necessary.
- External exposure screening was continued to be performed by the staff members of the public health center.
- Since the main city office building could not be used, the office work was performed at the temporary city office building. The Nuclear Emergency Response Office was established within the organization of the city to start decontamination work, air dose measurements, and other necessary measures to deal with radiation.
- In May, the general consultation contact point for residents concerning the earthquake disaster was opened. The city office workers, including the staff members of the public health center, worked for residents to issue "disaster victim certificates" and "disaster damage certificates" among other tasks.

3 Summary and measures to be taken in the future

Two months after the earthquake, when we were performing routine work as usual, was regarded as the starting point for reconstruction. We endeavor to, for example, perform health checkups using the same system same as in ordinary times. Our efforts to restore the usual working system refreshed the mental and physical condition of the staff members. However, since their own houses were damaged and they could find no opportunity to reduce their anxiety about radiation, their mental fatigue increased daily. It is necessary to ensure an opportunity and establish a department to take care of the mental health of the staff members.

 C **October 1, 2011 to March 31, 2012 (seven months to one year)**

1 Situation

- A large-scale indoor play space, "PEP Kids Koriyama," was opened.
- The Basic Resident Registration System was restored, which revealed the decrease in population (Figure 11-3).

2 Main activities

- Integrating dose meters were distributed to expectant mothers, young children, and elementary school pupils to start monitoring the external exposure dose. There were as many as 14,294 expectant mothers and preschool age children and young children for whom continuous measurements were made for 120 days from November 1, 2011 to February 29, 2012.
- In November, we commissioned four nuclear emergency response advisors of the city to give us advice

11 Measures Taken by the Koriyama City Public Health Center

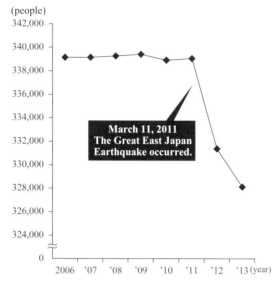

Figure 11-3 Change in the population of Koriyama City (Population of residents as of January 1 each year)

on the measures to be taken to deal with a radiation disaster.
- The inspection of radioactive substances contained in foods consumed in general households was started in 42 locations in the city.
- In December, the "Basic Policy for Reconstruction of Koriyama City" and the "Koriyama City Reproduction Decontamination Plan" were developed.
- In January 2012, the measurement of the radiation dose at personal residences and the lease of survey meters (scintillation type) and electronic integrating dose meters for individual people were started.

3 Summary and measures to be taken in the future

During the implementing of health programs, such as delivering maternal and child health handbooks and performing health checkup for babies, there were an increasing number of mothers and parents who expressed their anxiety about radiation. In this period, we started to consider radiation as one of factors surrounding our life and strongly feel the necessity of starting a program that could reduce the anxiety of parents.

 D April 1, 2012 to March 31, 2013 (one year and one month to about two years)

1 Situation

- The population continued to decline (Figure 11-3).
- Since indoor play spaces operated by the private sector were built and the "list of indoor play spaces" was posted on the website of the prefecture, parents could select a play space to use.

Chapter 2 | Initiatives of Public Administrations

2 Main activities

- In April, the Radiation Health Management Center was established in the public health center and internal exposure inspection was started using a whole-body counter.
- During the period from October to March in the following year, thyroid inspection (pilot inspection) in the Fukushima Health Management Survey was performed for all residents 18 years old or younger of Koriyama City.
- As in the previous year, integrating dose meters were distributed to expectant mothers, young children, and elementary school pupils for the second year to monitor the external exposure dose. There were as many as 7,474 expectant mothers and preschool age children and younger children for whom continuous measurements were made for 231 days from May 30, 2012 to January 15, 2013.
- During health checkups for babies, there were a number of mothers who mentioned that their children were playing outdoors less frequently. Consequently, a health program was implemented, whereby parents and children could take exercise together and parents could talk together.

3 Summary and measures to be taken in the future

- Thanks to the opportunities for parents to talk together and the classes where parents and children could take exercise together, they became better acquainted and developed improved communicate with one another. Parents reported, for example, "I can now communicate with my children in a more calm manner at more ease," and "We wanted to evacuate after we had been affected by the disaster, but we eventually decided to stay here for various reasons and have been feeling very anxious. However, I believe it was a good decision because we could get acquainted with various people." Stabilizing the mothers' mental condition led to relieving the anxiety of their children.
- People who had evacuated from municipalities in Futaba-Gun often visited the contact point of the city for consultation on life, health, and other matters. Assuming that public health services are supposed to resolve issues for people and communities from their region, it is considered necessary for the host municipality where evacuees from other municipalities now live to actively cooperate with the staff of the evacuees' municipality to support the health management of the evacuees.

(Koichi Abe, Keiko Saito)

12 Measures Taken by the Aizu Public Health and Welfare Office

1 Outline of the areas under jurisdiction

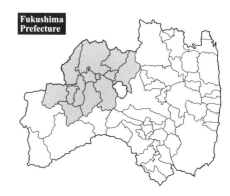

(1) Municipalities under jurisdiction

The following two cities, eight towns, and three villages are under the jurisdiction: Aizuwakamatsu City and Kitakata City, Kitashiobara Village, Nishiaizu Town, Bandai Town, and Inawashiro Town of Yama-Gun, Aizubange Town, Yugawa Village, and Yanaizu Town of Kawanuma-Gun, Mishima Town, Kaneyama Town, Showa Village, and Aizumisato Town of Onuma-Gun

(2) Population/population aging rate (as of January 1 each year)

	2011	2013
Population	261,592	255,980
Population aging rate	29.2	29.9

2 Damage situation caused by the earthquake and nuclear disaster in the areas under jurisdiction

(1) Damage situation (as of March 12, 2013)

Physical damage	Completely destroyed	Half destroyed	Partially destroyed
Residential buildings	24	162	6,756
Public facilities		34	
Others		1,904	

Human damage	Direct deaths	Associated deaths	Missing	Injured
	1	3	0	10

(2) Evacuation situation (as of March 12, 2013)

	End-March 2011	End-September 2011	End-March 2012	Latest
Installation of shelters	32	2		
No. of evacuees	4			
No. of evacuees accepted	3,775	6		
No. of residents living in temporary houses for residents and evacuees accepted				1,322 (as of end-August 2013)

(Emergency Response Headquarters of Fukushima Prefecture: Calculated based on the flash report on the damage situation caused by the 2011 off the Pacific coast of Tohoku Earthquake)

Chapter 2　Initiatives of Public Administrations

 March 11 to April 30, 2011 (up to one month)

1　Situation

- On March 11, 2011, an earthquake with a seismic intensity of 6 lower was observed in the Aizu District.
- The Emergency Response Headquarters of Fukushima Prefecture and the Local Emergency Response Headquarters of the Aizu District were established.
- The Aizu District Disaster Medical Care Coordination Headquarters was established. (The joint meetings of medical relief teams and health management teams were started.)
- The medical support system study meeting was held (participated in by medical institutions and municipalities).
- The Fukushima Disaster Medical Support Network was established. The submission of the medical support registration form was requested.
- Primary shelters were opened in the Aizu District.
- Naraha Town, Okuma Town, and Katsurao Village relocated their office functions to the Aizu District.
- Secondary shelters (hotels, Japanese-style inns, guest houses, and pensions) were opened in the Aizu District.
- Among primary shelters, those in prefectural high schools were closed.
- Applications to live in an emergency temporary house started to be accepted and the construction of emergency temporary houses were started in the Aizu District.

2　Main activities

- The Emergency Response Headquarters of Fukushima Prefecture, the Local Emergency Response Headquarters of the Aizu District, and the health and welfare team were established.

(Exposure screening)
- Emergency exposure screening was started. (The parties involved were the Aizu Public Health and Welfare Office (hereinafter referred to as "the public health center"), Fukushima Prefectural Aizu General Hospital, the Japan Association of Technologists, Hamamatsu University School of Medicine, the Fukushimaken Association of Radiological Technologists, Kyoto Prefecture, Kumamoto City, Miyagi Prefecture, University of Fukui, The University of Tokushima, Hokkaido, Osaka Prefecture, and the Federation of Electric Power Companies of Japan.)
- The scale of the inspection site was reduced and the inspection hours were changed. The inspection site had been Aidu Chuo Hospital on March 13. Subsequently, the site was changed and since April 25, inspection has been performed at the Aizu public health center.

(Monitoring of radioactive substances in drinking water)
- Monitoring was started for tap water.
- Consultation was provided on drinking water in response to requests.

(Medical relief activities)
- Visits to primary shelters were started to provide medical care (by the staff of Shiga Prefecture, Japanese Red Cross Society, Kyoto Prefecture, Kyoto Medical Association, the local medical association, and Fukushima Prefectural Aizu General Hospital), which we coordinated. Subsequently, visits to secondary shelters were started to provide medical care, which we also coordinated.
- Visits to the evacuated staff members of the municipalities were started to provide them with medical care, which we coordinated. Health management teams also started visits to shelters to provide support.

(Pharmaceutical product supply activities)
- The Aizu Pharmaceutical Association held a director meeting to clarify the agreed items (how to handle prescriptions and cooperation with the local medical institution).
- We provided the list of pharmaceutical products stored in the Aizu public health center.
- We developed a procurement transmittal form for pharmaceutical products and other goods and used the form.

(Health management activities)
- We started the health condition survey at primary shelters. Subsequently, we started an exhaustive survey at secondary shelters.
- Health management teams (of Fukushima Prefectural Aizu General Hospital, the Ministry of Health, Labour and Welfare, Fukushima Medical University, City of Sapporo, Nagano Prefecture, Hiroshima City, Aomori Prefecture, Kanagawa Prefecture, Okayama Prefecture, Yamaguchi Prefecture, Kawasaki City, and National Hospital Organization) started paying visits to provide support, for which we conducted coordination.
- Mental healthcare teams from the psychiatric medical institutions in the Aizu District (six teams), Fukui Prefecture, and Kyoto Prefecture started support activities, for which we conducted coordination, and we also participated in the "Aizu District mental healthcare team liaison meeting" formed by the psychiatric medical institutions in the Aizu District.
- We held a regular meeting every day and shared information to clarify issues.
- We conducted support and coordination activities to accept each medical institution.

(Social welfare activities)
- After participating in the Support Meeting for Affected Persons with Disabilities, we clarified the issues to be addressed and started matching the activities of the Council of Developmental Support Center, Japan with the needs of the Aizu District.
- We coordinated the operation to certify the need for long-term care (such as conducting the survey of the condition of the municipalities from which evacuees had come and the survey of the condition of the municipalities accepting evacuees and holding meetings with the relevant parties) and gave advice on the certification of long-term care needs.
- We visited the community general support center of the municipalities from which evacuees had come and the municipalities that had accepted evacuees.

(Measures taken to deal with damage to waterworks facilities)
- We started the survey of the damage and restoration of waterworks facilities in the municipalities under our jurisdiction.
- We coordinated the support request for and the dispatch of water trucks in the municipalities under our jurisdiction.

(Food sanitation support activities)
- We conducted a survey of the actual diet condition of each shelter using questionnaires.
- We distributed sanitary management pamphlets for hand-washing, disinfection, and cooking at each shelter and started visits to shelters to give sanitary guidance.
- We also started sanitary guidance on how to cook and store food.

(Disaster-affected pet protection activities)
- We supported the activities to temporarily keep dogs and cats.
- We provided support for the distribution of equipment to rear pets, such as cages, and feed to support the pets accompanying evacuees.
- We started the transportation of pets to shelters; transportation of dogs and cats to protect pets left in the warning zone.
- We started a survey of the actual condition of pets left in the warning zone.

| Chapter 2 | Initiatives of Public Administrations |

3 Summary and measures to be taken in the future

(Exposure screening)

- Without exposure screening, various restrictions were imposed on residents on various occasions; such as restricting moving into a shelter, visiting a medical institution, and moving into an apartment house. Issuance of an inspection completion certificate led to a sense of security for residents and other people concerned.
- It is essential to secure decontamination facilities as well as hot water shower facilities for decontamination.
- It is necessary to make people aware of the Fukushima Emergency Exposure Medical Activities Manual and conduct a study on how to utilize the same.

(Monitoring of radioactive substances in drinking water)

- It is necessary to comprehensively explain the inspection system as well as the inspection results.

(Medical relief activities)

- A liaison meeting was held before starting the activities, which made it possible to confirm the role of each member.
- It is necessary to have a meeting to avoid duplicated visits to shelters.
- Medical relief teams conducting activities were requested to submit the "medical support registration form," which facilitated coordination of the medical relief teams.
- Confusion could be avoided by using only the pharmaceutical products in the shelters of the prefecture and the medicines brought by each medical relief team and letting everyone thoroughly understand that prescriptions would not be issued.
- It is useful for evacuees to store their medical record.

(Pharmaceutical product supply activities)

- Pharmacists dispatched from inside and outside of the prefecture accompanied medical relief teams. This contributed to decreasing the time required to supply pharmaceutical products. Pharmacists are essential for the activities of medical relief teams.
- The consultation corner for medicines provided by pharmacists at each shelter brought a sense of security to the residents.
- The inventory of pharmaceutical products provided free of charge from across the country was controlled with the cooperation of each pharmaceutical association, which contributed to their proper control.

(Activities of health management teams)

- A survey to check the health condition of the residents must be immediately conducted.
- To provide support that meets the requirement of the affected municipalities, it is necessary to first decide on how to support and then establish the system that allows execution of the decision.
- To provide nutrition and diet support, it is necessary to cooperate with the staff members in charge of diet support activities.

(Social welfare activities)

- We conducted coordination for the certification of long-term care needs by quickly checking the actual situation and discussing specific matters.

(Food sanitation support activities)

- We visited each shelter to explain how to safely cook and store food at the shelter.

(Disaster-affected pet protection activities)

- The activities to protect pets that could not evacuate together with their owner and had to be left alone were conducted not only by the public administration but also by animal welfare groups. This lead to a significant issue of the dispersion of disaster-affected pets across the country as well as the dispersion of the relevant protection information.

- Even in the cases where evacuees could be together with their pets, there was a limitation to keeping pets, because of concerns about possible trouble with other evacuees in a temporary shelter. To protect disaster-affected pets, coordination is required in a series of stages, such as evacuation together with pets, management of pets at shelters, protection of pets left alone, management of protected animals, and handling of pets that cannot be returned to their owner.
- The contact point for support workers must be centralized.
- To share information on the details of support activities and clarify the issues, short meetings held on a daily basis are efficient.

B : May 1 to September 30, 2011 (two to six months)

1 Situation

- Fukushima Prefecture announced the implementation of the Fukushima Health Management Survey and its continuation for 30 years.
- Evacuees started brief visits to their home in the warning zone.
- Evacuees started moving into emergency temporary houses in the Aizu District.
- The primary shelters in the Aizu District started to close.
- The elderly people support center and the residents' salon were opened in temporary houses in the Aizu District.
- Temporary day service facilities for children were opened.
- The Niigata-Fukushima heavy rainfall disaster occurred.
- The secondary shelters in the Aizu District started to close.
- Okuma Town and Naraha Town established liaison councils to support evacuees.
- Residents in the planned evacuation zone started evacuation.
- The number of primary and secondary evacuees in the areas under the jurisdiction of the Aizu District peaked (9,559 people).
- The designation of an emergency evacuation-ready zone was comprehensively lifted.
- Katsurao Village relocated its office function to Miharu Town.

2 Main activities

(Exposure screening)
- Starting in September, inspection was performed only on weekdays.

(Monitoring of radioactive substances in drinking water)
- Monitoring of tap water was continued. The scope of inspection was expanded to include private water-works, water supply facilities, drinking water supply facilities managed by municipalities, and drinking water wells.
- Consultation was provided about drinking water in response to requests.

(Medical relief activities)
- Visits were paid to secondary shelters to provide medical care, which we coordinated, and we also distributed blood-pressure gauges to shelters with 50 or more evacuees.
- Based on the exhaustive survey results, we recommended evacuees to have medical examinations by the medical relief team.
- Visits to shelters to provide medical care were started with the staff members of the affected municipalities, which we coordinated.

Chapter 2 | Initiatives of Public Administrations

- At the end of June, visits to shelters to provide medical care were terminated and the Aizu District Disaster Medical Care Coordination Headquarters was dissolved.
- The activities to supply pharmaceutical products were concluded at the end of June.

(Activities of health management teams)

- Visits to secondary shelters and temporary houses were started.
- Support to affected municipalities was continued.
- Regular meetings were held twice a week and weekly reports were created to share information.
- Study meetings on support to residents and on the cases where support was required were held.
- Tokyo Metropolitan Government started direct support to the affected towns.
- Health management teams coordinated the activities of the support teams.
- Support was provided for evacuees to prepare meals by themselves.
- The Fukushima counselling and support specialist team (consisting of the members of Fukushima Care Manager Association, Fukushima Association of Certified Social Workers, Fukushima Medical Social Worker Association, Fukushima Association of Psychiatric Social Workers, Fukushima Physical Therapy Association, and Fukushima Association of Occupational Therapists) started its activities.
- Mental health education was started in secondary shelters.
- Mental health support was started for the staff members of affected municipalities.
- The mental health care staff of the Aizu public health center started their activities.
- Support for a cooking practice course and health consultations were provided before evacuees moved into a temporary house.
- The activities of the support teams from outside of the prefecture for health management teams were concluded.
- The volunteer group of clinical psychotherapists from Kyoto Prefecture started its activities.

(Social welfare activities)

- We provided the support after the conclusion of the "contract to commission the consultation and support program for children with disabilities affected by the disaster" between Fukushima Prefecture and the Council of Developmental Support Center, Japan.
- We coordinated the operation to certify the need for long-term care (such as conducting the survey of the condition of the municipalities from which evacuees had come and the survey of the condition of the municipalities accepting evacuees, holding meetings with the relevant parties, and reporting the situation and submitting the proposal of countermeasures to the main prefectural office) and gave advice on the certification of long-term care needs.
- We held an information exchange meeting of the community general support centers in the affected areas under the jurisdiction of the Aizu District.
- We held an information exchange meeting of all of the community general support centers in the Aizu District.

(Food sanitation support activities)

- We visited each shelter to give sanitary guidance.
- We gave sanitary guidance on how to cook and store food.

(Disaster-affected pet protection activities)

- We conducted a survey of the actual condition of pets left in the warning zone.
- We provided support to shelters (vaccinations and support for the management of rearing pets).
- We started disaster-affected pet protection activities associated with residents' brief visits to their homes.
- We started accommodating disaster-affected pets in animal hospitals in the Aizu District.
- We started activities to protect disaster-affected pets in the warning zone.
- We started the disaster-affected pet transfer program and the operation of host families for disaster-affected pets.

3 Summary and measures to be taken in the future

(Monitoring of radioactive substances in drinking water)
- It is necessary to comprehensively explain the inspection system as well as the inspection results.

(Medical relief activities)
- It is necessary to take proper exercise to prevent physical strength from declining.
- Visits together with the public health nurses of the affected municipalities were started, which spread a sense of security among the residents.
- Visits to the staff members of the affected municipalities were started to provide medical care.

(Health management activities)
- It is necessary to be involved in the support of the staff members of the affected municipalities and the staff members in charge.
- It is necessary to review the support system to meet the situation of the affected municipalities.
- It is necessary to provide information to continue support at the place where evacuees have relocated.

(Social welfare activities)
- Thanks to the cooperation of the local organizations and groups concerned, and the support of the Council of Developmental Support Center, Japan, rehabilitation facilities for children could be developed.
- In order to promptly communicate the demand for the certification of long-term care needs to the main prefectural office, it is necessary to check the current situation and clarify issues.
- Holding an information exchange meeting of the community general support centers made it possible to understand the current situation in other centers and review the individual centers' own activities.

(Food sanitation support activities)
- Stronger stress was put on sanitary guidance given in visits to each shelter so that sufficient attention might be paid to avoid food poisoning.

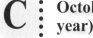

C October 1, 2011 to March 31, 2012 (seven months to one year)

1 Situation

- Thyroid inspection was started.
- The Consumer Affairs Center in Fukushima Prefecture started the inspection of food and other products free of charge using a simplified radiation analyze.
- The elderly support center in the Aizu District started day care services.
- Temporary shelters and secondary shelters in the Aizu District were closed.
- Evacuees moved into temporary houses and temporary subsidized rental houses.
- Naraha Town relocated its office functions to Iwaki City and the town office in the Aizu District became a branch office.

2 Main activities

(Exposure screening)
- Inspection was performed only on weekdays.

(Monitoring of radioactive substances in drinking water)
- Monitoring of radioactive substances in drinking water was continued.
- Consultation was provided on drinking water and food in response to requests.

Chapter 2 Initiatives of Public Administrations

(Inspection of radioactive substances in processed food)
- Inspection of radioactive substances in processed food was started.

(Health management activities)
- Regular meetings were held twice a week to share information.
- The exhaustive survey of evacuees was continued.
- Support to affected municipalities was continued.
- Health consultation and health education were provided in temporary houses and in exchange salons.
- Visits were paid to temporary houses and temporary subsidized rental houses.
- Study meetings on the cases where support was required, information exchange meetings of support groups, and liaison meetings to support affected people continued to be held.
- "Parent and child exchange meetings" for evacuees were held.
- Study meetings on support of residents were started with a focus on mental healthcare.
- Regular meetings with living support counselors as well as care meetings were started.
- The mental healthcare team of Kyoto University Hospital started its support.
- Support (mental health seminars, stress checks, mental health consultations, and relaxation seminars) for support workers, such as the staff members of affected municipalities and our public health center, was started.

(Social welfare activities)
- We held a seminar to study how to support elderly people in the event of a disaster.
- We held information exchange meetings of the community general support centers in the affected areas under the jurisdiction of the Aizu District (regular meetings).

(Food sanitation support activities)

(Disaster-affected pet protection activities)
- The same activities as those before September 30, 2011 were continued.

3 Summary and measures to be taken in the future

(Monitoring of radioactive substances in drinking water)
- It is necessary to elaborately explain the inspection system as well as the inspection results.

(Health management activities)
- In order to take measures meeting the requests of the affected municipalities, regular meetings were held to confirm their demands.
- To take care of mental health, a focus was placed on support for evacuees and support workers.

(Social welfare activities)
- Holding information exchange meetings of the community general support centers on a regular basis made it possible to share information.

D April 1, 2012 to March 31, 2013 (one year and one month to two years)

1 Situation
- Evacuees started to return to their affected municipalities.

2　Main activities

(Exposure screening)
- Inspection was performed only on weekdays.

(Monitoring of radioactive substances in drinking water)
- Monitoring of radioactive substances in drinking water was continued.

(Inspection of radioactive substances in processed food)
- Inspection of radioactive substances in processed food was continued.

(Health management activities)
- Regular meetings were held once a week and weekly reports were created.
- Health consultation and health education were provided in temporary houses and exchange salons.
- Visits were paid to temporary houses and temporary subsidized rental houses.
- Study meetings about the cases where support was required, information exchange meetings of support groups, liaison meetings to support affected people, and parent and child exchange meetings continued to be held.
- The Aizu District Center for Disaster Mental Health (Fukushima Center for Disaster Mental Health) started its activities.
- The mental healthcare team of Kyoto University for children started its activities.
- The volunteer group of clinical psychotherapists from Kyoto Prefecture continued its activities.
- Regular meetings with living support counselors as well as care meetings were continued.
- Publicity and education campaigns aimed to prevent suicide were run (involving those people, such as evacuees, staff members of affected municipalities, and living support counselors).

(Social welfare activities)
- We held information exchange meetings of the community general support centers in the affected areas under the jurisdiction of the Aizu District (regular meetings).

(Disaster-affected pet protection activities)
- Comprehensive protection activities were conducted.

3　Summary and measures to be taken in the future

(Health management activities)
- The staff members of the contact points for affected municipalities were assigned to their respective municipalities, which made it possible to promptly clarify the important issues.
- It is necessary to review the support system to meet the situation of the affected municipalities.
- It is necessary to conduct coordination of the activities of individual support organizations.

(Yukie Takahashi)

13 Measures Taken by the Minami-Aizu Public Health and Welfare Office

1 Outline of the areas under jurisdiction

(1) Municipalities under jurisdiction

The following three towns and one village are under the jurisdiction: Shimogo Town, Hinoemata Village, Tadami Town, and Minamiaizu Town of Minami-Aizu-Gun

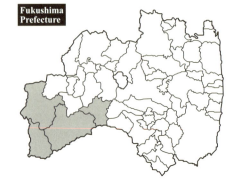

(2) Population/population aging rate (as of January 1 each year)

	2011	2013
Population	29,782	28,803
Population aging rate	36.8	37.2

2 Damage situation caused by the earthquake and nuclear disaster in the areas under jurisdiction

(1) Damage situation (as of March 12, 2013)

Physical damage	Completely destroyed	Half destroyed	Partially destroyed
Residential buildings	0	0	0
Public facilities		0	
Others		16	

Human damage	Direct deaths	Associated deaths	Missing	Injured
	0	0	0	1

(2) Evacuation situation (as of March 12, 2013)

	End-March 2011	End-September 2011	End-March 2012	Latest
Installation of shelters	7			
No. of evacuees				
No. of evacuees accepted	101			
No. of residents living in temporary houses for residents and evacuees accepted				

(Emergency Response Headquarters of Fukushima Prefecture: Calculated based on the flash report on the damage situation caused by the 2011 off the Pacific coast of Tohoku Earthquake)

13 Measures Taken by the Minami-Aizu Public Health and Welfare Office

 March 11 to April 30, 2011 (up to one month)

1 Situation

- On March 11, an earthquake with a seismic intensity of 5 lower was observed; however, there was neither human nor property damage.
- On March 14, primary shelters were opened at 27 locations in the areas under our jurisdiction. On and after March 15, a maximum of 223 evacuees were accepted at 10 locations from the warning zone within 30 km from the Fukushima Daiichi Nuclear Power Station of the Tokyo Electric Power Company.
- On April 4, secondary shelters, mainly guest houses, were opened at 136 locations broadly in the areas under our jurisdiction and evacuees relocated there from primary shelters.
- On April 26, the mental healthcare team of Gifu Prefecture started to be dispatched.

2 Main activities

- We conducted coordination with hospitals and other facilities to accept the patients from the hospitals located in the warning zone.
- We conducted coordination to determine where to accept those who had been accommodated in the facilities located in the warning zone.
- Public health nurses paid visits to shelters to provide consultations.
- We performed external exposure screening.
- We conducted coordination for external support (the child mental healthcare team of Kyoto Prefecture and the mental healthcare team of Gifu Prefecture) and the external support teams paid visits to shelters together with public health nurses to provide consultations.
- On the 14th, three staff members under the jurisdiction of other public health centers in the prefecture were dispatched.
- Study meetings on how to support evacuees were held with the towns from and to which the evacuees had relocated.

3 Summary and measures to be taken in the future

- Collaboration with the municipalities and the institutions concerned in routine work at ordinary times led to the development of the support system at an early stage.
- A flexible way of providing support was required under the circumstances where extremely limited information was available.
- There were an increasing number of elderly people who needed care due to the change in living environment after evacuation. It is necessary to establish welfare shelters at an early stage.
- Nighttime temperature was sometimes lower than -10°C and the chill from the floor was severe. It is necessary to take measures, particularly against cold, such as distribution of makeshift beds.

Chapter 2　Initiatives of Public Administrations

B　May 1 to September 30, 2011 (two to six months)

1　Situation

- On May 20, the number of evacuees in secondary shelter peaked at 797.
- On May 24, the dispatch of the mental healthcare teams of Gifu Prefecture ended.
- On September 20, primary shelters were closed.

2　Main activities

- The mental healthcare team of Gifu Prefecture paid visits to evacuees together with public health nurses and dietitians. Living support specialists and public health nurses accompanied the mental healthcare team on their visits.
- We ran publicity and education campaigns to prevent infectious diseases and heatstroke.
- We held lectures and consultation meetings on nutrition and mental health for evacuees in secondary shelters.
- A study was conducted with the towns from and to which the evacuees had relocated on how to support evacuees.
- Health education and individual consultations were provided by the Mental Health and Welfare Centre (psychiatrists and psychologists).
- We dispatched our staff members to conduct pet protection and support activities in the warning zone.
- We performed monitoring of radioactive substances in drinking water and processed food.

3　Summary and measures to be taken in the future

- Since guest houses and Japanese inns in a mountainous area remote from medical institutions and supermarkets were mainly used as secondary shelters, it was inconvenient for evacuees to visit medical institutions and purchase commodities.
- Some residents wanted information from the municipality from which they had come and if the staff members of the respective municipalities were stationed nearby, they could feel secure. However, the staff members had a significant mental and physical burden because they themselves were also affected by the disaster.

C　October 1, 2011 to March 31, 2012 (seven months to one year)

1　Situation

- On December 6, secondary shelters were closed.
- Evacuees (168 people in 52 households in the areas under our jurisdiction) eventually relocated to temporary subsidized rental houses.
- No temporary houses were built.

2 Main activities

- Public health nurses paid visits to shelters and also visited the residents living in temporary subsidized rental houses.
- We performed external exposure screening.
- Protection and support activities for pets in the warning zone were conducted.
- We dispatched our staff members to perform monitoring of radioactive substances in drinking water.
- We performed monitoring of radioactive substances in processed and other foods.

3 Summary and measures to be taken in the future

- During this period, evacuees led their lives apparently without any problems; however, they had a significant mental burden due to uncertain future prospects in their life. It is necessary to continue to provide support.
- It is necessary to provide life-related information because the pace of livelihood reconstruction varies depending on evacuees.

D : April 1, 2012 to March 31, 2013 (one year and one month to two years)

1 Situation

- There were no temporary houses. Evacuees moved into temporary subsidized rental houses (97 people in 45 households).

2 Main activities

- Public health nurses paid visits to all of the temporary subsidized rental houses.
- The staff members of the Fukushima Center for Disaster Mental Health in the Aizu District and public health nurses paid visits to temporary subsidized rental houses.
- We performed external exposure screening and implemented the child mental healthcare program.
- We performed monitoring of drinking water and inspection of radioactive substances in processed and other foods.

3 Summary and measures to be taken in the future

- As time elapses, issues confronting individual people vary; however, it is necessary to provide the opportunities and places where people can share their distress and be relaxed.
- Visits by public health nurses can provide a sense of security.

(Tomoko Yuda, Yumiko Toshima)

Chapter 3

Situation of and Countermeasures by Each Individual Municipality

14 Efforts of Tomioka Town

1 Situation of the municipality

(1) Demographics (as of January 1 of each year)

	2011	2012	2013
Population	15,839	14,686	14,536
Number of households	6,293	5,887	5,800
Average number of people per household	2.5	2.5	2.5
Number of births	133	96	
Birth rate	8.4	6.5	
Number of deaths	200	153	
Mortality	12.3	10.4	
Ratio of the elderly aged 65 or older	21.3	21.5	22.3

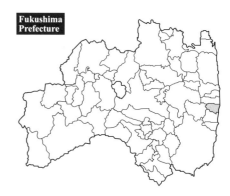

(2) Geographical features

Total area: 68.47 km^2 (approximately 12.3 km east-west; approximately 8.8 km north-south)

Distance from the Fukushima Daiichi Nuclear Power Station of the Tokyo Electric Power Company: approximately 9 km

Evacuation area: An evacuation order was issued to the entire town.

Transportation network: Joban Expressway; National Route 6; JR Joban Line; Ono-Tomioka Prefectural Road

2 Situation of damage by the earthquake, tsunami and the nuclear disaster

(1) Damage by the Great East Japan Earthquake (as of February 20, 2013)

Property damage	Completely destroyed	Half destroyed	Partially destroyed
House			
Public institution			
Other			

Human damage	Deaths by disaster	Disaster-related deaths	Missing persons	Injured persons
	23	146	1	Unknown

* The number of disaster-related deaths exceeds that of deaths by disaster.

* Detailed property damage is unknown due to the difficulty of confirmation.

(2) Situation of evacuation

① Evacuation centers inside the local municipality

	Number of evacuation centers	Number of evacuees	Available period
Residents	0	0	
Evacuees received	0	0	

* Because all the residents were evacuated outside the town, no evacuation centers were set up within the town.

② Approximate number of evacuees in evacuation centers outside the municipality (as of February 20, 2013)

	End/March 2011	End/September 2011	End/March 2012	Latest period
First evacuation center	2,900	344	0	0
Second evacuation center	0	107	0	0
Temporary housing	0	2,546	2,471	2,655
Municipally-subsidized housing	0	13,461	13,870	12,988

Chapter 3 — Situation of and Countermeasures by Each Individual Municipality

③ Approximate number of voluntary evacuees

Inside Fukushima Prefecture		Outside Fukushima Prefecture (number of evacuees & prefectures)	

Outlook of damage related to the nuclear disaster

- The Off the Pacific Coast of Tohoku Earthquake occurred on March 11, 2011, with its seismic center off the Sanriku coast. In Tomioka Town a seismic intensity of 6 or more and a maximum 21.1meter high tsunami were observed, taking many lives and damaging assets/properties of the residents. The JR Tomioka Station, railroads, sewage treatment plants, roads and many houses were swept away by the tsunami. The earthquake and the consequent tsunami also caused a nuclear power plant accident, resulting in an unprecedented nuclear disaster.
- On March 12, an evacuation order was issued to residents living within a 10-km range from the Fukushima Daiichi Nuclear Power Station of the Tokyo Electric Power Company (hereinafter referred to as the "Fukushima Daiichi Nuclear Power Station"). Following this evacuation order, the 6,000 residents of Tomioka Town were evacuated to nearby Kawauchi Village with a population of 3,000. However, some residents who were not able to be accommodated at evacuation centers in Kawauchi Village had to look for shelter on their own, and were wandering the streets.
- On March 15, an order to stay indoors was issued to residents living within a range of 20–30 km from the Fukushima Daiichi Nuclear Power Station, based on which both Tomioka and Kawauchi residents were evacuated to Koriyama City on March 16.
- The evacuation order issued to Tomioka Town has not been lifted yet because the entire town has been designated as a hazard area. Residents are not allowed to return to their homes, being forced to lead inconvenient lives as evacuees in unfamiliar areas. Inevitably, severe problems caused by the separation of family members, concerns about radioactive substances and health problems are increasingly becoming evident among them. To enable residents to return home without feeling anxiety, there remain many problems to be solved, such as full-fledged decontamination work and decommissioning/dismantling work of nuclear reactors, which will take several decades to complete.

3 Countermeasures against nuclear disaster (as of January 2013)

	Name of project	Division in charge	Number of targeted persons (households)	Expectant mothers	Nursing mothers	Babies	Young children	Elementary school students	Junior high school students	Senior high school students	People age 19 to 39	People age 40 or older	Remarks (major operations)
1	Distribution of cumulative dosimeters	Living Environment Division	All households	○	○	○	○	○	○	○	○	○	Distribution started in August 2012.
2	Lending of cumulative dosimeters	Health and Welfare Division	1,900 persons	○		○	○	○	○				Lending and collection of cumulative dosimeters as well as the aggregation of the results began in December 2011.
3	Refreshment for young children	Educational General Affairs Division/ Planning Division					○						Overnight exchange programs outside Fukushima Prefecture
4	Refreshments for elementary school and junior high school students							○	○				Gatherings for reunion and overnight exchange programs outside Fukushima Prefecture
5	Monitoring and measurement of the air radiation levels	Living Environment Division											Measurements at 72 monitoring posts within the town twice a month
6	Real-time measurement of the radiation dose (Ministry of the Environment)	Living Environment Division											
7	Measurement and mapping of the air radiation levels in the whole town	Town Development Division											
8	Replacement of the surface soil on the grounds in child education facilities and schools (Miharu School)	Educational General Affairs Division											Replacement started in September 2011, before classes were resumed.
9	Preceding decontamination work (Town Office) (Cabinet Office)	Town Development Division											

Countermeasures against external exposure

112

	No.	Item	Division	Target												Remarks
Countermeasures against internal exposure	10	Decontamination demonstration projects (Yoru-no-mori Park, the Second Junior High School, Refre Tomioka) (Cabinet Office)	Town Development Division													
	11	Monitoring prior to full-scale decontamination work (in paddy fields, residential land soil, etc.)	Town Development Division													
	12	Examination of breast milk	Health and Welfare Division				○									Examinations of breast milk have been implemented as part of baby consultation programs provided by Fukushima Prefecture. Also, they have been concurrently conducted with Whole Body Counter measurements at the Hirata Central Hospital.
	13	Whole Body Counter measurements (conducted by the town)	Health and Welfare Division	All residents	○	○		○	○	○	○	○	○	○		Measurements are commissioned to medical institutions. The Division conducts notification and publicity.
	14	Whole Body Counter measurements (conducted by Fukushima Prefecture)	Health and Welfare Division	All residents	○	○		○	○	○	○	○	○	○		Arrangement of measurement schedules and notification & publicity.
	15	Inspection of radioactive materials in food	Industry Promotion Division	All residents	○	○	○	○	○	○	○	○	○	○		Inspection and analysis at four sites, including the Tomioka Town Koriyama Office.
	16	Thyroid gland examination (conducted by Fukushima Prefecture)	Health and Welfare Division				○	○	○	○	○	○				Publicity
	17	Inspection of radioactive materials in well water, rivers, etc. (Ministry of the Environment)	Living Environment Division													
Others	18	Study sessions on radiation (Ministry of the Environment)	Health and Welfare Division										○	○		Targeted participants: parents/guardians of children attending to childcare institutions and after-school facilities
	19	Sampling of respondents for every survey under the Fukushima Health Management Survey	Health and Welfare Division	All residents	○	○	○	○	○	○	○	○	○	○		
	20	Cancer screening	Health and Welfare Division	Residents of designated ages	○								○	○		Stomach cancer, lung cancer, colorectal cancer, prostate cancer, cervical cancer and breast cancer
	21	Metabolic syndrome screening/ medical examinations	Health and Welfare Division	Residents aged 18 or older									○	○		Examinations in a group have been conducted within Fukushima Prefecture; examinations on an individual basis have been implemented at medical institutions outside Fukushima Prefecture.
	22	Medical examinations under the Fukushima Health Management Survey (conducted by Fukushima Prefecture)	Health and Welfare Division	All residents	○	○	○	○	○	○	○	○	○	○		Generally 20 to 22 items in one examination.
	23	Publication of disaster information magazines	Planning Division	All households	○	○	○	○	○	○	○	○	○	○		Issuance and distribution twice a month
	24	Issuance of a health management file (conducted by Fukushima Prefecture)	Health and Welfare Division	All residents	○	○	○	○	○	○	○	○	○	○		

Chapter 3 Situation of and Countermeasures by Each Individual Municipality

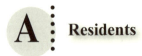
A Residents

1 Nutrition (meals/water)

a. Situation

(At evacuation centers in Kawauchi Village)
- It was especially difficult to secure foods during March 12 to 16.
- At a local public assembly hall, the heads of the administrative wards of the village, local community leaders and women's association members prepared warm *miso* soup and other simple foods to provide to residents evacuated from Tomioka Town. At schools, community centers and other public facilities, the town officials and women's association members of the village prepared rice balls and distributed them to the evacuees.
- Bread and other emergency relief supplies reached evacuees on and around March 14.

(At the Big Palette Fukushima)
- All the residents were evacuated again from Kawauchi Village to Koriyama City on March 16.
- At Koriyama City, residents took shelter in the Big Palette Fukushima (hereinafter referred to as "the Big Palette"), a local convention complex. Emergency relief supplies were continually carried into the Big Palette by cargo truck.
- Residents spent six months at the Big Palette, during which they were provided high-calorie and high-fat meals every day. Pre-packed meals in a *bento* style were most frequently distributed to them, but with insufficient vegetables, nutritionally unbalanced dishes and no hot food. Rice balls, high-calorie stuffed breads and milk were also distributed in the morning and evening. Other than three daily meals, residents were given rice with curry sauce and other relief foods prepared by volunteer staff members. In spite of such a dietary environment, most residents remained idle all day long, except for when they went to the toilet and lined up to receive relief supplies. Obviously, the residents had a lack of exercise and an excessive intake of nutrition.

(At temporary housing and municipally-subsidized housing)
- It may be surprising that there are some residents who were not able to cook their own daily meals after moving to temporary housing, due to a wide variety of reasons.
- Because evacuation centers, temporary housing and municipally-subsidized housing generally do not have gardens/fields, residents are unable to grow vegetables to eat, causing a decreased intake of vegetables. Additionally, residents have almost no opportunity to work in the fields, weed a garden or take a walk along a garden/field. They have nothing to do other than eating, and they just stay indoors all day long. The residents themselves are well aware of the need to improve their unbalanced diets and take more exercise.
- According to the results of medical examinations, all the obesity indices such as a body mass index (BMI), a blood sugar level, low-density lipoprotein cholesterol (LDL-C) and a neutral lipid levels have increased among residents. The results have also revealed an increase in cases of diabetes.

b. Responses (actual measures)
- At the first evacuation centers in Kawauchi Village, the town officials and local volunteers tried to make 4,000 rice balls, aiming to distribute them at one time to all residents. Although they started making rice balls in the morning, it was already evening when all of them were prepared. By the time residents ate

them, the rice balls had become cold and hard. Eventually, the town finally managed to provide meals to residents and to secure a food supply in a critically difficult situation. Thankfully, rice was provided by Kawauchi Village residents.

- When residents took shelter in the Big Palette, the town changed the supplier of *bento* meals and asked a new supplier to add more salad dishes to the meals. Responding to an earnest request for hot meals, the town officials boiled a large amount of water in the morning and placed it within the premises at each distribution point, so that residents could eat instant noodles.

- Nutritionists assigned to the Ken-poku Public Health and Welfare Office and the Ken-chu Public Health and Welfare Office (hereinafter collectively referred to as "a public health and welfare office") were entrusted with dietary instructions for diabetic patients, hypertension patients, and other residents in need of some dietary support programs.

c. Summary/measures in the future

- At evacuation centers in Kawauchi Village, the amount of food was restricted. In contrast, excessive *bento* meals, beverages and other emergency relief supplies were distributed to residents at the Big Palette, which inevitably led to overeating.

- Having nothing to do at evacuation centers, many residents spent a day just eating, sleeping after eating, then waking up after an announcement of food distribution and going to receive more food. As a result of such a daily life, many residents gained weight.

- Because evacuation centers are not equipped with test kitchens, nutritionists are not able to provide dietary instruction through cooking practices.

- It is important to ensure residents' well-balanced diets and healthy lives as much as possible at evacuation centers. However, actual conditions were so confused that it was impossible to systematically sort out emergency relief supplies and efficiently distribute them to residents. Also, there were no expert officials (professional personnel in dietetics) at evacuation centers.

- At evacuation centers, it is important to limit the amount of food distributed to each individual resident. The most important thing to be considered is a deliberate allocation of emergency relief supplies.

- Since residents left evacuation centers to live independently, dietary instruction programs have not often been conducted due to difficulties in finding a suitable venue. Even if an adequate venue is found, some residents have no means of transportation to get there. The nutritionists are looking for a solution to provide dietary instruction to residents in an effective manner and at the best suitable places.

2 Exercise (environmental improvement)

a. Situation

- Almost no detailed information on the earthquake and the nuclear power plant accident was available before moving to the Big Palette. Additionally, due to little knowledge of radiation, no precautions against radiation had been taken.

- Residents underwent radiation screening at the time of entering the Big Palette. The Big Palette continued serving as a radiation screening venue.

- At the Big Palette residents took a place, being scattered all over the premises; it was difficult to know where each individual resident was within the facility. Particularly, for medical staff members, it was quite hard to find and identify persons at high risk.

- As the first emergency relief support from other prefectures, Sugito Town of Saitama Prefecture, a friendship city of Tomioka Town, sent seven buses to Kawauchi Village on March 16 to help residents evacuate from the village to the Big Palette. On the next day, about 250 residents moved to Sugito Town by taking the seven buses. During the transfer of residents, public health nurses of Sugito Town also helped to check each resident's health condition.

- Fukushima Prefecture served as a liaison for emergency relief assistance teams dispatched from other municipalities such as Yokohama City, Fukuoka Prefecture and Shiga Prefecture.

- The town's Health Promotion Section returned to normal working operations on May 16. The section officials organized a team of four to answer inquiries from residents about medical examinations for young children and vaccination. They also provided health care support to residents staying at hotels and other secondary evacuation centers, in cooperation with emergency relief support members dispatched from outside Fukushima Prefecture.

- Medical examinations for adults and elderly residents living within Fukushima Prefecture have been commissioned to the Fukushima Preservative Service Association of Health, and group medical examinations have been conducted in Koriyama and Iwaki cities of Fukushima Prefecture. For residents taking shelter in other prefectures, medical examinations have been commissioned to the Association for Preventive Medicine of Japan; these residents are able to undergo individual medical examination at medical institutions in their host prefectures. Tomioka Town's public health nurses have arranged for and coordinated medical institutions to conduct necessary administrative procedures, and respond to any inquiries concerning medical examinations.

- In some temporary housing, residents have cultivated fields to grow vegetables and enjoyed walking in a group.

b. Responses (actual measures)
- The town officials in charge brought iodine tablets when taking evacuation to Kawauchi Village on March 12. They visited evacuation centers both inside and outside Kawauchi Village to provide the tablets to residents who wished to take them.

- After moving to Kawauchi Village, the town officials looked for stores in business outside the village and purchased medicines, portable blood pressure gauges and other necessary commodities. The purchased items were allocated to each individual evacuation center established within Kawauchi Village.

- The town officials set up an aid station in the convention hall of the Big Palette in cooperation with doctors and pharmacists who were also evacuated from Tomioka Town. They also strived to systematically allocate space to residents, placing a priority on young children, the elderly and persons with disabilities for staying within the convention hall.

- A map indicating where each individual resident stayed within the Big Palette premises was created, with the aim of immediately responding to the needs of residents at high risk. The map was updated over time.

- To help prevent the development of deep vein thrombosis/pulmonary embolism ("economy-class syndrome"), acupuncturists and massagers walked around of the Big Palette sites to encourage residents to do stretching exercises, showing them exercise examples. Moreover, staff members of Fukushima Medical University conducted a confirmation test to judge whether or not residents developed economy-class syndrome. To help prevent the development of this syndrome, they distributed stockings to residents and encouraged residents to wear them.

- The town's Health Promotion Section returned to normal working operations on May 16. After that, direct responses to inquiries from, and the needs of, residents taking shelter in evacuation centers were entrusted to emergency relief support members. The Health Promotion Section's officials were pressed with administrative duties and telephone counseling services concerning medical examinations and vaccinations.

- Debriefing meetings about the results of medical examinations conducted in 2012 were held at assembly rooms in temporary housing sites, at which residents received personal instructions on their health management.

- At assembly rooms in temporary housing sites, emergency relief assistance teams conducted a health care program called "*kenko salon*" once a month, encouraging residents to gather together to do exercise. This program continued to be held and fostered new programs, such as a muscular strength improvement program, which aims to help prevent the elderly from requiring nursing care.

- Livelihood support counselors from the Council of Social Welfare (hereinafter referred to as the "social welfare council") have encouraged residents to acquire the habit of going outdoors to do some exercises for their continued good health.
- A miniature golf course was established on the premises of Tomioka Town temporary housing located in Koriyama City.

c. Summary/measures in the future

- The Big Palette was not an adequate long term living environment.
- At evacuation centers, especially large-scale evacuation centers, it is important to improve the living environment so that residents can be as comfortable as possible. Additionally, in order to efficiently offer necessary support to residents, it is also indispensable to obtain the understanding and cooperation of the residents about well-ordered allocation of space.
- Living in evacuation centers was an unusual experience for residents, inevitably making them feel stressed and hesitant to do even their routine exercises. It is important to continue providing information on exercise programs to residents, encouraging them to join in group exercises.

3   Rest (mind, anxiety, suicide, etc.)

a. Situation

- Most residents initially thought that they could return home within a few days. Unfortunately, they were evacuated again from Kawauchi Village to the Big Palette. Facing a rapidly changing situation that became far more serious than they had imagined, residents increasingly felt strongly anxious about their future.
- Operations of the Health Promotion Section generally do not include stress management programs for residents.
- The number of identified alcohol dependence cases has increased compared to before the earthquake. It is difficult to find a solution to the alcohol abuse problems.

b. Responses (actual measures)

- For residents who are in need of mental health care in their host Iwaki City, nurses and public health nurses assigned to the Tomioka Town Iwaki Office as well as the staff members of the Fukushima Center for Disaster Mental Health have provided necessary support. For residents taking shelter in the suburban area of Koriyama City, the town's public health nurses and the staff members of the Fukushima Center for Disaster Mental Health have offered them necessary support. Mental health care for serious cases has been conducted in close collaboration with the staff members of the Ken-chu Public Health and Welfare Office.
- With the aim of maintaining good mental health conditions of the town officials, the General Affairs Division has commissioned a specialized commission to continuously offer counseling services to them and implement a questionnaire survey on their mental health condition once a year.
- As a preventive measure against suicide, pamphlets containing mental health care information and programs have been distributed to all the households twice a year.

c. Summary/measures in the future

- Some residents had developed alcoholic dependence before the earthquake; others have increased their

Chapter 3 | Situation of and Countermeasures by Each Individual Municipality

dependence on alcohol due to drastic changes in life style (unemployment, separation of a family, etc.), death of familiar or neighboring persons and various other difficulties caused by the earthquake. It seems that a dependence on alcohol is largely influenced by changes in living circumstances.

- Because the number of suicides has shown a rapid increase after the earthquake, it is urgently required that effective countermeasures be taken.

4 Others

a. Situation

- Following an evacuation order issued on March 12, residents headed to Kawauchi Village. However, the maximum capacity of evacuation centers in Kawauchi Village was 6,000 in total and some 10,000 residents had to find shelter in other municipalities on their own.
- Some residents, who were unable to be accommodated at evacuation centers, had to spend several days living in their own cars.
- When the evacuation order was issued, the town announced over the local wireless radio broadcasting the order and urged residents to take shelter. A local firefighting team's car and the town's publicity car also rushed around the town to call for evacuation. However, some residents were left behind because they could not clearly understand the broadcast/announcement.
- Although phone lines had worked in Kawauchi Village until March 13, they became unavailable after that date. In this situation, in which there was no way to connect with people outside the village, TV broadcasting was the only source of information for the residents.
- When evacuating to Kawauchi Village, residents thought they could return home within several days because they were not informed of the nuclear accident at the Fukushima Daiichi Nuclear Power Station.
- Residents who stayed in their cars judged that safety would not be secured in Kawauchi Village. They decided to independently evacuate the village and headed to safer places.
- The Fukushima Daiichi Nuclear Power Station was in an extremely serious situation for several hours from late in the night of March 14 to the early morning of March 15. Not knowing the situation, Tomioka Town and Kawauchi Village declared in the morning of the 15th the safety of the Fukushima Daiichi Nuclear Power Station and jointly announced a decision that both residents could continue staying in the village, with the aim of avoiding further confusion among residents. Meanwhile, at 11:00 a.m. on the same day, an order to stay indoors was issued to residents within a range of 20–30 km from the nuclear power plant.
- Residents of some municipalities were evacuated as early as on the 15th. However, Tomioka Town and Kawauchi Village missed an opportunity to evacuate residents on the 15th because of the announcement of the safety declaration. The town and village residents were finally evacuated on the 16th, but a delayed evacuation and a withdrawal of the safety declaration caused confusion among them.

b. Responses (actual measures)

- On March 11, the town started emergency response activities around 15:00 to 16:00, first setting up evacuation centers.
- An evacuation order was issued on the morning of the 12th to residents living within a 20-km range of the Fukushima Daiichi Nuclear Power Station, following which residents were evacuated to Kawauchi Village. At the village, residents were accommodated at local assembly halls, schools, community centers and other public facilities.
- On the 16th, residents were evacuated again to the Big Palette located in Koriyama City together with Kawauchi Village residents.
- By August 2011, the Big Palette accommodated a maximum of 2,500 evacuees from the disaster-stricken areas.

14 Efforts of Tomioka Town

B Expectant/nursing mothers and children

1 Nutrition (meals/water)

a. Situation
- Immediately after the earthquake, town officials were unable to respond to the needs of expectant/nursing mothers and children because they were pressed with emergency response activities at evacuation centers.
- When taking shelter in Kawauchi Village, artificial milk (milk powder) and disposable diapers were in extremely short supply.
- There was a few young children at the Big Palette; about 30 to 40 children of preschool-age and younger.
- Large amounts of emergency supplies, including milk powder and disposable diapers, were carried into the Big Palette.
- Large amounts of candy, snacks, cookies and other confections reached the evacuation centers. Because exposure to radiation was a great concern, children were unable to play outdoors and spent most of the day indoors instead. Inevitably they developed unfavorable habits of playing games all day long, eating too many snacks, soda beverages, and juice. Overeating of confections was a common tendency among children.
- As with the case of adults, *bento* style meals with high-calorie fried dishes and almost no vegetables were distributed to children.

b. Responses (actual measures)
- During the stay in Kawauchi Village, the town officials went to pharmacies to purchase milk powder, disposable diapers and other necessary commodities.
- It was impossible to respond to the needs of expectant mothers and children.
- Nutrition management of Tomioka Town's elementary school and junior high school (Miharu School) students is entrusted to nurse-teachers and school nutritionists.
- The school lunches for Tomioka Town's elementary school and junior high school (Miharu School) students had been served in the form of *bento* meals from a supplier. The town altered the supplier to a school lunch center located in Tamura City.

c. Summary/measures in the future
- School children in Fukushima Prefecture had originally shown an increasing tendency toward obesity. After the earthquake, the prefecture ranked first in the country in the number of obese students of a certain school grade. Some reports say that children in Fukushima Prefecture have been restricted to play outdoors to prevent exposure to radiation, thereby causing decreased exercise and an increase in the number of overweight children. It is necessary to comprehensively examine and improve children's daily activities, dietary habits and the quality of meals at evacuation centers.
- Importantly, instructions on how to spend time at an evacuation center (including self-management of diets) should be provided to residents when they are accommodated in their first evacuation center.

2 Exercise (environmental improvement)

a. Situation
- Because of the nuclear accident at the Fukushima Daiichi Nuclear Power Station, opportunities to play

119

outdoors decreased for children.

- Information on safe places where children can play is insufficient.
- School bus operations started after the earthquake, which resulted in decreased exercise among primary and junior high school students.

b. Responses (actual measures)

- It is necessary to provide information on safe playing spaces to residents, in cooperation with host municipalities.
- Measures for exercise and physical activities of Tomioka Town's elementary school and junior high school (Miharu School) students are entrusted to nurse-teachers.

c. Summary/measures in the future

- It is necessary to provide information on favorable exercise effects and radiation impact to parents/guardians of school children in an easy to understand format.
- It may be necessary to take some measures to prevent the development of lifestyle related diseases among children.

3 Rest (mind, anxiety, suicide, etc.)

a. Situation

- There are many students who were unable to adapt themselves to school in their host municipality and moved to another school.
- After the earthquake, the number of students who do not go to school and stayed at home, who have trouble with bullying at school and who go to school but just stay in a sickroom has increased.
- The results of medical examinations for young children revealed that the number of children who require a follow-up examination, such as infants who talk late and hyperactive children was increasing.
- Many families have faced difficulties in receiving help to raise their children because family members, relatives and friends took shelter separately, scattering all over Japan.
- Some parents said that they often feel hesitant to talk to local parents and children at playing spaces in host municipalities because they feel themselves to be "an outsider."

b. Responses (actual measures)

- Dedicated counselors were assigned to schools.
- In April 2013, the town's public health nurses and midwives resumed home-visiting services for parents having a baby.
- Support programs for parents with babies/toddlers were conducted in 2013 in Koriyama and Iwaki cities.
- Home-visiting services were implemented in collaboration with the Fukushima Center for Disaster Mental Health.

c. Summary/measures in the future

- It is necessary to exactly understand children's situations/problems at school in host municipalities and take adequate measures to solve them. This should be done in cooperation with the Educational General Affairs Division.
- It is urgently required to increase the number/frequency of home visits and telephone counseling services for expectant/nursing mothers and young children.

4 Others

a. Situation

- Examination of breast milk has been conducted by Fukushima Prefecture. Shortly after the nuclear accident, the town received inquiries from expectant/nursing mothers about where and how they can undergo the examination. Upon hearing an explanation that all the cost must be covered by an examinee and how much the approximate cost would be, they answered that they would not undergo examinations due to financial reasons.
- Expectant/nursing mothers might have felt anxiety, and had questions about; "Is it safe to let children play outdoors?", "Should children wear a mask?", and "Is it safe to hang laundry outdoors?". However because medical examinations for young children were commissioned to each host municipality, Tomioka Town officials in charge had no opportunity to directly answer their questions. It was difficult to accurately understand and directly respond to their anxiety and concerns.
- There has been tremendous pressure for mothers to protect their children from exposure to radiation and secure safe living environments.
- It is difficult to entrust host municipalities with all of the necessary follow-up medical examinations for young children; some necessary actions might be required.

b. Responses (actual measures)

- During January to March, study sessions on radiation were held for mothers nursing preschool children as part of programs conducted by the Ministry of the Environment. The purpose was to help expand their correct knowledge of radiation.
- Aiming to manage residents' daily dose, the town procured cumulative dosimeters for personal use in December 2011 as part of Fukushima Prefecture subsidized projects. The cumulative dosimeters have been lent to expectant mothers and young children (from babies to junior high school students).
- Dose measurements were conducted in each host municipality, using dosimeters (glass badges).

c. Summary/measures in the future

- The most urgent task is to secure and improve living conditions under which women can deliver a baby and nurse a child without feeling anxiety for the future.

C People requiring assistance during a disaster (vulnerable people in case of a disaster)

1 Nutrition (meals/water)

a. Situation

- Shortly after the earthquake, it was impossible to respond to the special needs of people requiring assistance during the disaster.

b. Responses (actual measures)

- It was staff members from various welfare facilities, not the town officials, who actually responded to the special needs of people requiring assistance during the disaster.

c. Summary/measures in the future

- In preparation for the occurrence of a new type of influenza, the town had stocked emergency foods for people requiring assistance during a disaster. However, the town officials failed to bring such food stocks

Chapter 3 | Situation of and Countermeasures by Each Individual Municipality

when taking shelter. As a future task, it is necessary to expand emergency food stocks, including enough food and commodities for people requiring assistance during a disaster.

2 Exercise (environmental improvement)

a. Situation
- There were many welfare facilities within the town, including nursing-care facilities for the elderly, group homes and facilities for developmentally disabled children.
- Residents of nursing-care facilities were also evacuated to Kawauchi Village, where two of them died.
- Although the town urged residents to take shelter using local wireless radio broadcasting, many residents, including people requiring assistance during a disaster, were left stranded within the town.
- Residents of Toyo Gakuen and the Koyo Aisei-En facilities for developmentally disabled children/ persons were evacuated to Kamogawa City of Chiba Prefecture and Gunma Prefecture, respectively.
- Because mentally disabled persons receiving care at home were evacuated with other residents, it was quite difficult to confirm who took shelter and who did not, and to identify their whereabouts.
- For residents who have mental disabilities and those with alcohol abuse problems, a public health nurse and a welfare section official in charge of persons with disabilities were paired to visit and support them.
- There are many elderly residents who have a sense of crisis, fearing that they may not return home if they become unable to stand and walk by their own. They have actively participated in a health care program named "*kenko salon*" and acquired the habit of taking a walk, thereby striving to manage/ maintain their good health.

b. Responses (actual measures)
- Some residents voluntarily helped their elderly neighbors who were living alone to take shelter. Welfare commissioners also supported and took care for their assigned elderly residents.
- The town set up an aid station in the convention hall of the Big Palette and gave a priority for staying within the hall to the residents of nursing-care facilities for the elderly, young children, elderly people and persons with disabilities.
- Doctors not only examined patients at the aid station but also went around to the premises of the Big Palette to check the health condition of each individual resident.

c. Summary/measures in the future
- Residents living in temporary housing include people requiring assistance during a disaster; such as those who have mental and other disabilities, the elderly, and persons who cannot move on their own.
- It is important to classify residents at an early stage of evacuation, into a group of healthy residents and a group of residents with special needs in times of disaster (young children, the elderly and persons with disabilities), then systematically allocating spaces at evacuation centers. Such a systematic separation of residents will enable effective emergency relief support for disaster vulnerable people.

3 Rest (mind, anxiety, suicide, etc.)

a. Situation
- As a general tendency, people requiring assistance during a disaster are sensitive to changes in sur-rounding environments. After the earthquake, many of them showed unstable health conditions and were hospitalized.

b. Responses (actual measures)

- From the end of March, staff members of the Asaka Hospital, which is located near the Big Palette, examined people requiring assistance during the disaster once a week at the Big Palette. For residents who were unable to take a bath due to their disabilities, the staff members provided a bathing service as well.

c. Summary/measures in the future

- A failure to urge all people requiring assistance during a disaster to take shelter is one of the points that the town can improve.
- People requiring assistance during a disaster were generally affected by changes in the surrounding environment. However, after moving to temporary housing where privacy was relatively secured, their health/mental conditions gradually became stable. For people requiring assistance during a disaster who entered temporary housing far from the Asaka Hospital, the town referred them to their nearest hospital, so that they can continue receiving treatment.
- Attentive care for children with developmental and other disabilities is indispensable.
- An official register of residents requiring assistance during a disaster must be developed and regularly updated based on which various emergency relief activities and support programs should be provided.

4 Others

- After the earthquake, many residents were forced to live separately from their family members. Therefore, there are many elderly persons who are living alone in temporary housing, which has caused the development or progress of a cognitive impairment. Wandering and other troublesome habits specific to cognitively impaired patients can be an obstacle to continue living in temporary housing. However, there are only a few cases where doctors determine the necessity of hospitalization because cognitively impaired elderly persons generally give a prompt reply and show relatively low aggression in front of a doctor. However, on returning to temporary housing, they tend to cause trouble.
- It is difficult to provide 24-hour care for the cognitively impaired elderly at temporary housing. The longer the evacuation period becomes, the greater the number of the elderly who cause trouble. The number of residents who require special assistance will also increase over time. In preparation for prolonged evacuation, some measures to effectively support them must be considered.

(Keiko Abe, Yuko Owada, Maimi Kato)

15 Efforts of Futaba Town

1 Situation of the municipality

(1) Demographics (as of January 1 of each year)

	2011	2012	2013
Population	7,099	6,649	6,541
Number of households	2,603	2,488	2,457
Average number of people per household	2.8	2.7	2.6
Number of births	45	51	40
Birth rate	3.6	4.4	3.5
Number of deaths	111	138	68
Mortality	1.56	2.07	1.03
Ratio of the elderly aged 65 or older	26.5	26.4	27.5

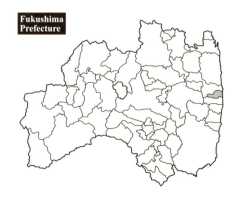
Fukushima Prefecture

(2) Geographical features

Total area: 51.40 km² (approximately 12.85 km east-west and approximately 5.50 km north-south)

Distance from the Fukushima Daiichi Nuclear Power Station of the Tokyo Electric Power Company: approximately 4 km to Town Office

Current evacuation areas: a difficult-to-return zone (where 96% of the residents resided) and an evacuation order lifting preparation zone (northeastern part of the town where 4% of the residents resided), based on the designation of May 28, 2013.

Transportation network: Joban Expressway running through the central part of the town; National Route 6 running in a north-south direction; National Route 288 running in an east-west direction

2 Situation of damage by the earthquake, tsunami and the nuclear disaster

(1) Damage by the Great East Japan Earthquake (as of February 25, 2013)

Property damage	Completely destroyed	Half destroyed	Partially destroyed
House	95	7	Unknown
Public institution			
Other			

Human damage	Deaths by disaster	Disaster-related deaths	Missing persons	Injured persons
	20	90	1	Unknown

(2) Situation of evacuation

① Evacuation centers inside the local municipality (as of October 25, 2013)

	Number of evacuation centers	Number of evacuees	Available period
Residents	0	0	0
Evacuees received	0	0	0

② Approximate number of evacuees in evacuation centers outside the municipality (as of February 25, 2013)

	End/March 2011	End/September 2011	End/March 2012	Latest period
First evacuation center	Unknown	759	345	137
Second evacuation center	0	0	0	0
Temporary housing	0	446	842	881
Municipally-subsidized housing	0	2,580	2,659	2,544

* Evacuation centers within Fukushima Prefecture only. Public housing included.

15 Efforts of Futaba Town

③ Approximate number of voluntary evacuees

Inside Fukushima Prefecture		Outside Fukushima Prefecture (number of evacuees & prefectures)	

Outlook of damage related to the nuclear disaster

- All the residents were evacuated.
- The number of residents taking shelter as of the end of August 2013
  Evacuees within Fukushima Prefecture: 3,825 (1,570 households)
  Evacuees outside Fukushima Prefecture: 3,069 (1,391 households)
  Evacuees at evacuation centers within Saitama Prefecture: 103 (66 households)
  Residents taking shelter in 40 prefectures throughout the country, including the above two prefectures.

3 Countermeasures against nuclear disaster (as of January 2013)

		Name of project	Division in charge	Number of targeted persons (households)	Expec- tant mothers	Nursing moth- ers	Babies	Young children	Elemen- tary school students	Junior high school students	Senior high school students	People age 19 to 39	People age 40 or older	Remarks (major operations)
Countermeasures against internal exposure	1	Lending of per- sonal dosimeters	Health and Welfare Division	4,725 persons	○	○	○	○			○	○	○	Distribution & collec- tion of personal dosim- eters and aggregation & analysis of results
	2	Lending of per- sonal dosimeters	Resident Life Divi- sion	All house- holds	○	○	○	○	○	○	○	○	○	Distribution and collection of personal dosimeters
	3	Refreshment for young children	Educational General Affairs Division											
	4	Refreshments for elementary school and junior high school students	Educational General Affairs Division											(Gatherings for reunion)
	5	Monitoring and measurement of the air radiation levels	Resident Life Divi- sion											Conducted at emergency temporary housing
	6	Real-time measurement of the radiation dose (Ministry of the Environment)	Ministry of the Environ- ment											
	7	Measurement and mapping of the air radiation levels in the whole town	Cabinet Office											Wide-area monitoring of a hazard area and a deliberate evacuation zone
	8	Examination of breast milk	Fukushima Prefecture			○								
	9	Whole Body Counter measure- ments (conducted by the town)	Health and Welfare Division	All residents	○	○		○	○	○	○	○	○	Arrangement of a venue & schedule, notification and publicity, examina- tions and analysis
Countermeasures against internal exposure	10	Whole Body Counter measure- ments (conducted by Fukushima Prefecture for children aged 4 to 18 and adults)	Health and Welfare Division	6,779 persons	○	○		○	○	○	○	○	○	Arrangement of a venue (other than host municipalities located in western Japan) & schedule, notification, publicity
	11	Food and water quality inspection	Industry Promotion Division	All residents	○	○	○	○	○	○	○	○	○	Inspection and analysis
	12	Thyroid gland examination (conducted by the town for residents under 40 years old)	Health and Welfare Division	2,956 persons	○	○	○	○	○	○	○	○		Notification and publicity, meetings with suppliers, contracts and bill payment
	13	Thyroid gland examination (for residents under 18 years old)	Fukushima Prefecture				○	○	○	○	○			Notification and publicity
	14	Urine examination for internal expo- sure to radiation	Health and Welfare Division	All residents	○	○	○	○	○	○	○	○	○	Notification and publicity, meetings with suppliers, contracts and bill payment
	15	Debriefing ses- sions for exposure dose measurement results	---											Announcement through the town's website and public relations magazines

Others					C1	C2	C3	C4	C5	C6	C7	C8	C9	
	16	Study sessions on radiation	Planning Division	Disaster Recon-struc- tion and Town Building Commit-tee										
	17	Cancer screening	Health and Welfare Division	Residents of des-ignated ages								○	○	Lung cancer, stomach cancer, colorectal cancer, prostate cancer, uterine cancer and breast cancer
	18	Lecture meetings on radiation	Health and Welfare Division	All residents	○	○	○	○	○	○	○	○	○	Lectures by local advisers on radiation, university professors and others (8 meetings in total)
	19	Sampling of respondents for a basic survey in the Fukushima Health Management Survey	Health and Welfare Division	All residents	○	○	○	○	○	○	○	○		
	20	Publication of disaster informa-tion magazines	Secretary and Public Relations Division	All residents	○	○	○	○	○	○	○	○	○	Issuance on a twice-a-month basis
	21	Issuance of citizen health cards (con-taining a column for recording radiation exposure levels)	Health and Welfare Division	All residents	○	○	○	○	○	○	○	○	○	Notification and publicity, meetings with suppliers, contracts and bill payment

A Residents

- On the next day after the earthquake, Futaba Town residents were evacuated to Kawamata Town.
- On March 19, about 2,000 residents were evacuated again to the Saitama Super Arena, which is located in Saitama City.
- The residents moved to Kazo City of Saitama Prefecture on March 30 and 31.
- As of November 2013, the number of evacuees from Futaba Town is 23 at the former Saitama Prefectural Kisai High School in Kazo City and 918 in total in evacuation centers throughout Saitama Prefecture. About half of the residents (approximately 900), who were evacuated to Saitama City, have already returned to Fukushima Prefecture. Some 1,600 residents are in Iwaki City.
- The majority of the residents taking shelter in evacuation centers in Kazo City are households with elder people and the elderly who were living alone. Their average age is 70 years old.
- The Futaba Town Office was initially relocated to Kazo City, where almost 80 officials worked. The office was relocated again to Iwaki City on June 17, 2013.

1 Nutrition (meals/water)

a. Situation

- On the night of March 11, 2011, the town asked staff members of special nursing care facilities for the elderly and health & welfare facilities to make rice balls for the residents. However, because the amount of rice was restricted, a priority was given to the elderly and children in distributing rice balls; inevitably there were some residents who did not receive them. The town officials were the lowest priority.
- Although it was initially planned to distribute two rice balls per person, the staff members had to change the number to one per person due the shortage of rice.
- Neighboring residents brought pastries and other foods to share them with residents at evacuation centers.
- Because there was no bottled water, the town's assembly members and residents worked together to carry in plastic containers of water for cooking use.
- Free meals were initially distributed *bento* style to the residents taking shelter in evacuation centers, while residents living in an apartment and other temporary housing had to pay for their daily meals. Inevitably a sense of unfairness grew among residents. To maintain impartiality, it was decided to charge a fee for *bento* meals.
- Because each room of the Kisai High School in Kazo City was not equipped with cooking facilities, residents cooked food on their own in a home economics room located on the 4th floor. This meant that most elderly persons, who stayed on the 1st floor due to difficulties in walking or standing up by themselves, had no choice but continue requesting *bento* meals even after a fee was charged. Including these elderly persons, a total 30 residents requested *bento* meals. There were also some residents who cooked simple meals in their own room, using an electric cooking stove.
- Although being aware that *bento* meals are nutritionally unbalanced, some residents purchased them at a convenient store.
- Residents' nutritionally unbalanced diet was one of the concerns. Because evacuation centers are designated as special food service facilities, the town received instructions from Saitama Prefecture to assign a nationally certified senior nutritionist at an evacuation center set up within the prefecture.
- There are many male residents who have been forced to live apart from their family members for the sake of their jobs. Some of them have no idea what to eat to maintain a nutritionally well-balanced diet.

Chapter 3 — Situation of and Countermeasures by Each Individual Municipality

b. Responses (actual measures)

- Aiming to remember meals at home, residents initiated and have continued a cooking program named "mental refreshment salon." The participating residents were highly pleased to eat warm rice served in a pottery bowl not in a plastic container, and using lacquered chopsticks not disposable ones, for the first time in the six months since evacuation. Although the menu in this cooking program was initially predetermined, participants have increasingly decided on the menu by a group decision. Fish meals were the most frequently requested menu items. Residents living in municipally-subsidized housing have also been encouraged to join in.
- Some residents have separately conducted unique cooking programs in a group.
- Aiming to help residents deepen their understanding of a nutritionally well-balanced diet, the town has requested a nutritionist to write an article for public relations magazines distributed to each household once a month.
- To assess the obesity indices of residents, a weight measurement program has been conducted by nutritionists every month.

c. Summary/measures in the future

- In a disaster response manual that had been prepared before the earthquake, it was recommended for residents to individually prepare food and water/beverages stocks for an emergency. However, under a situation where all the residents had to evacuate the town, they faced a desperate shortage of even a day's worth of hot meals and water/beverages.
- The purpose of the "mental refreshment salon" was to help residents recover a healthy and well-balanced diet as well as bring about a sense of togetherness among them.
- One resident said, "When the distribution of *bento* meals terminated in September, I thought that I might feel bothered by cooking food on my own. In fact, however, I felt rather reassured and realized a gradual return to my normal daily life." Listening to such a comment, the town officials were firmly determined to do their utmost to help residents restore their peaceful life in Futaba Town as early as possible.

2 Exercise (environmental improvement)

a. Situation

- Residents had an opportunity to exercise at evacuation centers under the instruction of a supporting group of volunteer members, physical therapists and doctors.
- It was surprising that volunteer members reached affected areas as early as from March 12 to 19. Their immediate response was appreciated because the town officials could not afford to request the dispatch of disaster-relief volunteers. Actually they had no idea how to request such help and where to make the contact. (It was Fukushima Prefecture that served as a contact liaison.)
- Several days after evacuation, some residents voluntarily gathered outside an evacuation center to do radio gymnastic exercises in a group.
- Some residents have borrowed fields to grow vegetables and have intentionally taken exercise; others have tended to be homebound all day long.

b. Responses (actual measures)

- At a temporary evacuation center's gymnasium, the town officials stood on the stage and encouraged residents to take exercise together. Along with singing, residents enjoyed exercising.
- To prevent the development of deep vein thrombosis/pulmonary embolism (economy-class syndrome) and other types of physical inactivity diseases (disuse syndrome), residents were encouraged to exercise to maintain healthy blood circulation.

| | 15 | Efforts of Futaba Town |

- Residents have regularly had an opportunity to take exercise together at both evacuation centers and temporary housing.

c. Summary/measures in the future

- A health management team has conducted exercise classes and nursing-care prevention classes, with the cooperation of the members of the Council of Social Welfare (hereinafter referred to as the "social welfare council"). It is important for the town to maintain a favorable relationship with the council.

3   Rest (mind, anxiety, suicide, etc.)

a. Situation

- Taking into consideration that Futaba Town residents have been forced into unusual circumstances after the earthquake, the town officials in charge of health care developed a mental health checklist to understand residents' mental condition. The checklist was used in health surveys for the residents taking shelter throughout the country. The results of the checklist revealed a higher ratio of residents with depression, compared to that identified in other reports.
- Some residents have complained of a sense of uneasiness due to changes in circumstances.
- As a general impression, the condition of residents suffering from post-traumatic stress disorder (PTSD) has increasingly improved thanks to regular support provided by a post-disaster mental health care center.
- Because there were some young residents who personally called a town official to ask advice on jobs and health-related problems, the town has initiated a health consultation line service for residents.
- According to the officials who provided home visit support to residents, an increasing number of residents are suffering from alcohol abuse and other alcohol-related problems, irrespective of whether they are working or not.

b. Responses (actual measures)

- For residents who had some problems with their mental health checklist results, the town officials in charge have regularly met and talked with them to help solve the problems.
- Some of the residents taking shelter in Kazo City and other municipalities within Saitama Prefecture are suspected of having depression. Among such residents, some may be at imminent risk of worsening and need immediate medical treatment. The town intends to gather them to provide a step-by-step cognitive behavioral therapy (CBT) in cooperation with a post-disaster mental health care center.
- There are residents who have not answered health-related questionnaire survey, and the town officials have repeatedly urged them to reply.
- Regarding residents whose mental health checklist results showed some abnormalities, the officials in charge have confirmed their intention to consult a specialist at their host municipality. With the consent of the residents, the officials have contacted health promotion sections of host municipalities to refer them to local medical institutions. The Futaba Town officials have also asked host municipalities to send back a consultation report of the residents.
- For residents who feel mental instability, the town officials in charge have discussed with the social welfare council and specialists of other fields how to offer necessary support for them.
- In cooperation with a post-disaster mental health care center, residents who have alcohol-related problems have been referred to a dedicated medical institution.
- As part of efforts to prevent suicide, the town officials have asked residents whether or not they could sleep well at night. Pamphlets containing information on mental consultation services have also been prepared and distributed to all the households.

Chapter 3 | Situation of and Countermeasures by Each Individual Municipality

c. Summary/measures in the future
- Whether or not residents have slept well at night is a fundamental concern.

4 Others

a. Situation
- Expecting to receive better social and health care services as evacuees, some residents have transferred a certificate of residence to a new address in the host municipalities. There were also some residents who were required to transfer their residence certificates to receive nursing care insurance at host municipalities.

(Health care personnel)
- Immediately after the earthquake, the town had three public health nurses. However the number has decreased over time and there was just one at the end of 2011. To address such a shortage, the town received help from other municipalities all over Japan, while at the same time employing newly commissioned and/or temporary nurses in 2011.
- In 2013 two nurses were officially registered in the town, organizing a team of three public health nurses.
- Currently three public health nurses are registered at the Futaba Town Fukushima Branch Office, which is located in Koriyama City (one commissioned nurse, one nurse transferred from Fukushima Prefecture under a fixed-term employment contract, and one nurse dispatched from the Japanese Nursing Association). Four to five temporary nurses are also assigned to the branch office.

(Health care operations)
- Before the enforcement of the Special Act on Measures concerning Nuclear Evacuees, residents were not able to receive vaccinations in their host municipalities without a request form issued by Futaba Town. Therefore, health care personnel had been pressed with hectic administrative procedures.
- Even after the enforcement of the Special Act on Measures concerning Nuclear Evacuees, health care personnel had been busily occupied with extra work. Because reports on medical examinations for young children and vaccinations in host municipalities are not immediately send back to Futaba Town officials, they have to check who underwent or did not undergo the examinations and vaccinations.
- Being occupied by administrative procedures relating to maternal & child health care services as well as nursing care insurance, health care personnel were not able to focus on their primary work; the provision of personal health care services to each individual resident.

(Management of evacuation centers)
- Each evacuation center has a residents' association. However, due to frequent changes in the number of residents taking shelter there, the association has been gradually losing its function. Detailed rules concerning the management of evacuation centers have not yet been fully established.
- Residents are not required to report of their absence from evacuation centers, which may cause a problem. In fact, because some victims were away from their evacuation centers without any notification, the town officials were very worried about their safety.
- Lights go out at a predetermined time at evacuation centers. Temporary staff members went round on patrol at night within the premises.
- Living in a group at evacuation centers tends to cause troubles among residents.

b. Responses (actual measures)

(Health care operations)

- At Kawamata Town, the town officials in charge of health care visited several evacuation centers over two days to provide health care consultation services to residents in cooperation with the officials of Kawamata Town. A maximum of 900 residents took shelter in the gymnasium of the Kawamata Town Iizaka Primary School.
- At Kawamata Town, the town officials in charge of health care went around to the evacuation centers to make a list of evacuees. However, it was difficult work because the number of evacuees at each shelter frequently changed.
- Due to a definite shortage of health care personnel, it was impossible for existing health care personnel to manage all the residents' health conditions alone. Therefore, the town called for help from residents having a qualification as a nurse, and two to three nurses working at the Fukushima Prefectural Ono Hospital and the Futaba Kosei Hospital voluntarily offered help. Commissioned welfare volunteers also responded to the call for help and assisted in providing health consultation service to residents.
- Meeting and conferences were held as needed among health care personnel, the members of the social welfare center, and the town officials in charge of welfare administration to discuss how to address serious cases. Moreover, as part of health care operations at an early stage of evacuation, the town requested a medical practitioner in Futaba Town and two doctors from the Medical Association of Kazo City to offer continued visits to evacuation centers (once a month and twice a month, respectively) to examine residents. For residents living in evacuation centers separately from their family members, these doctors took time after examinations to talk with their family members about conditions and necessary treatment.
- Volunteer staff meetings have been held regularly, aiming to promote information sharing among rehabilitation staff members, volunteer organizations, the town officials in charge of health management, the social welfare center, and the post-disaster mental health care center.

(Home-visiting support)

- In Fukushima and Saitama prefectures, home-visiting support has been offered to all the residents, irrespective of whether they are children or the elderly, and whether they live in temporary housing or municipally-subsidized housing.
- After home visits, a meeting/conference has been held to assess who should be given a priority for more frequent visits.
- For residents taking shelter within Fukushima Prefecture, a health management team of Futaba Town Fukushima Branch Office has provided home-visiting support and prepared and managed a list of residents requiring special health care. This was done in collaboration with livelihood support counselors and the social welfare council.
- A health management team of Futaba Town and the social welfare council have met together to share information on all the residents. They have compiled information on all households into one register and managed it.
- In Koriyama City, temporary public health nurses, nurses dispatched from the Japanese Nursing Association and prefectural officials employed under a fixed-term contract have organized a health care team to provide a health program named "*kenko salon*" for residents. In addition, the team has provided home-visiting support to understand the health condition of all residents.
- Information on all the households taking shelter in Kazo City has been obtained through home visits and complied into a register. When the Futaba Town Office, which was temporarily relocated to Kazo City, will move to Iwaki City in the future, information on residents who will be determined to have remained in Kazo City will be entrusted to Kazo City.

Chapter 3 Situation of and Countermeasures by Each Individual Municipality

c. Summary/measures in the future
(Management of evacuation centers)
- The longer the time spent as evacuees, the more selfish the residents become due to exhaustion from living at evacuation centers.
- When the number of residents who took shelter in Kazo City amounted to some 1,300, their possible death was their greatest concern.
- Information disseminated through the mass media strongly influenced residents in evacuation centers. To avoid the spread of unnecessary concerns and baseless rumors among residents at evacuation centers, it is important to promptly provide necessary information to residents.
- Because the Futaba Town Office was temporarily relocated to Kazo City, residents taking shelter in Kazo City frequently visited health management team members. It was natural for elderly persons to rely on the team members. However, too much reliance may deter their early independence from public support. Their heavy reliance was considered quite unusual.
- It is necessary to set out rules for the favorable management of evacuation centers.

(Health care operations)
- Decentralized operations are not efficient to offer high quality health care services to residents.
- Some residents were not able to receive even essential health services such as medical examinations for young children, vaccinations, and other medical checkups. Arrangement and coordination of these services are a time consuming process. How to promptly proceed with such time consuming work in an emergency situation is one of the future tasks for the town to consider.
- The application of the Special Act on Measures concerning Nuclear Evacuees must be fully implemented throughout the country so that disaster victims can immediately receive health care services such as medical examinations for young children and vaccinations in their host municipalities. It is also indispensable to develop a system to fully and accurately understand who have undergone medical examinations and who have been left behind by these services.
- Residents are legally obligated to notify the town of their removal from the host municipality when moving to other municipalities.
- Host municipalities have no legal obligation to report or provide information to Futaba Town on the implementation of medical examinations for residents evacuated from the town. However, if residents fail to undergo routine vaccinations within a prescribed fiscal year, they have to pay for the service. Therefore, the town will strive to identify residents who have not yet received the service and encourage them to undergo the procedures as early as possible.

B Expectant/nursing mothers and children

1 Nutrition (meals/water)

a. Situation
- On the night of the earthquake, the Health Care Futaba (a comprehensive health and welfare facility) faced a shortage of artificial milk (milk powder) and baby bottles.
- Gymnasiums of elementary and junior high schools that served as evacuation centers also had no milk powder and disposable diaper stocks for the emergency.

b. Responses (actual measures)
- On the night of the earthquake, pediatrics department staff of the Futaba Kosei Hospital adjacent to

15 Efforts of Futaba Town

Health Care Futaba thankfully shared their baby bottle and milk powder stocks for residents taking shelter in Health Care Futaba.
- Milk powder and disposable diapers were distributed to the elementary and junior high school gymnasiums as well as other evacuation centers.

c. Summary/measures in the future
- Before the earthquake, the town officials had considered preparing milk powder for babies with lactose intolerance and/or allergies in case of an emergency situation. However, when the earthquake happened, they could not afford to pay attention to those babies, and even milk powder for ordinary babies had not been stored in sufficient amounts.

2 Exercise (environmental improvement)

a. Situation
- Initially, children and expectant/nursing mothers were kept sitting all day long in a confined corner of the school gymnasium.

b. Responses (actual measures)
- The highest priority was to refer expectant mothers to medical institutions with an obstetrician-gynecologist.
- As with the case of other residents, expectant mothers were also encouraged to do some exercises according to their health conditions.

c. Summary/measures in the future
- At an early stage of evacuation, it is important to inform residents of the possible development of disuse syndrome, and encourage them to do some exercises.

3 Rest (mind, anxiety, suicide, etc.)

a. Situation
- Changes in their mental condition have recently been observed among children.
- There are some preschool children who show symptoms of selective mutism. As a characteristic symptom, they have difficulties in talking with others in a group at a nursery school, kindergarten, etc. However, because they have no problem with conversation with their family members at home, most of their mothers are not concerned about the symptom.
- After residents moved from the Saitama Super Arena Stadium to evacuation centers in Kazo City, school children were also transferred to local kindergartens and schools. There were some children who were considered to be at risk of becoming a truant from school.
- Although identification of developmentally disabled children was difficult even before the earthquake, delayed detection of such children has recently become more prominent. Two to three cases have occurred, where mental disabilities of children were identified by chance when the town officials conducted home visits to the family.

b. Responses (actual measures)
- In Futaba Town, there was a mental health care center for children before the earthquake. Children with selective mutism who had received treatment at the center were referred to a day-care facility for children in each individual host municipality. According to reports from such day-care facilities, children with

Chapter 3 Situation of and Countermeasures by Each Individual Municipality

selective mutism from Futaba Town seemed to be harmfully effected by the earthquake.

- Thanks to the assistance of the doctors of the Saitama Prefectural Mental Health Center, interviews and counseling services were able to be offered to residents at the Saitama Super Arena Stadium and shelters in Kazo City.

- The town's board of education members and school personnel provided necessary support to truant students from school in host municipalities. There was a case where a public health nurse brought a truant student to the pediatrics department of a medical institution.

- Aiming at an early detection of developmentally disabled children, the town has announced a schedule of medical examinations for young children through public relations magazines. The town has also encouraged children having developmental disabilities to consult a public health center in their host municipalities.

c. Summary/measures in the future

- It is necessary to obtain information on students truant from school and share it with their teachers in host municipalities.

- Home-visiting support to each individual household was a good opportunity to provide consultation for developmentally disabled children to their mothers.

- When a resident who received home-visiting support in Kazo City moved to Iwaki City, information on this resident and home-visit records were smoothly transferred to the Iwaki Office of the Soso Public Health and Welfare Center. As can be seen from this example, it is assuring and indispensable to keep close relationships with host municipalities, particularly among public health nurses.

4 Others

a. Situation

- As a recent problem, disparities in support programs between residents within Fukushima Prefecture and those taking shelter outside Fukushima Prefecture have become prominent.

- Over the long period of time, the town constantly received inquiries about maternity health-record books, vaccinations, and medical examinations for young children.

- Vaccinations for young children within Fukushima Prefecture has been managed by Futaba Town; young children taking shelter outside the prefecture have been allowed to have vaccinations in their host municipalities based on the Special Act on Measures concerning Nuclear Evacuees. The town has made various efforts to ensure that all the residents are fully informed of the details.

b. Responses (actual measures)

- Aiming to widely inform of health care support programs for expectant/nursing mothers and children, the town has announced detailed information in public relations magazines and disaster information magazines. The town has also inserted notes about health care service information into handouts distributed to each household.

(Iodine tablets)

- When it was decided to evacuate the town on the day after the earthquake, two public health nurses headed to Kawamata Town in advance, taking emergency iodine tablet stocks with them.

- Iodine for young children is prepared in the form of syrup. It is not to be given to young children without a doctor's prescription because the dose varies by age in months. However, thanks to the support of the President of the Fukushima Pharmacists Association, who was in Kawamata Town at that time, iodine syrup was promptly prepared and given to young children. Using a small measuring cup, the public

health nurses measured a dose in millimeters, exactly following the prescription. There was a problem that there was no water to wash a used cup after it was soaked in antiseptic solution.
- With the cooperation of several certified pharmacists, the public health nurses administered iodine tablets to residents individually, spending two days to visit all evacuation centers within Kawamata Town. For young children, an iodine was administered in the form of syrup.

(Expectant/nursing mothers)
- Expectant/nursing mothers were immediately referred to an obstetrician-gynecologist in Kawamata Town, enabling the town to keep contact with them.

c. Summary/measures in the future
- Regarding a cup used to administer iodine syrup to young children, although feeling hesitant, the public health nurses had no choice but to make repeated use of the cup after soaking it in antiseptic solution and wiping with gauze. From a sanitary point of view, it was a completely inappropriate process. However, they were urgently required to administer iodine tablets/syrup to all the residents in an emergency situation, and were not to be bothered by the reuse of the cup.
- Even after expectant/nursing mothers moved to other municipalities throughout the country, the town was able to obtain information on them. Before the enforcement of the Special Act on Measures concerning Nuclear Evacuees, expectant/nursing mothers wishing to receive medical treatment/services in their host municipalities had to pay all the costs. Because they contacted the town to inquire about procedures for a refund of the payment, it was relatively easy to know where they were.

C People requiring assistance during a disaster (vulnerable people in case of a disaster)

1 Nutrition (meals/water)

a. Situation
- Many elderly residents answered that they ate instant noodles for the first time in their lives at evacuation centers.
- When the distribution of the free *bento* meals was finished, provision of meals that were specially accommodated to the condition of each patient was also ended. After that, residents had to order "*bento* meals accommodated to each patient" from a supplier, as needed.

b. Responses (actual measures)
- A training camp that served as an evacuation center was equipped with a simple kitchen, where meals specially accommodated to the conditions of patients with hypertension, renal malfunction and diabetes had been prepared in a *bento* style. Staff members of the Health and Welfare Center of Kazo City and the Saitama Cooperative Hospital assisted in organizing menus and calculating nutrient balance of such special *bento* meals.
- A commissioned nutritionist was employed in 2012. Following a decision to impose a fee for *bento* meals after September, the *bento* meals specially accommodated to the condition of patients prepared by nutritionists was also ended.

c. Summary/measures in the future
- Eating instant noodles on a daily basis may have harmful effects on the health of the residents.
- Generally speaking, providing every meal to the elderly is not desirable for their dietary independence.

Chapter 3 — Situation of and Countermeasures by Each Individual Municipality

2 Exercise (environmental improvement)

a. Situation

- A lack of exercise, particularly among the elderly, was already prominent at the primary evacuation centers.

b. Responses (actual measures)

- The head office of the Council of Social Welfare is located in Kazo City; many social welfare staff members are assigned there. They have provided various exercise programs such as nursing care preventive classes and day-care programs for residents.

c. Summary/measures in the future

- It is impossible to provide necessary health care support for residents by a health management team alone. Usually, having a favorable and continuous relationship with relevant institutions is indispensable.

3 Rest (mind, anxiety, suicide, etc.)

a. Situation

- After residents were evacuated to the Saitama Super Arena Stadium, an elderly resident living alone and having integration dysfunction syndrome was hospitalized due to a worsening of mental stability. Upon hearing that the Town Office might move somewhere else and that evacuation centers might be closed, the patient became slightly upset. Although the doctor judged that it was impossible for the patient to live in an evacuation center, the patient now lives in a private room prepared at an evacuation center in Kazo City.

b. Responses (actual measures)

- Expecting that the patients may recover their mental stability by meeting/talking with a Futaba Town official, an official in charge of residents with disabilities and a public health nurse visited the hospital to see the patient. Telling the patient that "The Town Office will not abandon you" and "We will come to pick you up," they tried to make the patient feel secure. After the patient settled down, they went to the hospital again to take him/her back to an evacuation center.

c. Summary/measures in the future

- When surrounding circumstances change and emergency situations occur, elderly people tend to lose their mental stability. To prevent them from feeling uneasy and becoming upset, it is necessary to promptly communicate correct information to them.

(Sachiko Inoi)

16 Efforts of Okuma Town

1. Situation of the municipality

(1) Demographics (as of January 1 of each year)

	2011	2012	2013
Population	11,515	10,972	10,968
Number of households	4,240	4,072	4,023
Average number of people per household	2.7	2.6	2.7
Number of births	116	111	
Birth rate	10	10.1	
Number of deaths	122	132	
Mortality	10.5	12	
Ratio of the elderly aged 65 or older	19	19	19.9

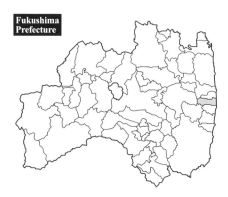

Fukushima Prefecture

(2) Geographical features

Total area: 78.70 km² (approximately 15.4 km east-west; approximately 6.7 km north-south)

Distance from the Fukushima Daiichi Nuclear Power Station of the Tokyo Electric Power Company: Four nuclear power units are located within the town

Evacuation area: an evacuation order lifting preparation zone; a restricted residence zone; a difficult-to-return zone (as of December 10, 2012)

Transportation network: National Route 6; JR Joban Line Ohno Station

2. Situation of damage by the earthquake, tsunami and the nuclear disaster

(1) Damage by the Great East Japan Earthquake (as of December 31, 2012)

Property damage	Completely destroyed	Half destroyed	Partially destroyed
House	48		
Public institution			
Other			

Human damage	Deaths by disaster	Disaster-related deaths	Missing persons	Injured persons
	11	72	1	

* Details cannot be confirmed due to the designation as a difficult-to-return district.

(2) Situation of evacuation

① Evacuation centers inside the local municipality

	Number of evacuation centers	Number of evacuees	Available period
Residents	0	0	
Evacuees received	0	0	

② Approximate number of evacuees in evacuation centers outside the local municipality (as of December 31, 2012)

	End/March 2011	End/September 2011	End/March 2012	Latest period
First evacuation center				
Second evacuation center				
Temporary housing			2,771	2,698
Municipally-subsidized housing			5,924	5,858

Chapter 3 | Situation of and Countermeasures by Each Individual Municipality

③ Approximate number of voluntary evacuees (as of December 31, 2012)

Inside Fukushima Prefecture	0	Outside Fukushima Prefecture (number of evacuees & prefectures)	0

Outlook of damage related to the nuclear disaster

- The Great East Japan Earthquake occurred on March 11, 2011. Immediately after the earthquake, the town officials were involved in disaster-relief activities at each individual evacuation center.
- An evacuation order was issued to the whole town on March 12, following which residents were evacuated to gymnasiums and other evacuation centers set up mainly in Tamura City. Establishing an earthquake emergency response headquarters within the sites of the Tamura City General Gymnasium, the town initiated disaster-relief operations at every evacuation center. After the explosion occurred at the Fukushima Daiichi Nuclear Power Station, hospitals and pharmacies were temporarily closed. Although they resumed activity before long, many residents, especially elderly residents, became ill and suffered from health problems. As a result, requests for an ambulance were continually made every day. At the end of March, the town officials were very busy taking   countermeasures against the spread of norovirus infection among residents.
- On April 3, residents moved to the secondary evacuation centers in the Aizu area. The Aizu Public Health and Welfare Office staff members (hereinafter referred to as the "the public health and welfare office") and other medical staff cooperated with each other to go around to the evacuation centers and examined residents.
- On April 5, the Okuma Town Office and its Aizu-Wakamatsu Branch Office were relocated to the Otemachi Office of the Aizu-Wakamatsu City Hall. After operations were resumed in the new office, the Okuma Town officials were fully occupied responding to the urgent needs of residents.
- In the middle of April, a health survey and health counseling for residents taking shelter in about 60 accommodation facilities located in Aizu, Kitakata and Kitashiobara areas were conducted.
- In late June, residents began moving to temporary housing. Health counseling services for residents were provided at assembly rooms within the temporary housing sites. For persons requiring assistance, home-visiting services were offered separately. Aiming to prevent residents from feeling helpless, a friendly gathering facility named "*Okuma salon –Yukkuri Suppe*" was also opened.
- In the middle of September, a nursing-care prevention class named "*Iki-iki Salon*" started.
- On October 11, the town opened the Iwaki Liaison Office within the temporary housing site prepared in the Iwaki City Yoshima Industrial Park.
- In late October, general medical examinations were initiated at the Aizu, Iwaki and Koriyama venues. Aiming to help the effective health management of residents, close coordination between other medical checkups implemented inside and outside Fukushima Prefecture was secured.

3 Countermeasures against nuclear disaster (as of May 2013)

		Name of project	Division in charge	Number of targeted persons (households)	Expect-ant mothers	Nursing moth-ers	Babies	Young children	Elemen-tary school students	Junior high school students	Senior high school students	People age 19 to 39	People age 40 or older	Remarks (major operations)
Countermeasures against external exposure	1	Lending of personal dosimeters (glass badges) (for kindergarten children to junior high school students)	Educational General Affairs Division					○	○	○				
	2	Lending of personal dosimeters (for expectant mothers and children under 18 year old)	Health Center		○		○	○	○	○	○			
	3	Refreshments for elementary school and junior high school students	Educational General Affairs Division						○	○				A gathering for reunion named "*Okumakko Minna Atsumare*"
	4	Monitoring and measurement of the air radiation levels	Environ-mental Measures Division											
	5	Measurement and mapping of the air radiation levels in the whole town	Environ-mental Measures Division											
	6	Real-time measurement of the radiation dose (Ministry of the Environment)	Ministry of the Environ-ment											
	7	Decontamination of houses (in model districts within the town)	Reconstruc-tion Projects Division											
	8	Examination of breast milk	Fukushima Prefecture			○								

138

Category	No.	Item	Division	Target	1	2	3	4	5	6	7	8	9	Remarks
Countermeasures against internal exposure	9	Whole Body Counter measurements	Health Center	All residents who are interested in the measurements	○	○		○	○	○	○	○	○	Schedule arrangement, notification and publicity
	10	Whole Body Counter measurements (conducted by Fukushima Prefecture for residents 4 to 18 years old)	Health Center					○	○	○	○			Arrangement of schedule & venue, notification and publicity
	11	Food and water quality inspection	Industry and Construction Division		○	○	○	○	○	○	○	○	○	
	12	Thyroid gland examination (conducted from May)	Health Center	All residents who are interested in the measurements	○	○		○	○	○	○	○	○	Schedule arrangement, notification and publicity
	13	Thyroid gland examination (conducted by Fukushima Prefecture)	Fukushima Prefecture	Residents aged under 18			○	○	○	○	○			
	14	Urine examination for internal exposure to radiation (conducted from May)	Health Center	Residents aged under 18			○	○	○	○	○			Schedule arrangement, notification and publicity
Others	15	Study sessions on radiation	Environmental Measures Division	All residents	○	○	○	○	○	○	○	○	○	
	16	Radiation classes	Educational General Affairs Division					○	○	○				The classes have been conducted as part of comprehensive studies at school
	17	Cancer screening	Health Center	Residents of designated ages								○	○	Lung cancer, stomach cancer, colorectal cancer, prostate cancer, uterine cancer and breast cancer
	18	Sampling of respondents for a basic survey to the Fukushima Health Management Survey	Health Center	All residents	○	○	○	○	○	○	○	○	○	
	19	Publication of disaster information magazines	General Affairs Division	All residents	○	○	○	○	○	○	○	○	○	Issuance of publicity magazine "Okuma" twice a month

* The town has commissioned the implementation of the Research Institute of Radiation Safety for Disaster Recovery Support.

Chapter 3 Situation of and Countermeasures by Each Individual Municipality

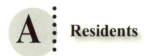

A Residents

1 Nutrition (meals/water)

a. Situation

- Because instant noodles and pastries constituted the majority of meals at primary evacuation centers, residents were at risk of becoming malnourished.
- Due to the risk of exposure to radiation, cargo trucks and other vehicles carrying emergency relief supplies were not allowed to reach evacuation centers. The relief supplies were unloaded at a transit stop nearby.
- At inns, hotels and other secondary evacuation centers, many residents were unhappy with the taste of dishes they were served. The dishes seemed to be more salty than their lightly flavored local meals.
- Although the contamination of foods by radiation was a great concern for residents, no food inspection system was available at that time. Inevitably, opinions on the intake of local rice, vegetables and water varied by person even within a family, resulting in disorganized family diets.

b. Responses (actual measures)

- When foods and other commodities were in short supply, the town distributed whatever stocks it had to residents to allow them to survive the critical situation.
- Information on facilities in host municipalities that conducted food quality inspection was conveyed to residents. Later, the town also established a system for food quality inspection on its own.

c. Summary/measures in the future

- In case distribution of emergency relief supplies and other commodities may stop due to baseless rumors, each household is advised to store several days' worth of food, artificial milk (powder milk), disposable diapers, bottled water, baby foods, etc.

2 Exercise (environmental improvement)

a. Situation

- Following an evacuation order issued to the whole town, residents took shelter in different municipalities within and outside Fukushima Prefecture. It was very difficult for the town to confirm the safety of all the residents.
- The primary evacuation centers were mainly a general gymnasium and other public facilities within Tamura City. The inferior living environment in the cold gymnasium caused the spread of norovirus infection, leading to an increased number of residents who became ill. Requests for ambulances were made continually every day.
- At medical institutions residents were first asked whether or not they had undergone radiation screening. Therefore, they were unable to receive prompt medical treatment.
- As secondary evacuation centers, approximately 60 accommodation facilities such as hotels and inns were prepared for residents in Aizu-Wakamatsu and Kitakata cities.
- Temporary housing was established mainly in Aizu-Wakamatsu and Iwaki cities. In Aizu-Wakamatsu City, residents formed a group by administrative ward to reside in temporary housing; conventional solidarity and relationships among local community members have been relatively well maintained. In contrast, because residents individually resided in temporary housing in Iwaki City, it seems that a sense

of helplessness has been growing among them.

- Each individual room within temporary housing sites is generally small and has thin walls. Residents have to pay constant attention not to make noise that would bother neighbors.
- The town has received many complaints from residents living in municipally-subsidized housing about bad accessibility to information and announcements from the town as well as about unequal distribution of necessary commodities.

b. Responses (actual measures)

- The town strived to disseminate information to residents through its public relations magazine "*Okuma*" and on a Blog.
- At the secondary evacuation centers, a health survey was conducted in cooperation with inns and hotels as well as public health and welfare offices, with the aim of understanding each individual resident's health condition. Home-visiting support was also provided to persons in need of assistance.
- Health care staff members went around to evacuation centers to offer health counseling services and medical care support to residents.

c. Summary/measures in the future

- Because residents have been forced to live for a prolonged period as evacuees, it is an urgent task to develop effective health management programs for them.

3 Rest (mind, anxiety, suicide, etc.)

a. Situation

- The primary evacuation centers for residents were mainly a general gymnasium and other public facilities within Tamura City. Because privacy was not secured at all under these inferior circumstances, many residents felt increasingly stressed at the primary evacuation centers. However, they were positively involved in volunteer work, thereby helping them to cope with their increased stress.
- After residents were evacuated to the secondary evacuation centers, private rooms were allocated at inns and hotels. While residents were able to have some extent of privacy, strong ties and the solidarity maintained among them at primary evacuation centers were broken up. Uncertainty about the future suddenly arose, causing many residents to become ill from insomnia, high blood pressure and other diseases.
- The more the details about the damage to the nuclear accident were brought to light, the more contradictory reports were made. Such a flood of complicated and differing information inevitably strengthened residents' anxiety and concerns.
- Residents are very worried about whether or not they were exposed to radiation. There exist some pessimistic opinions among them that "registered residents of Okuma Town" may not be able to marry in the future.
- Due to baseless rumors, some residents have been forced to conceal the fact that they are from Okuma Town (to avoid becoming a target of bullying, mischief and calumnies).
- There were some residents who did not want to let neighbors know that they are from Okuma Town; the town officials in charge of home visits were desperately asked not to be noticed by anyone when visiting them.
- After the earthquake, many residents lost their jobs and were forced to live separately from their family members. Extreme anxiety about the future increasingly posed serious health problems for them such as insomnia, depression, alcohol dependency, and abuse.
- Because many residents initially thought that they would be able to return home within a few days, they took shelter with the barest necessities. Unfortunately, whether or not and when they will be allowed

Chapter 3 | Situation of and Countermeasures by Each Individual Municipality

to return to the town is still far from certain. Residents are filled with anxiety about their future life.

- While recognizing that young children should not return to the town due to a high level of radiation observed, many elderly residents have a strong hope to spend their remaining lives in Okuma Town.

b. Responses (actual measures)

- At secondary evacuation centers, a health survey was conducted in cooperation with inns and hotels as well as public health and welfare offices, with the aim of understanding each individual resident's health condition. Home-visiting support was also provided to persons requiring assistance.
- In cooperation with the staff members of the Council of Social Welfare (hereinafter referred to as the "social welfare council") as well as volunteer members, a friendly gathering facility named *Okuma salon –Yukkuri Suppe*" was set up in a nearby area at the Aizu-Wakamatsu Branch Office. The purpose of this facility was to offer emotional support to residents to prevent them from experiencing a sense of helplessness.
- In collaboration with post-disaster mental health care teams dispatched from Fukushima and Kyoto prefectures, mental health counseling services and other health care programs were conducted. An "*Anmin Café*" program, which aims to help residents enjoy peaceful sleep, was also initiated.
- A questionnaire survey to assess each individual resident's health condition was conducted as part of general medical examinations by the town. If the survey and medical examination results identified residents who are supposed to be at high risk of having mental health problems, home visits were provided to them.

c. Summary/measures in the future

- Because residents have been forced to spend a prolonged period of time as evacuees, it is an urgent task to develop effective mental health care programs for them.
- The town intends to improve its health care services, with the collaboration of relevant institutions and residents' organizations; such as commissioned welfare volunteers, coordinators of dietary improvement, and health care volunteers.

4   Others

a. Situation

(Personnel)

- Three public health nurses had worked in Okuma Town (one at the regional comprehensive support center and two at the health care center). After the earthquake there was a lack of manpower and they could only to deal with immediate operations.
- Although several public health nurses were dispatched from Fukushima and other prefectures, the Okuma Town's three public health nurses had to provide detailed instructions to them, while on the other hand responding to an emergency situation.
- Because dispatched public health nurses worked on a one week shift basis, the Okuma Town's three public health nurses had to take time every week to report their activities.
- A dispatch of public health nurses from Miyoshi Town and Ogose Town (both in Saitama Prefecture) was appreciated. Because they were long-term dispatched nurses, health care operations could be confidently entrusted to them.
- Okuma Town also received a dispatch of public health nurses from Saitama, Aomori and Hokkaido prefectures.
- At evacuation centers, the town received tremendous support from volunteer residents, public health nurses of Tamura City and Miharu Town, nurses of the Ken-chu Public Health and Welfare Office, the

16 Efforts of Okuma Town

nurses of Japanese Nursing Association, and the nurses of the School of Nursing of Fukushima Medical University. Thankfully, many doctors and nurses from both Japan and abroad also assisted in offering health care operations to the victim residents.

(Increased administrative workload and the Special Act on Measures concerning Nuclear Evacuees)
- After the enforcement of the Special Act on Measures concerning Nuclear Evacuees, there was a flood of various inquires about the act from people within and outside of Fukushima Prefecture. In addition to answering such inquiries, the town officials were also required to keep close contact with host municipalities and provide explanation/notification of the act to residents, resulting in their significantly increased administrative workload. In case of vaccinations, for example, it took a long time to follow the necessary procedures such as contact with host municipalities, announcements to the residents, and requests for payment. Being fully occupied with such complicated administrative operations, the town officials were unable to focus on their regular duties, or personal services accommodating the needs of individual residents.
- After the Special Act on Measures concerning Nuclear Evacuees (hereinafter referred to as "special measures for evacuees") took effect, residents were allowed to have medical examinations for younger children and vaccinations at their host municipalities in a similar manner with local residents.
- The problem was that notification of the enforcement of the special measures for evacuees was insufficient. Because some host municipalities' divisions/sections in charge of medical examinations did not completely understand the special measures, the Okuma Town officials were unable to smoothly coordinate with them. There were also some host municipalities that were not able to afford to proceed with the necessary administrative operations for evacuee residents due to confusion after the earthquake. It seemed that there was a difference in response to and interest in, the special measures for evacuees among host municipalities.

(Nuclear power station/radiation)
- Radiation screening was conducted mainly at the Tamura City General Gymnasium. A certificate of completion was issued to residents who passed the screening. Without the certificate, residents were not allowed to enter evacuation centers and consult a doctor at medical institutions.
- Even when requesting an ambulance, residents were asked whether or not they had undergone the screening. They felt a profound resentment against the refusal to accept residents with no screening certificate, even in critical situations.
- Depending on which evacuation centers residents took shelter, some residents took stable iodine tablets/syrup and others did not. Because the administration of stable iodine tablets/syrup was not officially and accurately indicated, baseless rumors and inaccurate information further complicated the situation, thereby resulting in confusion and increased anxiety among residents.

(Health promotion activities)
- In conducting general medical examinations, it was difficult to secure venues and make announcements to the residents and respond to the needs of residents taking shelter outside Fukushima Prefecture.
- Coordination between general medical examinations conducted by the town and those implemented by the Fukushima Health Management Survey by the prefecture was poor. Residents did not know which examinations they needed to undergo.
- All of the administrative operations of the town have been temporally conducted at the Aizu-Wakamatsu Branch Office and the Iwaki Liaison Office. Currently, livelihood support counselors of the social welfare council provide home-visiting services to residents living in temporary housing and municipally-subsidized housing in the two cities. As a future task, health care services must be offered to residents

Chapter 3 — Situation of and Countermeasures by Each Individual Municipality

taking shelter in the Soma area and the Nakadori district as well.

b. Responses (actual measures)

(Health management activities)

- The town conducted medical examinations in Aizu-Wakamatsu, Koriyama and Iwaki cities for residents within Fukushima Prefecture. Regarding residents taking shelter outside Fukushima Prefecture, the implementation of group medical examinations has been entrusted to commissioned medical institutions.
- Health counseling services have been offered at assembly rooms in the temporary housing sites. At municipally-subsidized housing, *salon* programs (health-related gatherings) have been provided in cooperation with the social welfare council.
- In collaboration with the regional comprehensive support center, nursing-care prevention classes were regularly held.
- All of the administrative operations of the town have been temporally conducted at the Aizu-Wakamatsu Branch Office and the Iwaki Liaison Office. Currently, livelihood support counselors provide home-visiting services to residents living in temporary housing and municipally-subsidized housing in the two cities. For residents who are supposed to have some health problems, constant home visits have been provided even if the counselors in charge have changed.

(Nuclear power station/radiation)

- Fukushima Prefecture performed internal exposure dose inspections and thyroid gland examinations, using Whole Body Counters.
- Personal electronic dosimeters were distributed to expectant mothers and young children.
- Study sessions on radiation were held, inviting lecturers from the Education Center for Disaster Medicine of Fukushima Medical University.

c. Summary/measures in the future

- It is an urgent task to establish an effective system to obtain the latest information on all the residents' situation in host municipalities and implement a follow-up survey. Because residents have been taking shelter in different municipalities throughout the country, the town has no choice but to entrust personal care programs for the residents to each individual municipality. However, it is a town's obligation to understand the residents' entire situation and critical information. To end this, the town will strive to keep close contacts with all host municipalities.
- Some residents do not want to let neighboring people and others know that they are evacuees from Okuma Town; case-by-case responses will be required when providing home visits to them.
- From a resident perspective, more close collaboration between the town and Fukushima Prefecture is required to create a system that allows residents to smoothly undergo necessary medical examinations.
- An official of a supporting municipality said that "We really wanted to start disaster-relief operations at an early stage of evacuation, but we were not allowed to head to Okuma Town immediately after the explosion of the nuclear power station. It took a long time before we received detailed directions." Responding to this comment, an Okuma Town official said "We did not understand the situation and wondered why no relief supplies reached us." As can be seen from these remarks, a prompt and effective emergency support system among municipalities must be considered.

16 Efforts of Okuma Town

B ⋮ Expectant/nursing mothers and children

1 Nutrition (meals/water)

a. Situation

- Milk powder, water, and baby food were in short supply at the primary evacuation centers. It was also difficult to secure a place for feeding breast milk/milk powder to babies.
- Instant noodles and pastries constituted the majority of meals at the primary evacuation centers, causing a nutritionally unbalanced diet.
- Many nursing mothers were seriously concerned about food safety. There were many inquiries from them such as "Is it safe to feed breast milk?" and "Is it safe to feed home-grown vegetables to children?"

b. Responses (actual measures)

- After emergency relief supplies reached evacuees, milk powder, water, and baby foods were immediately distributed to babies and young children.
- In distributing necessary items to young children, it was almost impossible to consider their age and condition. The town officials could only distribute to them what appeared to be what was suitable for their age.

2 Exercise (environmental improvement)

a. Situation

- At the primary evacuation centers, nursing mothers had no choice but to let their crying babies cry in the spacious, yet crowded gymnasium. Because children were not allowed to play outdoors and had to spend all day long staying in a confined corner at evacuation centers, they felt increasingly stressed.
- Living in a group in the cold gymnasium resulted in the spread of norovirus infection among residents. Many infected residents suffered from symptoms such as diarrhea and vomiting.
- Implementation of all medical examinations for young children was entrusted to each individual municipality.
- Residents taking shelter in the Aizu area, where a relatively low radiation dose has been observed, were seemingly not worried about exposure to radiation. On the other hand, nursing mothers taking shelter in areas with high radiation doses showed a great concern, not letting children play outdoors.
- There are many mothers who are hesitant to or are unable to become familiar with neighbors in temporary housing because their babies frequently cry at night.
- Many families were forced to separate after the earthquake. Fathers had to live in apart for the sake of jobs, while mothers and children were unable to move to other places because of school.

b. Responses (actual measures)

- Fukushima Prefecture provided consultation services inside the prefecture. Receiving full cooperation from the Japan Midwives Association, the prefecture offered telephone counseling and baby-visiting services to expectant/nursing mothers.
- Childcare counseling services and cooking classes were conducted at a friendly gathering facility "*Okuma salon –Yukkuri Suppe*" and assembly rooms within temporary housing sites.
- Since the resumption of classes in late April, 2011, kindergartens, elementary and junior high schools have strived to communicate correct knowledge about radiation to students.

Chapter 3 | Situation of and Countermeasures by Each Individual Municipality

- Personal dosimeters (glass badges) were distributed to kindergartens, elementary and junior high schools. For young children, nursing mothers and children under 18 years of age, electronic dosimeters for personal use were distributed, at their request.

c. Summary/measures in the future
- It is urgently required to identify residents whose children have not yet undergone medical examinations and encourage them to receive the examination as early as possible.
- It is indispensable to organize data on mothers and children and systematically store and manage the data.

3 Rest (mind, anxiety, suicide, etc.)

a. Situation
- Child-rearing in unfamiliar areas caused serious stress to mothers, resulting in a trend toward increased child abuse problems.
- There were many consultations from expectant mothers about their unborn babies and possible pregnancy. Such consultations included "When I became pregnant, my husband had been working at the nuclear power station. Is there no affect to the fetus?" and "Is it safe to feed breast milk after delivering a baby?"
- Many younger generation couples rearing a child are determined not to return to Okuma Town because a high radiation dose is observed there. They feel uneasy about their uncertain future.
- Some nursing mothers are suffering from baseless rumors in host municipalities. For example, when they tell that they come from Okuma Town, they were sometimes avoided by local mothers.
- There were many concerns about the results of thyroid ultrasound examination (A2 grade) and whole body measurements.
- Some nursing mothers are worried that they and their children might have been exposed to radiation.
- Mothers have faced hardships to rear children in unfamiliar places.
- A mother was worried about her child's mental health, saying that her child might be emotionally hurt because neighboring children gradually moved to a new school.
- There are some children suffering from the trauma of the earthquake. They often cry and become nervous when aftershocks occur.

b. Responses (actual measures)
- The town distributed questionnaires at the time of the announcement of medical examinations for young children. The questions on child-rearing included: "Do you have someone in your host municipality from whom you can ask advice about childcare?", "Do you know where to go in your host municipality to ask advice about childcare?" and "Have you ever received childcare services from the municipalities?" Based on the questionnaire survey results, home visits and telephone counseling services were offered, as needed, to those requiring some follow-up support.
- Fukushima Prefecture's consultation services and full cooperation from Japan Midwives Association were greatly appreciating for supporting expectant/nursing mother.
- Health counseling services and exchange programs for mothers and children such as a gathering for children named "*Kumanoko Gakkyu*," cooking classes and a baby massage program were offered, thanks to the cooperation from public welfare and health offices, the Japan Midwives Association and a post-disaster mental health care team dispatched from Kyoto.
- Dedicated counselors were assigned to schools. Students and parents requiring some support were referred to public counseling staff members.
- When residents who need some follow-up support were identified, necessary treatment and support were

146

entrusted to public health nurses of their host municipalities.

c. Summary/measures in the future
- Because the implementation of medical examinations for young children was entrusted to host municipalities, it has increasingly become difficult for the town over time to offer face-to-face, attentive services to each individual resident. It is necessary to establish a system to ensure that residents can continue receiving necessary support and services at host municipalities during a prolonged period of evacuation.

 ## C People requiring assistance during a disaster (vulnerable people in case of a disaster)

1 Nutrition (meals/water)

a. Situation
- At the primary evacuation centers, it was impossible to separately cook soft meals for residents with special needs.
- Some elderly residents are not concerned at all about the radiation dose and eat home-grown vegetables.
- Some residents living alone did not have regular and well-balanced meals. In some cases, they developed alcohol dependency.

b. Responses (actual measures)
- When foods and other commodities were in short supply, the town distributed whatever stocks it had to residents to allow them to survive the critical situation.
- Information on facilities in host municipalities that conducted food quality inspection was conveyed to residents. Later, the town also established a system for food quality inspection on its own.

c. Summary/measures in the future
- In case the distribution of commodities may stop due to baseless rumors, each household is advised to store several days' worth of food, artificial milk (milk powder), disposable diapers, bottled water, baby food, etc.

2 Exercise (environmental improvement)

a. Situation
- Persons requiring assistance during a disaster were not fully informed of where to take shelter in an emergency.
- Because doctors and pharmacy staff were also evacuated, residents were not able to get any medical care.
- Most elderly residents desperately desire to return to Okuma Town because they consider the town to be their home for the rest of their lives. Even when their family members moved to other municipalities, they preferred to share the town's fate. Inevitably, the number of elderly people living apart from their family members increased.
- In municipally-subsidized housing, some households of elderly persons have difficulties in communicating with other residents and are mentally isolated from local neighbors.
- In providing home-visiting services, service providers must be careful to protect each resident's privacy because some residents do not appreciate the service and show their opposition, saying "Why do you visit me? How did you know I am living here?"
- There are some residents who absolutely refuse home visits and any other support from the town.

Chapter 3 | Situation of and Countermeasures by Each Individual Municipality

b. Responses (actual measures)

- Separate home-visiting services for residents with disabilities have been entrusted to the Aizu-Wakamatsu Branch Office and the Iwaki Liaison Office.
- As part of nursing care prevention efforts, a regional comprehensive support center started an exercise class named *Iki-iki Kyoshitsu* in areas with temporary housing. The center is now striving to expand the classes in other areas.

c. Summary/measures in the future

- Although some municipalities established welfare shelters, residents were not well informed about the shelters. If they had been more clearly informed, more residents with special needs would be accommodated at the shelters.
- Some persons requiring assistance during a disaster were not able to respond to the town's questionnaire survey and to ask for some support/services on their own. It is urgently required to understand their current situation. To this end, the town initiated an effort to have some connections with those left uncared of.
- Requirements for confidentiality of private information have constituted an obstacle for smooth health care operations. It is likely that the town failed to notice some residents who have remained in critical situations.
- For residents who cannot be contacted by phone, there may be no way but to ask their host municipalities to provide them home visits and necessary support.

3   Rest (mind, anxiety, suicide, etc.)

a. Situation

- For details, please refer to the section of "A. Residents."

b. Responses (actual measures)

- Regarding persons requiring assistance whose safety has not been confirmed, the town officials have repeatedly made phone calls to ask their situations.
- Home visits and other separate services are entrusted to the staff members of branch offices located in Aizu-Wakamatsu and Iwaki cities.

c. Summary/measures in the future

- Regarding persons requiring assistance who have been staying shut up at home, it is essential to develop and take effective measures for offering necessary support.
- It is desirable that the Special Act on Measures concerning Nuclear Evacuees applies not only to medical examinations but also to follow-up support programs for residents.

(Yumiko Sawada)

17 Efforts of Kawauchi Village

1 Situation of the municipality

(1) Demographics (as of January 1 of each year)

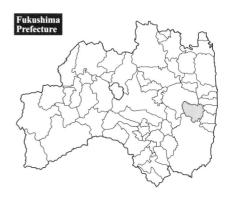

	2011	2012	2013
Population	3,031	2,887	2,820
Number of households	1,135	1,123	1,122
Average number of people per household	2.67	2.57	2.51
Number of births	15	10	
Birth rate	5.2	3.5	
Number of deaths	47	55	
Mortality	16.3	19.5	
Ratio of the elderly aged 65 or older	34.6	34.8	34.9

(2) Geographical features

Total area: 197.38 km² (approximately 15 km east-west; approximately 13 km north-south)

Distance from the Fukushima Daiichi Nuclear Power Station of the Tokyo Electric Power Company: approximately 24 km

Evacuation areas: a 20-km range from the Fukushima Daiichi Nuclear Power Station; a restricted residence zone; an evacuation order lifting preparation zone

Transportation network: Approximately 75 minutes by car from the JR Koriyama Station; Approximately 40 minutes by car from Banetsu Expressway Ono I.C.

2 Situation of damage by the earthquake, tsunami and the nuclear disaster

(1) Damage by the Great East Japan Earthquake (as of February 1, 2013)

Property damage	Completely destroyed	Half destroyed	Partially destroyed
House	4	511	160
Public institution	0	1	0
Other	0	0	0

Human damage	Deaths by disaster	Disaster-related deaths	Missing persons	Injured persons
	0	50	0	0

(2) Situation of evacuation

① Evacuation centers within the local municipality (as of February 1, 2013)

	Number of evacuation centers	Number of evacuees	Available period
Residents	1	200	3/14-16
Evacuees received	20	8,000	3/12-16

② Approximate number of evacuees in evacuation centers outside the local municipality (as of February 1, 2013)

	End/March 2011	End/September 2011	End/March 2012	Latest period
First evacuation center	295	0	0	0
Second evacuation center	506	20	0	0
Temporary housing	0	720	929	885
Municipally-subsidized housing	0	1,193	1,251	1,157

Chapter 3 | Situation of and Countermeasures by Each Individual Municipality

③ Approximate number of voluntary evacuees (As of August 5, 2011)

Inside Fukushima Prefecture	2,375

Outside Fukushima Prefecture (number of evacuees & prefectures)	617 persons in 26 prefectures

Outlook of damage related to the nuclear disaster

①When the Great East Japan Earthquake occurred on March 11, 2011, a seismic intensity of 6 or lower was observed in Kawauchi Village. Despite of such a high seismic intensity, damage in the village was not very serious. Although some roads were cracked, there were no impassable roads within the village. No housing property was destroyed and all the residents survived from the earthquake and the tsunami.

②On March 12, some 8,000 residents of Tomioka Town came into to the village to take shelter and they stayed for five days. On March 16, residents of both Tomioka Town and Kawauchi Village were evacuated together to Koriyama City.

③On April 22, the designation as "an indoor evacuation zone" of the village based on its location within a 20–30 km range from the Fukushima Daiichi Nuclear Power Station was altered to "an evacuation-prepared zone." However, judging from relatively low radiation dose in the village and a low risk of another explosion of the nuclear power station, the designation as "an evacuation-prepared zone" of the village was called off on September 30.

④In January 31, 2012, the village made a declaration of "returning home," based on its post-disaster recovery and reconstruction plan. First, the village officials returned to the village at the end of March and resumed all administrative operations from the FY2012. As of April 2012 170 residents returned to the village. Since then, the number has steadily increased; permanent returnees as of April 2013 numbered 505. Together with temporary returnees who stay in the village for over four days per week, the number totals 1,299. Although some residents have been leading a dual life in Kawauchi Village and host municipalities, approximately 40% of all residents have returned.

⑤Designation as a hazard area within a 20-km range from the Fukushima Daiichi Nuclear Power Station was called off on March 31, 2012. After the review of evacuation zones on April 1, 2012, the village was divided into two zones according to radiation dose: an evacuation order lifting preparation zone (equivalent to areas where 313 persons in 145 households resided); a restricted residence zone (equivalent to areas where 40 persons in 15 households resided).

⑥The number of residents taking shelter as of July 2013 is 1,249 persons in Koriyama City, 377 persons in Iwaki City and 396 persons in municipalities outside Fukushima Prefecture.

③ Countermeasures against nuclear disaster (as of January 2013)

		Name of project	Division in charge	Number of targeted persons (house-holds)	Expect-ant mothers	Nursing moth-ers	Babies	Young children	Elemen-tary school students	Junior high school students	Senior high school students	People age 19 to 39	People age 40 or older	Remarks (major operations)
Countermeasures against external exposure	1	Measurement by personal dosimeters	Educational Affairs Division/ Health and Welfare Division	Expectant mothers as well as junior high school students or younger	○	○	○	○	○	○				Distribution, collection, notification of results, and analysis
	2	Refreshments for elementary school and junior high school students	General affairs division, Education Bureau						○	○				Overnight exchange programs during summer and winter vacations
	3	Monitoring and measurement of the air radiation levels	Recon-struction Promotion Division	1,195 house-holds	○	○	○	○	○	○	○	○	○	Measurements of the air radiation levels were conducted for all the households from October to November 2011.
	4	Real-time measurement of the radiation dose (Ministry of the Environ-ment)	Recon-struction Promotion Division	27 mea-surement spots within the village	○	○	○	○	○	○	○	○	○	Measurement by real-time dosimeters at 72 measuring posts within the village
	5	Measurement and mapping of the air radiation levels in the whole village	Recon-struction Promotion Division	Mesh survey within a range of 2 km	○	○	○	○	○	○	○	○	○	Mapping based on the monitoring results conducted by the Ministry of Education, Culture, Sports, Science and Technology in July 2011
	6	Replacement of the surface soil on the grounds in childcare facilities, child education facilities and schools	Recon-struction Promotion Division	Three educa-tional institu-tions				○	○	○				Decontamination work of childcare facilities and elementary & junior high schools was conducted by March 2012

Category	No.	Item	Division	Target	1	2	3	4	5	6	7	8	9	Remarks
Countermeasures against internal exposure	7	Decontamination of houses	Reconstruction Promotion Division	1,195 households	○	○	○	○	○	○	○	○	○	Decontamination of houses (The decontamination work was completed in 1,159 households as of January 31, 2013)
	8	Decontamination of public and medical institutions	Reconstruction Promotion Division	Thorough decontamination of public institutions	○	○	○	○	○	○	○	○	○	Decontamination work of all public facilities was outsourced.
	9	Whole Body Counter measurements (conducted by the village)	Health and Welfare Division	All residents	○	○	○	○	○	○	○	○	○	Measurements based on agreements between medical institutions have been conducted for residents age 4 years and older, at residents' request. Announcement, acceptance, coordination and analysis of results
	10	Whole Body Counter measurements (conducted by Fukushima Prefecture for children 4 to 18 years old)	Health and Welfare Division					○	○	○	○			Notification and guiding
	11	Food and water quality inspection	Rural Development Promotion Division/ Resident Affairs Division	All households	○	○	○	○	○	○	○	○	○	Food inspection: procurement of equipment and measurement at 11 spots within the village Water quality inspection: monitoring inspection of drinking water once a week
	12	Thyroid gland examination (conducted by Fukushima Prefecture)	Health and Welfare Division					○	○	○	○			
	13	Inspection of school meals	Educational Affairs Division					○	○	○				Inspection of both each individual ingredients for meals and meals as a whole offered at childcare facilities and elementary & junior high schools
	14	Thyroid gland examination, lecture meetings on radiation and health counseling (conducted by the village)	Health and Welfare Division					○	○	○	○	○		Planning, arrangement of lecturers and publicity
	15	Debriefing sessions for measurement results of exposure dose	Health and Welfare Division									○	○	Planning, arrangement of lecturers and notification
	16	Cancer screening	Health and Welfare Division									○	○	
Others	17	Replacement of the surface soil in rice paddies	Rural Development Promotion Division	Decontamination of rice paddies, vegetable fields and grassland	○	○	○	○	○	○	○	○	○	Decontamination work is now underway in 432 ha of rice paddies, 182 ha of vegetable fields and 95 ha of grassland.
	18	Measurement and mapping of the radiation dose in the soil in the whole village	Rural Development Promotion Division	Soil survey in rice paddies	○	○	○	○	○	○	○	○	○	Soil survey at 218 spots
	19	Study sessions on radiation	Health and Welfare Division	All residents								○	○	Health counseling has also been held simultaneously.
	20	Sampling of respondents for a basic survey in the Fukushima Health Management Survey	Health and Welfare Division											Conducted by Fukushima Prefecture (The village conducts publicity activities.)
	21	Publication of disaster information magazines	General Affairs Division	For both evacuated and returned residents	○	○	○	○	○	○	○	○	○	Preparation of articles, printing, distribution and sorting out

Chapter 3 Situation of and Countermeasures by Each Individual Municipality

A Residents

1 Nutrition (meals/water)

a. Situation

- Because rice balls and pastries initially constituted the majority of meals at evacuation centers, a nutritionally unbalanced diet was a great concern.
- Some residents purposely kept an excessive amount of personal emergency relief supplies (foods) at evacuation centers, which caused food sanitation-related problems.
- A prolonged stay at evacuation centers and uncomfortable living conditions at temporary housing inevitably resulted in residents' decreased motivation to cook. There were many residents who did not cook themselves, purchasing *bento* meals and other ready-prepared foods every day.
- A worsening of their metabolic syndrome screening results was found in some residents.
- At the evacuation centers, many residents with lifestyle related diseases were not able to continue self-treatment and self-control of their lifestyle.
- Because the village had no waterworks, concerns about well water contamination by radioactive materials increased among residents.
- Despite feeling some anxiety about soil contamination by radiation, returnees started growing vegetables on their own because there were only a few stores within the village and returnees had difficulties in procuring their daily food stuffs.

b. Responses (actual measures)

- Food quality inspection was conducted at assembly rooms in evacuation centers.
- Water inspection was conducted.
- Lecture meetings on radiation and counseling on radiation were held.
- Nationally certified senior nutritionists provided nutritional guidance and cooking programs for residents.

c. Summary/measures in the future

- Effective dietary management at evacuation centers, particularly for residents with diseases, needs to be discussed.
- It is necessary to take long-term measures to prevent the development of lifestyle related diseases.

2 Exercise (environmental improvement)

a. Situation

- At evacuation centers residents were initially forced to live in a confined space, and were feeling anxious about the emergency situation they faced, exposure to radiation and the future. Inevitably, residents had a lack of exercise, generating a great concern about physical malfunctions and the development of physical inactivity diseases (disuse syndrome) such as deep vein thrombosis/pulmonary embolism (the so-called "economy-class syndrome").
- After moving to the secondary evacuation centers and temporary housing, there were many residents who started taking walks with friends. However, the entire amount of exercise and activity in their daily lives were decreased compared to before the earthquake.

17 Efforts of Kawauchi Village

b. Responses (actual measures)
- Care prevention prevention classes were held at assembly rooms within the temporary housing sites.

c. Summary/measures in the future
- It is necessary to ensure that residents fully understand the importance of exercise and effective exercise examples, thereby preventing them from needing nursing-care support and developing lifestyle related diseases.
- Nursing-care and lifestyle related disease prevention programs are scheduled to be held in each individual residential ward by health care support volunteers.

3 Rest (mind, anxiety, suicide, etc.)

a. Situation
- Residents in municipally-subsidized housing tended to feel helplessness due to the lack of exchanges with local neighbors.
- Many residents experienced growing stress due to concerns about the future and a sudden change in family structure (breaking up of family units).
- After administrative operations were resumed in Kawauchi Village, many of the residents taking shelter in other municipalities tended to feel left behind.

b. Responses (actual measures)
- Home-visiting services were offered to attentively listen to concerns and problems of each individual resident.
- Staff members of a post-disaster mental health care team/center conducted home visits.
- Post-disaster mental health care programs were conducted (tips for good sleep, music therapy, etc.).
- Training programs to attentively listen to residents were carried out mainly for commissioned welfare volunteers.
- Lecture meetings and counseling programs on radiation were conducted.

c. Summary/measures in the future
- Continued mental health care programs and home-visiting services are necessary.
- It is necessary to create a system that enables local community members such as commissioned welfare volunteers, women's association members, and other supporting volunteers to effectively support and attentively listen to the residents.

B Expectant/nursing mothers and children

1. Nutrition (meals/water)

a. Situation
- Many expectant/nursing mothers and children were evacuated to outside Fukushima Prefecture shortly after the earthquake. Among residents who took shelter with the village officials, there were young children in need of artificial milk (milk powder) and baby foods.
- Because rice balls and pastries initially constituted the majority of meals at evacuation centers, the intake of sugar and snacks inevitably increased. Undesirable dietary habits and unregulated rhythms of daily lives were found among residents.

Chapter 3   Situation of and Countermeasures by Each Individual Municipality

- Due to increased opportunities to eat ready-prepared meals, many children increasingly preferred strong-tasting foods.
- There were residents who felt anxious about food contamination (water and vegetables) and breast milk contamination by radiation.

b. Responses (actual measures)
- After emergency relief supplies reached evacuation centers, milk powder and baby foods were immediately distributed to young children, as needed.
- At the time of medical examinations for young children, counseling programs were also provided.

c. Summary/measures in the future
- It is necessary to include milk powder, baby foods and disposable diapers into stockpiles for an emergency.

2   Exercise (environmental improvement)

a. Situation
- Because children were not initially allowed to play outdoors, their activity levels decreased. As a result, a decline in their body strength was observed.

b. Responses (actual measures)
- Play corners for kids were set up within the sites of evacuation centers.
- Personal dosimeters (glass badges) were distributed.
- Lecture meetings on radiation were conducted.
- Decontamination work was conducted both inside and outside all school buildings and school zones within the village.
- Monitoring posts (equipment to monitor radiation dose in the environment) were installed in the village.

c. Summary/measures in the future
- Club activities at school and other outdoor activities were resumed after the completion of decontamination work. Therefore, the amount of exercise has gradually increased for students.
- Lectures on radiation and lifestyle related diseases were held, in cooperation with schools.
- Based on the results of medical examinations, the village intends to intensify cooperation with schools to take adequate measures for health care of students.

3   Rest (mind, anxiety, suicide, etc.)

a. Situation
- Living in a group at evacuation centers caused unregulated rhythms of daily lives. As a result, an increasing number of children showed mental instability and frequent thumb-sucking.
- There were many parents/guardians who showed anxiety about radiation effects on the health of their children.
- Sudden changes in family environments caused nursing mothers and children to feel increasing stress.
- Residents were very confused by the flood of information, not knowing what to trust.

b. Responses (actual measures)
- The village made arrangement so that residents can undergo medical examinations and vaccinations in

their host municipalities.
- Certified clinical psychologists organized lecture meetings and gatherings mainly for residents taking shelter in other municipalities.
- Medical examinations for young children and counseling programs were implemented.
- Lecture meetings on radiation were held.

c. Summary/measures in the future

- Home-visiting services are very important as an opportunity to listen carefully to each individual resident.
- It is necessary to provide more opportunities (such as medical examinations) for parents/guardians to exchange information with each other.
- Early dissemination of correct information is indispensable to prevent residents from being confused and seized with anxiety by the flood of information they might experience.

C People requiring assistance during a disaster (vulnerable people in case of a disaster)

1 Nutrition (meals/water)

a. Situation

- Because meals were indiscriminately supplied to residents at evacuation centers, it was impossible to respond to special needs of the elderly and persons with diseases.
- Some residents did not take shelter even after the entire village was designated as a hazard area. Water, food, and other commodities were provided to them once a week.
- Because the village had no waterworks, concerns about the contamination of well water by radioactive materials increased among residents.

b. Responses (actual measures)

- A request was made to supply more healthy and well-balanced meals to residents at evacuation centers.
- Instruction programs to prevent food poisoning were provided to residents.
- In cooperation with dietetic associations, rice porridge was offered to residents, as needed.
- Nutritionists offered group education programs. They also visited each home to provide dietary guidance.
- At the time of returning medical examination results to residents, personal nutritional guidance was also offered, as needed.

c. Summary/measures in the future

- It is indispensable to include food and other commodities for persons with special needs into stockpiles for an emergency.
- It is necessary to secure special meals for patients undergoing artificial dialysis and/or having diabetes.

2 Exercise (environmental improvement)

a. Situation

- At evacuation centers residents initially were forced to live in a confined space, feeling anxious about the emergency situation they faced, exposure to radiation, and the future. Inevitably residents did not get enough exercise, generating a great concern for the development of economy-class syndrome and a decline in their physical strength.

Chapter 3 | Situation of and Countermeasures by Each Individual Municipality

- Immediately after evacuation, residents who had received nursing-care services were temporarily not able to get necessary day-care services at a dedicated facility. As a result, their physical activity decreased.
- At evacuation centers and in host municipalities, persons with special needs were unable to receive nursing care support and faced a decline in their physical function. As a result, an increasing number of residents with special needs applied for permission to receive public nursing care support or to reside in nursing-care facilities.

b. Responses (actual measures)
- The village's health care officials helped a diaper exchange.
- Nursing-care services by dedicated staff members and other volunteer members were coordinated.
- Various programs were conducted in an effort to prevent the development of economy class syndrome.
- In collaboration with exercise-related volunteer members, nursing-care prevention programs were conducted.
- Nursing-care prevention classes were provided at assembly rooms in temporary housing sites.

c. Summary/measures in the future
- To prevent residents from needing nursing-care support and developing economy class syndrome, it is necessary to take effective measure as early as possible to ensure that residents fully understand the importance of exercise. Securing dedicated staff members and fostering volunteer members are also indispensable steps.

3　Rest (mind, anxiety, suicide, etc.)

a. Situation
- Many residents were terribly anxious about aftershocks, radiation and the future, feeling severely stressed due to living in a group at evacuation centers.
- Because of the sudden change in the living environment at evacuation centers and in host municipalities, as well as being anxious about uncertainties about the future and about radiation, many residents became ill from insomnia and depression.
- Many residents experienced a change in family structure (breaking up of family members units) after evacuation and returning to their village, thereby feeling considerably anxious and stressed.
- After the village resumed administrative operations in Kawauchi Village, many residents taking shelter in host municipalities experienced a feeling that they were left behind.

b. Responses (actual measures)
- Home-visiting services were offered to attentively listen to concerns and problems of each individual resident.
- Staff members of a post-disaster mental health care team/center provided home visits.
- Post-disaster mental health care programs were conducted (tips for good sleep, music therapy, etc.).
- Lecture meetings and counseling programs on radiation were conducted.

c. Summary/measures in the future
- Because evacuees are eager to talk to others, it is necessary to provide home visits to listen to them.
- It is important for the village to collect information on medical institutions and have closer collaboration with them.

D Others

- Arrangements for medical examinations and vaccinations for evacuees were conducted.
- Nursing-care prevention classes and various types of salon (gatherings) programs were implemented.
- Social gatherings for residents were conducted.
- Health counseling services were offered after examinations for internal exposure to radiation and thyroid gland examinations that were both conducted by Fukushima Prefecture.
- Lecture meetings on radiation, mainly by health management advisers, and gatherings for information exchange were held.
- Pharmacists provided health education programs and counseling services.
- Mental health management measures by the village:
  - It is necessary to establish an official register of residents requiring assistance and regularly provide evacuation drill programs for them in case of an emergency.
  - It is important to have the latest contact information about residents (for example, a register of evacuees) to confirm their safety and their health conditions.
  - The administrative workload of the village officials has increased due to the arrangement of supporting staff members, health investigation programs and other operations.

(Keiko Ikari)

18. Efforts of Naraha Town

1. Situation of the municipality

(1) Demographics (as of January 1 of each year)

	2011	2012	2013
Population	8,027	7,701	7,655
Number of households	2,892	2,801	2,780
Average number of people per household	2.78	2.75	2.75
Number of births	59	39	
Birth rate	7.35	5.06	
Number of deaths	137	69	
Mortality	17.06	8.96	
Ratio of the elderly aged 65 or older	25.8	25.49	26.61

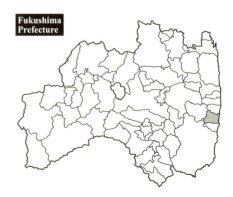

Fukushima Prefecture

(2) Geographical features

Total area: 103.45 km²

- Naraha Town is located in an area facing the Abukuma mountain range in the west and the Pacific Ocean in the east. The Ide and Kido rivers run through the town. With a temperate climate all the year round, the town has almost no snowfall in winter.

Distance from the Fukushima Daiichi Nuclear Power Station of the Tokyo Electric Power Company: within a 20-km range

Distance from the Fukushima Daini Nuclear Power Station: within an 8-km range.

Initially, almost 80% of the total town area was designated as a hazardous area. Based on the revision of hazardous areas on August 10, 2012, the town has been designated as an evacuation order lifting preparation zone.

Transportation network: JR Joban Line (Tatsuta Station and Kido Station); National Route 6; Iwaki-Namie Line of Prefectural Road 35

"Michi-no-eki Naraha," a rest stop characterized by an *onsen* facility for one-day visitors, is one of the sights of the town.

- Focusing on the fostering of football players and promotion of sport and health industries, Naraha Town established the "J Village," a complex to train national football players, and a medical center in the vicinity of the complex. The town has also actively promoted the tourist industry based on its abundant natural environment, by establishing *onsen* facilities, places for *ayu* (sweetfish)/salmon fishing, seaside swimming areas and campgrounds.

2. Situation of damage by the earthquake, tsunami and the nuclear disaster

(1) Damage by the Great East Japan Earthquake (as of October 1, 2013)

Property damage	Completely destroyed	Half destroyed	Partially destroyed
House	7.8	789	351
Public institution			
Other			

Human damage	Deaths by disaster	Disaster-related deaths	Missing persons	Injured persons
	11	79	2	5

* Damage to houses is still under investigation.

* An estimated 10.5 meter high tsunami was observed in the town, causing some 2.87 km² of area including residential land and rice paddies to be flooded. The number of houses that have so far been confirmed to have been swept away or were flooded by the tsunami is 125. In addition to direct damage by the earthquake and tsunami, indirect damage must be considered. A prolonged evacuation has resulted in further damage to houses due to wear and tear from moisture and leaks in the roof. Burglary and invasion by wild and livestock animals have also caused houses to be run-down.

18 Efforts of Naraha Town

(2) Situation of evacuation

① Evacuation centers within the local municipality (as of January 1, 2013)

	Number of evacuation centers	Number of evacuees	Available period
Residents	0	0	
Evacuees received	0	0	

② Approximate number of evacuees in evacuation centers outside the local municipality (as of April 1, 2013)

	End/March 2011	End/September 2011	End/March 2012	Latest period
First evacuation center	Unknown	24	0	0
Second evacuation center	Unknown	73	5	0
Temporary housing	0	1,211	2,840	3,049
Municipally-subsidized housing	0	1,344	3,888	3,771

③ Approximate number of voluntary evacuees (As of April 1, 2013)

Inside Fukushima Prefecture	0		Outside Fukushima Prefecture (number of evacuees & prefectures)	None

---

Outlook of damage related to the nuclear disaster

① A massive earthquake with a magnitude of 9 occurred at 14:46 on March 11, 2011. Immediately after the earthquake, a warning of a giant tsunami was issued to residents living in coastal areas. Following the warning, town officials guided the residents to evacuation centers located on higher grounds. They spent the whole night there.

② At 08:00 on March 12, the town used the local wireless radio broadcasting system to order all residents to take shelter to the south. Following the order, residents shared cars to drive to a total of eight evacuation centers within Iwaki City. Some residents headed to other municipalities throughout the country, counting on staying with their close friends or relatives. For the evacuation of some 120 residents living in nursing-care facilities within the town, official vehicles and buses were used to drive them to evacuation centers in Iwaki City. For the elderly residents living in nursing-care welfare/health facilities, residents living in group homes for persons with mental and intellectual disabilities, and the elderly residents regularly visiting day-care facilities, the town officials drove them to evacuation centers in Iwaki City. At 16:00 on that day, the town established a disaster response headquarters in the premises of Iwaki City Chuo-dai Minami Elementary School. A maximum of 5,771 residents took shelter in evacuation centers within Iwaki City.

③ Because the distribution of commodities stopped due to the explosion of the Fukushima Daiichi Nuclear Power Station of Tokyo Electric Power Company (hereinafter referred to as the "Fukushima Daiichi Nuclear Power Station"), food, gasoline and other commodities were in short supply. Moreover, because residents of Iwaki City were also evacuated to other municipalities, evacuees from Naraha Town were unable to consult medical institutions and pharmacies. Dispatch of health management assistance teams from other prefectures was also halted. Under such a critical situation, a growing fear of death and feeling of anxiety were rapidly spread among officials and residents. In an effort to mediate the effects of exposure to radiation, the officials distributed stable iodine tablets/syrup to each evacuation center and made them ready for administration at any time.
Based on "a mutual cooperation agreement on disaster prevention and disaster relief" concluded with Aizumisato Town, the town decided on March 16 to evacuate residents to Aizumisato Town. Priority of evacuation was given to, in order, expectant mothers, children and the elderly. A total of some 1,000 residents were evacuated to Aizumisato Town in seven stages. (Some residents chose to stay in evacuation centers in Iwaki City.)

④ Radiation exposure screening at evacuation centers started on March 14, 2011. A certificate of completion was issued to the residents who underwent the screening test. Without the certificate, residents were not allowed to enter inns, guesthouses, public facilities and other evacuation centers. However, there were some residents who had difficulties in going to the screening venues due to a lack of gasoline and no means of transportation.

⑤ A strong aftershock occurred on April 11, 2011, making residents taking shelter in Iwaki City frightened and extremely uneasy.

⑥ In April 2011, the town began evacuating residents to inns, hotels and other secondary evacuation centers located in the Aizu area (33 sites) and Iwaki City (4 sites). The officials not only supported residents' evacuation but also resumed their regular duties such as administrative procedures for vaccinations and medical examinations for expectant mothers. However, because residents were scattered all over Japan, administrative duties and contact/coordination work were terribly complicated, causing the officials' workload to increase many times over.

⑦ In June 2011, residents began moving to temporary housing (one in Aizumisato Town and 13 in Iwaki City). After the movement, home visits were provided with the aim of understanding each individual resident's condition.
Furthermore, from September 2011 the town sequentially set up; one support center and one group home within the temporary housing site in Aizumisato Town, and two support centers and two group homes (one for persons with disabilities) within the temporary housing sites in Iwaki City. At these facilities, a wide variety of programs were offered to accommodate the immediate needs of, mainly, young children, the elderly, and persons with disabilities. Such programs included short-term day care support for young children, gatherings for nursing mothers, nursing-care prevention classes, and short-term stays at nursing-care facilities for the elderly.
In April 2012, Naraha Town's elementary school and junior high school resumed classes at temporary school buildings. *Kodomoen*, a facility serving as both a kindergarten and a day nursery, was also resumed in January 2013.

159

Chapter 3 Situation of and Countermeasures by Each Individual Municipality

⑧ As a result of the revision of hazardous areas, the town was designated as an evacuation order lifting preparation zone on August 10, 2012. Because daytime return was permitted in the zone, an increasing number of residents went back to the town during the day to clean and fix their houses.

⑨ After temporary housing was established in Iwaki City, residents taking shelter in the Aizu area and other municipalities outside Fukushima Prefecture increasingly moved to Iwaki City. Therefore, the town office was also relocated to Iwaki City to offer effective and prompt administrative support to the residents. Given that residents will be forced to continue to be evacuees, it is urgent for the town to find a way to receive full cooperation from host municipalities in offering necessary administrative services to the residents. At the same time, keeping close cooperative relationships with other municipalities displaced due to the disaster will also be indispensable. To these ends, a new organizational framework that enables the adequate managing of administrative duties must be established. It is also a pressing issue to develop; livelihood support programs for the affected residents (particularly programs that help residents can feel fulfilled, community fostering programs, etc.), health management programs concerning possible exposure to radiation, preventive measures against disuse syndrome and lifestyle related diseases. Regarding support programs for children, it is necessary to conduct a follow-up survey over time to examine how their physical and mental development was effected by their unstable life as evacuees, sudden changes in family structures and exposure to radiation. Long term support based on the follow-up survey results must be offered.

Moreover, facing the sudden separation due to the evacuation, many families have had difficulties in supporting and caring for their elderly family members living apart. To address this serious problem, the town is urgently required to develop a new health-care/welfare/medical support system, thereby effectively responding to the immediate needs of residents.

⑩ Aftershocks sometimes occur, even now, causing residents to feel anxiety and frightened. Additionally, reports by the mass media about the accidents at the Fukushima Daiichi Nuclear Power Station always make residents become fearful, and some residents exhibit post-traumatic stress symptoms.

⑪ It is said that it takes several decades to complete decommissioning work. Because many residents are supposed to be involved in the decommissioning work in the future, the town is required to closely cooperate with personnel working at many other duties to provide adequate health management and medical programs for such residents.

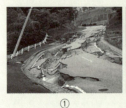
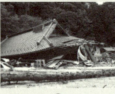
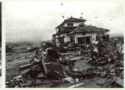
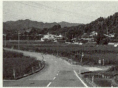

① ② ③ Damage by the earthquake and the tsunami

Tall goldenrod growing thick all over the paddy fields in the town

3 Countermeasures against nuclear disaster (as of January 2013)

		Name of project	Division in charge	Number of targeted persons (households)	Expectant mothers	Nursing mothers	Babies	Young children	Elementary school students	Junior high school students	Senior high school students	People age 19 to 39	People age 40 or older	Remarks (major operations)
Countermeasures against external exposure	1	Measurement by personal dosimeters (glass badges)	Radiation Measures Division	All residents	○	○	○	○	○	○	○	○	○	Procurement, distribution, calibration and management
	2	Lending of Geiger counters	Radiation Measures Division	Companies and returnees										Procurement, lending, calibration and management
	3	Lending and distribution of air dosimeters	Radiation Measures Division	All households and residents	○	○	○	○	○	○	○	○	○	Procurement, distribution, lending, calibration and management
	4	Monitoring and measurement of the air radiation levels	Radiation Measures Division											Procurement, management, recording and public announcement
	5	Real-time measurement of the radiation dose (Ministry of the Environment)	Radiation Measures Division											Conducted by the Ministry of the Environment
	6	Measurement and mapping of the air radiation levels in the whole town	Radiation Measures Division											Conducted by the Ministry of the Environment
	7	Replacement of the surface soil on the grounds in childcare facilities, child education facilities and schools	Radiation Management Division											Conducted by the Ministry of the Environment

	No.	Item	Division	Target	1	2	3	4	5	6	7	8	9	Remarks
Countermeasures against internal exposure	8	Decontamination of houses (Ministry of the Environment)	Radiation Measures Division	All households	○	○	○	○	○	○	○	○	○	Conducted by the Ministry of the Environment
	9	Decontamination of public and medical institutions (Ministry of the Environment)	Radiation Measures Division											Conducted by the Ministry of the Environment
	10	Examination of breast milk	Radiation Measures Division	50 persons		○								Measurement of a radiation dose
	11	Whole Body Counter measurements (conducted by the town)	Radiation Measures Division	All residents	○	○	○	○	○	○	○	○	○	Schedule arrangement, notification of results, contracts, publicity, guiding and shuttle bus service
	12	Whole Body Counter measurements (conducted by Fukushima Prefecture for children aged 4 to 18)	Radiation Measures Division	900 residents aged 4 to 18	○	○	○	○	○					Notification, guiding and publicity
	13	Food and water quality inspection	Radiation Measures Division	All residents	○	○	○	○	○	○	○	○	○	Procurement of equipment and measurement
	14	Thyroid gland examination (examined by Fukushima Prefecture)	Resident's Welfare Division	400 persons			○	○	○	○	○			Publicity (Implementation is conducted by Fukushima Prefecture)
	15	Blood test (conducted by Fukushima Prefecture)	Resident's Welfare Division	All residents	○	○	○	○	○	○	○	○	○	Publicity, notification of results, implementation and aggregation of results
	16	Inspection of school meals	Board of Education				○	○	○	○				Procurement of equipment, inspection and training of school personnel
	17	Debriefing sessions for measurement results of exposure dose	Radiation Measures Division	All residents	○	○	○	○	○	○	○	○	○	Notification and publicity
	18	Study sessions on radiation	Radiation Measures Division	All residents	○	○	○	○	○	○	○	○	○	Publicity and implementation
Others	19	Cancer screening (for residents aged 20 to 39, at their request)	Resident's Welfare Division	2,000 persons								○		Publicity, implementation and notification of results
	20	Replacement of the surface soil in rice paddies	Industrial Promotion Division											Conducted by the Ministry of the Environment
	21	Measurement and monitoring of the radiation dose in the soil in the whole town	Radiation Management Division											Conducted by the Ministry of the Environment
	22	Lecture meetings on radiation	Radiation Measures Division	All residents	○	○	○	○	○	○	○	○	○	Publicity, implementation and request for lecturers
	23	Sampling of respondents for a basic survey in the Fukushima Health Management Survey	Resident's Welfare Division	All residents	○	○	○	○	○	○	○	○	○	
	24	Publication of disaster information magazines	Environment Protection and Disaster Prevention Division	All households			○	○	○	○	○	○	○	In public relations magazines
	25	Issuance of citizen health cards (containing a column for recording radiation exposure levels)	Resident's Welfare Division	All residents	○	○	○	○	○	○	○	○	○	Conducted by Fukushima Prefecture
	26	Distribution of protective clothing	Environment Protection and Disaster Prevention Division	Returned residents and residents who request the distribution							○	○	○	Off-site Center
	27	Planting test	Industrial Promotion Division											Planning and implementation

Chapter 3 Situation of and Countermeasures by Each Individual Municipality

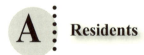

A Residents

1 Nutrition (meals/water)

a. Situation

(From March to April 2011)
- Residents had only two meals per day. Due to high-carbohydrate and high-salt diet, an increasing number of residents complained of hypertension, hyperglycemia and constipation.

(From April to July 2011)
- Residents were able to have three well-balanced meals per day after they moved to inns and hotels.

(After August 2011)
- Residents began moving to temporary housing and municipally-subsidized housing. Some family members were forced to live separately, constituting small-scale households. As a result of such sudden changes in a living environment, the number of residents who did not cook for themselves increased. Most of them purchased ready-prepared dishes and pre-packed *bento* meals at convenience stores and supermarkets or dined out.

b. Responses (actual measures)
- The town strived to secure three meals per day, by combining relief foods and *bento* meals. Nutritionists visited each evacuation center to provide nutritional advice to residents.
- Nutritional advice was provided at inns and hotels.

c. Summary/measures in the future
- Diet environments have drastically changed after the earthquake, causing residents to purchase ready-prepared dishes and eat out frequently. Many residents eat alone of unvarying foods such as high-calorie, nutritionally unbalanced and strong taste meals that are sold in a single serving. The greatest concern caused by such diets was the development/worsening of lifestyle related diseases, increased mental stress and other severe health problems. It is indispensable to offer effective diet support for residents, according to their actual conditions and living environments.

2 Exercise (environmental improvement)

a. Situation
- A cold virus spread among the residents during the first month after the earthquake. There were some elderly residents who were hospitalized due to the development of pneumonia.
- Immediately after the earthquake, there was an increase in number of cases of hypertension among town officials and firefighters.
- After moving to secondary evacuation centers such as hotels and guesthouses, privacy was secured thanks to private rooms. However, because most residents stayed in their own room during the day, it became difficult for the town to understand their situations.
- Some residents did not have anything to do during the day because of unemployment and sudden changes of residential/living environments. Inevitably, their total exercise taken and physical activities decreased.

| | 18 | Efforts of Naraha Town |

- Various medical examination results revealed that an increasing number of residents gained weight and experienced higher blood sugar levels and increased blood pressure, compared to before the earthquake. This trend was particularly prominent among residents in their fifties and sixties.
- After the designation as a hazard area was canceled on August 10, 2012, daytime return was allowed. Many residents went back to the town during the day to clean and fix their houses.

b. Responses (actual measures)

- Medicines were prescribed at the time of health checks by medical staff members who went around to evacuation centers or they were prepared based on each individual resident's drug diary (maximum three days' worth of medicines). Remedies for colds as well as other medical and sanitary supplies were secured and provided, as needed.
- Immediately after evacuation, the town focused on the medical treatment and health management of the town officials and firefighting members.
- At an early stage of evacuation, residents were encouraged to gather at a reception hall of hotels and other evacuation centers to do exercise together. After moving into temporary housing and municipally-subsidized housing, weekly nursing-care prevention classes and exercise classes were conducted at assembly rooms in temporary housing sites and nearby vacant stores. Radio gymnastic exercise programs were also conducted every morning at an assembly room in all temporary housing, leading to a regular habit of exercise among residents.
- Effects of nursing-care prevention classes and exercise classes were evaluated based on the results of physical fitness tests. The town advised staff members at these classes to attentively respond to the needs and situations of each individual resident.
- Since the designation as a hazard area was canceled and daytime return was allowed, the town has measured a radiation dose in water, finished products and farm products of Naraha Town five days in a week. The town has also lent radiation meters/air dosimeters to residents who wish to measure air levels both inside and outside a house and the radiation dose of the laundry hung indoor and of daily commodities.

c. Summary/measures in the future

- The development of physical inactivity diseases (disuse syndrome) at evacuation centers must be prevented. To this end, it is required to encourage residents at an early stage of evacuation to do some physical activities, depending on their situation and physical condition. It is also indispensable to improve and ensure an exercise environment in which residents can take a walk and exercise during the period of evacuation.

3 Rest (mind, anxiety, suicide, etc.)

a. Situation

(March 11 to April, 2011)

- The city was deluged with daily protest calls about unsatisfactory services from residents, arising from their anxiety about radiation, concerns about health, fear, resentment and anger. There were also some residents who were strongly tortured by a feeling of sadness and felt guilty about leaving their pets and livestock animals at home.

(After May 2011)

- Because of unemployment and uncertainty for the future, residents were filled with deep resentment, dissatisfaction and nostalgia.
- After the relocation to temporary housing and municipally-subsidized housing, strong dissatisfaction

Chapter 3 | Situation of and Countermeasures by Each Individual Municipality

arose among residents in municipally-subsidized housing and among those taking shelter in other prefectures because they felt unfairness in accessibility of necessary information, commodities and services, compared to residents in temporary housing. Residents also increasingly suffered from the heavy stress of unfamiliar residential environments, sudden changes in their lifestyle, new relationships with others and sleeplessness. Moreover, residents were differently damaged by the earthquake, the tsunami and the nuclear power plant accident. Inevitably, residents had different feelings and opinions, causing a growing sense of inequality and discrimination among them.

- With the prolonged period of evacuation, many residents lost their roles at home and in society, and began suffered from declined motivation, apathy, and a sense of loss.

- Residents suffered from an excessive amount of mental stress, a decline in their concentration/memory, uneasiness, a lack of confidence, sleeplessness and other problems caused by anxiety for the future and by unstable surrounding conditions. As a result, an increase in the frequency/amount of drinking alcohol and habitual drinking in the morning were observed among male residents. For female residents, a frequent intake of sleeping pills was a common tendency.

- Many elderly residents showed a decline in their physical & mental function and developed cognitive impairment. As a result, severe burdens of nursing-care support have been imposed upon their family members.

- There is a wide gap in opinions among generations over residents' return to Naraha Town. Even among a family, a sharp divergence of opinion exists. Some residents are concerned about their future, while others are filled with extreme anxiety about their livelihood in the future. As another remarkable change after the earthquake, an increasing number of residents consulted with friends about their concerns and anxiety, not their family members. It must also be mentioned that some residents have been unable to consult with anyone after the earthquake.

b. Responses (actual measures)

- Post-disaster mental care team members went around at the primary/secondary evacuation centers to check the health condition of each individual resident and offer counseling services.

- In September 2011, a survey on evacuees' behavior and a study session on radiation were conducted, in cooperation with Fukushima Medical University.

- After residents moved to temporary housing, *"Otoko Meshi,"* a cooking program for alcohol-dependent residents and male residents living alone, was held every month.

- Comprehensive medical examinations (general medical checkups and cancer screenings) were implemented in July and September 2011. Medical examinations for residents taking shelter outside Fukushima Prefecture were conducted in December. Follow-up instructions and briefing sessions started in November 2011. Moreover, health management guidance for residents with metabolic syndrome also started in November 2012.

- Aiming to promote health improvement and active exchanges among residents, health counseling and a health-related program named *"kenko-salon"* have been provided at temporary housing sites.

- Before the earthquake, the town had planned a talk & concert event named *"Kokoro-no Talk & Concert"* as part of its suicide prevention initiatives. With almost two years since the planning, the event was finally held on March 9 and 10, 2013. Many residents energetically took part in this event from planning to the preparatory processes. Taking the opportunity of this talk and concert event, a CD song with a theme of great nostalgia for Naraha Town was released under the title *"Furusato-kara-no Tegami Naraha-yori* (a letter from hometown Naraha)" from HN Corporation and Pulana Music, Inc.

- Temporary housing liaison personnel and livelihood support counselors have offered regular visits to residents in temporary housing and municipally-subsidized housing to understand their living and health conditions. For residents who are supposed to need some support, special care and services have been

provided, as needed, by nurses, public health nurses, certified clinical psychologists and psychiatrists.
- The town officials and other counselors are also earthquake victims; they are supposed to have been under tremendous mental stress. Therefore, mental health care programs, study sessions and various programs exclusively for such "support providers" have been conducted.

c. Summary/measures in the future
- Home visits by temporary housing liaison personnel and livelihood support counselors were useful in accurately understanding the current situation of residents in temporary housing/municipally-subsidized housing and immediately responding to their needs and problems. Additionally, because these staff members have systematically organized the records of home visits and held regular meetings to discuss adequate nursing-care support, they have promptly responded to the needs of residents by sharing information and cooperating with each other.
- Because the town officials and other counselors are also the earthquake victims, they are also under tremendous mental stress. It is indispensable to provide mental health care programs, study sessions and various other support programs exclusively for them at an early stage after a disaster.
- Because residents' feelings and opinions vary by generation, sex, living environment, and damage incurred by the earthquake, different residents have different mental problems. It is required to attentively and separately support them, according to their situations.

B Expectant/nursing mothers and children

1 Nutrition (meals/water)

a. Situation
(From March 11 to 15, 2011)
- After an emergency evacuation order was issued, the town quickly secured artificial milk (milk powder), baby bottles and disposable diapers for young children.

(After April 2011)
- Because medical examinations for young children were entrusted to each individual host municipality, it was impossible to understand the living conditions of young children taking shelter in other municipalities. However, at the time of an interview and counseling session for young children and their parents conducted one year after the explosion at the Fukushima Daiichi Nuclear Power Station, most parents answered that they made sure to purchase drinking water and pay attention to the origins of any food products, feeling anxious about their children's internal exposure to radiation.

b. Responses (actual measures)
- Artificial milk (milk powder), baby bottles and disposable diapers were procured from drug stores and pharmacies. Because the town had secured water before a cutoff, the town was able to provide boiled water to make milk.
- When school lunches were resumed at schools and "*Kodomo-en*" (a facility serving as both a kindergarten and a day nursery), the town purchased radiation meters to check the radiation dose of each food product. School lunches were offered after safety confirmation by the radiation meters.

c. Summary/measures in the future
- It is necessary to include milk powder, water for making milk, baby bottles, disposable diapers and baby

food into stockpiles for an emergency.
- Children's diets (including baby foods) and dietary habits changed as a result of the earthquake. It is necessary to accurately understand the actual conditions and take adequate measures to improve children's dietary environment.

2   Exercise (environmental improvement)

a. Situation
(After April 2011)
- Due to a fear of possible exposure to radiation, children were not allowed to play outdoors, being forced to stay in a confined corner of evacuation centers. As a result, opportunities to exercise were considerably decreased.

b. Responses (actual measures)
- A hands-on experience program of straw sandal making was conducted at temporary housing sites (Figure 18-1).
- Gatherings for young children and their parents/guardians were held at a support center, with the aim of promoting exchanges among children and providing a play space for them.

c. Summary/measures in the future
- Shortly after the explosion at the Fukushima Daiichi Nuclear Power Station, there were only a few young children who wore a mask. The reason might be attributed to the fact that residents were not informed about radiation effects. They also had a lack of awareness about possible exposure to radiation. It is necessary to regularly hold education programs about radiation, thereby contributing to the residents' increasing awareness of radiation.
- Playing outdoors and the habit of taking adequate exercise are indispensable to promote the physical development of young children. One of the future tasks for the town is how to secure and improve environments in which children can enjoy physical activities without feeling anxious about exposure to radiation.

3   Rest (mind, anxiety, suicide, etc.)

a. Situation
(March 12, 2011)
- The explosion at the Fukushima Daiichi Nuclear Power Station created great concerns among residents

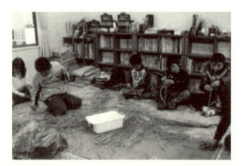

Figure 18-1   A hands-on experience program of straw sandal making at the temporary housing site

about the possible exposure to radiation and the future consequences on their lives. They suffered severely from mental and physical stress, while at the same time facing various difficulties in the society.

(After May 2011)

- Although daytime return was permitted, children were not allowed to step into the town. Therefore, it was difficult for some parents to return to the town and fix their houses because they were not able to find someone to look after their children while they were away.
- There were some students who had bullying problems at school or became a truant from school in host municipalities.

b. Responses (actual measures)

- On March 15, 2011, stable iodine tablets/syrup were secured and distributed to residents. Explanation about the administration of them was also provided. However, residents did not take them.
- During April to June 2011, post-disaster mental health care team members dispatched from Kyoto offered personal counseling programs for residents every week at the evacuation centers.
- In August 2011, radiation dose measurements using Whole Body Counters were implemented for children age 4 to 18 years old at the Hirata Central Clinic in Tokai Village.
- In November 2011, the town purchased personal dosimeters (glass badges) to lend them to households with an expectant mother and young children. Study sessions on radiation were also held. Lending of the dosimeters to all the households started in April 2012.
- In November 2011, Fukushima Prefecture started a thyroid gland examination for children age 4 to 18 years old.
- Since June 2012, counseling sessions for parents/guardians of young children have been held every month. The purpose is to check each individual child's development and maturity level as well as to receive general inquiries from parents/guardians about dietary problems, oral health care, mental problems, childcare and, radiation. Dentists, podiatrists, doctors of Fukushima Medical University, public health nurses, dental hygienists, dietitians, certified clinical psychologists and childcare workers have answered inquiries from participating residents.
- Since June 2012, children's post-disaster mental health care team members dispatched from Kyoto (a joint team of specialists in medical and educational fields such as psychiatrists, certified clinical psychologists, and licensed psychiatric social workers) have visited elementary and junior high school students of Naraha Town for three days every two weeks to have an interview and offer advice for them. The team members have also provided training and counseling programs for teachers and other school staff members.

c. Summary/measures in the future

- Because stable iodine for young children is prepared in the form of syrup not tablets, the use and storage of it are quite difficult and it must be always kept tightly covered. The distribution and administration of stable iodine syrup are also extremely difficult because it is generally not prepared per dose and the dose varies by age. Moreover, there was no official in Naraha Town who had received training on the administration of stable iodine syrup to young children. Although some officials of Fukushima Prefecture had undergone the training, they did not provide a smooth respond to the urgent needs for stable iodine in an emergency situation. It must also be mentioned that the training program had not prepared for a wide variety of situations. As a lesson learned from the nuclear disaster, it is important to ensure that every resident can easily and promptly take stable iodine tablets/syrup in any emergency situation. For example, it may be desirable to distribute iodine in advance to residents, encouraging residents to store it on their own and make ready for adequate and prompt administration in an emergency situation. From

Chapter 3 Situation of and Countermeasures by Each Individual Municipality

a safety perspective, it is essential for residents to obtain an accurate knowledge of stable iodine tablets/syrup. Parents are strongly urged to understand what allergies their children have, so as not to introduce side effects by taking stable iodine syrup.
- It is necessary to ensure that all the residents have a well-founded knowledge of countermeasures against exposure to radiation such as the measurement of radiation dose and wearing of a mask or protective clothing.
- For truant students and students having bullying problems, it is generally quite difficult to immediately address their situation by cooperating with the board of education of their host municipalities. As a future task, it is indispensable to establish a collaborative system with host municipalities, thereby immediately and adequately responding to the needs of students in any situation.

C People requiring assistance during a disaster (vulnerable people in case of a disaster)

1 Nutrition (meals/water)

a. Situation
(From March 12 to 16, 2011)
- Liquid foods for the elderly residents living in a dedicated nursing care facility were in short supply.
- It was impossible to use water for cooking due to a cutoff of the water supply. Pastries, rice balls and other emergency foods were distributed every day. Due to protein-poor and vegetable-poor diets as well as an excessive intake of carbohydrates, an increasing number of residents suffered from high blood sugar levels and constipation.

b. Responses (actual measures)
- The town strived to prepare liquid foods.
- Combining *bento* meals and foods cooked at an emergency kitchen, the town strived to secure and provide well-balanced diets for the residents.

c. Summary/measures in the future
- Vegetable juice is effective to help compensate for a lack of vegetables in daily diets.
- To immediately accommodate the needs of persons requiring nursing care during a disaster, liquid food stocks for an emergency need to be prepared.

2 Exercise (environmental improvement)

a. Situation
(From March 12 to 16, 2011)
- The health conditions of the elderly residents living in a dedicated nursing care facility worsened.

(From March 12 to May, 2011)
- A cold spread among the residents during the first month after the earthquake. There were some elderly residents who were hospitalized due to the development of pneumonia.
- A lack of exercise generated a great concern about the development of physical inactivity diseases (disuse syndrome) and pulmonary deep vein thrombosis/thromboembolism (economy-class syndrome).

(After May 2011)
- Facing a decline in physical and mental functions as well as serious stress caused by a sudden change in the living environment, many elderly residents wished to receive necessary support and assistance at day care facilities. As a result, the number of nursing care recipients (particularly those who were certified as nursing necessary level 1 or 2) increased.

b. Responses (actual measures)
- Residents were reminded to make sure to wash their hands and gargle conscientiously. Sanitary conditions at toilets and other public spaces at evacuation centers were improved, aiming to prevent the spread of infectious diseases among residents.
- A decision on which hotels, guesthouses and temporary housing should be allocated to residents with disabilities was made based on the level of their disabilities.
- While staying at the primary evacuation center, residents took radio gymnastic exercises and other rhythmic gymnastics to music every day. After they moved to hotels and guesthouses, health counseling programs, health-related gatherings, and exercise instructions were conducted every week at hotels and assembly rooms of the temporary housing facilities.(Figure 18-2)
- Since September 2011, nursing care prevention classes have been held at a newly established support center (five days per week) and an assembly room of each temporary housing site (once a week). Physical strength tests have also been implemented, aiming to not only evaluate individual resident's physical strength level but also instruct them on adequate exercise.
- Oral health care for the elderly has constituted an integral part of nursing care classes.
- Makeshift beds were carried into evacuation centers for residents with physical disabilities. When they move to temporary housing, the town discussed with them finding most suitable type of housing for them. As needed, the town lent makeshift beds to them after leaving evacuation centers.

c. Summary/measures in the future
- As physical strength test results indicate, it is important to take some measures to prevent the development of disuse syndrome among residents at an early stage of evacuation.
- Due to concerns about a decline in physical/mental functions and severe stress caused by a sudden change in the living environment, there were many elderly residents and their family members who wished to receive necessary support at a dedicated day care facility. As a measure to help reduce the number of nursing care recipients, the town is required to independently conduct nursing care prevention classes other than similar classes/projects recommended under the Long-Time Care Insurance Law.

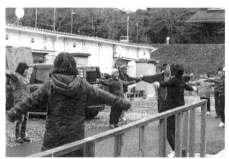
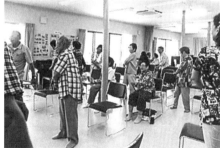

Figure18-2 Residents taking exercise at an emergency center

Chapter 3 — Situation of and Countermeasures by Each Individual Municipality

3 Rest (mind, anxiety, suicide, etc.)

a. Situation

(From March 12 to 15, 2011)
- Due to a water cutoff in Iwaki City, artificial dialysis was not able to be performed.
- Although residents with mental disabilities showed symptoms such as insomnia and auditory hallucinations, it was almost impossible to secure the necessary medicines for them.
- At evacuation centers, it gradually became quite difficult to look after residents in need of nursing care by only the few staff members available.
- Because dedicated hospitals for children with mental retardation and residents with mental disabilities became inaccessible due to evacuation, these outpatients had to find new hospitals.

(After February 2012)
- A group home for the persons with disabilities was established. However, this facility accommodated both residents with mental disabilities and intellectual disabilities regardless of their sex, causing frequent problems and troubles among residents. Moreover, the staff members of the facility also struggled with unfamiliar working conditions.

b. Responses (actual measures)
- On March 12 and 13, the town offered a shuttle service to medical institutions located in Iwaki City so that patients could undergo artificial dialysis. After March 14, these patients were evacuated to medical institutions inside/outside Fukushima Prefecture for continuation of their dialysis treatments.
- Residents who had lived in dedicated nursing-care facilities were returned to their families or relatives. Some were transferred to other dedicated hospitals and facilities located inside and outside of Fukushima Prefecture.
- The town helped mentally disabled residents to make contact with and go to psychiatric hospitals.
- In April 2011, the town strived to confirm the safety and current situation of elderly residents, while at the same time offering a counseling line service for them.
- The elderly residents requiring nursing care, who were supposed to face difficulties in spending time at evacuation centers, were accommodated with their family members at public facilities in host municipalities. In host municipalities, they received 24-hour support from staff members of the Council of Social Welfare.
- Post-disaster mental health care team members regularly provided counseling and advice to both the residents living in a group home for persons with disabilities and the staff members.

c. Summary/measures in the future
- Prescription and administration of medicines for psychiatric diseases are difficult; support from psychiatrists at an early stage of evacuation is indispensable.
- For residents who had regularly utilized their own drug diary and brought it when taking shelter, necessary medicines were smoothly prescribed and administered even in an emergency situation. The importance of drug diaries was reconfirmed.

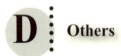

D Others

- In early April 2011, expectant mothers and children began moving to various municipalities throughout the country to take shelter. With the aim of supporting them, the town resumed its legal duties relating to medical examinations for expectant mothers and young children and vaccination services. To be specific, the town requested host municipalities to conduct vaccinations and medical examinations for evacuees from Naraha Town, while at the same time encouraging the expectant mothers and children to receive these services in their host municipalities. Because the records of medical examinations and vaccinations had been stored in the form of register and electronic data, the officials were able to promptly proceed with necessary procedures. The "wide-area vaccination" and "wide-area medical examination for expectant mothers" systems that had been implemented in municipalities within Fukushima Prefecture also contributed to smooth administrative operations.

- In September 2011, a support center for temporary day care and a children's hall were established, for the purpose of looking after young children during after-school hours and during a long-term holiday period.
- In November 2011, a questionnaire survey for parents/guardians of young children on their living conditions and problems in their daily lives was conducted, aiming to effectively respond to their needs.
- To support schoolchildren who may fall behind in their studies due to a prolonged evacuation, a learning support program was started in April 2012. In this program, volunteer staff helped schoolchildren's studies with nighttime classes held three times a week and classes during long-term holidays.
- In the early May 2011, public health nurses of towns/villages located in the Futaba area gathered together to hold a liaison meeting and exchanged information on medical examinations and vaccination services in their own municipality. To share information and discuss how to address urgent problems, the meeting has been regularly conducted.
- In the early April 2011, the city was deluged with protest calls from residents about services. While responding to their anger, resentment, dissatisfaction and complaints, the officials suffered from severe mental distress, with growing stress and overwork. In light of such a situation, the town entrusted to mental care specialists support for the town officials and the members of the social welfare council who are in a position to offer social services and support to residents.
- Aiming to offer effective and prompt social services to residents, the town frequently conducted the relocation of the office, administrative reorganization, and reshuffling of personnel, according to where most residents took shelter. Inevitably, the town officials also had to change their places of residence and assume duties with different groups of personnel, aiming to have flexibly to respond to the circumstances. Moreover, each individual official was required to play two or more roles, being forced to take on both regular and emergency duties.
- Immediately after the earthquake and the nuclear accident at the Fukushima Daiichi Nuclear Power Station, public health nurses became actively involved in disaster relief activities at large-scale evacuation centers with an accommodation capacity of several hundred persons. During such an early stage of on-site relief activities, they strived to understand actual conditions & problems associated with health-care support for the victims, which enabled developing successful and efficient disaster-relief operations. Specifically, they developed a mechanism to coordinate town officials' operations at evacuation centers and disaster relief activities by health-care management team members dispatched from other prefectures and other volunteers. The mechanism also enabled systematic management of medical prescriptions, from requests, distribution to each resident, to confirmation of administration.
- After health-care and welfare support specialists were dispatched, the town's public health nurses strived to develop a system/mechanism enabling information sharing and close collaboration with them, which were both indispensable for effective health management of residents. They also held a daily meeting at the primary/secondary evacuation centers. Even after residents moved to temporary housing, public health nurses continued a weekly meeting to discuss health-care support programs for residents. Moreover, they had frequent opportunities to talk with temporary housing liaison personnel, livelihood support counselors, and commissioned child welfare volunteers, with the aim of keeping close contact with them.
- The disaster response headquarters assigned the town's managerial officials as the head of each evacu-

Chapter 3 Situation of and Countermeasures by Each Individual Municipality

ation center. With the aim of developing a prompt and adequate support system, these heads reported actual conditions of evacuation centers every day and posed immediate problems at headquarters meeting. They also made daily schedules and ensured that all staff members of each evacuation center were informed of the schedule, so that relief operations could be smoothly conducted.

- At the primary evacuation centers, doctors and other medical staff members went around the premises to check the health condition of residents. After the examination, the officials in charge collected/gathered medical prescriptions written by the doctors, went to a pharmacy to prepare medicines for residents and distributed the medicine to each individual resident. After the on-site examination by doctors was terminated in May 2011, the town operated a shuttle bus between evacuation centers and local medical institutions, so that residents were able to consult their nearest medical institution.
- As part of mental care efforts for those who are in a position to offer social support to residents, the town conducted mental counseling services and learning programs to livelihood support counselors and temporary housing liaison personnel.
- To measure radiation levels within the town, the officials carry radiation meters. To prevent the risk of exposure to radiation for unborn babies, female residents under 40 years old are currently restricted in their employment within Naraha Town.
- The health care officials conducted a survey on actual living conditions of residents at inns, guesthouses, temporary housing and municipally-subsidized housing. Based on the results they offered repeated home visits to residents/households that required some support, as needed.

(Yukie Tamane)

19. Efforts of Namie Town

1 Situation of the municipality

(1) Demographics (as of January 1 of each year)

	2011	2012	2013
Population	20,869	19,360	19,082
Number of households	7,198	6,799	6,755
Average number of people per household	2.9	2.8	2.8
Number of births	171	135	137
Birth rate	8.2	7.0	7.2
Number of deaths	266	468	233
Mortality	12.7	24.2	12.2
Ratio of the elderly aged 65 or older	26.6	26.9	27.8

* A total 7 public health nurses work in Namie Town (one in charge of radiation, two in charge of nursing care, four in charge of health management)

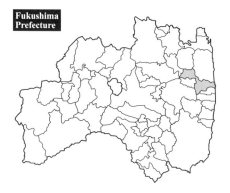
Fukushima Prefecture

(2) Geographical features

Total area: 223.10 km^2

Distance from the Fukushima Daiichi Nuclear Power Station of the Tokyo Electric Power Company: approximately 4 to 35 km (the easternmost town in Fukushima Prefecture)

Transportation network: JR Joban Line; National Route 6; National Route 114

2 Situation of damage by the earthquake, tsunami and the nuclear disaster

(1) Damage by the Great East Japan Earthquake (as of March 13, 2013)

Property damage	Completely destroyed	Half destroyed	Partially destroyed
House	644 (586 by the tsunami and 58 by the earthquake)		
Public institution			
Other			

Human damage	Deaths by disaster	Disaster-related deaths	Missing persons	Injured persons
	182	254		

* The 182 deaths by the disaster include 33 missing persons.

* Other than completely-destroyed and severely-destroyed properties, the degree of damage to properties was not judged.

(2) Situation of evacuation

① Evacuation centers inside the local municipality

	Number of evacuation centers	Number of evacuees	Available period
Residents			
Evacuees received			

② Approximate number of evacuees in evacuation centers outside the municipality (as of March 13, 2013)

	End/March 2011	End/September 2011	End/March 2012	Latest period
First evacuation center	2,851			
Second evacuation center				
Temporary housing			4,476	4,500
Municipally-subsidized housing			9,270	9,170

Chapter 3 | Situation of and Countermeasures by Each Individual Municipality

③ Approximate number of voluntary evacuees

| Inside Fukushima Prefecture | | Outside Fukushima Prefecture (number of evacuees & prefectures) | |

Outlook of damage related to the nuclear disaster

- On March 11, 2011, a nuclear accident occurred at the Fukushima Daiichi Nuclear Power Station of the Tokyo Electric Power Company (hereinafter referred to as the "Fukushima Daiichi Nuclear Power Station"), resulting in a release of radioactive materials to the natural environment. On March 12, an evacuation order was issued to residents living within a 10-km range of the Fukushima Daiichi Nuclear Power Station, under the name of the Prime Minister. Following the evacuation order, almost all the Namie Town residents were evacuated to the Tsushima district. The town office was also relocated to the Tsushima district.
- Because it was expected that areas affected by the release of radioactive materials would be further expanding, an evacuation order was issued on March 15 to areas within a 20-km range of the Fukushima Daiichi Nuclear Power Station. Based on the order, the Mayor of Namie Town decided to evacuate all town residents. The town office was relocated to Nihonmatsu City.

3 Countermeasures against nuclear disaster (as of March 2013)

		Name of project	Division in charge	Number of targeted persons (house-holds)	Expect-ant mothers	Nursing moth-ers	Babies	Young children	Elemen-tary school students	Junior high school students	Senior high school students	People age 19 to 39	People age 40 or older	Remarks (major operations)
Countermeasures against external exposure	1	Personal dose measurements	Health and Insurance Division	All resi-dents	○	○	○	○	○	○	○	○	○	Measurement of exter-nal exposure dose every three months, distribu-tion & collection of personal dosimeters and aggregation & analysis of the measurement results
	2	Refreshments for elementary school and junior high school students	Livelihood Support Division of the Board of Education Secretariat						○	○				
	3	Monitoring and measurement of the air radiation levels	Livelihood Support Division of the Preparation Office for Returning to Namie Town											
	4	Measurement of the air radiation levels in the whole town	Preparation Office for Returning to Namie Town											
	5	Decontamination of houses	Hometown Recon-struction Division											
	6	Decontamination of public and medical facilities	Hometown Recon-struction Division											
	7	Inspection and calibration of per-sonal dosimeters (glass badges)	Health and Insurance Division	All house-holds										
Countermeasures against internal exposure	8	Examination of breast milk	Fukushima Prefecture			○								
	9	Whole Body Counter measure-ments (conducted by the town)	Health and Insurance Division	All resi-dents	○	○		○	○	○	○	○	○	Arrangement of measurement venues & schedules, notification & publicity, examina-tion and analysis
	10	Whole Body Counter measure-ments (conducted by the town for children aged 4 to 18)	Health and Insurance Division					○						Arrangement of measurement venues & schedules, notification & publicity, examina-tion and analysis
	11	Food and water quality inspection	Livelihood Support Division											Conducted by the town for residents ages 19 to 40 years old.

174

Others	12	Thyroid gland examination (conducted by the town)	Health and Insurance Division		○	○	○	○	○	○	○	○		Annual examination conducted by the town for residents under 18 years old. Arrangement of venues & schedules, notification & publicity, examination and analysis
	13	Measurement of initial exposure dose	Health and Insurance Division				○	○	○	○	○			Chromosome testing, arrangement of venues & schedules, notification and aggregation of examination results
	14	Debriefing sessions for measurement results of exposure dose	Health and Insurance Division											
	15	Study sessions on radiation	Environmental Measures Division	All residents										
	16	Cancer screening	Health and Insurance Division	Residents of designated ages								○	○	Stomach cancer, colorectal cancer, prostate cancer, uterine cancer, and breast cancer
	17	Sampling of respondents for a basic survey in the Fukushima Health Management Survey	Tax Division	All residents	○	○	○	○	○	○	○	○	○	
	18	Issuance of citizen health cards (containing a column for recording radiation exposure levels)	Health and Insurance Division	All residents	○	○	○	○	○	○	○	○	○	Distribution, publicity, contracts, procedures for reissuance of health cards and an explanatory meeting for the usage of health cards
	19	Health Management Review Committee	Committee members from the Health and Insurance Division											Holding of a review meetings, preparation of the health management outline, announcements to the review committee members, and provision of remuneration
	20	Namie Town Temporary Emergency Clinic	Health and Insurance Division	All residents	○	○	○	○	○	○	○	○	○	Arrangement of a monthly schedule of doctors and nurses, administrative procedures for insurance claims, and issuance of written passing permissions.

Chapter 3 Situation of and Countermeasures by Each Individual Municipality

A Residents

1 Nutrition (meals/water)

a. Situation
- At the primary evacuation centers, high-carbohydrate foods such as rice balls and breads constituted the majority of meals, causing unbalanced diets among residents.
- At some primary evacuation centers, local volunteer members cooked simple foods for evacuees.
- Plastic bottles of water were the only available beverage at the primary evacuation centers.

b. Responses (actual measures)
- It is necessary to establish a system that enables residents and other volunteer members to actively cooperate with each other to secure enough food in an emergency situation.
- In a case where all the town residents are evacuated, it is difficult to secure enough food and relief supplies to be distributed to all residents by the town alone. Therefore, the town ensures that each resident individually stores three day's worth of foods for an emergency.
- Although it is a responsibility of the town to prepare a minimal amount of food stocks for an emergency, it is difficult to maintain a large amount of food for a long period of time due to the expiration date. Therefore, the town needs to intensify its collaboration with the private sector and other municipalities by, for example, concluding a mutual cooperation agreement on disaster prevention and emergency relief activities.

2 Exercise (Environmental improvement)

a. Situation
- Residents spent most of the day indoors due to anxiety about exposure to radiation. Inevitably, a lack of exercise was observed among residents.
- At some evacuation centers, residents took radio gymnastic exercises every morning. Whether or not residents actively took some exercises varied by evacuation center.
- It was after residents moved to temporary housing that the town could afford to take overall measures to solve a lack of exercise among residents.

b. Responses (actual measures)
- Indicating that the development of physical inactivity diseases (disuse syndrome) among residents was only a matter of time, nonprofit organizations (NPOs) pointed out the necessity for some exercises for residents. Following their advice, the town asked the NPO members to conduct exercise programs at the primary evacuation centers. The exercise programs have been continuously conducted after residents moved to the secondary evacuation sites, such as hotels and inns as well as temporary housing, to prevent residents from becoming nursing-care recipients.

c. Summary/measures in the future
- The town intends to continue offering exercise programs based on the residents' living conditions.
- The exercise programs are not only for residents living in temporary housing but also for those in municipally-subsided housing.

3 Rest (mind, anxiety, suicide, etc.)

a. Situation

- At the primary evacuation center, it was relatively easy to confirm the safety of residents and understand their living conditions. However, after residents moved to the secondary evacuation centers such as hotels and inns, it became difficult for the town to know their situation because they spent most of the day in their private rooms. There were some residents who refused to receive home visits by the officials.
- At hotels and inns, residents who had lived alone were asked to form a group of four to share a room. Although some were able to get along with group members, others could not, feeling an increasing stress from human relationships. There were some residents who had no alternative but to stay in the lobby all day due to bullying by roommates or other human relationship reasons.
- For a family that had lived in a large house, life as evacuees in a narrow space was unbearable. The lack of privacy caused each family member to feel severely stressed.
- The town obtained the cooperation of private volunteers for attentively listening to residents, as well as the efforts of psychologists and psychiatrists from universities/postgraduate schools located outside Fukushima Prefecture in offering mental health care support to residents.
- Although the town provided mental health counseling programs to residents, it was often the case that residents suffering from severe mental problems did not, or were unable to participate in the programs. Therefore, home-visiting counseling services were indispensable to maintain the mental health of such residents. However, it is challenging for mental health care staff members to build mutual trust with such residents in just 1 to 2 months.
- There was a resident who repeatedly made bitter complaints about radiation to the town officials. In fact, the repeated unusual complaints were attributed to the resident's severe mental problems, not anxiety about the exposure to radiation.

b. Responses (actual measures)

- Mental health nurses went around to each room of hotels and inns to identify residents suffering from heavy stress from human relationships. As needed, the nurses provided frequent visits to those who are under severe stress and strived to listen to them.
- In some cases, the town allocated another room to residents who were unable to get along with roommates at inns and hotels.
- To address a severe stress among family members, it may be effective to make the elderly members and younger members stay in separate spaces at an evacuation center.
- Mental health nurses and public health nurses went around to the evacuation centers to identify residents at high risk of stress-related problems. As needed, the nurses made a request, through the public health and welfare office (hereinafter referred to as the "health office"), to post-disaster mental health care teams for home visits for such residents.

c. Summary/measures in the future

- Residents commented that they felt reassured by having an opportunity to talk with mental health nurses, public health nurses and other medical workers about not only their health problems but also anxiety, concerns and other mental problems.
- A cooperative relationship with post-disaster mental health care teams was quite helpful for the town officials in providing effective mental health and welfare services to the residents. When the officials identified residents who were supposed to have some mental problems, they were promptly referred to the team to receive necessary treatment.
- Fukushima Prefecture is advised to take the leadership in conducting regular simulations of emergency

Chapter 3 | Situation of and Countermeasures by Each Individual Municipality

response activities, based on the cooperation among municipalities within the prefecture. From the perspective of mental health care of disaster victims, it is desirable to establish a network of mental health care teams within the prefecture so that the team members can share necessary information and promptly initiate home-visiting care and other vital mental support activities in times of disaster.

- After the improvement of symptoms of physical health problems, other symptoms specific to mental problems were observed among residents. It is essential to concurrently provide both physical and mental health management programs to disaster victims.

4 Others

a. Situation

- Disposable diapers for adults, adhesive bandages and disinfectants were in short supply on the first day of evacuation. Such medical supplies were donated to evacuees from drug stores located near the town's head office.
- Dead bodies were gathered together and examined at a gymnasium in the Tsushima district where a high radiation dose was observed. Because the examination work was hard and continued from morning to evening, some examiners became sick and suffered from post-traumatic stress disorder (PTSD) symptoms.
- Evacuation centers were flooded with similar types of mental care, exercise, and medical team volunteer members that rushed to the area from throughout the country. Moreover, there were some disaster relief volunteer groups that came to evacuation centers without prior contact with the town. Therefore, the town officials, who had been busily occupied with the response to the immediate needs of residents, could not afford to coordinate with such volunteer members to systematically provide emergency response activities for residents.
- Under an emergency situation in which all the residents were forced to evacuate the town, the town officials were unable to bring critical documents, data sources and important tools stored at the town office. The official register of residents was also absent, so the town officials had to develop a handwritten register based on a survey of each resident at the primary evacuation centers. Therefore, it took a long time before personal support and services for each individual resident started. Confirmation of the safety of the residents was also inadequate at the primary evacuation centers.
- Because the local council of social welfare (hereinafter referred to as the "social welfare council") did not work at all due to the earthquake, it was impossible to coordinate welfare volunteers and caretakers.
- Some medical team members handed medicines to residents by just judging from their symptoms, without confirming each individual resident's regular medicines. Because such medical staff did not give any instruction on administration to residents, it was often the case that some residents who received medicines did not remember what the medicine were for.
- Multiple medical teams conducted separate medical activities at the evacuation centers, which caused many residents to receive similar medicines from different medical staff members. For example, when a resident complained of sleeplessness, a medical team member passed sleeping pills to the resident. Then, another medical team member came and asked about the health condition of the same resident. When the resident again complained of sleeplessness, the second medical team member also passed the resident sleeping pills. Moreover, feeling considerably anxious and fearful that they might not be able to consult a doctor and continue receiving medicines in the future, many residents intentionally received the same type of medicines from different medical team members and stored them.
- Before the earthquake, members of the social welfare council and the Japanese Red Cross Society had regularly carried out drills on the preparation of emergency food and the distribution of emergency relief supplies. However, their experiences in the drills were in vain, under a situation where all residents had

to evacuate the town.

b. Responses (actual measures)
- Thanks to the cooperation of the Japanese Consumer Co-operative Union (COOP), the town was able to distribute emergency relief supplies to the residents.
- Residents were unable to properly brush their teeth at the evacuation centers due to the lack of toothpastes, toothbrushes and other necessities. Members of the Dental Hygienists' Association checked the oral conditions of residents and provided advice to elderly residents not to choke on food.

c. Summary/measures in the future
- Based on collaborative relationships with local pharmacies and stores, the town needs to establish a system that secures the supply of food and other commodities for the residents in times of disaster.
- To secure the distribution of emergency relief supplies in times of disaster, it is not sufficient to maintain collaborative relationships with only private companies operating within the town because such companies will also be required to evacuate the town when a disaster occurs. Establishment of partnerships with private companies operating in other municipalities inside and outside of Fukushima Prefecture is also necessary.
- In securing emergency relief supplies during a disaster, too much reliance upon a partnership with only local private companies is not desirable for the town. It is advised that "mutual cooperation agreements on disaster prevention and disaster relief" be concluded among municipalities throughout the country so that they can help each other in times of disaster, in terms of the provision of relief supplies and funding support.
- Examiners of dead bodies suffered from severe mental problems due to heavy work. To reduce their mental stress as much as possible, they should work in shifts.
- As part of disaster preparedness efforts, data files of the official register of the residents need to be stored on an external server computer.
- A lack of collaboration among volunteer staff members inevitably results in unorganized emergency relief activities in affected areas. Therefore, the town is required to secure personnel who coordinate volunteer staff members in times of disaster.
- To immediately respond to an emergency situation, it is very important to call for help from residents having a qualification as a nurse and other professional licenses.
- As a lesson from the fact that Fukushima Prefecture was not able to respond to the urgent needs of the disaster victims on its own, the establishment of a nation-wide emergency relief system is desirable. For example, if it is agreed upon among municipalities throughout the country that "X Town will provide necessary support to Y Town in times of disaster," more effective and immediate emergency response activities will be achieved.

B Expectant/nursing mothers and children

1 Nutrition (meals/water)

a. Situation
- Mothers who took shelter in the town's head office on the day of the earthquake (March 11) requested the provision of artificial milk (milk powder), disposable diapers and baby wipes. Responding to the request, the town asked local pharmacies to provide the requested items.
- Due to a lack of detergent to wash baby bottles and the cutoff of the water supply, mothers were not

Chapter 3 | Situation of and Countermeasures by Each Individual Municipality

able to prepare milk for babies.

- Milk powder, disposable diapers and baby wipes did not immediately reach the town as emergency relief supplies.
- No baby food was available. It seemed that mothers individually managed to secure some food for their babies.

b. Responses (actual measures)

- Based on the requests from mothers taking shelter in the town's head office, the officials asked a nearby pharmacy to provide necessary items for babies.
- The town officials boiled bottled mineral water in an electric kettle so that mothers could prepare milk for their babies.
- Because a little milk powder remained in some nursery schools, the town officials collected it and distributed it to nursery schools with no milk powder stock. Milk powder provided from the local pharmacy was also distributed, as needed. There remained some powder after the distribution, and the officials brought it when they evacuated.
- After the town's head office was relocated within the building of the Towa Branch Office of the Nihonmatsu City Hall, the supply of milk powder brought from Namie Town was almost depleted. Therefore, the town officials went to Fukushima City and Koriyama City, both located in the Nakadori area, to purchase milk powder from pharmacies.

c. Summary/measures in the future

- It is impossible to stock a large amount of milk powder for an emergency. The town is required to maintain a cooperative relationship with local pharmacies, drug stores, etc., as part of its disaster preparedness efforts.
- In preparing emergency food stocks, the town focused on elderly residents and persons with disabilities, without paying special attention to the needs of young children.
- Milk powder, baby foods and baby bottles need to be added to the town's stockpiles for emergencies.
- It is necessary to deepen each individual resident's awareness of disaster preparedness.

2 Exercise (Environmental improvement)

a. Situation

- Young children were not allowed to play outdoors due to possible exposure to radiation.
- There were many young children who ran around, making noise in the lobbies of inns.
- The town officials could not afford to look after young children and check their health conditions at evacuation centers.

b. Responses (actual measures)

- The town secured play/study spaces for young children at the primary evacuation centers.
- The town also secured study rooms at the secondary evacuation centers.

c. Summary/measures in the future

- Early announcements of radiation dose measurement results to the residents must have relieved their anxiety about the risk of exposure to radiation.
- The town is required to ask local child care organizations to secure victim children's access to playing spaces, toys, and picture books.
- It is necessary to secure volunteer teachers who can visit evacuation centers and provide learning sup-

19 Efforts of Namie Town

port to evacuee students.

3   Rest (mind, anxiety, suicide, etc.)

a. Situation

- Responses to the needs of young children varied by evacuation centers. At some evacuation centers, nursery school childcare workers read picture books to young children.
- Feeling hungry and fearful in the dark and cold evacuation centers, young children increasingly lost mental stability and started crying. Every time young children cried, mothers had to cradle them in their arms outside in the cold. Mothers were forced to spend many sleepless nights.
- The town officials did not pay careful attention to young children's mental condition. Because young children managed to play with each other at evacuation centers, the officials automatically assumed that they had no severe mental problems.

b. Responses (actual measures)

- At the secondary evacuation centers, town-owned nursery school childcare workers planned and provided a friendly gathering for mothers and young children at a room within a hotel.
- With the aim of understanding the situation of mothers and their children who were mentally isolated from other evacuees, the town's public health nurses provided home visits to them.

c. Summary/measures in the future

- Mental problems of young children were gradually brought to light after residents moved to temporary housing or municipally-subsidized housing. The town had almost no trained personnel to provide mental health care support for victim children, resulting in a failure to take early responses to young children having mental health problems.
- It is necessary for the town to always secure officials who can immediately provide necessary mental health care support and services to young children in times of disaster.
- The town officials' focus was to address the health problems of elderly residents and persons requiring assistance during a disaster. As a point that the town must reconsider, if the town had taken appropriate measures and provided necessary mental health care support to young children at an early stage of evacuation, some of the current problems such as truants from school or students staying shut up at home might have been prevented.
- The town must develop a system that enables prompt mental support for young children in times of disaster.

4   Others

a. Situation

- After the town's head office was relocated to a building of the Towa Branch Office of the Nihonmatsu City Hall, the town officials immediately confirmed whether children had taken shelter or not.
- After taking shelter in the Tsushima district, some households with expectant/nursing mothers and young children individually took shelter outside Fukushima Prefecture to avoid the risk of exposure to radiation. It was difficult for the town to identify their whereabouts.

b. Responses (actual measures)

- The town officials asked children who came to the office to undergo a radiation dose measurement using a Whole Body Counter, "What route did you come here to undergo the examination?"

181

Chapter 3 Situation of and Countermeasures by Each Individual Municipality

- Because most schools did not know students' emergency contact information other than their fixed phone numbers at home, it took a long time before school personnel confirmed the safety of all students. For preschool children and expectant/nursing mothers, the town was unable to confirm their safety.

c. Summary/measures in the future
- It is necessary that the town officials bring a register of young children and expectant/nursing mothers when evacuating, so that the safety and situations of such residents can be confirmed as early as possible after a disaster.

C People requiring assistance during a disaster (vulnerable people in case of a disaster)

1 Nutrition (meals/water)

a. Situation
- Priority for receiving emergency food supplies was given to people requiring assistance during a disaster.
- At a gymnasium that served as the primary evacuation center, rice and breads constituted the majority of meals. Such meals were unpopular among elderly residents because rice and breads were difficult to swallow. Because an increasing number of elderly residents refused to eat them, the leftover rice balls with roasted sesame and salt were piled in a corner of the gymnasium. The same situation was observed for a certain period of time at other primary evacuation centers, where no simple food was cooked by volunteer members.

b. Responses (actual measures)
- Many elderly residents tried to drink as little water as possible because they wanted to reduce the frequency of going to a toilet at evacuation centers. To prevent elderly residents from getting dehydrated, the town officials encouraged them to make sure to take plenty of water.
- As a general tendency, elderly residents individually kept rice balls, breads and other distributed foods for a long time at evacuation centers. The town officials strived to collect outdated food from them to prevent elderly residents from becoming ill by eating spoiled foods.
- It was regrettable that the town was unable to offer hot dishes to residents. During a period of evacuation in the cold winter, water was the only available beverage for residents.
- Liquid foods were prepared at hospitals.

c. Summary/measures in the future
- It is necessary for the town to secure nutrition supplement drinks, vegetable juice and other easy-to-take food stocks for emergencies.

2 Exercise (Environmental improvement)

a. Situation
- The number of physical therapists, occupational therapists and allied health care professionals was insufficient. Due to the lack of manpower for nursing-care preventive efforts, the number of nursing-care recipients increased.

b. Responses (actual measures)
- Various nonprofit organizations (NPOs) conducted a variety of nursing-care initiatives for elderly

residents. The town's public health nurses were mainly involved in the coordination of such different initiatives.

c. Summary/measures in the future

- The shortage of care workers is a critical problem. If the number of nursing-care recipients increases, their health inevitably becomes worse because they do not receive adequate necessary care. It is essential to offer various nursing-care preventive programs at evacuation centers at an early stage of evacuation.

3 Rest (mind, anxiety, suicide, etc.)

a. Situation

- For details, please refer to the section of "A. Residents."

b. Responses (actual measures)

- As part of efforts to support the elderly residents and residents with mental disabilities taking shelter alone, the town officials and neighboring residents strived to be mindful of the needs of such vulnerable people in times of disaster.
- The town officials formed several groups to conduct health checks of elderly people and persons requiring daily assistance. The daily health checks were quite useful in understanding the health conditions of vulnerable people in times of disaster and facilitated smoothly responding to their urgent needs.

c. Summary/measures in the future

- At an early stage of evacuation, residents were asked to form groups and collectively watch over group members. The watch-over system within a group contributed to the residents' increased awareness of the importance of mutual assistance during a disaster.

4 Others

a. Situation

- At evacuation centers, persons with disabilities were left alone in their own excrement.
- Although there were approximately 40 residents who were in need of artificial dialysis treatment, they faced difficulties in finding medical institutions for the continuation of treatment. In some hospitals, the residents had no choice but to undergo the treatment in the night due to a low capacity for handling dialysis cases. There were also some hospitals that were filled with patients evacuated from other municipalities, and refused the acceptance of Namie Town's patients in need of artificial dialysis.
- Because no insulin was available, residents had to go to Fukushima Medical University (hereinafter referred to as the "prefectural medical university") to receive insulin injections.
- Stoma devices were in short supply. There was a resident who was unable to use a stoma device and suffered from an inflammation of their stoma. The inflammation had already eased when the resident consulted the town's public health nurse. Although the town obtained a kit of stoma devices and provided them to the resident, some of the devices were not suitable for the resident.
- Mentally-disabled inpatients were taken to and temporarily left at the evacuation center. Although being able to stand and walk on their own, these inpatients did not even know their own name and had no idea whether they had been in a mental hospital or a nursing-care facility. Because there was no medical record of prescriptions for these inpatients, the town was at a loss as to what kinds of medicines should be administer to them.
- Late-night wandering was observed among the cognitively impaired elderly.

Chapter 3 | Situation of and Countermeasures by Each Individual Municipality

b. Responses (actual measures)

- The town allocated temporary housing located near a hospital to residents in need of artificial dialysis treatment. The town officials, by rotation, took some of the residents to the hospital by bus every day so that these residents could have artificial dialysis treatment.
- The town officials took residents who needed an insulin injection to Fukushima Medical University every day.
- Special nurses for stomas and other volunteer nurses walked around the evacuation centers to maintain stoma devices in good condition.
- The town hospitalized mentally-disabled inpatients that were left at evacuation centers in other medical institutions.
- The town looked into the backgrounds of unidentified mentally-disabled inpatients that were left at evacuation centers after hospitalizing them. There were inquiries about unidentified mentally-disabled inpatients from several municipalities.
- The town officials provided 24-hour care for the cognitive impaired elderly with late-night wandering problems.
- Some elderly residents did not bring their dentures when evacuating. Taking into consideration that most of their dentures were swept away by the tsunami and that elderly residents were inconvenienced in their daily lives by the loss, the association of dentists gave them priority for consultations at a relatively early stage of evacuation.

c. Summary/measures in the future

- The town had not assumed a critical situation in which hospitals became inaccessible. As part of disaster preparedness efforts in the future, the town should take some measures that enable an urgent response to patients requiring artificial dialysis, insulin injections and stoma devices.
- Making a list of inpatients with mental disabilities and supporting their evacuation in times of disaster are beyond the range of administrative operations. Each medical institution is strongly advised to be well-prepared for a disaster and take responsibility of all the inpatients' evacuation.
- It must be ensured that residents always bring their own drug diary for an emergency situation.

(Ryoko Yoshida, Kimie Yoshida, Mihoko Suzuki, Chikako Kai, Takayo Nemoto)

20 Efforts of Katsurao Village

1 Situation of the municipality

(1) Demographics (as of January 1 of each year)

	2011	2012	2013
Population	1,567	1,524	1,517
Number of households	477	475	471
Average number of people per household			
Number of births		5	6	10 (estimated)
Birth rate			
Number of deaths	17	22	11
Mortality			
Ratio of the elderly aged 65 or older	31.5	32.1	33.0

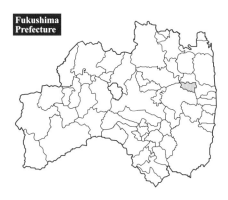
Fukushima Prefecture

(2) Geographical features

Total area: 84.23 km² (approximately 15 km east-west; approximately 8 km north-south)

Distance from the Fukushima Daiichi Nuclear Power Station of the Tokyo Electric Power Company: 31 km in a west-northwest direction to Kaminogawa-aza-Kaminogawa; 25 km in west-northwest direction to Ochiai-aza-Ochiai; 21 km in a northwest direction to Katsurao-aza-Noyuki; 21 km in a west-northwest direction to Ochiai-aza-Oohanachi.

Evacuation area: The village was initially divided into a planned evacuation zone and a hazard zone. At 0:00 on March 22, 2013, the village was reorganized into a preparatory zone for lifting the evacuation order, a restricted residence zone and a difficult-to-return zone.

Transportation network: By bus operated by Fukushima Transportation or bus operated by Katsurao Village from the Funehiki Station of JR Banetsu-to Line; approximately 40 minutes by car from Banetsu Expressway Funehiki Miharu I.C (from Funehiki Miharu I.C through National Route 288 to National Route 399).

2 Situation of damage by the earthquake, tsunami and the nuclear disaster

(1) Damage by the Great East Japan Earthquake (as of May 1, 2012)

Property damage	Completely destroyed	Half destroyed	Partially destroyed
House	5	2	241
Public institution	(Under investigation)		
Other			

Human damage	Deaths by disaster	Disaster-related deaths	Missing persons	Injured persons
	1	16	(1)	Unknown

* The person recorded as a "missing person" is supposed to have died from the tsunami. On the family register, the person is recorded as "the dead."

(2) Situation of evacuation

① Evacuation centers within the municipality (as of May 1, 2012)

	Number of evacuation centers	Number of evacuees	Available period
Residents	2	96	3/12 - 14
Evacuees received			

Chapter 3 — Situation of and Countermeasures by Each Individual Municipality

② Approximate number of evacuees in evacuation centers outside the municipality (as of May 1, 2012)

	End/March 2011	End/September 2011	End/March 2012	Latest period
First evacuation center	179			
Second evacuation center	431			
Temporary housing		897	881	809
Municipally-subsidized housing		554	544	526

③ Approximate number of voluntary evacuees (as of May 1, 2012)

Inside Fukushima Prefecture	79

Outside Fukushima Prefecture (number of evacuees & prefectures)	86 persons in 16 prefectures

Outlook of damage related to the nuclear disaster

In the evening of March 11, the village officials tried to confirm all residents' safety, using an Internet telephony system (fiber optic communications). For residents whose safety was not confirmed by the phone, the village officials formed four groups and looked for them.

On March 12, evacuation centers were set up for residents evacuating from areas within a 20-km range of the Fukushima Daiichi Nuclear Power Station. Because blankets and food were in short supply, the village called for the provision of blankets, foods and other emergency supplies, using the local wireless radio broadcasting system. In the night of March 12, residents living in areas within a 20-km range of the nuclear power station were accommodated at the evacuation centers. Women's association members cooked simple emergency food for the evacuees.

Meals for the evacuees were also cooked by the women's association members on March 13.

On March 14, aiming to evacuate all the residents outside the village, the officials identified residents with no means of transportation and discussed how to evacuate them outside the village. Although the village asked Fukushima Prefecture to help find host municipalities, the prefecture refused the mediation work, with an excuse that the prefecture had no instruction for mediation from the national government. Helplessly, the village had to decide where to evacuate on its own. At 21:15 on the same day, the village broadcasted an announcement of evacuation to residents, following which residents took shelter at Azuma Sports Park (located in Fukushima City) and other various areas.

On March 15, the village received an offer from the disaster response headquarters of Aizu-Wakamatsu City to accommodate the village residents at evacuation centers in Aizubange Town in the city. After explaining about the offer to the residents, the village residents were finally accommodated in the primary evacuation centers such as the Kawanishi Community Hall and the Aizu Nature Center.

On March 17, radiation screening was implemented. On March 18, the Basic Residents Registration Network System was back in use.

On March 23, because of the bitter cold weather, the village displaced residents, particularly elderly residents, to a welfare and health facility *Ginzan-so*.

In late March, residents began moving to the secondary evacuation centers.

On April 21, the village set up the Bange Branch Office and resumed normal working operations.

On June 14, the village opened the Miharu Office. On June 26, residents began moving to temporary housing set up in Miharu Town. Temporary housing was allocated to residents by administrative-ward group.

20 Efforts of Katsurao Village

③ Countermeasures against nuclear disaster (As of May 2013)

		Name of project	Division in charge	Number of targeted persons (households)	Expectant mothers	Nursing mothers	Babies	Young children	Elementary school students	Junior high school students	Senior high school students	People age 19 to 39	People age 40 or older	Remarks (major operations)
Countermeasures against external exposure	1	Personal dose measurements (personal cumulative dosimeters)	Residents and Livelihood Division	1,509 persons	○	○	○	○	○	○	○	○	○	Distribution of the dosimeters to all the village residents. Measurement, as needed.
		Personal dosimeters (glass badges)	Residents and Livelihood Division	65 persons			○	○	○	○				Distribution, collection, notification of the results and analysis
		Personal dosimeters (measurements of air levels and personal dose by electronic dosimeters)	Residents and Livelihood Division	12 persons	○	○								Distribution and collection & analysis of the measurement results
	2	Monitoring and measurement of the air radiation levels	Regional Promotion Division	13 posts										
	3	Measurement and mapping of the air radiation levels in the whole village	Regional Promotion Division											The results are announced every month in public relations magazines.
	4	Replacement of the surface soil on the grounds in childcare facilities, child education facilities and schools	Board of Education											
	5	Decontamination of houses	Regional Promotion Division	471 households	○	○	○	○	○	○	○	○	○	Started in FY2013
	6	Decontamination of public and medical institutions	Regional Promotion Division											
Countermeasures against internal exposure	7	Whole Body Counter measurements (conducted by the village)	Residents and Livelihood Division	1,509 persons	○	○	○	○	○	○	○	○	○	Based on an agreement between the Hirata Central Hospital, Whole Body Counter measurements and thyroid gland examinations are implemented at the same time.
	8	Whole Body Counter measurements (conducted by Fukushima Prefecture for children aged 4 to 18)	Residents and Livelihood Division					○	○	○				
	9	Food and water quality inspection	Regional Promotion Division	471 households	○	○	○	○	○	○	○	○	○	
	10	Thyroid gland examination (conducted by Fukushima Prefecture)	Residents and Livelihood Division	1,509 persons	○	○	○	○	○	○	○	○	○	Based on an agreement between the Hirata Central Hospital, Whole Body Counter measurements and thyroid gland examinations are implemented at the same time.
	11	Inspection of school meals	Board of Education	19 persons					○	○				
Others	12	Cancer screening	Residents and Livelihood Division										○	Targeted residents: those who 20 years or older for uterine cancer screening; 50 years or older for prostate cancer screening; 30 years or older for other cancer screenings
	13	Measurement and mapping of the radiation dose in the soil within the whole village	Regional Promotion Division											
	14	Sampling of respondents for a basic survey in the Fukushima Health Management Survey	Residents and Livelihood Division	1,509 persons	○	○	○	○	○	○	○	○	○	

Chapter 3 Situation of and Countermeasures by Each Individual Municipality

Katsurao Village residents were evacuated immediately after the disaster and moved later to the secondary evacuation centers and temporary housing. This article describes the residents' situation and efforts by the town, according to the following three durations and host municipalities:
- At Katsurao Village immediately after the disaster (since March 14, 2011)
- At Aizubange Town where residents took shelter in the secondary evacuation centers (from March 15 to June, 2011)
- At Miharu Town where residents moved to temporary housing (since June 2011). The Katsurao Village Office was relocated to Miharu Town.

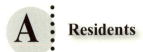

A Residents

1 Nutrition (meals/water)

a. Situation

(Katsurao Village)
- Some families had an enough food stocks because their houses are located far from stores. In addition, because most families had rice paddies and fields, they reserved a large amount of rice, vegetables, simmered Japanese butterbur sprouts, *tsukemono* pickles and other preserved foods. There was no imminent shortage of food.
- The supply of electricity and gas did not stop after the earthquake. Some households experienced a cutoff of their water supply due to a failure of water pipes, but the pipe failure was repaired in one day.

(Aizubange Town)
- Shortly after evacuation, nutritionally-unbalanced foods such as pastries and instant noodles constituted the majority of meals.
- Unsanitary conditions caused the development of norovirus infection among residents.
- Residents received daily meals at Inns and other secondary evacuation centers.
- Residents who forgot to bring their dentures when evacuating were unable to eat a proper diet. Residents' oral hygiene was poor due to the absence of toothbrushes.

(Miharu Town)
- Most households purchase drinking water because they are not only worried about radioactive contamination of water supplies but also not accustomed to drink tap water. (They had drawn drinking water from mountain streams.)
- After moving to temporary housing, there were some residents who frequently purchased ready-prepared meals due to sudden changes of the living environment. During a long evacuation period of three to five months, residents also showed less motivation to cook on their own.

b. Responses (actual measures)

(Aizubange Town)
- Countermeasures to prevent the development/spread of norovirus and influenza virus infections were taken.

(Miharu Town)
- Nutritionists and dental hygienists dispatched from the Ken-chu Public Health and Welfare Office provided home visits to conduct nutritional and oral instructions for residents.

20 Efforts of Katsurao Village

- Home-visiting services for residents living in municipally-subsidized housing started.

c. Summary/measures in the future

- Each household is advised to individually prepare food stocks for an emergency, being fully aware that the distribution of foods and other commodities may stop in times of disaster.
- A community hall adjoining to the gymnasium, in which residents took shelter, was equipped with a simple kitchen. It was fortunate that residents were able to eat hot dishes in a cold gymnasium, by cooking the distributed foodstuffs in the kitchen.
- It generally takes a long time to make a denture. It is necessary to remind residents to include dentures in their stockpile for emergencies.
- Some residents gained weight after the earthquake. Because it is quite difficult to make them lose weight by dietary instructions only, some more effective measures need to be developed.

2　Exercise (Environmental improvement)

a. Situation

(Katsurao Village)

- After an order to stay indoors was issued on March 12, a decreased amount of physical activity was observed among residents.
- There were some evacuees from coastal areas who were counting on staying with their relatives living in Katsurao Village. The village received many telephone inquiries about the safety of such evacuees from coastal areas.

(Aizubange Town)

- Radiation exposure screening tests were conducted at the Aizu Dome. Because many residents were not able to bring their dentures, eyeglasses and regular medicines, the village officials had to help such residents to smoothly undergo the screening test and other health checks.
- The town officials confirmed each individual resident's safety, using mobile phones.

(Miharu Town)

- There were some residents who actively took walks and did some exercises. However, compared to their previous farm work in the fields, the entire amount of their physical activity decreased. Inevitably, weight gain was observed as a common tendency among residents.
- After moving to temporary housing, residents had an increased opportunity to do work using their hands at assembly rooms within the sites. However, because of decreased physical activities outside the housing sites, many residents (particularly male residents) showed a decline in muscular strength.
- Some residents borrowed a farm filed to grow vegetables.

b. Responses (actual measures)

(Katsurao Village)

- According to the monitoring posts (air radiation level monitoring equipment) that were installed in front of the village office, no abnormality in air radiation levels was observed. Therefore, the village used a local wireless broadcasting system to announce to the residents that there was no need to worry about radiation. However, because an indoor evacuation order was issued to the village, the village also called for residents to stay indoors.
- The village officials confirmed the safety of residents, using mobile phones. After that, as preparation work to evacuate all residents outside the village, the village officials visited each household to confirm

189

Chapter 3 | Situation of and Countermeasures by Each Individual Municipality

whether or not the family members had a means of transportation to evacuate the village. The officials also confirmed if there were some evacuees from other municipalities within the village.

- After the evacuation on March 14, the officials went round within the village to confirm that no one was left behind.

(Aizubange Town)

- As part of measures against the development/spread of norovirus infection, the village reminded the residents to make sure to always wear a mask and wash their hands and gargle before eating.
- In cooperation with public health nurses and other nurses from inside/outside of Fukushima Prefecture, the village officials conducted home-visiting services for residents staying in gymnasiums, inns and other evacuation centers.
- Thanks to the cooperation of exercise instruction volunteer members from Aizubange Town, exercise programs were conducted for residents at gymnasiums.

(Miharu Town)

- As part of nursing-care prevention initiatives, the village gathered residents by an administrative-ward group and provided exercise instructions to them.
- At the time of home visits by the town officials, residents received exercise instructions by physical therapists, as needed.
- To prevent the elderly residents from requiring nursing-care support, staff members of a village's mutual-support center embarked on conducting some exercise programs for the elderly.

c. Summary/measures in the future

- When a disaster occurs, the village should not count solely on the emergency support by Fukushima Prefecture. Without developing an original disaster preparedness plan at a local municipality level, the village will not be able to promptly respond to the urgent needs of the residents in an emergency situation.
- It is necessary to conclude "a mutual cooperation agreement on disaster prevention and disaster relief" with municipalities inside and outside of Fukushima Prefecture.
- To reduce residents' stress caused by a lack of privacy at evacuation centers, it is necessary to partition off the space.

3 Rest (mind, anxiety, suicide, etc.)

a. Situation

(Katsurao Village)

- Physical damage by the earthquake was not so severe in the village. However, the more the details about the damage by the nuclear accident were brought to light, the more differing information was communicated through the media. Such a flood of controversial information caused confusion among residents.
- Although the village expected to receive some directions on emergency responses from Fukushima Prefecture, no direction or information were given. The village had no choice but to judge the criticality of the situation and conduct emergency response activities on its own, based on limited information obtained from the local fire stations and Kawauchi Village.

(Aizubange Town)

- During a prolonged stay at inns and other evacuation centers, many residents experienced growing stress due to concerns about an uncertain future livelihood and a sudden change in living environment that caused an increasing number of cases of sleeplessness and high blood pressure. Particularly, livestock farmers, who were forced to slaughter their livestock animals because of the animals' possible exposure to radiation, suffered from severe stress caused by a feeling of sadness and guilt.

- Many residents were filled with extreme anxiety about uncertain future livelihood. Because the residents were desperately eager to get someone to listen to their uneasy feelings and to know when they will be allowed to return to the village, the majority of complaints that the village received from the residents was that, "The village's public health nurses have not provided frequent home visits to me. I want them to listen to my concerns."

(Miharu Town)
- Temporary housing was allocated to residents by an administrative-ward group. Therefore, residents were able to feel at ease and secured surrounded by their old friends and acquaintances at temporary housing. However, with the prolonged period of evacuation, resident felt increasingly stressed in a confined space, thereby causing a growing number of troubles between neighbors.

(Aizubange and Miharu towns)
- Because residents had nothing to do at evacuation centers and temporary housing, an increase of habitual alcohol drinking in the daytime was observed among them.

b. Responses (actual measures)
(Aizubange Town)
- There were many residents who became ill and suffered from health problems. A case-by-case response to the needs of each individual resident was required.
- In cooperation with the staff members of the Disaster Medical Assistance Team (DMAT) and post-disaster mental health care teams, medical examinations and the prescription of medicines were provided to the residents.
- In cooperation with public health nurses and other nurses from inside/outside of Fukushima Prefecture, the village officials conducted home-visiting services for residents at gymnasiums, inns and other evacuation centers.
- Residents were anxious about exposure to radiation and grief for people killed by the tsunami. Moreover, a flood of differing information made them confused and caused concerns about an uncertain future. To share their uneasy feeling and prevent further concerns about the future, the village officials attentively listen to the residents.

(Miharu Town)
- Post-disaster mental health care team members started home-visiting programs for the residents in FY2011. For mentally unstable residents, continued home-visiting services were entrusted to a post-disaster mental health center in FY2012.
- Counseling programs by a certified clinical psychologist, which had been regularly conducted before the earthquake, was resumed.

c. Summary/measures in the future
- Not knowing what information to trust and what responses to take, the village officials were also confused. The village needs to develop its own disaster preparedness manual that enables immediate emergency responses on a local level in case of disasters.
- Village officials could not afford to offer post-disaster mental health support for residents who took shelter in their parents' home or in relative's houses. Rightfully, such residents must have felt extremely uneasy about their uncertain future and have been mentally exhausted from life as evacuees in unfamiliar living environments. To help them adapt themselves to a new life in host municipalities, a comprehensive

manual that describes not only local government level support programs but also collaboration efforts throughout the country needs to be established.

 B **Expectant/nursing mothers and children**

1 Nutrition (meals/water)

a. Situation
(Katsurao Village)
- At evacuation centers that accommodated residents living within a 20-km range of the Fukushima Dai-ichi Nuclear Power Station, disposable diapers and artificial milk (milk powder) were in short supply.
- Some families had an enough food stocks because their houses are located far from stores. There was no imminent shortage of food.

(Miharu Town)
- Most households purchase drinking water because they are not only worried about radioactive contamination of water supplies but also not accustomed to drink tap water. (They had drawn drinking water from mountain streams.)
- As one of the problems caused by a sudden change in living environments after evacuation, nutritionally-unbalanced diets were increasingly observed among many families.

b. Responses (actual measures)
(Katsurao Village)
- Evacuees from other municipalities made a request to the village for boiled water to make milk for babies. Responding to the request, the village officials secured boiled water and a milk-feeding corner at evacuation centers.

(Aizubange Town)
- Because foods and other commodities were in short supply at evacuation centers, the village made a list of necessary relief supplies and asked Fukushima Prefecture to send them to the residents. However, it took a long time before the requested relief supplies reached the residents.

(Miharu Town)
- Nutritionists have held a series of gatherings for expectant/nursing mothers and babies. For example, participating mothers received instructions on baby foods from the nutritionists.
- Playing programs for young children named "*asobi-no-kyoshitsu*" were conducted. Snacks and others refreshments were offered to participating young children.

c. Summary/measures in the future
- Each household is advised to individually prepare food stocks for an emergency. Because the distribution of commodities may stop in times of disaster, the village is also required to maintain adequate stockpiles in case of disasters.

2 Exercise (Environmental improvement)

a. Situation

(Aizubange Town)

- Radiation exposure screening tests were conducted at the Aizu Dome.
- So as not to bother neighbors at evacuation centers and to evacuate as far away as possible to avoid the risk of exposure to radiation, many families with young children changed evacuation destinations; such as their parents' home and relative's houses.

(Katsurao Village and Aizubange Town)

- Because there was a risk of exposure to radiation, residents were advised not to go outdoors unnecessarily. As a result, their physical activity was inevitably decreased.
- Young children were not allowed to play outdoors due to possible exposure to radiation. Because young children had no choice but to play indoors, their physical activity was decreased.

(Aizubange and Miharu towns)

- Young children experienced a decreased opportunity to play with each other.

b. Responses (actual measures)

(Katsurao Village)

- According to the monitoring posts (air radiation level monitoring equipment) installed in front of the village office, no abnormality in air radiation levels was observed. Therefore, the village used a local wireless broadcasting system to announce to residents that there was no need to worry about radiation. However, because an indoor evacuation order was issued to the village, the village also called for residents to stay indoors.

(Aizubange Town)

- As part of measures against the development/spread of norovirus infection, the village reminded the residents to make sure to wear a mask and to wash their hands and gargle before eating.

(Miharu Town)

- At gatherings for expectant/nursing mothers and babies, baby massage programs and other exercise programs were conducted.
- Nursery school childcare workers conducted play programs for young children in a dedicated room named "*asobi-no kyoshitsu*." The purpose of the programs was to support the healthy development of young children and secure a play space for them.

(Aizubange and Miharu towns)

- The village encouraged the residents to undergo vaccinations.

c. Summary/measures in the future

- When a disaster occurs, the village should not count on emergency support solely provided by Fukushima Prefecture. Without developing a disaster preparedness plan at a local municipality level, the village will not be able to promptly respond to the urgent needs of residents in an emergency situation.
- It is necessary to conclude "a mutual cooperation agreement on disaster prevention and disaster relief" with municipalities inside and outside of Fukushima Prefecture.
- To reduce residents' stress caused by a lack of privacy at evacuation centers, it is necessary to partition

Chapter 3 | Situation of and Countermeasures by Each Individual Municipality

off the space.

● With decreased opportunities to play outdoors at evacuation centers, young children have gradually developed various mental and physical health problems. The continuation of follow-up support is indispensable for the sound development of their bodies and minds.

3 Rest (mind, anxiety, suicide, etc.)

a. Situation

(Katsurao Village)

● Physical damage by the earthquake was not severe in the village. However, as more details about the nuclear accident were revealed, the more differing information was reported through the media. Such a flood of controversial information caused confusion among residents.

(Aizubange Town)

● Due to concerns about uncertainty for the future and growing stress of living in a group, many residents complained of sleeplessness at evacuation centers.

● Children cheerfully played with their brothers/sisters and friends at gymnasiums, inns and other evacuation centers. Whenever they saw their children playing, mothers felt sorry that their children caused annoyance to other residents. Inevitably, the mothers felt increasingly stressed.

● To avoid possible exposure to radiation, some families with expectant mothers and young children evacuated outside Fukushima Prefecture.

(Katsurao Village, Aizubange Town and Miharu Town)

● Many parents showed anxiety about radiation effects on the health of their children.

b. Responses (actual measures)

(Aizubange Town)

● The village officials made a phone call to residents to ask whether or not they had any emergency health problems due to inaccessibility to medical institutions.

(Miharu Town)

● One of the purposes of gathering programs for expectant/nursing mothers and babies is to promote information exchange among mothers, thereby helping mothers solve the problems of child rearing.

● Nursery school childcare workers conducted play programs named "*asobi-no kyoshitsu*" for young children and their mothers. Not only playing/exercise programs for young children, but mental and childcare counseling for mothers were also offered at these programs.

● To offer post-disaster mental health support, a certified clinical psychologist conducted counseling programs.

● In cooperation with the staff members of the DMAT and a post-disaster mental health care team, village officials offered home-visiting services to understand each individual resident's mental condition.

c. Summary/measures in the future

● Not knowing what information to trust and what responses to take, the village officials were confused. The village needs to develop its own disaster preparedness manual that enables immediate emergency responses on a local government level in case of disasters.

● For residents who took shelter in their parents' home or relative's houses, the village officials could not afford to offer post-disaster mental health support. Rightfully, such residents must have felt extremely uneasy about uncertainty for the future and have been mentally exhausted from life as evacuees in unfamiliar living environments. To help them adapt themselves to their new life in host municipalities, a comprehensive manual that describes not only local government level support programs but also collaboration efforts throughout the country needs to be established.

People requiring assistance during a disaster (vulnerable people in case of a disaster)

1 Nutrition (meals/water)

a. Situation

(Katsurao Village)
- Because many households in the village had drawn drinking water from mountain streams, residents were not affected by a cutoff of the water supply.
- It was lucky for the residents that the supply of electricity and gas was not stopped after the earthquake.

(Aizubange Town)
- Residents who forgot to bring their dentures when evacuating were unable to eat a proper diet. Residents' oral hygiene was poor due to the absence of toothbrushes.

(Miharu Town)
- Persons requiring assistance showed a slight decline in their physical strength, along with the decline in their social functioning ability.

b. Responses (actual measures) (Katsurao Village)
- Although the village added toothbrushes to a list of relief supplies to be requested to Fukushima Prefecture, the supplying of toothbrushes was delayed.

(Aizubange Town)
- Doctors dispatched from other municipalities examined residents. As needed, the doctors referred residents to medical institutions and administered medicines.
- Measures against the development/spread of norovirus and influenza virus infection were taken.

(Aizubange Town and Miharu Town)
- Closely communicating with the staff members of a regional mutual assistance center, the village officials strived to check each individual resident's health condition. When residents with a poor health condition were identified, home visits were immediately provided. Moreover, the village provided necessary welfare and health services to such residents, in cooperation with the social welfare council staff members.

c. Summary/measures in the future
- It is difficult to offer emergency relief support by each local municipality alone. To ensure the prompt provision of necessary assistance and support to disaster victims, a cooperative system with various other private organizations needs to be established.
- It generally takes a long time to make a denture. It is necessary to remind residents to include dentures into stockpiles for an emergency.

Chapter 3 | Situation of and Countermeasures by Each Individual Municipality

2 Exercise (Environmental improvement)

a. Situation

(Aizubange Town)

- Radiation exposure screening tests were conducted at the Aizu Dome. There were some residents who did not evacuate and stayed within Katsurao Village for several days.
- Residents, who took shelter in the Azuma Sports Park (located in Fukushima City) and evacuation centers within Aizubange Town, received radiation exposure screening tests. Because many residents were not able to bring their dentures, eyeglasses and regular medicines, the village officials had to help such residents undergo the screening test.
- Having nothing to do in a cold gymnasium with no heating equipment, many residents spent a day just lying in a blanket.
- Before evacuating all the residents outside the village, the officials confirmed the safety of residents and identified those who had no means of transportation to evacuate. After that, the officials discussed how to evacuate them outside the village.

(Miharu Town)

- Some residents became homebound, gaining weight due to a lack of exercise. There were many residents who faced difficulties in adapting themselves to a new living environment.

(Katsurao Village, Aizubange Town, and Miharu Town)

- Because there was a risk of exposure to radiation, residents were advised not to go outdoors unnecessarily. Their physical activity was inevitably decreased.

b. Responses (actual measures)

(Katsurao Village)

- According to the monitoring posts (air radiation level monitoring equipment) installed in front of the village office, no abnormality in air radiation levels was observed. Therefore, using a local wireless broadcasting system, the village announced to the residents that there was no need to worry about radiation. However, because an indoor evacuation order was issued to the village, the village also called for residents to stay indoors.
- The officials went round within the village to confirm that no one was left behind.

(Aizubange Town)

- As part of measures against the development/spread of norovirus infection, the village reminded the residents to make sure to wear a mask and to wash their hands and gargle before eating.
- In cooperation with public health nurses and other nurses from inside/outside of Fukushima Prefecture, the village officials conducted home-visiting services for residents at gymnasiums, inns, and other evacuation centers.

(Miharu Town)

- In collaboration with a support center for persons with disabilities, the village offered an opportunity for residents with disabilities to do work using their hands.
- A mental health program named "*hidamari-kai*" was resumed. The purpose of the program is to encourage mentally disabled persons to take more exercise and prevent them from staying shut up at home.

(Aizubange Town and Miharu Town)
- The village urged residents to have influenza and pneumococcal vaccinations.
- At evacuation centers that accommodated a large number of elderly residents, the village officials conducted a daily stretching exercise program, using a towel, for the elderly residents.

c. Summary/measures in the future
- It is difficult for each local municipality to offer emergency relief support. To ensure the prompt provision of necessary assistance and support to disaster victims, a cooperative system with various other private organizations needs to be established.
- To promptly respond to the urgent needs of the residents in an emergency situation, it is necessary for the village to develop an original disaster preparedness plan.
- It is necessary to conclude "a mutual cooperation agreement on disaster prevention and disaster relief" with municipalities inside and outside of Fukushima Prefecture.
- A long period of evacuation at a facility not equipped with heating apparatus will inevitably worsen the health condition of elderly residents and persons with disabilities. To maintain their favorable health conditions, it is necessary to install heating devices in evacuation centers or move them to facilities equipped with a heating system at an early stage of evacuation.

3 Rest (mind, anxiety, suicide, etc.)

a. Situation
(Katsurao Village)
- Physical damage by the earthquake was not so severe in the village. However, the more the details about the damage by the nuclear accident were brought to light, the more differing information was reported through the media. Such a flood of controversial information caused confusion among residents.

(Aizubange Town)
- There was an increase in the number of the elderly who developed cognitive impairment due to a sudden change in the living environment.
- The worsening of health conditions of residents with mental disease was attributed not only to sudden changes in the living environment but also to the unavailability of their regular medicines.

b. Responses (actual measures)
(Aizubange Town)
- There were many residents who became ill and suffered from health problems. A case-by-case response to the needs of each individual resident was required.
- In cooperation with public health nurses and other nurses from inside/outside of Fukushima Prefecture, the village officials conducted home-visiting services for residents at gymnasiums, inns and other evacuation centers.
- Residents were filled with anxiety about exposure to radiation and grief for people killed by the tsunami. Moreover, a flood of contradictory information made them confused and caused a growing concern about uncertain livelihood in the future. To share their uneasy feeling and prevent further concerns about the future, the town officials attentively listened to the residents.

(Miharu Town)
- A mental health program named "*hidamari-kai*" was resumed. The purpose of the program is to encourage mentally disabled persons to take more exercise and prevent them from being homebound.

Chapter 3 | Situation of and Countermeasures by Each Individual Municipality

- In collaboration with a support center for persons with disabilities, the officials strived to accommodate urgent needs of each individual disabled resident.
- In cooperation with the staff members of the DMAT and a post-disaster mental health care team, the village officials offered home-visiting services to understand each individual resident's mental condition.

c. Summary/measures in the future

- The village is required to ensure that all residents include their regular medicines into stockpiles for an emergency. The village also should check after evacuation whether or not each individual resident maintained their regular medication schedule.
- There were some residents who stayed shut up at home all day long. As needed, the village encouraged them to go outdoors and take exercise.
- It is very important for persons with disabilities to consult a medical staff member and receive appropriate treatment at an early stage of evacuation.
- Some residents completely lost their mental stability after the earthquake. There were some cases in which such residents regained their composure by participating in a mental health program.

(Tomoko Matsumoto)

21. Efforts of Hirono Town

1. Situation of the municipality

(1) Demographics (as of January 1 of each year)

	2011	2012	2013
Population	5,509	5,308	5,219
Number of households	1,969	1,921	1,902
Average number of people per household	2.80	2.76	2.74
Number of births	41	31	40
Birth rate	7.4	5.8	7.7
Number of deaths	75	59	74
Mortality	13.6	11.1	14.2
Ratio of the elderly aged 65 or older	22.9	23.1	

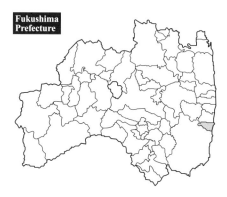

Fukushima Prefecture

(2) Geographical features

Total area: 58.39 km^2 (approximately 13 km east-west; approximately 7 km north-south)

Distance from the Fukushima Daiichi Nuclear Power Station of the Tokyo Electric Power Company: approximately 21- 28 km

Evacuation area: The whole town was initially designated as an evacuation-prepared zone.

Transportation network: Joban Expressway Hirono I.C; JR Joban Line Hirono Station; National Route 6

2. Situation of damage by the earthquake, tsunami and the nuclear disaster

(1) Damage by the Great East Japan Earthquake (as of May 8, 2012)

Property damage	Completely destroyed	Half destroyed	Partially destroyed
House	113	216	1,590
Public institution	2		
Other			

Human damage	Deaths by disaster	Disaster-related deaths	Missing persons	Injured persons
	2	27	1	

* Half-destroyed properties include 35 significantly destroyed houses, town-managed collective housing (15 households) and a sewage treatment plant.

(2) Situation of evacuation

① Evacuation centers within the municipality (as of March 15, 2011)

	Number of evacuation centers	Number of evacuees	Available period
Residents	5	300	3/11 - 14
Evacuees received		40	3/11 - 14

* All residents were evacuated outside the town.

② Approximate number of evacuees in evacuation centers outside the municipality (as of April 17, 2013)

	End/March 2011	End/September 2011	End/March 2012	Latest period
First evacuation center				
Second evacuation center				
Temporary housing				1,538
Municipally-subsidized housing				1,925

③ Approximate number of voluntary evacuees

Inside Fukushima Prefecture		Outside Fukushima Prefecture (number of evacuees & prefectures)	

Chapter 3 | **Situation of and Countermeasures by Each Individual Municipality**

Outlook of damage related to the nuclear disaster

- The Fukushima Prefecture Disaster Prevention Information System and all other means of communications were cut off due to the earthquake. TV programs that could be viewed using an in-house generator were the only available source of information for the residents.
- The town received a notification of the situation of the Fukushima Daini Nuclear Power Station of the Tokyo Electric Power Company (hereinafter referred to as the "Fukushima Daini Nuclear Power Station"), based on Article 10 (a provision regarding a notification obligation of radiation dose above the limit specified by Cabinet Order) and Article 15 (a provision regarding instructions as to nuclear emergency situation response measures) of the Act on Special Measures Concerning Nuclear Emergency Preparedness. However, the town was not notified of any information on the situation of the Fukushima Daiichi Nuclear Power Station.
- An evacuation order issued to areas within a 10-km range of the Fukushima Daini Nuclear Power Station was also applied to some parts of the town. However, after deliberation at the town's disaster response headquarters, the town decided to evacuate all residents from the town to secure the safety of all residents.
- When announcing that all residents need to be evacuated, specific host municipalities had not yet been decided upon. Therefore, the town could only urge residents to take evacuation "in a westerly or southerly direction."
- For residents who did not have their own car and were not able to evacuate on their own, the town briefly gathered them at public facilities within the town, then drove them outside the town by a town bus and other public vehicles.
- Although the town made a request to the Fukushima Prefecture Disaster Response Headquarters for emergency evacuation buses for residents, it took almost 24 hours before the buses arrived at the town because of a delay in the arrangement of buses and bad traffic conditions. In fact, when the buses reached the town, most residents had already been evacuated. The town used only two buses to evacuate the remaining residents.
- Town officials, firefighting team members and Self-Defense Force officials visited each household to identify residents who needed assistance during evacuation. After the identification, the town asked the national government and Fukushima Prefecture to assist with prompt evacuation of such residents.

3 Countermeasures against nuclear disaster (as of January 2013)

	Name of project	Division in charge	Number of targeted persons (households)	Expectant mothers	Nursing mothers	Babies	Young children	Elementary school students	Junior high school students	Senior high school students	People age 19 to 39	People age 40 or older	Remarks (major operations)
1	Distribution and collection of personal dosimeters	Welfare Environment Group Residents' Health Management Group	About 1,900 households	○	○	○	○	○	○	○	○	○	Distribution of dosimeters to all households, acceptance, distribution and collection for calibration
2	Distribution of dosimeters (badges)	Residents' Health Management Group	About 120 persons					○	○				Coordination with schools, announcements to parents/guardians and notification of results
3	Real-time measurement of the radiation dose (Ministry of the Environment)	Welfare Environment Group	28 posts										Response to inquiries from residents
4	Decontamination of public facilities	Decontamination Work Group	All residents	○	○	○	○	○	○	○	○	○	Monitoring and decontamination work
5	Monitoring and Measurement of the air radiation levels in the whole town	Decontamination Work Group	All residents	○	○	○	○	○	○	○	○	○	Aggregation and announcements of the measurement results
6	Decontamination and replacement of the surface soil on the grounds in nursery schools, kindergartens, primary schools and junior high schools	Childcare Group of the Board of Education Decontamination Work Group				○	○	○	○				Monitoring and decontamination work
7	Shuttle bus operation for elementary school and junior high school students	Board of Education						○	○				An explanatory meeting for parents/guardians, review of the shuttle bus route, contracts and announcements
8	Decontamination of all houses	Decontamination Work Group	All residents	○	○	○	○	○	○	○	○	○	Monitoring and decontamination work
9	Whole Body Counter measurements	Residents' Health Management Group	All residents			○	○	○	○	○	○	○	Acceptance of application, notification of the measurement results, reports to Fukushima Prefecture (A clinic within the town conducts the measurement.)

200

No.	Activity	Group	Target										Remarks
10	Thyroid gland examination (conducted by Fukushima Prefecture)	Residents' Health Management Group	All residents				○	○	○	○			Schedule arrangement and notification
11	Inspection of the radiation dose of school meals	Childcare Group of the Board of Education	About 160 persons			○	○	○	○				Purchase of equipment, measurement and announcements of the inspection results
12	Food and water quality inspection	Industry Group	All residents	○	○	○	○	○	○	○	○	○	Purchase of equipment, acceptance, measurement, notification and announcements of the inspection results
13	Lecture meetings on radiation	Residents' Health Management Group	All residents	○	○	○	○	○	○	○	○	○	Request for lecturers and announcements to the residents
14	Study sessions of radiation (for elementary school and junior high school teachers)	Board of Education	About 50 persons										Request for lecturers
15	Sampling of respondents for a basic survey in the Fukushima Health Management Survey	Residents' Health Management Group	All residents	○	○	○	○	○	○	○	○	○	
16	Decontamination of farmland (deep plowing and spraying of chemicals)	Industry Group	All residents	○	○	○	○	○	○	○	○	○	Monitoring and decontamination work
17	Measurement and mapping of the radiation dose in the soil within the whole town	Industry Group											
18	Maintenance and management of emergency temporary housing set up inside and outside the town	Welfare Environment Group	About 1,500 persons	○	○	○	○	○	○	○	○	○	Response to various inquiries from residents living in emergency temporary housing
19	Information dissemination to residents taking shelter in host municipalities	All Divisions	All residents	○	○	○	○	○	○	○	○	○	Sending of public relations information magazines twice a month

Chapter 3 Situation of and Countermeasures by Each Individual Municipality

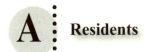

A Residents

- Immediately after the earthquake, Hirono Town residents took shelter in four municipalities; namely, Ono Town, Ishikawa Town, Hirata Village, and Iwaki City.
- Residents began moving to the secondary evacuation centers on April 9.

1 Nutrition (meals/water)

a. Situation
- Residents were accommodated at four evacuation centers. At one of the evacuation centers, residents had only two meals per day for a certain period of time due to a shortage of food. However, in general, enough emergency food supplies were distributed to residents at the four evacuation centers.
- A large-scale earthquake with an epicenter directly under Iwaki City occurred on April 11, causing severe damage to the secondary evacuation centers set up within the city. Because the supply of water was cut off and distribution of food supplies stopped for several days after the earthquake, evacuation centers, where many food supplies had already arrived, shared the distributed foods with other evacuation centers within the city.
- Information such as "cold rice balls were distributed at some evacuation centers, while warm rice balls and *miso* soup were prepared at other evacuation centers" was easily exchanged among residents through cell-phone messages. Inevitably, a growing sense of inequality caused residents to feel dissatisfied.
- Food poisoning occurred due to rice balls distributed from Fukushima Prefecture. The rice balls were prepared by suppliers in the Aizu area and were temporarily gathered at Koriyama City to sort out before distributing to each evacuation center. The time-consuming process from preparation to distribution was the cause of food poisoning.

b. Responses (actual measures)
- At one of evacuation centers in the host village, the village officials, women's association members and other local volunteers cooked in turn almost every day for evacuees from Hirono Town. Deeply appreciating the kindness of such local people and feeling ashamed for just receiving and eating every meal without doing anything by themselves, some Hirono Town female residents and licensed chefs also helped cooking in turn. On the other hand, there were some evacuation centers where Hirono Town officials took the leadership in cooking for the residents.
- The town paid careful attention to allocate food supplies to all evacuation centers as equally as possible.
- Foodstuffs were sent from all over Japan to the residents. Moreover, thanks to the support at host municipalities, residents were able to secure food supplies.

c. Summary/measures in the future
- Despite of all the difficulties caused by an exceptional level of the earthquake and the tsunami, large amounts of food supplies promptly reached the affected areas. Japan's distribution system and the Japanese people's spirit of mutual assistance were admirable.
- A system that Fukushima Prefecture used to gather rice balls from many suppliers and distribute them to the affected areas is not desirable. With the aim of reducing the risk of food poisoning and backing up local suppliers, Fukushima Prefecture is advised to conclude an outsourcing contract with local suppliers, thereby enabling a prompt distribution of rice balls.
- It is necessary for the town and each household to store several days' worth of emergency food and be

21 Efforts of Hirono Town

sure to bring them when undertaking evacuation.

2 Exercise (Environmental improvement)

a. Situation
- At a gymnasium that served as a primary evacuation center, pet dogs and cats also stayed with their owners.

b. Responses (actual measures)
- Following advice from a veterinarian of the Fukushima Prefecture Public Health Center, the town strived to systematically allocate space to residents at the gymnasium. To be specific, the warm second floor of the gymnasium was allocated to residents at high risk for various infectious diseases caused by pet animals. Residents who had no problem with sharing a space with animals stayed on the first floor.
- Under the leadership of the head of the dietary improvement promotion council, volunteer members from each host municipality were divided into a "cooking group," a "cleaning group" and a "distribution group" and were involved with their assigned work. Thanks to the systematic volunteer work, aid/medical team members were able to focus on their emergency relief activities at evacuation centers. Each municipality's responsible volunteer workers were regularly gathered together and asked to ensure that necessary information was shared among all volunteer staff members.
- Residents voluntarily formed a "trash group" and a "toilet cleaning group" to maintain good hygiene in evacuation centers. At evacuation centers with a relatively large number of Hirono Town officials, most cleaning work was conducted by the officials.

c. Summary/measures in the future
- Staying in a confined space of evacuation centers might cause deep vein thrombosis/pulmonary embolism (the economy-class syndrome). With the aim of preventing the development of such diseases due to a lack of exercise, residents gathered together every morning to take radio gymnastic exercises at evacuation centers.
- It is necessary to take some measures for residents who take shelter with pet animals.
- Because all evacuees are forced to share spaces at evacuation centers in an emergency situation, it is essential to take effective measures to prevent the spread of infectious diseases among them.

3 Rest (mind, anxiety, suicide, etc.)

a. Situation
- Residents increasingly felt impatient as they worried about possible effects of invisible radiation and did not have correct information on damage by the tsunami. Aftershocks that occurred almost every day also caused residents to become terribly frightened.
- Many residents complained of sleeplessness at evacuation centers.

b. Responses (actual measures)
- Medical consultation was provided to residents.
- Mental health care officials went around to the evacuation centers to offer counseling services.
- TV programs and the Internet were main sources of information for the residents. Most residents had their own mobile phones.

Chapter 3 | Situation of and Countermeasures by Each Individual Municipality

c. Summary/measures in the future

● One resident commented, "Because I felt severely stressed by inconvenient living at evacuation centers and was filled with extreme anxiety about my livelihood in the future, mental care support by the officials reassured me very much."

● It is necessary to establish a system that enables prompt communication of correct information to residents immediately after a disaster.

● "Support providers" are required to have some knowledge of mental health care and receive practical training.

4 Others

a. Situation

● After the tertiary evacuation to Iwaki City, the town finally resumed normal working operations and started full-fledged disaster response activities.

● After the earthquake, the town conducted special medical examinations. Although the duration was one day shorter than that of regular medical examinations, residents (including those who were taking shelter outside Fukushima Prefecture), equivalent to approximately 80% of regular examinees, underwent the special medical examinations.

● Some residents, who returned from host municipalities outside Fukushima Prefecture, answered that they were not very worried about exposure to radiation because air radiation levels were monitored by monitoring posts (monitoring equipment).

● There are some residents who regularly check radiation levels in and around their houses, using portable dosimeters that were distributed to each individual household.

b. Responses (actual measures)

● Upon deciding on the resumption of school from September (a month when the second semester starts in Japan), the town held explanatory meetings, lecture meetings on radiation, and radiation-related counseling sessions for parents/guardians, aiming to smoothly proceed with the resumption.

● After the resumption of school, the town regularly inspected the radiation dose in ingredients of school lunches and air levels within the premises of each individual school and school lunch center. The inspection results were regularly circulated among relevant parties. The town also announced numerical results of decontamination through public magazines.

● Lecture meetings on radiation and workshops conducted by an advisory group from Fukushima Medical University have been regularly held.

● Monitoring posts (air radiation level monitoring equipment) were installed at each assembly hall and other public facilities so that residents can easily confirm air radiation levels on their own.

● Thanks to the host town's physicians who promptly visited gymnasiums and other evacuation centers, Hirono Town residents were able to receive some medicines and other medical supplies at an early stage of evacuation.

● Residents at some evacuation centers participated in a "shopping tour on a bus" that was conducted as part of support programs for disaster victims.

c. Summary/measures in the future

● After the tertiary evacuation to Iwaki City, the town resumed regular working operations in the city. Because the majority of Hirono Town residents began concentrating in temporary housing prepared in the city, the town was able to offer effective health management programs to residents.

● Special medical examinations conducted after the earthquake constituted a good opportunity for residents to share necessary information with others. Additionally, before and after the examinations, many residents visited the town's temporary office set up in Iwaki City to go through various necessary procedures.

- Initially, residents considered evacuation centers as just "a place to take shelter" during the time a higher air radiation level is observed. However, they now recognize how significant it is to secure evacuation centers as "a safety net" for an emergency.

- At a gymnasium where residents took shelter, relief activities were systematically conducted by a "medical care team," a "general support team," and other specific teams. Therefore, medical care officials were able to focus on conducting a survey on the health conditions of the residents. If all staff members had conducted relief activities independently, effective and smooth medical care support might not be offered to the residents.

- The strong social solidarity in a host town was very impressive. In such a town, emergency response activities were conducted based on a firmly-established cooperative relationship with the Fukushima Prefecture's Health and Welfare Office. Self-reliance Support Council members were also actively and voluntarily involved in emergency assistance programs. Hirono Town had much to learn.

- Hirono Town feels gratitude to all municipalities inside and outside of Fukushima Prefecture, particularly to municipalities with which the town had almost no close previous relationship, for their assistance and generous support for the victim residents.

- Some residents are extremely worried about the exposure to radiation, while others are not. There exists a sharp divergence of opinions on radiation among residents. Even if the town announces correct radiation information, some pessimistic residents do not trust the information. Because radiation is invisible and its effects on health do not show up immediately, it is very difficult for the town to address each individual resident's anxiety, concerns, and opinions.

- Initially, as many as eight municipalities had actively taken part in a series of nuclear disaster drills conducted by Fukushima Prefecture. However, the drills gradually became one of the local programs of Futaba and Okuma towns where nuclear power units are located, on the assumption that a nuclear disaster will not occur in real life. As can be seen from our experience, however, a nuclear disaster will not only cause severe damage to host towns of power units; a wider surrounding area will also be affected by the disaster. Moreover, even if appropriate measures against a nuclear disaster are developed, they cannot work effectively without the residents' awareness of nuclear disaster preparedness. Both effective nuclear disaster prevention plans and region-wide awareness of disaster preparedness are indispensable in the future.

- If a nuclear disaster occurs at the Hamadori district again, Fukushima Prefecture is strongly advised to make phone calls to all municipalities within the prefecture to promptly receive evacuees from the district.

- Because the national government's response to the nuclear disaster lacked consistency, Hirono Town residents feel doubts about their safety from radiation and are hesitant to return to the town.

- Although Fukushima Prefecture had established the Off-Site Center (OFC) in Okuma Town as a local base facility for disaster response activities, the center did not function due to the damage done by the earthquake and the tsunami. Therefore, the prefecture temporarily displaced the local base to the Fukushima Prefecture Community Hall, which led to a delay in initiating prompt emergency relief activities. Fukushima Prefecture needs to review its disaster management base strategy.

- It is a responsibility of the Governor of Fukushima Prefecture to hear various opinions from medical personnel and radiation specialists and immediately judge the necessity of taking iodine tablets/syrup. The judgment results and other vital information obtained through the System for Prediction of Environmental Emergency Dose Information (SPEEDI) should be promptly disseminated to each individual municipality under the name of the Governor. Without such information and instructions from the prefecture, local municipalities are not able to conduct appropriate emergency relief activities.

Chapter 3 Situation of and Countermeasures by Each Individual Municipality

- The town is required to secure host municipalities in advance and ensure that all residents are informed of where to take shelter in an emergency situation.

B Expectant/nursing mothers and children

1 Nutrition (meals/water)

a. Situation
- Many residents purchased drinking water and paid careful attention to the origins of any food products.
- Although disposable diapers and artificial milk (milk powder) were in short supply and were not sold anywhere immediately after the earthquake, they were distributed in large amounts later.
- When resuming classes at school, the town supposed that many parents may have doubts about the safety of foodstuffs in school lunches.

b. Responses (actual measures)
- A resident living in Ishikawa Town donated disposable diapers and one of her two cans of milk powder to babies evacuated from Hirono Town.
- For school lunches, inspection of the radiation level in foodstuffs was conducted to confirm the safety of school meals. The inspection results were reported to parents/guardians in an easy-to-understand format.
- Decontamination and repair work of school lunch centers was completed prior to the resumption of school. Therefore, the town was able to resume both classes and school lunches at the same time.

c. Summary/measures in the future
- Emergency relief supplies may not reach disaster victims immediately after an earthquake. Because babies have no source of nutrition other than milk powder, it is critically important to maintain milk powder stocks for babies for use during an emergency.

2 Exercise (Environmental improvement)

a. Situation
- Some junior high school students attending a baseball club moved to other schools outside of the town to continue their club activities. There were also students who had decided not to return to Hirono Town for the continuation of their club activities.
- Decontamination work of school grounds and parks was conducted, so that young children can play outdoors.

b. Responses (actual measures)
- Indoor playing programs for young children were conducted, with the aim of providing playing spaces for young children and encouraging information exchange among parents/guardians.
- Air radiation level monitoring equipment was installed within the town.
- Repeated decontamination work was conducted in outdoor sports facilities, educational facilities and school zones.

c. Summary/measures in the future
- Because young children have had their outdoors play restricted, it is necessary to secure indoor playing spaces for them.

21 Efforts of Hirono Town

- Aiming to improve the environment in which young children can play and enjoy exercise without feeling anxious about the possible exposure to radiation, decontamination work of outdoor sports facilities must be completed as early as possible.

3　Rest (mind, anxiety, suicide, etc.)

a. Situation
- After evacuation, it was difficult for mothers to find a hospital when young children caught a cold or babies kept crying at night due to some health problems.

b. Responses (actual measures)
- After the resumption of classes at school, some parents sought advice of the town officials about their children's truancy from school. The town officials visited their schools to understand the current situation. As needed, the town officials and board of education members conducted home visits to talk with truant students and provide advice for their parents.
- According to a student, Hirono Town's teachers and board of education members attended students at the school bus and conducted friendly conversation with the student; such as "Good morning. How are you?" and "How was your day at school today?"
- If medical examination results identified young children, newborn babies and parturient women who were supposed to need some follow-up support, the town's public health nurses provided home-visiting services. In some cases, home visits and other necessary support were entrusted to public health nurses of such residents' host municipalities.
- School counselors have visited junior high schools every week.
- The town offered a school bus service for students taking shelter far from school. The town officials, who were well acquainted with each individual student, served as school bus drivers. Because the bus drivers carried on friendly conversation with the students and enjoyed the conversation, they were popular with both students and their parents.

c. Summary/measures in the future
- To maintain existing mental health follow-up programs for elementary school and junior high school students, close collaboration among the town officials, school personnel, and board of education members needs to be established.
- The town is required to ensure that young children, newborn babies, and their mothers undergo necessary medical examinations, aiming at the early detection of their physical and mental health problems. If some problems are identified, the town should offer continued follow-up support in collaboration with the public health nurses, doctors, and relevant medical institutions.

4　Others

a. Situation
- Shortly after the earthquake, the town advised many expectant mothers to take shelter outside Fukushima Prefecture and deliver a baby in the host municipalities. Therefore, the town initially received many requests for a refund of overpayment of childbirth expenses.
- In an evacuation center, there was a family with a baby who had been born one month before the earthquake. To help ensure the baby's health and safety, the town allocated to the family a room apart from other residents and gave priority to the family for using a bathroom.
- Soon after the earthquake, because milk powder was in short supply within Fukushima Prefecture, many

Chapter 3 Situation of and Countermeasures by Each Individual Municipality

families with babies and toddlers took shelter in other prefectures.

- After the end of the spring vacation, elementary school, junior high school, and high school students moved to the secondary evacuation centers.
- It was possible that high school students could go to local school within Iwaki City after the end of the spring vacation.
- Because the majority of Hirono Town residents began concentrating in Iwaki City, the town received permission to use some classrooms within the premises of the local elementary school and junior high school in Iwaki City and resumed classes for students evacuated from Hirono Town.
- In late April 2012, a town official found an expectant mother gathering *warabi* shoots within Hirono Town. She explained to the official that "I am going to deliver a baby outside Hirono Town" and "I am just taking a walk because the air radiation level is relatively low today." The official advised her to be sure to wear a mask when taking a walk and never eat the gathered *warabi* shoots because they may be contaminated with radiation.
- Although there are not many junior high school teachers in the town, they attentively listened to concerns and anxiety of each individual student and provided necessary follow-up support to them. Such efforts by the teachers successfully created a good relationship of trust among teachers, students, and parents/ guardians.
- Hirono Town's elementary school and junior high school teachers made strenuous efforts to always be considerate of students' feelings. They frequently visited local schools in host municipalities to understand the physical and mental health conditions of students evacuated from Hirono Town and supported the students' mental stability.

b. Responses (actual measures)

- The town officials made contact with all expectant mothers, including those who took shelter outside of Fukushima Prefecture, to understand their situations. Expectant mother evacuating in other prefectures did not express many concerns about radiation.
- In allocating secondary evacuation centers to residents, the town considered easy accessibility to school for each individual family.
- Because some students had to walk 7 to 8 km to go to school, the town decided to operate a school bus for them, using a town bus.
- The town has distributed personal dosimeters (glass badges) to elementary school and junior high school students, at their parents' request. In 2013, personal dosimeters were distributed to about 70 to 80 % of elementary school students and almost 50% of junior high school students.

c. Summary/measures in the future

- Surprisingly, personal dosimeters have not been distributed to 100% of school students. This fact indicates that there are some parents who are not much concerned about their children's possible exposure to radiation.
- The greatest concern of parents after the disaster was early resumption of classes for children. Therefore, the town received many requests from parents to converge all of the Hirono Town's school functions in one municipality to resume school as early as possible. In fact, it is difficult in an emergency situation to secure an appropriate place/facility having enough capacity to resume classes in a host municipality. However, school is symbolic of the local community and serves a central role in fostering children who will become the driving force of the future society. As a lesson from the disaster, if a similar disaster occurs somewhere in the future, each local municipality is advised to focus on the convergence of school functions in one place and resume classes at an early stage of evacuation.

21 Efforts of Hirono Town

C People requiring assistance during a disaster (vulnerable people in case of a disaster)

1 Nutrition (meals/water)

a. Situation
- For residents who missed an opportunity to evacuate and stayed in their homes, it was difficult to secure water and food because the supply of water was cut off and stores within the town were closed.
- When offering meals at evacuation centers, no special attention was paid to residents who had difficulties in eating/swallowing. For such residents, it was difficult to eat the same food as those offered to ordinary residents.

b. Responses (actual measures)
- Self-Defense Force officials distributed foods and water to the residents staying in their own homes.
- Rice porridge in a retort pouch was offered to residents, as needed.

c. Summary/measures in the future
- Special meals for residents requiring nursing care should be included into emergency relief food supplies.

2 Exercise (Environmental improvement)

a. Situation
- Because persons requiring assistance were accommodated within the same space with ordinary residents at the primary evacuation centers, both parties felt inconvenience.

b. Responses (actual measures)
- The town asked dedicated facilities to accept mentally disabled residents and the bedridden elderly.
- Many elderly residents were accommodated in an evacuation center equipped with floor heating.

c. Summary/measures in the future
- Due to the limitation of manpower, the number of residents with disabilities who could be accepted at dedicated facilities was also limited. On the other hand, it is almost impossible that persons requiring assistance and other ordinary residents live together, sharing a space. As a future task for the town, it is necessary to both expand the accommodation capacity of welfare facilities and improve living environments of each evacuation center.
- It is necessary to secure places where persons requiring assistance can take shelter in times of disaster.

3 Rest (mind, anxiety, suicide, etc.)

a. Situation
- Some residents were forced to take shelter separately from their family members.

b. Responses (actual measures)
- Town officials and neighbors paid close attention to and helped care for residents requiring assistance.
- Residents who have a certificate as a caregiver or nurse also looked after their neighboring residents

Chapter 3 | Situation of and Countermeasures by Each Individual Municipality

who required assistance.

c. Summary/measures in the future

- A system that enables the continuation of services for residents requiring nursing care and other special assistance must be established.
- It is essential for the town to build a cooperative relationship with nursing care facilities and other welfare facilities within the town.
- Each administrative ward of the town is advised to identify residents requiring assistance in advance and intensify cooperative ties with various welfare-related organizations. This as part of local level disaster preparedness efforts.

4　Others

a. Situation

- In Iwaki City, it was difficult to perform artificial dialysis due to a cutoff of the water supply. Although Minami Tohoku Hospital located in Koriyama City offered to provide artificial dialysis treatments of outpatients from Hirono Town, the shortage of gasoline was a critical problem to drive to the hospital even a few days in a week. To address such a problem, the hospital provided conveniences for the outpatients; allowing them to stay within the premises of the hospital in the daytime and lending vacant beds to them at night. In cooperation with a urology hospital in Iwaki City, serious patients were transferred to a medical institution in Tokyo by the hospital's patient transfer bus.
- It was more than one month after the evacuation to Iwaki City that the local urology hospital accepted artificial dialysis patients evacuated from Hirono Town.
- Because some residents who were in need of artificial dialysis treatment did not have mobile phones and the town officials had no way of making contact with them, they delayed undergoing necessary treatments.
- Thanks to the mediation of a regional comprehensive support center in a host town, some residents with disabilities were able to receive necessary support at day care facilities.
- Because the local council of social welfare (hereinafter referred to as the "social welfare council") was temporarily dissolved after evacuation, the elderly residents who had received support at the social welfare council and other welfare centers came to the town's public health center to ask for continuation of nursing-care support.
- Some elderly residents who developed low blood pressure at a gymnasium (one of the evacuation centers) were hospitalized. After their health condition improved, these elderly residents were accommodated in a welfare facility for the elderly located in Ishikawa Town. Arrangements were made through the mediation of a regional comprehensive support center in each individual host municipality.
- Medical institutions in the Nakadori district provided an advanced level of medical treatment. This was exemplified by a Hirono Town resident who was confined to a wheelchair. After evacuating to the district, the resident consulted a local orthopedic surgeon to have an artificial joint and an artificial femoral head implanted. The implantation surgery enabled the resident to stand up and walk on his own. As another example, there was also a Hirono Town resident who escaped death thanks to cardiac surgery in the Nakadori district.
- The town asked the Self-Defense Force officials to regularly confirm how many residents did not take shelter and stayed in their own homes. The number was more than 30 at the very least. Every time the officials looked for them, the residents concealed themselves so as not to be found.
- There was an 80-year-old resident who left an evacuation center and returned home at his own discretion. He lived alone and remained active, waking up with the sun, doing all necessary things during the

day and going to sleep at sundown.

b. Responses (actual measures)

- As a substitute for a denture case, the town officials cut off the upper half of plastic bottles. The plastic bottles and denture cleaning agents were distributed to residents, as needed, for the purpose of maintaining the oral health condition of residents.
- Because there were many residents at high risk of infection at evacuation centers, the town strenuously strived to prevent the development/spread of norovirus infection and infectious gastroenteritis among residents.
- In preparing temporary housing, the town also set up a temporary support center within the premises to provide day-care services for the elderly residents. However, the capacity of the temporary support center was less than that of the facility managed by the regional comprehensive support center in the town. Aiming to enable more residents to receive necessary support, the regional comprehensive support center resumed its day-care service operations after residents returned to the town.
- The town officials distributed food and other commodities to residents who did not take shelter.

c. Summary/measures in the future

- Immediately after the earthquake, residents in need of artificial dialysis treatment felt anxious as to whether or not they could receive continued treatment.
- Essentially, it was a role of the members of Fukushima Prefecture's Medical Treatment and Pharmaceutical Affairs Group to respond to the immediate needs of dialysis patients in times of disaster. However, because the earthquake brought devastating damage to a wide area of eastern Japan, the Group members were not able to promptly fulfill their role. Hirono Town hopes that Fukushima Prefecture will review the Group's emergency response system, learning a lesson from the failure to fulfill its role after the Great East Japan Earthquake.
- Before the earthquake, the town's welfare center staff members had discussed how to conduct emergency response activities in times of disaster. The staff members had intended to create a route map, similar to the one prepared by a local welfare facility, that could be used when carrying patients on a stretcher or transferring patients to a hospital. However, the route map created by the welfare facility was found useless in an emergency situation.
- After the earthquake, problems concerning the elderly residents were gradually brought to light. To prevent elderly persons' physical/mental functions from declining, the town needs to make continued efforts to take nursing-care prevention measures.
- When moving to temporary housing or municipally-subsidized housing, some elderly residents were forced to live apart from their family members. Inevitably, with no assistance from their children and grandchildren with meals and room cleaning, such elderly residents gradually wanted to be hospitalized or accommodated in a welfare facility. Even for the elderly residents who can go to the toilet on their own and cook for themselves at home, it was difficult to look after themselves in an unfamiliar environment, resulting in an increased number of nursing-care recipients among them. There were also many elderly people who were possessed with the idea that "I cannot do anything on my own in such an unstable living condition as an evacuee." Such pessimistic thinking also caused a decline in both the physical and cognitive abilities of the elderly residents.
- The greatest concern for the town is home nursing care of the elderly by male family members. For example, as a general trend, a situation in which a son has to provide nursing care for his mother due to the absence of any female family members often results in elder abuse. To help prevent elder abuse in households without female members, support from local community members is indispensable.
- The town officials are fully aware of how important it is to make residents, particularly the elderly resi-

Chapter 3 | Situation of and Countermeasures by Each Individual Municipality

dents, return to their normal life in Hirono Town as soon as possible.
- All of the elderly residents who returned to Hirono Town have good health. In contrast, elderly residents who have been forced to continue to take shelter in host municipalities show a decline in their physical and cognitive abilities.

(Shigeru Nemoto, Kazuma Komatsu, Marie Monma, Keiko Sakuma)

22 Efforts of Iitate Village

1 Situation of the municipality

(1) Demographics (as of January 1 of each year)

	2011	2012	2013
Population	6,544	6,361	6,357
Number of households	1,963	1,958	1,932
Average number of people per household	3.3	3.3	3.3
Number of births	50	37	52
Birth rate	7.6	5.8	8.1
Number of deaths	73	90	92
Mortality	11.2	14.1	14.5
Ratio of the elderly aged 65 or older	30	29.1	29.4

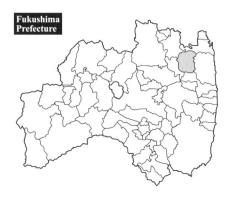

(2) Geographical features

Total area: 230.13 km² (approximately 15.2 km east-west; approximately 16.8 km north-south)

Distance from Fukushima Daiichi Nuclear Power Station of the Tokyo Electric Power Company: approximately 40 km

Evacuation area: Evacuation order lifting preparation area: 4 administrative districts; restricted habitation area: 15 administrative districts; difficult-to-return area: 1 administrative district

Transportation network: National Route 399; Prefectural Route 12

2 Situation of damage by the earthquake, tsunami and the nuclear disaster

(1) Damage by the Great East Japan Earthquake (as of March 31, 2013)

Property damage	Completely destroyed	Half destroyed	Partially destroyed
House	0	0	331
Public institution	0	0	8
Other			

Human damage	Deaths by disaster	Disaster-related deaths	Missing persons	Injured persons
	0	42	0	0

(2) Situation of evacuation

① Evacuation centers inside the local municipality (as of March 16, 2011)

	Number of evacuation centers	Number of evacuees	Available period
Residents	1	150	March 16 to May 15
Evacuees received	6	1,610	March 12 to 20

② Approximate number of evacuees in evacuation centers and other sites outside the local municipality

	End/March 2011	End/September 2011	End/March 2012	Latest period
First evacuation center	0	0	0	0
Second evacuation center	0	0	0	0
Temporary housing	0	1,217	1,219	1,175
Municipally-subsidized housing	0	3,553	3,795	3,980

③ Approximate number of voluntary evacuees

Inside Fukushima Prefecture		Outside Fukushima Prefecture (number of evacuees & prefectures)	

Chapter 3　Situation of and Countermeasures by Each Individual Municipality

▬▬ **Outlook of damage related to the nuclear disaster** ▬▬

①On March 11, the Nuclear Emergency Response Headquarters was established immediately after the Great East Japan Earthquake.
The whole staff was involved in disaster-relief activities from the following day.

②From March 19 to April 30, a total of approximately 500 residents, who consisted of voluntary evacuees from the village and evacuees from outside the village, were evacuated in groups to Kanuma City, Tochigi Prefecture.

③On April 22, the whole village was designated as a deliberate evacuation area, and all residents were required to be evacuated. It took a great number of personnel and significant amount of time to secure residences in evacuation destinations and provide evacuation guidance to residents.

④On May 21, health checkups and consultations on radiation were conducted, targeting residents living in three areas where a high radiation dose was detected.

❸ Countermeasures against nuclear disaster (as of January 2013)

		Name of project	Division in charge	Number of targeted persons (house-holds)	Expect-ant mothers	Nursing moth-ers	Babies	Young children	Elemen-tary school students	Junior high school students	Senior high school students	People age 19 to 39	People age 40 or older	Remarks (major operations)
Countermeasures against external exposure	1	Distribution of dosimeters	Business Promotion and Decon-tamination	All house-holds	○	○	○	○	○	○	○	○	○	Lending a dosimeter per household at its request
	2	Refreshment for expectant mothers (relaxation in low-dose areas)	Education Division											
	3	Refreshment for young children	Education Division					○						
	4	Refreshment for elementary school and junior high school students	Education Division						○	○				Planning programs, recruiting participants and accompanying them, as needed
	5	Monitoring of air levels	Business Promotion and Decon-tamination											Distributing air dosim-eters to all households
	6	Real-time measurement of radiation dose (Ministry of the Environment)												
	7	Measurement of air levels in the whole city & creation of maps												
	8	Replacement of the surface soil on the grounds in childcare facilities, child education facilities and schools	Education Division					○	○	○	○			Replacing the surface soil in temporary hous-ing sites in evacuation destinations
	9	Decontamination of houses	Business Promotion and Decon-tamination	All house-holds										Planning to conduct decontamination in all areas in 2013 and 2014
	10	Decontamination of public and medical institu-tions												Village Office
Countermeasures against internal exposure	11	Examination of breast milk				○								Introducing examina-tion institutions only to those who are interested
	12	Whole Body Counter measure-ments (conducted by Iitate Village)	Health and Welfare Division		○	○	○	○	○	○	○	○	○	
	13	Whole Body Counter measure-ments (conducted by Fukushima Prefecture, target-ing those age 4 to 18)	Health and Welfare Division					○	○	○	○			
	14	Food and water quality inspection	Business Promotion and Decon-tamination	All house-holds	○	○	○	○	○	○	○	○	○	

	#	Activity	Division	Target										Notes
	15	Thyroid gland examination (conducted by Iitate Village)	Health and Welfare Division				○	○	○	○	○			Conducting examinations every year; targeting all kindergarteners and elementary and junior high school students in the village; collecting consent forms
	16	Thyroid gland examination (conducted by Fukushima Prefecture)	Education Division				○	○	○	○	○			
	17	Inspection of school meals	Education Division				○	○	○	○				
	18	Debriefing sessions for measurement results of exposure dose	Health and Welfare Division											
	19	Study sessions on radiation (kindergartens, elementary and junior high schools)	Education Division/ Health and Welfare Division					○	○	○				
	20	Cancer screening (those age 19 to 39)	Health and Welfare Division									○		
	21	Replacement of the surface soil in rice paddies	Business Promotion and Decontamination											
	22	Measurement of radiation dose in soil in the whole city & creation of maps	Business Promotion and Decontamination											
Others	23	Lecture meetings on radiation	Health and Welfare Division	All households	○	○	○	○	○	○	○	○	○	
	24	Sampling of respondents for a basic survey in the Fukushima Health Management Survey	Health and Welfare Division	All households	○	○	○	○	○	○	○	○	○	
	25	Publication of disaster information magazines	Planning Division/ Public Relations	All households										
	26	Publication of risk communication newspapers (Subjects related to radiation)	Health and Welfare Division	All households	○	○	○	○	○	○	○	○	○	Publishing newspapers six times a year; holding editor meetings
	27	Issuance of citizen health cards (containing a column for recording radiation exposure levels)	Health and Welfare Division	All households	○	○	○	○	○	○	○	○	○	

Chapter 3 Situation of and Countermeasures by Each Individual Municipality

With agriculture as its main industry, Iitate Village determined not to participate in the Heisei grand municipal merger. It has been involved in regional development for 30 years, centering on more than 20 administrative districts (residents' associations and neighborhood associations).

Accordingly, local communities have become empowered and have supported village development, agriculture promotion and local health and welfare activities.

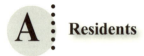
A Residents

1 Nutrition (meals/water)

a. Situation

- Due to the nuclear power station accident, 1,200 people were evacuated from the Coastal Region to the village. The village worked to establish evacuation centers and prepare meals outdoors, in cooperation with fire companies and women's associations. However, since radiation was reported to be dispersed even in the village, it was busy taking countermeasures.
- Since contamination was identified in water from a small water-supply system, restrictions on the use of water were imposed. Since a large amount of bottled water was brought in to the village every day through the cooperation of the Self-Defense Forces, staff members were busy distributing the water to residents. Although restrictions on the use of water were lifted on May 20, residents requested to have bottled water continuously distributed due to concerns about the possible health effects of water.
- Since transportation of goods was disrupted due to a fuel shortage, the amount goods sold at stores were decreasing daily.

b. Responses (actual measures)

- The village received evacuees from other municipalities and provided them with support for their diet and livelihood.
- Due to radioactive contamination in the tap water, the village distributed bottled water to individual households.
- Due to a shortage of commodities caused by fuel scarcity, the village procured relief supplies and distributed them.

c. Summary/measures in the future

- It is necessary to inspire people to store emergency provisions, artificial milk (milk powder), diapers and other necessaries, in case of emergencies and natural disasters such as earthquake.

2 Exercise (Environmental improvement)

a. Situation

- Since the whole village was designated as an evacuation area, residents were forced to live indoors. Consequently, an increase in lifestyle-related diseases, such as obesity, hypertension, dyslipidemia and hyperglycemia, was recognized.
- From June 22, the administrative operations of the village office were carried out outside the village.
- Educational activities were conducted through public relations magazines to communicate the importance of engaging in exercise and physical activities in evacuation destinations.
- Fukushima Prefecture also gradually organized a system in which residents could undergo an examination for internal exposure, and conducted examination of those who were interested.

22 Efforts of Iitate Village

b. Responses (actual measures)
- The village made arrangements so that residents could move to Kanuma City, Tochigi Prefecture, when they desired to.
- Since the whole village was designated as a deliberate evacuation area on April 22, the village struggled to ensure evacuation destinations for residents.
- From June 22, the administrative operations of the village office were carried out in Iino Town, Fukushima City.
- Fukushima Prefecture conducted an examination for internal exposure (at the National Institute of Radiological Sciences and the Tokai Village, or through onboard equipment.)

c. Summary/measures in the future
- Even after evacuation of residents was completed, the village was busy taking various measures and was unable to immediately develop a favorable environment where residents could exercise.

3 Rest (mind, anxiety, suicide, etc.)

a. Situation
- In some areas, mental health care centers were prepared at an early stage, which regularly held friendly gatherings in assembly rooms in temporary housing sites to provide mental consultation to residents.
- Seventy percent of the residents were evacuated to municipally-subsidized housing, while 30% of the residents, who were mainly elderly people, were evacuated to temporary housing. The village was very busy providing consultation in evacuation destinations.

b. Responses (actual measures)
- Mental consultation was offered to residents through hook-ups with mental health care centers.
- Nursing staff was temporarily employed to provide health consultation to residents in municipally-subsidized housing.

c. Summary/measures in the future
- Since health damage due to radiation is somewhat unclear, residents feel highly anxious about it. In addition, the national government kept changing its criteria for evacuation. Consequently, many parents with young children often became bewildered. It is necessary to clarify the criteria for evacuation in advance.

B Expectant and nursing mothers & children

1 Nutrition (meals/water)

a. Situation
- On March 20, water quality inspection was conducted for water from a small water-supply system in the village. The inspection results showed that 965 Bq of radioactive materials, which exceeded the standards of 300 Bq, was detected in the water.
- Due to no distribution of goods caused by fuel scarcity, no commodities were sold at any stores. In addition, vegetables grown and stored at home were unable to be eaten because they were damaged by radioactive materials. Consequently, residents were very anxious about not being able to procure food.

Chapter 3 — Situation of and Countermeasures by Each Individual Municipality

b. Responses (actual measures)
- From March 21, all staff members began to distribute bottled water to all households. The village continued to distribute water through the directors of administrative districts and at the village office until residents were evacuated.

c. Summary/measures in the future
- It is necessary to inspire people to store emergency provisions, artificial milk (milk powder), diapers and other necessaries, in case of emergencies and natural disasters such as an earthquake.

2 Exercise (Environmental improvement)

a. Situation
- Since residents were ordered to stay indoors as much as possible after the nuclear power station accidents, they continued to live indoors, which inevitably led to their lack of exercise. Moreover, in some evacuation destinations with high radiation levels; residents also had a lack of exercise.
- On April 21, schools were resumed at part of the school facilities outside the village, which were borrowed by the village.

b. Responses (actual measures)
- The village secured temporary evacuation destinations for expectant mothers and young children at inns outside the village, and encouraged them to move there.
- After all residents were ordered to be evacuated from the village, the village worked to move them to evacuation destinations, with the top priority placed on households with expectant mothers and children.

c. Summary/measures in the future
- Even after evacuation of residents was completed, the village was busy taking various measures and was unable to immediately develop a favorable environment where residents could exercise.

3 Rest (mind, anxiety, suicide, etc.)

a. Situation
- Since health damage from radiation caused by the nuclear power station accident was unclear, residents were anxious about the health of expectant mothers and children. Consequently, many mothers and children were voluntarily evacuated at first.
- Simple thyroid gland examination was conducted for junior high school students and younger children due to the concerns about the impact of spreading radioactive iodine (^{131}I) on thyroid glands. (Figure 22-1)

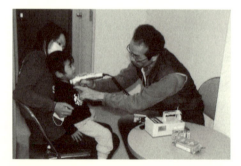

Figure 22-1 A child undergoing thyroid gland examination

b. Responses (actual measures)

- The village held lecture meetings on radiation several times by inviting specialists. However, since the national criteria for evacuation were not easily established before evacuation orders were given to residents, some residents had doubts about the contents of the lectures. The village keenly realized the difficulty of correctly informing residents about radiation.

c. Summary/measures in the future

- Even in a confusing situation, it is the most important to convey information correctly. In particular, the situation of radiation contamination, which contained a risk of threatening human health, should have been reported in a correct and timely manner.

People requiring assistance during a disaster (vulnerable people in case of a disaster)

1 Nutrition (meals/water)

a. Situation

- Nursing care establishments became unable to offer their services. Consequently, the elderly with higher-level nursing care needs were forced to move to nursing facilities inside and outside Fukushima Prefecture.

b. Responses (actual measures)

- The village deliberated over how to arrange nursing services for those who require nursing care and provide support to them in evacuation destinations in uncertain circumstances after the earthquake. The village tried to comply with the wishes of residents as much as possible.
- In a situation where drinking water was also contaminated, staff members individually visited elderly people living alone and residents on welfare to confirm their safety and provide health consultation, while distributing food and bottled water.

c. Summary/measures in the future

- Under a situation where the capacity of nursing facilities in the whole Fukushima Prefecture, which received new residents, exceeded permissible limits, staff at individual facilities made serious efforts to receive as many people as possible.
- Fukushima Prefecture should make arrangements to secure evacuation destinations in advance as a countermeasure against disaster.

2 Exercise (Environmental improvement)

a. Situation

- After the evacuation of all residents was completed, staff members visited elderly people who were in poor physical condition in their homes on a preferential basis and introduced exercises that could be done at home to prevent disuse syndrome.

b. Responses (actual measures)

- The village asked some local governments where residents were evacuated to hold regular exercise classes for residents living in temporary housing in the same way as they did for local residents. Consequently, residents living in temporary housing improved their strength.

Chapter 3 Situation of and Countermeasures by Each Individual Municipality

- From FY2012, similar exercise classes began to be held in all of the 11 temporary housing sites. For residents living in municipally-subsidized housing, the village also held exercise classes at facilities that it borrowed. However, since municipally-subsidized houses were located over a wide area, the village faced difficulties securing venues for the classes and found it difficult to take effective measures due partly to the lack of manpower.

c. Summary/measures in the future
- Although most of elderly people had lived in a large family, such as a three-generation family, before the earthquake, they were unable to live with their family members due to housing conditions in evacuation destinations. More elderly people moved to temporary housing, while seeking communication with others.
- Many elderly people, who were evacuated to municipally-subsidized housing with their family members, were unable to tolerate being alone during the day, when other family members work outside of the home, in unfamiliar areas and chose to move to temporary housing.

3 Rest (mind, anxiety, suicide, etc.)

a. Situation
- In some areas, mental health care centers were established in an early stage, which regularly held friendly gatherings in assembly rooms in temporary housing sites to watch over elderly people.

b. Responses (actual measures)
- Since many elderly people were evacuated to temporary housing, at first the village frequently provided health consultation for them. After they became more settled, the village provided health consultation once a month, and staff members visited them in their homes as needed.
- The village asked evacuees in collective housing, such as housing for government employees and company housing, to establish residents' associations to provide health consultation once a month.
- Since residents living in municipally-subsidized housing were located over a wide area, the village checked their health condition through home visits, in cooperation with livelihood support counselors from social welfare councils.
- The ratio of evacuation to temporary housing and municipally-subsidized housing was 30% and 70%, respectively. Although staff members watched over the health of residents in municipally-subsidized housing through home visits, visits to these houses were not time-efficient because of the time required to move between individual houses.

c. Summary/measures in the future
- At the beginning of evacuation, many residents reported that they suffered from a sense of loss because they lost their places in society, their purposes in life and their communities.
- Fortunately, in cooperation with the Fukushima Center for Disaster Mental Health, the village was able to respond to residents both as a group and individually depending on their situation.
- Since a certain number of residents lived together in temporary housing sites, the village easily provided health consultation to them. Meanwhile, since residents in municipally-subsidized housing were located over a wide area, staff members had to determine where the residents lived before their first visit. Accordingly, the first visit to residents took longer than subsequent visits.

D Others

- From FY 2012, the village began to provide an opportunity to promote risk communication by inviting experts on radiation to comment in the publication "*Kawara-ban Michishirube*" (Figure 22-2), a newspaper magazine about radiation, which was directed at a limited readership.
- In July 2012, the national government reorganized the districts in the village based on consultation with the village. As a result, the village was regionalized into 20 administrative districts: one difficult-to-return district where residents would be unable to return for six years after the disaster; 15 restricted habitation districts where they were unable to return for three to five years; and four evacuation order lifting preparation districts.
- The village will promote reconstruction work with the aim of declaring that all residents can return to the village, while taking into account the progress of full-fledged decontamination implemented by the national government, development of infrastructure and reconstruction plans. The village aims to have individual residents return to their normal lives through its reconstruction work. It intends to offer as much support as possible to residents regardless of whether they will return to the village or not.
- However, the village, which has less than 70 regular staff members, will need more than an ordinary effort to continue to provide equal services to residents who return to the village and those who do not. Currently, the village offers support for reconstruction, decontamination and livelihood of evacuated residents, while obtaining the cooperation of approximately 120 persons, including temporary workers from national, prefectural and municipal governments and emergency hire employees. However, it is facing great challenges to offer administrative services after it declares that all residents can return to the village and to secure the necessary human resources.
- The village realizes that it should provide health and welfare services to residents living both inside and outside the village. In this case, the village will be required to bear higher costs of administrative services than it does for residents living in evacuation destinations.

(Kumiko Matsuda)

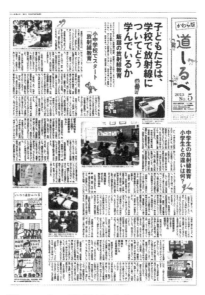

Figure 22-2   "*Kawara-ban Michishirube*," a newspaper magazine directed at a limited readership for risk communication

23 Efforts of Minamisoma City

1 Situation of the municipality

(1) Demographics (as of January 1 of each year)

	2011	2012	2013
Population	71,554	67,055	65,807
Number of households	23,890	23,021	22,913
Average number of people per household	3.0	2.9	2.8
Number of births	580	511	327
Birth rate	8.1	7.6	5.0
Number of deaths	818	1,533	718
Mortality	1,143.2	2,286.2	1,091.1
Ratio of the elderly aged 65 or older	26.0	26.7	28.1

* Birth rate: per 1,000 people; mortality: per 100,000 people

Fukushima Prefecture

(2) Geographical features

Total area: 398.50 km² (approximately 40 km east-west; approximately 50 km north-south)

Distance from Fukushima Daiichi Nuclear Power Station of the Tokyo Electric Power Company: approximately 25.5 km (Minamisoma City Hall)

Transportation network: National Route 6; JR Joban Line (5 stations); Prefectural Route 12

2 Situation of damage by the earthquake, tsunami and the nuclear disaster

(1) Damage by the Great East Japan Earthquake (as of February 1, 2013)

Property damage	Completely destroyed	Half destroyed	Partially destroyed
House	1,229	732	2,389
Public institution	17		16
Other			

Human damage	Deaths by disaster	Disaster-related deaths	Missing persons	Injured persons
	631	305	3	59

* Flooded area by tsunami: approximately 10% of the whole area of the city

(2) Situation of evacuation

① Evacuation centers inside the local municipality (as of March 14, 2012) From then onward: 3 sites

	Number of evacuation centers	Number of evacuees	Available period
Residents	37	8,261	March 11 to Dec. 28
Evacuees received			

* Evacuation centers set up immediately after the earthquake March 12: 37 sites; 7,935 people
March 13: 27 sites; 7,596 people
March 14: 23 sites; 8,261 people
March 15 – commencement of evacuation: 154 people on March 25 (minimum)

② Approximate number of evacuees in evacuation centers and other sites outside the local municipality (As of February 1, 2013)

	End/March 2011	End/September 2011	End/March 2012	Latest period
First evacuation center	194	78	0	0
Second evacuation center		1,181	23	0
Temporary housing		4,642	6,020	6,454
Municipally-subsidized housing		26,739	24,249	21,707

23 Efforts of Minamisoma City

③ Approximate number of evacuees (As of February 1, 2013)

Inside Fukushima Prefecture	17,496

Outside Fukushima Prefecture (number of evacuees & prefectures)	10,666 persons; 43 prefectures

Outlook of damage related to the nuclear disaster

①Due to the nuclear power station accident, Odaka Ward and the southern part of Haramachi Ward (approximately 107 km²) was designated as a restricted area within a 20-km range; the rest of Haramachi Ward and part of Kashima Ward (approximately 181 km²) as a deliberate evacuation area and an evacuation-prepared area within a 30-km range; and the rest of Kashima Ward (approximately 111 km²) as an area outside the 30 km zone. Thus, the city was divided into three parts.

②Many residents were evacuated voluntarily on an individual basis or in a group by bus to Katashina Village, Kusatsu Town and Higashi-Agatsuma Town in Gunma Prefecture, and Nagaoka City, Joetsu City, Sanjo City and Ojiya City in Niigata Prefecture. Other residents were voluntarily evacuated to Miyagi Prefecture, Yamagata Prefecture and other areas throughout Japan. Consequently, the population of the city was decreased to nearly 10,000 people at the end of March, 2011. The city, with deserted streetscapes, looked like a ghost town.

③Residents in medical institutions and nursing care insurance facilities were also forced evacuate, and many of them became ill on the way to evacuation destinations and after arriving there.

④Vulnerable people who were unable to transfer independently stayed in the city. Under the situation where daily commodities and food were in a short supply and public assistants from outside the city did not come, the delivery of goods was supported chiefly by individual volunteers. Although supporters did not come, medical support was eventually provided in April to people requiring assistance during a disaster (vulnerable people in case of a disaster) under the Disaster Relief Act by Nagasaki Prefecture and Nagasaki University.

⑤At first, people on the spot were able to obtain information on the actual situation of nuclear disaster only through the mass media.

⑥The city began to measure radiation in the air independently in May 1, 2011 to determine the actual levels of radiation in the city in detail.

❸ Countermeasures against nuclear disaster (as of January 2013)

		Name of project	Division in charge	Number of targeted persons (households)	Expectant mothers	Nursing mothers	Babies	Young children	Elementary school students	Junior high school students	Senior high school students	People age 19 to 39	People age 40 or older	Remarks (major operations)
Countermeasures against external exposure	1	Personal dose measurement	Health Promotion Division	7,420	○	○	○	○	○	○	○			Distribution, collection, notification of results, and analysis
	2	Lecture meetings on radiation	Health Promotion Division	All residents	○	○	○	○	○	○	○	○	○	Notification of results of personal dose measurements
	3	Refreshment for young children	Early Childhood Education Division											Not planned
	4	Refreshment for elementary school and junior high school students	School Education Division											Not planned
	5	Monitoring of air levels	Consumer and Environmental Protection Division											Measurement, record, and publication
	6	Radiation mesh survey	Consumer and Environmental Protection Division											Conducted only in FY2011; not planned in FY 2013
	7	Air level rate and soil survey in farmland	Agriculture, Forestry and Radiological Countermeasure Division	Farmland owners: 6,365 persons										Targeted farmland: 62.7 km²; water channels: 1,053 km; and farm roads: 156.7 km
	8	Measurement of air levels in the whole city & creation of maps	Consumer and Environmental Protection Division											Conducted in FY 2011 and FY 2012; not planned in FY 2013
	9	Replacement of the surface soil on the grounds in childcare facilities, child education facilities and schools	Educational Affairs Division				○	○	○	○				Replacement of the surface soil on grounds, etc.

223

Chapter 3 — Situation of and Countermeasures by Each Individual Municipality

	No.	Item	Division/Section	Target/Number	C1	C2	C3	C4	C5	C6	C7	C8	C9	Remarks
Countermeasures against internal exposure	10	Decontamination of houses	Decontamination Measures Section	19,132 households	○	○	○	○	○	○	○	○	○	Decontamination of roads, houses, business buildings, etc.
	11	Whole Body Counter measurements (conducted by Minamisoma City)	Health Promotion Division		○	○		○	○	○	○	○	○	Arrangement of WBC examination (hospitals), notification and coordinating of examination, contact to applicants, and management of results
	12	Whole Body Counter measurements (conducted by Minamisoma City)	Health Promotion Division		○	○			○	○	○	○	○	Arrangement of acceptance of applications, creation of name lists, delivery, aggregation, and report to the prefecture
	13	Whole Body Counter measurements (conducted by Fukushima Prefecture, targeting those age 4 to 18)	Health Promotion Division		○	○			○	○	○			Notification of WBC examination to evacuees outside the prefecture and coordinating of applications; not planned in FY 2013, because it is conducted by the prefecture
	14	Monitoring of radioactive materials in tap water	Waterworks											Three times per week (concluding agreements related to operations and paying the amount to be borne)
	15	Monitoring of radioactive materials in well water	Consumer and Environmental Protection Division											
	16	Concentration of radioactive materials in agricultural products	Agriculture, Forestry and Radiological Countermeasure Division	Many kinds of agricultural products										Survey of concentration of radioactive materials
	17	Monitoring of radioactive materials in school meals and other meals	School Education Division	3,462				○	○	○				Measurement, record, and publication
	18	Monitoring of radioactive materials in meals provided in nursery schools	Early Childhood Education Division			○	○							Measurement, record, and publication
	19	Simple analysis of radiation in food supplied for personal consumption	Consumer and Environmental Protection Division											Measurement, notification of results, and partial publication of results
	20	Cancer screening	Health Promotion Division		○	○						○	○	Arrangement of acceptance of applications, sending of checkup cards, notification of results, aggregation, and analysis
	21	Replacement of the surface soil in rice paddies	Agriculture, Forestry and Radiological Countermeasure Division											Under survey
	22	Sampling of respondents for a basic survey in the Fukushima Health Management Survey	Health Promotion Division									○	○	Request for sampling of respondents to the Information Policy Office, and report on the respondents to the prefecture
	23	Publication of disaster information magazines	Reconstruction Planning Department											Publication of the "Living Guidebook" and the "Situation of Minamisoma City after the Great East Japan Earthquake"
	24	Outpatient departments for health counseling on radiation	Minamisoma City Hospital	All residents	○	○	○	○	○	○	○	○	○	Provision of counseling

23 Efforts of Minamisoma City

A ⋮ Residents

1 Nutrition (meals/water)

a. Situation

- The living environment as well as the dietary environment changed due to evacuation. This caused many problems, such as concerns about food safety, decreased motivation for cooking, diminished intake of vegetables and unbalanced intake of food.

b. Responses (actual measures)

- The city promoted a campaign, "Healthy diet and bowl movements," to build up the health of residents so that they might be less affected by radiation. The city incorporated the following points into its health education and tried disseminating them to residents:
  - Eating food that has undergone radiological examination
  - How to remove radioactive materials from food by ways to cook
  - How to take food to improve immunity and healing ability
  - Preventing constipation

Specifically, the city focused on the "1:1:2 exercise campaign," which it had been conducting even before the earthquake occurred to recommend an ideal combination of food – one staple food, one main dish and two side dishes – as a healthy meal. Moreover, it held various cooking classes to overcome the residents' decreased motivation to cook and improve men's cooking techniques, with the aim of having them enjoy eating.

c. Summary/measures in the future

- Suffering from an unprecedented disaster, a nuclear power station accident, the city was caught in a difficult situation where information was so conflicting that it was difficult to figure out what information should be followed as the basis for taking action. The city became acutely aware of the importance of promptly providing residents with accurate information that they could understand and make decisions for themselves. Moreover, it is important to obtain valid information by analyzing data and checking its reliability before transmitting information.

2 Exercise (Environmental improvement)

a. Situation

- Residents were evacuated outside the city as they obtained information on the nuclear power station accident. Consequently, the population of the city decreased from 70,000 to nearly 10,000.
- In April, residents who were once evacuated outside the city began to gradually return home.
- Since public facilities, such as community centers, had become unavailable, group activities were unable to be resumed.
- There were concerns even about walking outdoors for exercise in fear of exposure to radiation.
- The city was flooded with inquiries about a community health examination, which was planned to be conducted in FY 2011, from residents in the city as well as in evacuation destinations outside the city.
- The city was deluged with protest calls about services. The complaints varied depending on evacuation destinations.

Chapter 3 Situation of and Countermeasures by Each Individual Municipality

b. Responses (actual measures)

- Aside from its public relations magazines, the city published "*Health Newsletter*" on an irregular basis.
- Around July, the city responded to a request for health education from a senior citizens' club.
- In July, the city conducted an examination for internal exposure to radiation.
- In August, a peer group for health promotion began to resume its activities.
- In November, the city resumed its activities to support the promotion of healthy exercise.
- The city began to hold an exercise class "*ichi ni no skip (one, two and skip)* ♪," targeting residents around their 50s. (twice per month)

c. Summary/measures in the future

- Fukushima Prefecture and other institutions should properly arrange their support services so that they are offered equally to individual local governments that were subject to disaster.
- The city will provide support to peer groups that have resumed their activities as well as promote the cooperation with them.

3 Rest (mind, anxiety, suicide, etc.)

a. Situation

- On March 15, the order to stay indoors was issued. The city began to evacuate residents by large buses according to its out-of-town emergency evacuation plan. Some residents were evacuated by family car.
- Since the city was divided into three parts and residents were forced to be evacuated, local communities were broken.
- Support was not offered during the month of March 2011. From April 4, 2011, support began to be provided by other prefectures and the Self-Defense Forces in accordance with Disaster Relief Act.
- Family members consisting of younger generations were evacuated and only elderly members stayed in the city, which led to a change in the family structure. Consequently, more people developed a feeling of isolation and complained about their poor mental condition.
- In 2012, a questionnaire survey conducted by a business institution in the city showed that there was a tendency towards a higher percentage of male residents in their prime who had no one to confide in and had thoughts of suicide within the previous year.

b. Responses (actual measures)

- The city conducted health examinations for residents living in temporary housing and municipally-subsidized housing.
- The city visited residents in their homes to care for their emotional and spiritual needs.
- The city held lecture meetings on mental health.
- The city conducted training for developing gatekeepers (those who provide support to, and watch over, people who are distressed).

c. Summary/measures in the future

- More residents may commit suicide in the future due to concerns about the uncertainty of the future. The city should not only implement administrative efforts but also take measures to prevent suicide. These can encourage self-awareness, and mutual support and relationships in local communities (regional development).

23 Efforts of Minamisoma City

B : Expectant and nursing mothers & children

1 Nutrition (meals/water)

a. Situation

- Immediately after the earthquake, the city could only manage to supply rice balls and pastries to residents.
- The nuclear power station accident stopped the distribution of goods. Consequently, residents faced difficulties procuring anything.
- Many residents came to health centers to seek artificial milk (milk powder).
- After the nuclear power station accident, expectant and nursing mothers and children were evacuated outside the city.
- Immediately after the nuclear power station accident, radioactive materials were temporarily detected in water reservoirs.
- There was high anxiety about local food materials.

b. Responses (actual measures)

- Since expectant and nursing mothers and children were evacuated outside the city, the city asked local governments in their evacuation destinations to respond to their needs.
- For evacuees (evacuation centers) in neighborhood areas, public health and welfare offices ("public health center") and dietetic associations in evacuation destinations provided support in cooperation with the city.
- Bottled water was temporarily distributed to children.

c. Summary/measures in the future

- The city was affected not only by the earthquake but also by the nuclear power station accident. Consequently, it is important to insure food safety. The city needs to improve the food inspection system and announce food safety. To this end, it is important for the city to encourage collaboration and discussions with relevant institutions, even during ordinary times.

2 Exercise (Environmental improvement)

a. Situation

- Immediately after the earthquake, most expectant and nursing mothers and children were evacuated outside the city.
- At first, the city did not know how many children stayed in the city.
- Staff members in charge were unable to be involved in regular activities for mothers and children, because they were busy engaging in disaster work, including providing support for residents in evacuation centers.
- The city received many inquiries from evacuees outside the city and was busy responding to them.
- Health examinations for young children showed that there were many young children who could not play outside and were restless.

b. Responses (actual measures)

- In June, health examinations for young children were resumed (Approximately 20% of the young

227

Chapter 3 | Situation of and Countermeasures by Each Individual Municipality

children originally targeted underwent the examinations). The city had trouble securing places for the checkups outside the 30 km zone (It borrowed spaces in kindergartens).

- Volunteer psychologists provided consultation to mothers in health examinations for young children.
- The city created documents that were necessary for young children to receive vaccination and health examinations for young children in evacuation destinations outside the city.
- In October, the city held the "*Nakayoshi Hiroba*" event four times to offer a place where children could play indoors.
- In October, the city distributed approximately 5,600 personal dosimeters (glass badges) to measure external exposure to radiation.
- In November, the city began to lend watch-type dosimeters solely to 100 expectant mothers.

c. Summary/measures in the future

- Since the Special Act on Measures concerning Nuclear Evacuees had not become effective, the city asked individual local governments to respond flexibly to the needs of mothers and children, including permitting them to receive vaccination and health examinations for young children without request forms.
- In many cases, individual local governments made decisions at their own discretion. This was because the national government and Fukushima Prefecture were unable to make necessary judgments and work out effective measures, even if the local governments sought their advice.

---

3 Rest (mind, anxiety, suicide, etc.)

a. Situation

- After the city ordered residents to evacuate the city, most expectant and nursing mothers and children were evacuated outside the city.
- As schools and kindergartens were resuming their activities, children gradually returned to the city.
- Many guardians were anxious about the impact of radiation. They felt stressed about the fact that they had to wear masks whenever leaving home and were unable to have children play outside. In addition, they felt uneasy about all aspects of their lives, including when they dried the laundry and the bedding outdoors and used air conditioners.
- There were many mothers/children who were forced to live apart from their husbands/fathers. Such an unstable living environment put stress on them.

b. Responses (actual measures)

- From July 11, 2011, the city commenced the internal exposure measurement program.
- From October 1, 2011, the city commenced the external exposure measurement program.
- The city held lecture meetings on radiation.
- The city conducted an individual consultation by psychologists based on Mental Health interview sheets of mothers and children in health examinations for young children and counseling sessions. (The number of psychologists was increased.)
- The city provided an opportunity for mothers to talk with each other (Refresh Mama Program, Maternity Family Seminar, etc.).

c. Summary/measures in the future

- The city should make sure the residents can obtain accurate knowledge about radiation, especially the impact of long-term exposure to low-dose radiation, so that they can choose their behavior and made decisions based on such knowledge. To this end, the city needs to repeatedly give a detailed explanation to individual residents to relieve their concerns about radiation.

People requiring assistance during a disaster (vulnerable people in case of a disaster)

1 Nutrition (meals/water)

a. Situation

- The nuclear power station accident caused food shortages. In particular, people had difficulty obtaining tube feeding nutrients and dietary supplements.
- The city was concerned about how to support those who were left behind at home.
- Immediately after the earthquake, medical institutions lost their function and continued to be unable to respond to people. Although some vulnerable people lost weight and became malnourished, the city had trouble responding to them because it was unable to procure food and goods to improve their physical condition.

b. Responses (actual measures)

- Based on information from public health nurses and medical teams, the city offered nutritional guidance at home when needed.
- Social welfare councils and other organizations provided assistance, including delivering food to individual homes.
- The city asked the Fukushima Prefecture Disaster Response Headquarters and the Japan Dietetic Association to provide the necessary goods.

c. Summary/measures in the future

- The cooperation with relevant institutions is crucial for the city to promptly grasp the situation of people requiring assistance during a disaster and take necessary measures for them. Moreover, since special foods, such as tube feeding nutrients, became hard to be procured, the city should store necessary quantity of the foods that may be needed in case of an emergency. In addition, it is important for the city to have these people promptly evacuated and secure evacuation destinations for them, as is the case with expectant and nursing mothers and children.

2 Exercise (Environmental improvement)

a. Situation

- As information on the nuclear power station accident was spreading, younger generations were evacuating from their home. Meanwhile, elderly people remained in their homes (or returned to their homes although they had been once evacuated). Accordingly, the number of households with elderly people living alone and only elderly people increased.
- There was news that people who were evacuated outside the prefecture caused trouble because they were unable to become accustomed to group living.
- Medical institutions in the city closed at the end of March. Some people were not only forced to stop taking medicine due to lack of availability but also unable to receive appropriate medical treatment.
- At the end of May, people began to move into emergency temporary housing that was built outside the 30 km zone (with the priority placed on elderly people and disabled people). In association with this, more people returned to the city from evacuation destinations.
- It was increasingly reported that elderly people who had nowhere to go, gradually began to be homebound and become immobile.

Chapter 3 | Situation of and Countermeasures by Each Individual Municipality

- In July, due to prolonged stays in evacuation centers in the city, more elderly people complained of their poor physical condition.
- In September, the city grasped the situation that people living in municipally-subsidized housing suffered from a feeling of isolation.

b. Responses (actual measures)

- From April 4 to May 27, the city visited a total of 595 homes to provide medical care. These visiting care services were realized thanks to medical support from the Nagasakiken Medical Association and Nagasaki University Hospital and in cooperation with the Self Defense Forces, health nurses from public health centers, and staff of Minamisoma City Hospital. The city's appropriate action for those who continued to live in their homes and who returned from evacuation destinations to their homes in poor physical condition contributed to improving their health.
- City employees in cooperation with nurses from Minamisoma City Hospital were dispatched to evacuation centers inside and outside the city to respond to difficult cases.
- The city conducted a health survey for those living in temporary housing and municipally-subsidized housing, and regularly held conferences between those involved using the survey results to resolve existing problems.
- From November, city employees began to implement a care prevention program ("*Tentomushi Kyoshitsu*," a free-for-all friendly gathering) as many times as possible.
- The city held exercise classes in assembly rooms in temporary housing sites.

c. Summary/measures in the future

- The city was embarrassed by the order that uniformly instructed residents to evacuate the area within a 30-km range after the nuclear power station accident. Since the city was unable to immediately build temporary housing and resume operation of welfare facilities, many people were forced to live in evacuation centers and live in evacuation destinations outside the city over a prolonged period. There is some question as to the validity of such uniform restrictions. However, individual local governments will need to create disaster response manuals in anticipation of such a situation.

3   Rest (mind, anxiety, suicide, etc.)

a. Situation

- On March 15, the order to stay indoors was issued. The city began to evacuate residents by large buses according to its out-of-town emergency evacuation plan. Some residents were evacuated by family car.
- Support was not offered during the month of March 2011. From April 4, 2011, support began to be provided by other prefectures and the Self-Defense Forces in accordance with Disaster Relief Act.
- Medical institutions, including departments of psychiatry, were closed and drugs became unavailable.
- Family members consisting of younger generations were evacuated and only elderly members stayed in the city, which led to a change in the family structure. Consequently, more people developed a feeling of isolation and complained about their poor mental condition.

b. Responses (actual measures)

- Staff members visited elderly people and disabled people who voluntarily stayed at home or who were unable to be evacuated to confirm their safety and check their means of transportation when evacuation orders were issued again.
- The city conducted health examinations for residents living in temporary housing and municipally-subsidized housing.

- The city visited residents in their homes to care for their emotional and spiritual needs.
- The city held lecture meetings on mental health.

c. Summary/measures in the future
- Since many of vulnerable people are unable to transfer independently, the city needs to prepare various name lists of these individuals and renew the lists as needed, while checking their situation.
- Medical institutions may lose their ability to provide medical care, and drugs may become unavailable. Accordingly, the city should take measures for those whose medical condition is likely to become worse due to termination of treatment, such as those who receive transportation fees for hospital visits under a System of Medical Payment for Services and Supports for Persons with Disabilitiesand those who receive mental disability certificates.

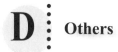

D Others

(Support from Nagasaki Prefecture; cooperation with Fukushima Prefecture and the Public Health Center)
- Some people remained in the city because they were unable to be evacuated against their will or did not want to leave their homes. Medical institutions, nursing care establishments and supermarkets were all closed. Staff at the Longevity Welfare Division worked hard to respond to people requiring assistance during a disaster and people requiring support despite the shortage of manpower. In addition, disaster volunteers working at social welfare councils made efforts to deliver goods. However, people requiring assistance and support were forced to live an inconvenient life under the situation where drugs and goods were lacking, and nursing services were not provided.
- Staff members would have liked to have communicated with the Deputy Director of the Soso Public Health Center, who had provided support even before the earthquake, to ask for advice. However, early during the disaster phones were dead. Moreover, they were busy with their emergency response responsibilities and were unable to cooperate with each other during the month of March.
- In April, medical support for disaster relief was provided by Nagasaki Prefecture (The rescue was made according to the Fukushima Prefecture Disaster Relief Act). At the same time, support was provided by Hospitals Bureau in Fukushima Prefecture, Fukushima Medical University, the Self-Defense Forces, fire-fighting organizations and the Soso Public Health Center. Eventually, the city was able to begin to visit people requiring assistance and support in their homes to provide medical care (in the medical and dental field). Moreover, doctors from local medical associations and dental associations also offered assistance.

(Mariko Oishi, Hitomi Shigihara, Chiharu Okazaki, Yukiko Sugimoto, Yukiko Iga)

24 Efforts of Tamura City

1 Situation of the municipality

(1) Demographics (as of January 1 of each year)

	2011	2012	2013
Population	39,594	39,489	38,858
Number of households	11,935	11,820	11,768
Average number of people per household	3.32	3.34	3.3
Number of births	261	245	
Birth rate	6.6	6.2	
Number of deaths	605	527	
Mortality	1528.0	1334.5	
Ratio of the elderly aged 65 or older	28.0	28.1	28.7

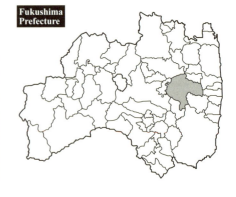

* The mortality rate per 100,000 persons.

(2) Geographical features

Total area: 458.3 km² (approximately 31 km east-west; approximately 29 km north-south)

Distance from the Fukushima Daiichi Nuclear Power Station of the Tokyo Electric Power Company: approximately 15–46 km

Evacuation area: Miyakoji Town of Tamura City

Transportation network: six stations of the JR Banetsu-to Line; one I.C of the Banetsu Expressway

2 Situation of damage by the earthquake, tsunami and the nuclear disaster

(1) Damage by the Great East Japan Earthquake (as of February 1, 2013)

Property damage	Completely destroyed	Half destroyed	Partially destroyed
House	19	196	4,137
Public institution			208
Other			850

Human damage	Deaths by disaster	Disaster-related deaths	Missing persons	Injured persons
	1	0	0	5

* Basic utilities and life lines within the city were not damaged by the earthquake and the tsunami.

(2) Situation of evacuation

① Evacuation centers inside the local municipality (as of March 12, 2011)

	Number of evacuation centers	Number of evacuees	Available period
Residents	4	291	March 12 to 16
Evacuees received	12	7,005	March 12 to August 10

* On the day following the earthquake, Tamura City began receiving evacuees from municipalities inside and outside of the city. An evacuation order was issued to the city's Miyakoji area (3,001 persons in 994 households), which is located within a 20–30 km range from the Fukushima Daiichi Nuclear Power Station. The city accommodated a maximum of 8,359 residents/evacuees at 18 evacuation centers set up within the city.

② Approximate number of evacuees in evacuation centers outside the municipality (as of February 28, 2013)

	End/March 2011	End/September 2011	End/March 2012	Latest period
First evacuation center	1,058	0	0	0
Second evacuation center		160	159	10
Temporary housing		918	918	2
Municipally-subsidized housing		493	776	292

③ Approximate number of voluntary evacuees (as of December 1, 2012)

Inside Fukushima Prefecture	14

Outside Fukushima Prefecture (number of evacuees & prefectures)	71 persons in 17 prefectures

Outlook of damage related to the nuclear disaster

- The number of residents accommodated at evacuation centers set up within Tamura City (as of January 11, 2013) 926 persons in temporary housing 665 persons in public housing, municipally-subsidized housing, etc. 629 returnees
- The number of evacuees from other municipalities to Tamura City (as of January 11, 2013) 49 persons in temporary housing 545 persons in employment promotion housing, municipally-subsidized housing, etc. A total of 594 persons

① Distribution of commodities such as gasoline and food products stopped due to the dispersion of radioactive materials. Some medical institutions were temporarily closed because staff members were unable to secure a means of transportation to their workplace and patient transfer cars were also unavailable because of a lack of gasoline.

② During the first week after the earthquake, the city announced information on availability of medical institutions within the city to the residents, using its wireless radio broadcasting system.

③ Radiation exposure screening tests started on March 13 at the city's general gymnasium. Measurements of the air radiation levels were also initiated on March 15. Over the wireless radio broadcasting system, the city cautioned residents to make sure to pay attention to the measurement results before they go outside.

④ The city prepared to distribute stable iodine tablets/syrup to the residents. However, because no instructions were issued from the national government or Fukushima Prefecture, the city did not distribute them to the residents.

⑤ The city resumed medical examinations for young children and other normal working operations in April 2011. Visiting services for residents staying in evacuation centers were continued until all evacuees moved to temporary housing.

3 Countermeasures against nuclear disaster (as of January 2013)

		Name of project	Division in charge	Number of targeted persons (households)	Pregnant women	Parturient women	Babies	Young children	Elementary school students	Junior high school students	Senior high school students	People age 19 to 39	People age 40 or older	Remarks (major operations)
Countermeasures against external exposure	1	Personal dose measurements	Health Management Division	5,500	○		○	○	○	○				Distribution, collection and notification & analysis of the measurement results
	2	Lending of electronic cumulative dosimeters (from FY2012)	Health Management Division		○						○			Development of the project's outline, lending of the dosimeters at any time at the City Hall and each branch office.
	3	Debriefing sessions for measurement results of cumulative personal dose (FY2011)	Health Management Division	Residents who underwent the measurement and their parents/guardians	○		○	○	○	○				
	4	Monitoring and measurement of the air radiation levels	Living Environment Division	81 spots										Measurement at 191 monitoring spots and announcements of the results
	5	Real-time measurement of the radiation dose from March 2012 (Ministry of the Environment)		110 spots										
	6	Replacement of the surface soil on the grounds in childcare facilities, child education facilities and schools	Educational General Affairs Division				○	○	○	○				Outsourcing
	7	Decontamination (starting from priority areas)	Living Environment Division	Within the whole city	○	○	○	○	○	○	○	○	○	Outsourcing
	8	A basic survey in the Fukushima Health Management Survey (conducted by Fukushima Prefecture)		All residents	○	○	○	○	○	○	○	○	○	

233

	No	Measure	Division	Target										Work
Countermeasures against internal exposure	9	Whole Body Counter measurements (conducted by the city)	Health Management Division	All residents (40,775 persons)	○	○		○	○	○	○	○	○	Installation of equipment, calibration, schedule arrangements, notification, measurement, debriefing, aggregation of the measurement results, and outsourcing of shuttle vehicles
	10	Whole Body Counter measurements (residents in an evacuation area by priority)	Health Management Division	The number of residents who underwent the measurement: 828 persons				○	○	○	○			Arrangement of venues & schedules, and notification of the measurement results
	11	Food and water quality inspection	Agriculture and Forestry Division	All households (11,768 households)	○	○	○	○	○	○	○	○	○	Acceptance of inspection, examination and notification of the inspection results
	12	Thyroid gland examination (conducted by Fukushima Prefecture)	Health Management Division				○	○	○	○	○			Sampling of examinees, arrangement of venues & schedules and guiding at the time of examination
	13	Inspection of school meals	Educational General Affairs Division	Elementary school and junior high school students				○	○	○				Purchase of equipment, measurement and announcements
	14		Social Welfare Division	Nursery schools, kodomoen and others			○	○						Purchase of equipment, collection of samples, examination and announcement of the results (collection of sampling in kodomoen and other facilities)
	15	Exposure to radiation prevention classes for mothers and young children conducted in May 2011	Health Management Division	All residents	○	○	○	○	○	○	○	○	○	Planning, publicity, and implementation
	16	Free medical examinations and cancer screening tests (FY2011)	Health Management Division									○	○	Publicity
	17	Special medical examinations and health counseling after the disaster (FY2011)	Health Management Division											Planning, publicity, and implementation
	18	A detailed health survey in the Fukushima Health Management Survey (conducted by Fukushima Prefecture)												Sampling of respondents to the survey
Others	19	Study sessions on radiation	Health Management Division Living Environment Division	All residents	○	○	○	○	○	○	○	○	○	Planning, publicity, and implementation
	20	Post-disaster mental health care projects (conducted in FY2011 by Fukushima Prefecture)	Health Management Division	Residents living in temporary housing										Publicity and implementation
	21	Home-visiting services for residents living in temporary housing	Health Management Division	Residents living in temporary housing										Schedule arrangements, implementation, and identification of problems
	22	Home-visiting services for residents staying at home within the evacuation area	Health Management Division	Residents staying at home within the Miyakoji district										Schedule arrangements, implementation, and identification of problems
	23	A health-related gathering program "kenko salon" (FY2012)	Council of Social Welfare	Residents living in temporary housing										Health counseling services, etc.
	24	Exercise classes for young children (a project by Fukushima Prefecture)	Health Management Division				○	○						Sampling of participants, arrangement of venues & schedules, and implementation

A ⋮ Residents

1 Nutrition (meals/water)

a. Situation

- Immediately after the earthquake, stores within the city were temporarily closed due to property damages and a delay in the distribution of commodities. After the stores reopened, residents were increasingly worried about radioactive contamination of water supplies, leading to a growing demand for bottled water. However, restrictions were imposed on the purchase of bottled water due to the shortage of supply.
- In some areas, residents had to depend on water supply trucks because well water, water drawn from a stream, and tap water became muddy after the earthquake.
- There was a divergence of opinion within families as whether to eat home-grown rice and vegetables. In most families, parents did not allow their children to eat home-grown food.
- At the primary evacuation centers, emergency foods that were cooked at a distant place caused the outbreak of food poisoning.
- Before measurement of the radiation levels in food started, many residents reframed from purchasing fresh foods and other food products that were produced within Fukushima Prefecture.

b. Responses (actual measures)

- The city announced water quality inspection results to the residents every day, using the wireless radio broadcasting system.
- The city conducted study sessions on radiation and food, with the aim of providing correct information to the residents.
- The city's emergency response headquarters regularly announced measurement results of the radiation levels in food in public relations magazines.

c. Summary/measures in the future

- Unlike farm households that have some vegetables and other food stocks, many general households are likely to rush to stores to buy up any food products for fear that stores may be closed in an emergency situation. To avoid such a chaotic situation and concerns about a lack of food, residents are strongly advised to prepare one week's worth of food/beverages for an emergency.
- To prevent the outbreak of food poisoning, it is desirable to cook emergency foods in an emergency kitchen within the evacuation centers or places as near as possible to evacuation centers.
- Because food/water safety is the greatest concern among the residents, information on daily necessities should be promptly sent out to the residents in an appropriate manner. For example, Tamura City made the best use of its wireless radio broadcasting system as a tool to disseminate safety information to residents.

2 Exercise (Environmental improvement)

a. Situation

- Due to a confined living space at evacuation centers, the amount of physical activity of residents was decreased. A decline in muscular strength was one of concerns for the residents.
- Before the earthquake, many elderly residents had grown vegetables in a garden and had developed long and close contact with neighbors. However, after moving to temporary housing, such elderly residents

Chapter 3 | Situation of and Countermeasures by Each Individual Municipality

were unable to grow vegetables on their own and lost their ties with their close acquaintances.

- Some elderly residents stayed at home, not taking shelter. However, because most of their neighbors evacuated to other places, their opportunities to go outdoors to do physical activities in the local community were decreased, resulting in diminished physical strength. Inevitably, an increasing number of such elderly residents became nursing-care service recipients.

b. Responses (actual measures)

- In an effort to prevent a lack of exercise among residents, post-disaster mental health care team members at evacuation centers led exercise programs at a predetermined times every day.
- Aiming to encourage residents to take exercise, the city's health office initiated a health-related gathering program named "*kenko salon*" at assembly rooms within the temporary housing sites. Gaining popularity among residents, the "*kenko salon*" program was regularly conducted.
- In collaboration with the social welfare council, the city started a health-related friendly gathering program "*fureai kenko salon*" in each administrative ward for elderly residents staying at home.

c. Summary/measures in the future

- Health support exercise programs to maintain the residents' muscular strength should be started as early as possible after each resident secures a living space at evacuation centers. Exercise programs are also expected to promote friendly exchanges among participating residents.
- *Salon* programs (friendly gatherings) to prevent residents from remaining being homebound should be conducted at assembly rooms within temporary housing sites, in cooperation with volunteer members. Such programs are also effective in relieving residents' metal stress and maintaining close ties and solidarity among local community members.
- The city is required to create "social resources" that are accessible by residents to meet their various needs, through collaborative relationships with public health and welfare offices (health office), the social welfare council, a regional comprehensive support center, and home-care support providers and other organizations.

---

3 Rest (mind, anxiety, suicide, etc.)

a. Situation

- It was often the case that residents with mental diseases were unable to adapt themselves to living with other evacuees at evacuation centers, developing a tendency towards troublesome behavior. In some cases, surrounding residents felt a growing stress due to such troublesome behavior.
- Some residents who were unable to adapt themselves to an unfamiliar living environment at evacuation centers complained about sleeplessness. A lack of privacy at evacuation centers caused health problems even among healthy residents.
- After moving to temporary housing in July 2011, residents complained about voices and noise from neighboring rooms.
- Residents, who remained in their houses within a former "evacuation-prepared zone," were very worried about the collapse of the local community due to evacuation. They also felt a growing sense of loneliness because there were almost no returnees to the areas.

b. Responses (actual measures)

- In cooperation with clinic doctors, "special medical examinations and health counseling after the disaster" was conducted at 9 venues within the city, including an "evacuation-prepared zone." (Please refer to Table 24-1.)

24 Efforts of Tamura City

Table 24-1 Outline of the Special Medical Examination (FY2011)

Implementation guidelines of the special medical examinations and health counseling

1. Purpose

Since the Great East Japan Earthquake and the nuclear power station accident within Fukushima Prefecture, the residents of Tamura City have been seriously concerned about the risk of exposure to radiation and possible other health problems. It is projected that it may take another six to nine months to conclude the severe nuclear accident problems. In light of such a situation, Tamura City has decided to conduct special medical examinations and health counseling mainly for residents in the "evacuation-prepared zone," prior to conventionally-scheduled regular medical examinations. The purpose of the special medical examinations is to help ensure a safe and secured life for the residents.

2. Organizer

Tamura City

3. Schedule

14:00 - 16:00 on May 4 (Wed.) at the Miyakoji Health Center (for residents in the Furumichi district)
9:30 - 11:30 on May 12 (Thru.) at the Kami-Iwaisawa Livelihood Support Center (for residents in the Iwaisawa district)
13:30 - 15:30 on May 12 (Thru.) at the Hotta Assembly Hall (for residents in the Hotta district)
14:00 - 16:00 on May 14 (Sat.) at the Yamane Annex of Tokiwa Community Hall (for residents in Yamane district)
9:30 - 11:30 on May 19 (Thru.) at the Yokomichi Assembly Hall (for residents in the Yokomichi district)
14:00 - 16:00 on May 19 (Thru.) at each health center (for residents within the jurisdiction of Ogoe Branch Office)
14:00 - 16:00 on May 26 (Thru.) at each health center (for residents within the jurisdiction of Funehiki Branch Office)
9:30 - 11:30 on June 2 (Thru.) at each health center (for residents within the jurisdiction of Tokiwa Branch Office)
14:00 - 16:00 on June 30 (Thru.) at each health center (for residents within the jurisdiction of Takine Branch Office)

4. Venue

Local assembly halls, health centers and other facilities

5. Details of the examinations

Interview with public health nurses and nutritionists Examination with a stethoscope by physicians
Oral care instructions by dentists Health counseling

6. Method of Publicity

Through the local wireless radio broadcasting system

7. Others

Aiming to adequately address residents' health concerns, the city will cooperate with relevant institutions/organizations and will:

①send an announcement of a recommended medical examination to each individual resident;
②announce mental health counseling scheduled to be conducted from May 2 to 5 at the Funehiki Community Hall;
③announce exposure to radiation prevention classes to be held on May 14 in Tokiwa and Ogoe districts and on May 22 in Funehiki and Takine districts;
④announce the implementation of comprehensive medical examinations

---

- Before residents moved to temporary housing or municipally-subsidized housing in July 2011, the city's public health nurses visited evacuation centers every day to check the health condition of each individual resident and provide "social resources" and information that were necessary to meet the various needs of residents.

- A talk-show event named "Save your Life" was held jointly by Tamura City and its neighboring two municipalities, inviting Minoru KAMATA (a physician) as a lecturer.

- In October 2011, home-visiting services were provided to all households within a former "evacuation-prepared zone."

- In collaboration with the city's disaster response headquarters, the Health Management Division held radiation classes.

- In October 2012, the city started health-related *salon* programs and announcements of the programs to residents within a former "evacuation-prepared zone."

c. Summary/measures in the future

- To set residents' minds at ease as much as possible in an emergency situation, it is effective for munici-palities to collaborate with private-sector organizations and institutions to promptly provide necessary support programs to victim residents. For example, Tamura City obtained cooperation from clinic physi-

Chapter 3 Situation of and Countermeasures by Each Individual Municipality

cians and dentists to provide health management support to the residents.
- Several issues were identified by home visits to all the residents living in temporary housing or living at home in the Miyakoji district. Aiming to address such issues, the city officials and other parties concerned have continually discussed necessary support programs and activities.

To provide effective support programs to residents, it is important to define a restoration vision for each area and set both short-term and long-term goals to realize the vision (see Figure 24-1).

4 Others

- Some parts of the Miyakoji district of Tamura City were temporarily designated as an "evacuation zone" and an "evacuation-prepared zone." Inevitably, residents in the district are divided into two groups: a

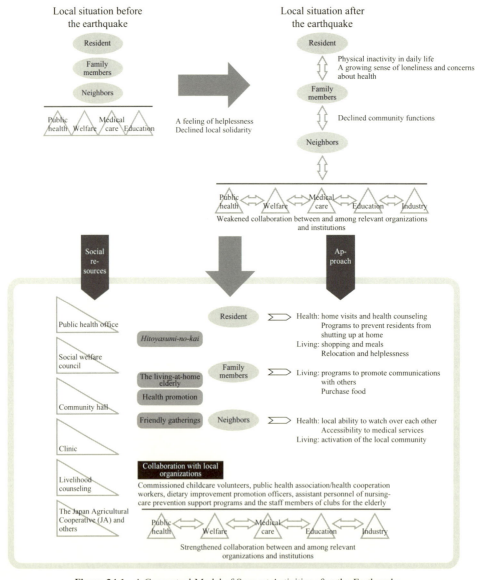

Figure 24-1 A Conceptual Model of Support Activities after the Earthquake

group of residents who took shelter in evacuation centers and then moved to temporary housing or municipally-subsidized housing; a group of residents who remained at home after the earthquake. A sudden change of the structure of the local community caused various problems to the residents in this district.

- The city held a monthly meeting to discuss effective support programs for residents remaining at home within the Miyakoji district.

B ⋮ Expectant/nursing mothers and children

1 Nutrition (meals/water)

a. Situation

- Initially, the city received many inquiries from residents about delayed distribution of commodities and the safety of breast milk, water and food products.
- For the first several days after the earthquake, foodstuffs were in short supply and simple foods were cooked for evacuees at evacuation centers. After emergency relief supplies reached them, there was a tendency for residents to receive the same types of food.

b. Responses (actual measures)

- Drinking water was distributed to expectant mothers, babies under the age of 12 months and breastfeeding mothers.
- The city announced information on institutions where mothers can undergo an examination of their breast milk.
- Nutritionists visited each evacuation center to provide instructions on milk powder formula and diets for babies.

c. Summary/measures in the future

- As a lesson learned from the fact that it took about one week before the distribution of commodities was resumed, residents are advised to stock one week's worth of water and food products for an emergency.

2 Exercise (Environmental improvement)

a. Situation

- Because it was impossible to take a bath at evacuation centers, evacuees faced difficulties in maintaining their personal hygiene.
- Because it was difficult to secure exercise/playing spaces at evacuation centers, some evacuees complained of being irritated by loud children. Particularly, children with developmental disabilities were not comfortable anywhere within evacuation centers.

b. Responses (actual measures)

- Thankfully, some volunteer residents offered to receive expectant mothers and young children in their houses so that such evacuees could take a bath and have accommodations. Some midwives also voluntarily provided health/exercise instructions to expectant mothers.
- From March to April 2011, the city strived to secure a playing space at evacuation centers. At the playing space, volunteer members read a picture book to young children.
- The city resumed medical examinations for young children in April 2011. At the medical examinations,

Chapter 3 Situation of and Countermeasures by Each Individual Municipality

the town officials attentively listened to parents/guardians who were filled with anxiety and concerns about their children's possible exposure to radiation and other child rearing problems. The city also distributed booklets containing information on radiation and other necessary information at the medical examinations for young children.

- As part of external exposure dose measurement programs in August 2011, the city started the distribution of personal dosimeters (glass badges) to children under 15 years old and expectant mothers.
- Monitoring results of the air radiation levels were announced to the residents several times a day, using a local wireless radio broadcasting system.
- The Ministry of Education, Culture, Sports, Science and Technology embarked on the installation of monitoring posts at public facilities within the city.
- In collaboration with the board of education, the city conducted an explanatory meeting for parents and guardians about the distribution of personal dosimeters to children and the replacement of the surface soil on the grounds of nursery schools, kindergartens and educational facilities. After the explanatory meeting, the surface soil of the grounds in nursery schools, kindergartens and educational facilities was replaced.

c. Summary/measures in the future

- At the primary evacuation centers, the city needs to take some effective measures to maintain personal and public hygiene, thereby preventing the spread of infectious diseases among evacuees.
- At the explanatory meeting about the distribution of personal dosimeters to children and the replacement of the surface soil of the grounds in nursery schools, kindergartens and educational facilities, the city received many questions from parents and guardians such as "We are confused by a lot of contradictory information and do not know what information to trust." Because the meeting was jointly held by the board of education, the city officials and the board of education members were able to appropriately answer their questions.
- Municipalities within Fukushima Prefecture strived to communicate each other by phone to share information on the distribution of personal dosimeters. Based on the information obtained, each municipality initiated the distribution to residents at its own discretion. To smoothly proceed with the distribution of personal dosimeters, Fukushima Prefecture should have organized relevant information and sent it to each municipality.
- Thanks to a radiation/health advisory group set up by Fukushima Prefecture, residents were able to consult a reliable adviser for their concerns and anxiety. It must have been difficult for the city to secure such advisers on its own and entrust to them with consultation services.

3 Rest (mind, anxiety, suicide, etc.)

a. Situation

- The city received an increasing number of consultations from residents about concerns about child rearing and overall living environments. The severity of concerns and anxiety varied considerably from person to person.
- Residents were filled with pent-up resentment, arising from anxiety and fear about radiation. Attentively listening to such complicated feelings among residents, the city officials also suffered from severe distress and overwork.

b. Responses (actual measures)

- To reduce parents' anxiety about radiation, exposure to radiation prevention classes for mothers and young children were held at four venues within the city, under the sponsorship of the National Institute of Radiological Sciences. (Please refer to Table 24-2 for details.)

- In cooperation with post-disaster mental health care teams, the city officials were able to provide professional counseling services to residents.
- After the notification of personal dose measurement results, the Health Management Division conducted study sessions on radiation to expand residents' knowledge about radiation.

c. Summary/measures in the future

- When a nuclear disaster occurs, an indoor evacuation order will be issued to the affected area and distribution of commodities such as foods and gasoline may stop, causing residents to feel a growing sense of uneasiness.
- When a disaster occurs, the city officials have to respond to residents' expression of strong dissatisfaction, resentment and other complaints. To prevent the officials from suffering from severe distress and mental problems, support programs to maintain their sound mental health are essential.
- To take effective countermeasures against radiation, the city needs to seek advice from specialists.

4 Others

- The city had been fully prepared for distribution of stable iodine tablets/syrup and had also run a simulation of the distribution. However, the city did not distribute them to the residents because no instruction

Table 24-2 Publicity on study sessions on radiation for mothers and children (FY2011)

The Exposure to Radiation Prevention Class for Mothers and Young Children in Tamura City
(Open Seminar by the National Institute of Radiological Sciences)

It is said that six to nine months may be necessary to conclude the severe nuclear accident problems at the Fukushima Daiichi Nuclear Power Station.

Under the sponsorship of the National Institute of Radiological Sciences, the city will hold an open seminar on radiation. The aim will be to provide an opportunity for nursing/expectant mothers to know how to ensure a safe and secure life in Tamura City. The lecturers will provide clear explanations of radiation, food contamination, and radiation effects on human health. The details of the seminar are as follows:

Organizer: the National Institute of Radiological Sciences

Dates & Venues:

10:45 to 12:15 on May 14 (Sat.) at Tokiwa Bunka-no-Yakata
13:30 to 15:00 on May 14 (Sat.) at Ogoe Branch Office
10:45 to 12:15 on May 22 (Sun.) at Funehiki Health Center
13:30 to 15:00 on May 22 (Sun.) at Tenchijin University in Takine

Lectures:

On May 14 (Sat.)
    "Basic knowledge about the effects of radiation"
    By Reiko KANDA, a senior researcher of the Research Center for Radiation Protection
    "Soils and foods in the future---tips for safe and secure diets"
    By Keiko TAGAMI, a head researcher of the Research Center for Radiation Protection
On May 22 (Sun.)
    "Basic knowledge about the effects of radiation"
    By Yoshiya SHIMADA, the leader of the Radiobiology for Children's Health Research Program
    "Soils and foods in the future---tips for safe and secure diets"
    By Keiko TAGAMI, a head researcher of the Research Center for Radiation Protection

---

<Contact phone number>

Health Management Division, Tamura City Office 81-22xx
Residents' Affairs Division, Takine Branch Office 78-12xx
Residents' Affairs Division, Ogoe Branch Office 79-21xx
Residents' Affairs Division, Miyakoji Branch Office 75-21xx
Residents' Affairs Division, Tokiwa Branch Office 77-21xx

Chapter 3 Situation of and Countermeasures by Each Individual Municipality

was issued from Fukushima Prefecture.
- In collaboration with the city's disaster response headquarters, the Health Management Division posted the personal dose measurement results in public relations magazines to be distributed to each household. Moreover, based on the personal dose measurement results, the division also discussed with the city's disaster response headquarters how to take necessary measures against radiation.

C People requiring assistance during a disaster (vulnerable people in case of a disaster)

1 Nutrition (meals/water)
- For details, please refer to the section of "A. Residents."

2 Exercise (Environmental improvement)

a. Situation
- Evacuees from other municipalities included patients requiring artificial dialysis treatment and persons undergoing home oxygen therapy. However, the city faced difficulties in finding hospitals that could receive such patients. Oxygen cylinders were also difficult to be secured.
- Because nursing-care services became unavailable immediately after the earthquake, a decline in their physical and mental functions was a great concern for nursing-care recipients.

b. Responses (actual measures)
- Doctors of the Tamura Medical Association and medical institutions outside Tamura City as well as other volunteer doctors visited the primary evacuation centers to examine the health conditions of residents.
- After the volunteer doctors prescribed medicines for residents at the primary evacuation centers, the city officials took the prescriptions to a pharmacy to have the necessary medicines prepared. Upon receiving the prepared medicines, the officials passed them to residents at evacuation centers.
- The city officials provided home visits to residents to identify and collect information on persons requiring nursing care.

c. Summary/measures in the future
- There were many residents who did not bring their regular medicines when evacuating or those who were out of regular medicines after evacuation. To be able to secure and provide necessary medicines to residents, the town needs to establish a cooperative system with local medical associations and pharmacist association.
- It is essential for the city to discuss "cooperative assistance in times of disaster" with all the relevant parties, thereby realizing a system to provide prompt responses to residents in an emergency situation.

3 Rest (mind, anxiety, suicide, etc.)

a. Situation
- While most of the younger residents took shelter in evacuation centers, many elderly residents and home-care service recipients remained in their houses. For elderly residents who were unable to be evacuated due to physical conditions, the greatest concern was a change in living environments, not the risk of exposure to radiation.

- There were many elderly residents who complained about a sense of loneliness because most of their neighbors evacuated to other places and they had no opportunity/place to communicate with others.
- It is often the case that elderly people living alone cannot fully understand announcements sent by mail from the city.
- Residents who were suffering from mental diseases or had alcohol abuse problems became the subject of discussion at evacuation centers and temporary housing.

b. Responses (actual measures)
- Immediately after the earthquake, the city officials provided home visits to residents requiring assistance who had been registered on a list made by officials in charge of welfare and nursing care. The aim was understanding their situation and responding to their urgent needs and concerns.
- The city conducted home visits to all residents staying within "an evacuation-prepared zone" in October 2011, identifying residents who were supposed to need some special support. For such identified residents, public health nurses, a regional comprehensive support center, post-disaster mental care team members, and commissioned welfare volunteers have collaborated in providing the continued support.

c. Summary/measures in the future
- It is generally difficult to ensure that persons requiring assistance are fully informed of important information disseminated from the city. Even if the city sends documents to them, such residents often do not fully read and understand the information on their own. To avoid their having a lack of information, the city needs to ask their neighbors to support them in acquiring and understanding important administrative information in case of an emergency.

4 Others

- Home visits and other attentive public services during a disaster are essential, particularly for persons requiring assistance who have difficulties in accessing necessary administrative information. Beginning with the preparation of a list of potential recipients of such support services, the city is required to develop a system that enables prompt responses to the urgent needs of persons requiring assistance in times of disaster.

(Ikuko Watabe)

25 Efforts of Kawamata Town

1 Situation of the municipality

(1) Demographics (as of January 1 of each year)

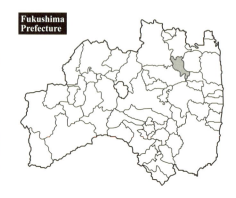

	2011	2012	2013
Population	15,530	15,178	14,789
Number of households	5,190	5,124	5,091
Average number of people per household	2.99	2.96	2.9
Number of births	62	75	
Birth rate	6.7	5.0	
Number of deaths	248	241	
Mortality	16.3	16.2	
Ratio of the elderly aged 65 or older	31.6	31.9	33.1

(2) Geographical features

Total area: 127.66 km² (approximately 12 km east-west; approximately 20 km north-south)

Distance from the Fukushima Daiichi Nuclear Power Station of the Tokyo Electric Power Company: approximately 45 km

Evacuation area: Yamakiya district of the town was designated as a "deliberate evacuation zone" on April 22, 2011.

Transportation network: National Route 114; National Route 349 running through in a north-south direction

2 Situation of damage by the earthquake, tsunami and the nuclear disaster

(1) Damage by the Great East Japan Earthquake (as of March 1, 2013)

Property damage	Completely destroyed	Half destroyed	Partially destroyed
House	28	30	1,287
Public institution	1	0	3
Other	52	118	236

Human damage	Deaths by disaster	Disaster-related deaths	Missing persons	Injured persons
	0	0	0	0

(2) Situation of evacuation

① Evacuation centers within the municipality (as of March 12, 2011)

	Number of evacuation centers	Number of evacuees	Available period
Residents	1	449	March 11 to 26
Evacuees received	11	48,967	March 12 to August 5

* The number shows cumulative evacuees because it is difficult to identify double-counted evacuees.

② Approximate number of evacuees in evacuation centers outside the municipality (as of March 13, 2013)

	End/March 2011	End/September 2011	End/March 2012	Latest period
First evacuation center				
Second evacuation center				
Temporary housing		415	414	398
Municipally-subsidized housing		649	651	649
Others (housing of relatives, friends etc.)		175	169	175

* The number includes residents who moved into the town and were born outside the town. The number of deaths is not included.

25 Efforts of Kawamata Town

③ Approximate number of voluntary evacuees (as of September 17, 2013)

Inside Fukushima Prefecture	25

Outside Fukushima Prefecture (number of evacuees & prefectures)	235 persons in 30 prefectures

Outlook of damage related to the nuclear disaster

- Although the town did not suffer severe property and human damage from the earthquake, residents experienced a shortage of commodities due to the nuclear power station accident.
- The national government and Fukushima Prefecture did not disseminate to each municipality sufficient information on what nuclear emergency responses should be taken. Due to the lack of information, a growing anxiety about radiation rapidly spread among the town residents.
- On March 17, the town started the measurement of the air radiation levels. The measurement results were announced to the residents in the town's disaster information magazines.
- About one month after the earthquake, the national government designated the Yamakiya district as a "deliberate evacuation zone." Following the evacuation order, all the residents were evacuated from the district by the end of June 2011.

❸ Countermeasures against nuclear disaster (as of January 2013)

		Name of project	Division in charge	Number of targeted persons (house-holds)	Expect-ant mothers	Nursing moth-ers	Babies	Young children	Elemen-tary school students	Junior high school students	Senior high school students	People age 19 to 39	People age 40 or older	Remarks (major operations)
Countermeasures against external exposure	1	Personal dose measurements	Child Education Division Health and Welfare Division	2,000	○	○	○	○	○	○				Distribution, collection, measurement, announcements of measurement results and analysis
	2	Refreshments for young children and their parents	Health Manage-ment Center	480			○	○						Planning, contract, notification, collection of participants and guiding
	3	Refreshments for elementary school and junior high school students	Child Education Division	900				○	○	○				Implementation of out-of- school activities for kindergarten and nursery school children as well as elementary school students
	4	Monitoring and measurement of the air radiation levels		All residents	○	○	○	○	○	○	○	○	○	Purchase of equipment, measurements, recording and announcements
	5	Real-time measurement of the radiation dose (Ministry of the Environment)		33 spots										
	6	Measurement and mapping of the air radiation levels in the whole town	Nuclear Disaster Counter-measures Division	All residents	○	○	○	○	○	○	○	○	○	Measurement results are provided to Fukushima Prefecture, after which the results are announced through the prefecture's publicity system
	7	Replacement of the surface soil on the grounds in childcare facilities, child education facilities and schools				.	○	○	○	○				Outsourcing, measurement, recording and analysis
	8	Decontamination of houses		All residents	○	○	○	○	○	○	○	○	○	Monitoring and decontamination
	9	Decontamination of public and medical institutions		All residents	○	○	○	○	○	○	○	○	○	Monitoring and decontamination
	10	Whole Body Counter measurements (conducted by the town)	Health Manage-ment Center	All residents				○	○	○	○	○	○	Installment of equipment, calibration, schedule arrangements, outsourcing of measurement & analysis, notification, management of a register of personal names and management of the measurement results

245

	No	Measure	Division	Target											Notes
Countermeasures against internal exposure	11	Whole Body Counter measurements (conducted by Fukushima Prefecture for children aged 4 to 18)	Health Management Center	1,200					○	○	○				Arrangement of venues & schedules, publicity and announcements
	12	Food and water quality inspection	Nuclear Disaster Counter-measures Division	All residents	○	○	○	○	○	○	○	○	○	○	Purchase of equipment, measurement, recording and announcements
	13	Thyroid gland examination (conducted by Fukushima Prefecture)	Health Management Center	All residents					○	○	○				Arrangement of venues & schedules and notification
	14	Inspection of school meals	Child Education Division					○	○	○	○				Implementation of ingredient monitoring of school meals to be offered at nursery facilities and elementary & junior high schools
Others	15	Debriefing sessions for measurement results of exposure dose	Child Education Division		○	○	○	○	○	○	○				Arrangement of venues & schedules and notification
	16	Study sessions on radiation		All residents	○	○	○	○	○	○	○	○	○	○	Dispatch of lecturers
	17	Cancer screening	Health Management Center	Residents age 20 years old or older									○	○	Arrangement of venues & schedules, notification & announcements and management of results
	18	Replacement of the surface soil in rice paddies	Nuclear Disaster Counter-measures Division	1,200 persons from the Yamakiya district	○	○	○	○	○	○	○	○	○	○	Conducted by the national government
	19	Measurement and mapping of the radiation dose in the soil within the whole city	Nuclear Disaster Counter-measures Division												
	20	Lecture meetings on radiation		All residents	○	○	○	○	○	○	○	○	○	○	Dispatch of lecturers
	21	Sampling of respondents for a basic survey in the Fukushima Health Management Survey	Health Management Center	All residents	○	○	○	○	○	○	○	○	○	○	Arrangement of venues & schedules
	22	Publication of disaster information magazines	General Affairs Division	All residents	○	○	○	○	○	○	○	○	○	○	Editing of papers and sending of magazines
	23	Issuance of a health management file to each individual Fukushima Prefecture resident	Health Management Center	All residents	○	○	○	○	○	○	○	○	○	○	Sending
	24	Reduction of the radiation dose in farmlands	Industry Division	All residents	○	○	○	○	○	○	○	○	○	○	Notification, publicity, distribution, measurement of radiation dose, and the management of measurement results

25 Efforts of Kawamata Town

A Residents

1 Nutrition (meals/water)

a. Situation

- Because radioactive materials were detected in water running from taps, residents had increasing concerns about the safety of water. A growing anxiety about the safety of local home-grown vegetables was also spread among residents.

b. Responses (actual measures)

- The town installed water-purifying devices at taps in the town's health office and distributed purified water to residents free of charge. The town also initiated, and has continued, the monitoring inspection of food.
- Food/water monitoring inspection results have been announced to the residents in public relations magazines on disaster information.

c. Summary/measures in the future

- The town intends to continue free distribution of purified water to the residents and monitoring inspection of food and water.
- To ensure residents' security and safety, the town will continue the announcement of radiation dose measurement results via the town's website and in public relations magazines on disaster information.

2 Exercise (Environmental improvement)

a. Situation

- After moving to temporary housing, residents who had been involved in farm work lost the opportunity to take physical activities outdoors. A lack of exercise was observed as a common tendency among residents.

b. Responses (actual measures)

- Exercise instructors conducted brain training and muscular strength improvement training programs at assembly rooms within the sites of temporary housing.

c. Summary/measures in the future

- It is desirable to continue various exercise programs at assembly rooms of temporary housing sites.
- A certain generation of residents and male residents seldom participated in exercise programs. It is necessary to develop special exercise classes for such non-participants so that more residents can take part in various exercise programs to maintain their good health.

3 Rest (mind, anxiety, suicide, etc.)

a. Situation

- Because residents in a deliberate evacuation zone took shelter in various places within and outside the town, social ties among them were broken.
- With the prolonged period of evacuation, an increasing number of evacuees felt uneasy about their

uncertain future and suffered from health problems.

b. Responses (actual measures)
- In cooperation with Fukushima Prefecture, the town officials provided home-visiting services to all evacuees.
- Information exchange and communication programs for residents in municipally-subsidized housing and temporary housing were conducted.
- An explanatory meeting of mental support programs for evacuees from the Yamakiya district was conducted.

c. Summary/measures in the future
- In collaboration with livelihood support counselors of the social welfare council, the town is required to continue the home-visiting services to persons requiring assistance.
- It is important to hold a lecture meeting on radiation and physical and mental health counseling by specialists, as needed.

4 Others

- With the aim of taking necessary measures and actions to promptly respond to the urgent needs of victim residents, the town established the Nuclear Disaster Countermeasures Division consisting of the Decontamination Section and the Resident Support Section.

B Expectant/nursing mothers and children

1 Nutrition (meals/water)

a. Situation
- Because radioactive materials were detected in water running from taps, residents had increasing concerns about the safety of water.
- It was difficult to secure daily commodities. Even artificial milk (milk powder) was in short supply.
- Because breastfeeding mothers were not able to have a well-balanced diet, some of them were worried about the possible malnutrition of their babies.

b. Responses (actual measures)
- In addition to the distribution of bottled water to households with young children, the town installed water-purifying devices at taps in the town's health office and distributed purified water to residents free of charge.
- The town distributed artificial milk (milk powder) to households with babies.
- Food inspection results have been announced to the residents in public relations magazines on disaster information.

c. Summary/measures in the future
- As part of disaster preparedness efforts, the town should develop a system that enables efficient and effective distribution of water and milk powder to residents in times of disaster.

2 Exercise (Environmental improvement)

a. Situation

- The Yamakiya district was the only district within the town that was designated as a deliberate evacuation zone.
- Concerns about possible contamination by radioactive materials rapidly spread among all the residents in the town.
- Because evacuees were restricted in outdoor activities during a prolonged evacuation period, they experienced a decreased amount of exercise and showed a tendency toward obesity.

b. Responses (actual measures)

- The national government took the initiative in conducting decontamination work in the Yamakiya district that had been designated as a deliberate evacuation zone.
- Kawamata Town also conducted decontamination work within the town at its own discretion. In conducting decontamination work, the town decided the priority of facilities/places to be decontaminated, based on the air radiation levels observed and the number of families within the area.
- The town installed air dosimeters in nursery schools and kindergartens within the town, while at the same time measuring air radiation levels at 53 monitoring spots located within the town.
- To measure external exposure to radiation, the town distributed personal dosimeters (glass badges) to residents.
- In cooperation with nursery schools, kindergartens and elementary schools, the town conducted a "happy school program" (refreshment program) in 2011 and 2012 in a suburban area of the town. The purpose of the program was to provide an opportunity for young children and students to play outdoors amidst rich natural settings, thereby making them feel refreshed. As another initiative, the town also started an *oyako-nobinobi* refreshment program in 2012 for parents and young children age 1 to 6 years old. Because of its great popularity, the target of this refreshment program was expanded to children age 1 to 18 years old in 2013.
- As part of exercise promotion programs, exercise instructors (other than school personnel) devised indoor exercise programs and schedules suitable for each individual school's students.
- In an effort to reduce radiation doses, the town implemented decontamination work of school grounds and school buildings in 2011 and 2012.

c. Summary/measures in the future

- The number of residents coming to the health center to measure a cumulative radiation dose has been declining over time. It can be said that the more the residents understand their personal radiation dose trend, the less attention they pay to regular measurements.
- Indoor playing spaces must be secured so that young children can enjoy physical activities without feeling anxious about the risk of exposure to radiation.

3 Rest (mind, anxiety, suicide, etc.)

a. Situation

- Because residents in the deliberate evacuation zone took shelter in various places within and outside the town, social ties among them were broken.
- Some of the residents living in districts other than a deliberate evacuation zone voluntarily took shelter in other municipalities within and outside of Fukushima Prefecture.
- There was a considerable concern about air radiation levels among nursing mothers.

Chapter 3 Situation of and Countermeasures by Each Individual Municipality

b. Responses (actual measures)
- To prevent a delay in providing administrative services such as medical examinations and vaccinations to young children taking shelter in other municipalities, the town strived to keep close contact with host municipalities.
- Not only parents but also some school students felt anxious about exposure to radiation.

c. Summary/measures in the future
- The happy school program was quite useful in helping young children feel both physical and mental refreshment.
- As part of mental health care support programs for school children and parents/guardians, the town assigned a dedicated social worker to each school.
- The town intends to continue these mental health care support programs for residents.

4 Others
- The town has distributed personal dosimeters (glass badges) to children age 18 or younger, encouraging them to continue measuring radiation. For expectant mothers, personal dosimeters have been distributed at the time of the issuance of a mother/child health handbook. The town has advised the continuation of personal dose measurement after delivering a baby.

C People requiring assistance during a disaster (vulnerable people in case of a disaster)

1 Nutrition (meals/water)

a. Situation
- Because distribution of commodities stopped after the earthquake, households with/of persons with disabilities faced difficulties in securing daily necessities.
- Because radioactive materials were detected in water running from taps, residents inevitably had increasing concerns about the safety of water.

b. Responses (actual measures)
- Commissioned welfare volunteers, care helpers and nursing-care specialists (care managers) strived to confirm the safety of each individual person with disabilities. After the confirmation, persons with disabilities received food supplies and water, as needed.
- The town officials confirmed what commodities were in short supply at nursing-care facilities, homes for elderly people requiring special care, health service facilities for the elderly group homes and nursing homes for the elderly. Based on the confirmation, daily necessities such as disposable diapers, towels, water, and food products were distributed to these facilities.

c. Summary/measures in the future
- It is particularly advisable for households with people requiring assistance during a disaster (vulnerable people in case of a disaster) to stock some amount of daily necessities for an emergency.

2 Exercise (Environmental improvement)

a. Situation

- After moving to temporary housing, residents who had been involved in farm work lost the opportunity to take physical activities outdoors. A lack of exercise was common among residents.
- Out-of-home day care facilities temporarily became unavailable immediately after the earthquake. Gasoline to be used by pickup cars for such facilities was also in short supply. Therefore, nursing-care recipients were unable to receive necessary services.

b. Responses (actual measures)

- Exercise instructors conducted brain training and muscular strength improvement training programs at assembly rooms within the sites of temporary housing.
- The town gave priority to out-of-home nursing care facilities for securing a supply of gasoline. With the cooperation between the town and staff members of nursing-care facilities, out-of-home day care services were resumed at a relatively early stage of evacuation.

c. Summary/measures in the future

- It is desirable to continue the exercise programs at assembly rooms of temporary housing sites.

3 Rest (mind, anxiety, suicide, etc.)

a. Situation

- Residents continually complained of concerns about the uncertain situation at the nuclear power stations.
- Anxiety about radiation effects on health increasingly spread among residents.

b. Responses (actual measures)

- The town officials strived to attentively listen to residents' concerns and anxieties to make them feel at ease.
- A registry of the elderly and vulnerable people in case of a disaster that had been made by commissioned welfare volunteers was useful in confirming the safety of such residents.
- The absence of correct information about radiation caused a growing fear of exposure to radiation among residents. To disseminate accurate information to residents, the town conducted various explanatory and lecture meetings on radiation and issued public announcements about radiation.

c. Summary/measures in the future

- As part of the town's disaster preparedness efforts, a system that ensures prompt evacuation of persons requiring assistance during a disaster should be established.
- As a general trend, elderly residents living alone experience a growing feeling of anxiety when a disaster occurs. To prevent them from becoming excessively uneasy, the town needs to offer mental support programs and ensure that elderly residents can gather together, share necessary information, and consoled each other. It is also essential to help elderly residents maintain their ties with local community members.
- Immediately after the earthquake, commissioned welfare volunteers, care managers, and nursing-care providers promptly responded to the urgent needs of persons requiring assistance, which was quite helpful to town officials. Because the importance of maintaining close relationships with local nursing-care providers and other parties concerned was reconfirmed, the town will make continued efforts to build a collaborative network with local communities.
- In December 2012, the town distributed "an emergency medical treatment information kit" to residents

Chapter 3 | Situation of and Countermeasures by Each Individual Municipality

living alone and to households of persons with disabilities.
- The number of *salon* facilities and friendly gathering programs in each administrative ward should be increased, with the aim of further strengthening solidarity among local community members.

4 Others

- To ensure that at-home nursing care providers and other nursing-care service providers can continue offering planned nursing-care programs and provide pickup services for nursing-care recipients during the disaster, the town gave a priority to such providers in securing a gasoline supply. Medical institutions also were a priority for receiving gasoline.

(Yuko Saito)

26. Efforts of Date City

1. Situation of the municipality

(1) Demographics (as of January 1 of each year)

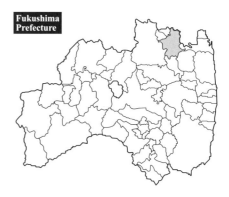

	2011	2012	2013
Population	65,902	64,603	63,571
Number of households	20,879	20,753	20,876
Average number of people per household	3.16	3.11	3.05
Number of births	405	328	
Birth rate	6.1		
Number of deaths	828	845	
Mortality	12.5		
Ratio of the elderly aged 65 or older	28.1	28.4	29.4

(2) Geographical features

Total area: 265.1 km^2 (approximately 13.3 km east-west; approximately 19.8 km north-south)

Distance from the Fukushima Daiichi Nuclear Power Station of the Tokyo Electric Power Company: approximately 45 km

Evacuation area: None

Transportation network: JR Tohoku Line (one station); Abukuma Express (10 stations); National Route 4; National Route 115

2. Situation of damage by the earthquake, tsunami and the nuclear disaster

(1) Damage by the Great East Japan Earthquake (as of August 6, 2012)

Property damage	Completely destroyed	Half destroyed	Partially destroyed
House	26	247	953
Public institution	0	0	187
Other			

Human damage	Deaths by disaster	Disaster-related deaths	Missing persons	Injured persons
	0	1	0	3

(2) Situation of evacuation

① Evacuation centers within the municipality (by July 31, 2011)

	Number of evacuation centers	Number of evacuees	Available period
Residents	13	993	Until April 18
Evacuees received	8	1,728	Until July 31

* The number of evacuees during the peak period are shown.

② Approximate number of evacuees in evacuation centers outside the municipality (as of March 1, 2013)

	End/March 2011	End/September 2011	End/March 2012	Latest period
First evacuation center	0	0	0	0
Second evacuation center	0	0	0	0
Temporary housing	0	0	0	0
Municipally-subsidized housing	0	0	0	0

Chapter 3 | Situation of and Countermeasures by Each Individual Municipality

③ Approximate number of voluntary evacuees (as of February 28, 2013)

Inside Fukushima Prefecture	21	Outside Fukushima Prefecture (number of evacuees & prefectures)	783 persons in 34 prefectures

Outlook of damage related to the nuclear disaster

- On April 11, one month after the nuclear power station accident, the national government designated areas where an annual cumulative dose may reach 20 mSv as a "deliberate evacuation zone." Although having a risk of 20 mSv, the Ishida Hojizawa ward of Ryozen Town, Date City, was not designated a deliberate evacuation zone. However, Date City individually began evacuating the residents of Ishida Sakanoue and Yagihei wards of Ryozen Town. Later, on June 30, a total of 113 households in 104 spots located within Ishida, Kami-oguni and Shimo-oguni wards of Ryozen Town, as well as Aiyoshi ward of Tsukidate Town, were designated as "specific spots recommended for evacuation." The designation was not legally binding. In addition to these wards, on November 25 15 households in 13 spots located within the Tomizawa ward of Hobara Town and Ishida and Shimo-oguni wards of Ryozen Town were also designated as specific spots recommended for evacuation because a relatively high radiation dose was observed in these areas.
- Environmental contamination by radiation due to the nuclear power accident was not limited to residents' living areas; farmland, mountains/forests, and rivers were also contaminated by radioactive materials. Particularly, agriculture, a key industry of Date City, was seriously affected by radiation. Baseless rumors also caused significant damage to the reputation of even industrial products manufactured in the city. To address such a severe situation, the city embarked on decontamination work in 2011, mainly in schools and other public facilities as well as areas where a relatively high radiation dose was observed. Moreover, the city conducted various health management efforts such as the distribution of personal dosimeters (glass badges) to residents, food quality inspection, and measurement of the internal exposure dose by Whole Body Counters. As a next step to cope with the severe situation, the city will focus on the continuation of decontamination work throughout the city, expansion of various health management programs, and measures to compensate for damages incurred by residents as a result of the nuclear accident.

3 Countermeasures against nuclear disaster (as of January 2013)

		Name of project	Division in charge	Number of targeted persons (households)	Expectant mothers	Nursing mothers	Babies	Young children	Elementary school students	Junior high school students	Senior high school students	People age 19 to 39	People age 40 or older	Remarks (major operations)
Countermeasures against external exposure	1	Personal dose measurements	Health Promotion Division	All residents (65,000 persons)	○	○	○	○	○	○	○	○	○	Measurement of all residents' personal exposure dose were continued from July 2012 to June 2013.
	2	Refreshment for young children	Educational General Affairs Division											
	3	Refreshments for elementary school and junior high school students		998 persons (FY2012)				○	○					Planning, coordination, collecting the participants and guiding
	4	Monitoring and measurement of the air radiation levels	Environment and Disaster Prevention Division	19 spots										Purchase of equipment, measurement, recording, and announcements
	5	Real-time measurement of the radiation doses (Ministry of the Environment)	Environment and Disaster Prevention Division	104 spots										
	6	Measurement and mapping of the air radiation levels in the whole city	Environment and Disaster Prevention Division	All over the city	○	○	○	○	○	○	○	○	○	Outsourcing, measurement, aggregation, creation of a map, and distribution (every three month)
	7	Replacement of the surface soil on the grounds in childcare facilities, child education facilities and schools	Radiation Countermeasures Division	All facilities			○	○	○	○				
	8	Decontamination of houses	Radiation Countermeasures Division	All over the city	○	○	○	○	○	○	○	○	○	The city is classified into three areas (A, B and C areas) according to radiation dose. Decontamination methods are different from area to area.
	9	Decontamination of public and medical institutions	Radiation Countermeasures Division	All over the city	○	○	○	○	○	○	○	○	○	
	10	Whole Body Counter measurements (conducted by the city)	Health Promotion Division	64,000 persons	○	○		○	○	○	○	○	○	Announcements to all the residents over 4 years old

	No.	Measure	Division	Scope										Remarks
Countermeasures against internal exposure	11	Whole Body Counter measurements (conducted by Fukushima Prefecture for children aged 4 to 18)	Health Promotion Division					○	○	○	○	○		Implemented only in FY2011
	12	Food quality inspection	Agriculture and Forestry Division	15,187 cases										15 inspection sites within the city. Acceptance of inspection and issuance of public announcement papers
	13	Thyroid gland examination (conducted by Fukushima Prefecture)	Health Promotion Division				○	○	○	○	○			Arrangement of venues in FY2011
	14	Inspection of school meals	School Lunch Center	All facilities				○	○	○				Introduction of inspection equipment, daily measurements and announcements of the results to parents/guardians
Others	15	Debriefing sessions for measurement results of exposure dose	Health Promotion Division	All residents	○	○	○	○	○	○	○	○	○	Coordination of lecturers & venues for debriefing sessions for measurement results of external exposure dose, announcements and management
	16	Study sessions on radiation	Health Promotion Division	All residents	○	○	○	○	○	○	○	○	○	Coordination of lecturers & venues, announcements, and management
	17	Measurement and mapping of the radiation dose in the soil within the whole city	Agriculture and Forestry Division	All over the city										Ordinary cultivated land
	18	Lecture meetings on radiation	Health Promotion Division	All residents	○	○	○	○	○	○	○	○	○	Coordination of lecturers & venues, announcements, and management
	19	Sampling of respondents for a basic survey in the Fukushima Health Management Survey	Health Promotion Division	All residents	○	○	○	○	○	○	○	○	○	Outsourcing
	20	Publication of disaster information magazines	Secretariat and Public Relations Division	All residents	○	○	○	○	○	○	○	○	○	Issuance twice a month

Chapter 3 Situation of and Countermeasures by Each Individual Municipality

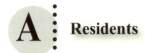

A Residents

1 Nutrition (meals/water)

a. Situation
- Because a combination of "rice and *tsukemono* pickles" or "pastries and juice" constituted the majority of meals after the earthquake, residents under treatment of lifestyle-related diseases were worried about a worsening of their diseases.
- A worsening of metabolic syndrome screening results was found in some residents.
- Due to a media report that radioactive substances were detected in tap water in the Tsukidate district, the city was flooded with inquiries about water quality inspection and with complaints from residents who were filled with fear of exposure to radiation.
- Basic utilities were damaged and distribution of commodities stopped after the earthquake. Residents staying in their own houses rushed to evacuation centers, seeking food and beverages.

b. Responses (actual measures)
- In cooperation with the members of the local medical association, specialist personnel of Fukushima Prefecture and Date City went to evacuation centers to provide counseling for nutrition and medical problems. The local association of dietitians also conducted an investigation to understand the current nutritional condition of residents at evacuation centers.
- The city officials offered home visits and educational programs on health problems, aiming to provide residents with instructions on well-balanced diets.
- After a while, residents, by rotation, independently began cooking vegetable-rich meals at evacuation centers.

c. Summary/measures in the future
- The city needs to maintain a nutritional balance in preparing stockpiles for an emergency.
- Long-term treatment measures for patients with lifestyle-related diseases must be taken by the city.

2 Exercise (Environmental improvement)

a. Situation
- Immediately after the nuclear power station accident, outdoor activities were severely restricted. As a trend that has been observed for a long period of time, the amount of outdoor exercises and other physical activities in daily lives has been decreasing among residents.

b. Responses (actual measures)
- The city encouraged residents to maintain good ventilation at evacuation centers. Residents were also advised to take radio gymnastic exercises every day.
- The Red Cross Volunteers from the Japanese Red Cross Society conducted games and light exercise programs at evacuation centers.
- Health promotion exercise classes and muscular strength improvement programs for elderly residents were resumed.
- Instructions on how to prevent the development of deep vein thrombosis/pulmonary embolism (the "economy-class syndrome") were given to residents at evacuation centers.

● Exercise instructors conducted some exercise programs for residents at evacuation centers.

c. Summary/measures in the future
● As a common tendency among residents, metabolic syndrome screening results have been worsening after the earthquake. If a disaster occurs, long-term measures to prevent the worsening of metabolic syndrome must be taken at evacuation centers at an early stage of evacuation.

3 Rest (mind, anxiety, suicide, etc.)

a. Situation
● Being confused by a flood of contradictory information, residents became increasingly worried about farmland contamination by radiation.
● The city was flooded with many inquiries from residents about the safety of local farm crops.
● Because outdoor activities were restricted, many residents were not able to go out, for example, to gather wild plants. As a result of such restrictions, an increasing number of residents showed being homebound or symptoms of depression.

b. Responses (actual measures)
● A health counseling program named "*ocha-nomini-koransho*" was held at assembly halls within areas designated as a specific spot recommended for evacuation.
● Counseling programs by certified clinical psychologists were conducted.

c. Summary/measures in the future
● It is important to offer mental health counseling for residents at an easy-to-access location (such as local assembly halls and evacuation centers) as early as possible after a disaster.
● For residents who are supposed to need some special support, home-visiting services by specialists should be offered.

B Expectant/nursing mothers and children

1 Nutrition (meals/water)

a. Situation
● After the nuclear power station accident, the distribution of commodities stopped due to baseless rumors about radiation. The city received many inquiries from expectant/nursing mothers about the supply of artificial milk (milk powder) and disposable diapers.
● On March 22, 2011, 120 Bq/kg of radioactive iodine (^{131}I) was detected in tap water in the Tsukidate district where a private water-supply system is used. In response to the detection, the city placed a restriction on an intake of water from the supply system and urged nursing mothers not to give tap water to babies. The restriction was lifted at 12:00 on April 1, 2011.
● A growing anxiety about contamination of water, vegetables, and other foods, as well as breast milk, was rapidly spread among residents. Although the city established a food/water quality inspection and monitoring system, interest in the system varied by persons. There were some households in which meals for mothers and young children and meals for other family members were prepared separately.

Chapter 3 | Situation of and Countermeasures by Each Individual Municipality

b. Responses (actual measures)

- The city called for donation of milk powder and disposable diapers from pharmacies and nursery schools within the city.
- In the administrative wards using a private water supply system, bottled water was distributed to households with babies and young children.
- For inquiries from residents about breast milk contamination by radiation, the city officials introduced the residents to the breast milk inspection institutions of Fukushima Prefecture.
- The city announced water and food quality inspection results in its newsletter "Disaster Management."
- The city made a request to the Fukushima Prefecture Disaster Response Headquarters for immediate distribution of milk powder and disposable diapers to the evacuees.

c. Summary/measures in the future

- As a lesson learned from the nuclear disaster, the city's disaster response headquarters and each individual household are strongly advised to maintain full stockpiles and to be well-prepared for any disasters in the future.
- Although residents have been increasingly paying attention to the measurement of the radiation in home-grown vegetables, their level of interest in the measurement of radiation in food varies by the type of foods and season. The city is required to further raise residents' awareness of the measurement.
- Taking the dispersion of radioactive substances, regional disparities in radiation levels and hot-spot areas into consideration, the city will continue the measurement of radiation in food.

2 Exercise (Environmental improvement)

a. Situation

- Because some areas were designated as a specific spot recommended for evacuation, parents and guardians became increasingly worried about their children's possible exposure to radiation in school zones and from outdoor activities.
- There were many young children who wore long-sleeved clothes and a mask even in the summer season.
- Outdoor activities and swimming in a pool were not allowed at schools.

b. Responses (actual measures)

- The first issue of the city's original "Disaster Management" newsletter was published on March 21, 2011. The purpose of the newsletter is to announce measurement results of the air radiation levels and disseminate other necessary information on radiation to the residents.
- To reduce a risk of exposure to radiation in school zones, school bus services were offered for students who travel a long distance to school.
- Replacement of the surface soil on the grounds in nursery schools, kindergartens, primary schools and junior high schools within the city was implemented.
- Swimming pool decontamination work was conducted at primary schools within the city.
- The city lent portable survey meters (Geiger counters) to residents.
- Simultaneous measurement and mapping of air radiation levels within the city was conducted. The measurement results and a created map were announced to the public.
- The city set up indoor playing spaces.
- Air conditioners were installed at all the primary schools and junior high schools located within Date City.

c. Summary/measures in the future

- When a nuclear disaster occurs, emergency response activities by the national government and Fukushima Prefecture will be concentrated in areas where the evacuation order is issued, thereby causing delayed responses to other affected areas. Therefore, each local municipality is strongly advised to quickly assess a critical situation and individually respond to the urgent needs of residents at its own discretion.
- The city intends to continue the monitoring and measurement of air radiation levels, using monitoring posts (air radiation level measurement equipment) installed within the city.
- To avoid residents' unnecessary exposure to radiation, the city will strive to effectively disseminate critical information such as the situation of the nuclear power station accident, real-time radiation levels, and indoor evacuation instructions, as needed.
- It is desirable to establish a system in which specialists and parents/guardians cooperate with each other in securing indoor playing spaces for young children and developing effective playing programs to prevent them from having a lack of exercise.

3 Rest (mind, anxiety, suicide, etc.)

a. Situation

- The more the details about the damage from the nuclear accident were brought to light, the more differing information was disseminated to residents. Such a flood of complicated information inevitably caused residents to become upset and confused.
- It was also quite difficult for the city to obtain correct information on the nuclear power station accident.
- Due to contradictory reports on radiation hot spots and differing safety/security information, a growing distrust and confusion arose among residents.
- Irrespective of age, all residents living within the city felt increasing concerns about exposure to radiation, becoming quite nervous about all aspects of daily life such as going outdoors, preparing meals, and hanging the laundry.

b. Responses (actual measures)

- Taking the highest priority to secure the safety of residents, the city asked several radiation specialists to serve as advisors and provide advice to residents about preventive measures against radiation.
- The city explained about the designation as a "specific spot recommended for evacuation" to the residents concerned and conducted an explanatory meeting for households wishing to evacuate the designated areas.
- Lecture meetings on radiation were held in every administrative ward within the city.
- The city distributed personal dosimeter (glass badges) to expectant mothers and young children to measure their external exposure to radiation. Measurement of their internal exposure to radiation was also implemented, using Whole Body Counters. Later, all the residents became the subject of both external and internal exposure measurements.
- Study sessions on radiation for parents/guardians were held.
- Friendly gatherings in which parents and young children can enjoy playing with each other were provided. Parents also participated in a group meeting to exchange information and share problems with each other.

c. Summary/measures in the future

- When basic utilities and other life lines are damaged by a nuclear disaster, necessary information will be obtainable only through limited sources. To ensure that residents, particularly expectant mothers and

young children, can calmly respond to an earthquake and other disasters, it is required for the city to develop and review its disaster preparedness manual.
- Safety confirmation sent to both expectant mothers and mothers rearing young children was relatively easy because their contact numbers (fixed phones/mobile phones) were filled in on a written notification of pregnancy or examinee sheets that were filed when receiving medical examinations for young children. For persons requiring assistance, data files of their contact information must be regularly updated and backed up.
- Because details of mental counseling differ from person to person, it is necessary for the city to develop collaborative relationships among mental health care team members, aiming to systematically manage and share case-by-case information with them.
- The city entrusted to several radiation specialists the provision of advice to residents about preventive measures against radiation, radiation effects on the immune system, diets, decontamination, mental health care and others issues.

C People requiring assistance during a disaster (vulnerable people in case of a disaster)

1 Nutrition (meals/water)

a. Situation

(Patients transferred from Futaba Hospital)
- Most patients transferred from Futaba Hospital (a hospital for mentally disabled people located in the Soso region) to evacuation centers of the city were bed-ridden or almost bed-ridden inpatients. It was unknown how many days they had had no meals.

b. Responses (actual measures)
- The city secured a supply of isotonic beverages, rice porridge in retort pouches, straws and spoons.
- The city asked doctors to examine the patients transferred from Futaba Hospital. Based on the doctors' judgment, meals were provided to them.
- The city officials assisted the patients transferred from Futaba Hospital to drink water and eat rice porridge.
- The city made the arrangement for nursing-care staff members to assist patients transferred from Futaba Hospital.

c. Summary/measures in the future
- It is necessary to include liquid foods for persons with difficulties swallowing into stockpiles for emergencies.
- If evacuees include many residents requiring nursing care, dedicated nursing-care staff members should be assigned.
- A minimum amount of water required to maintain life must be secured.

2 Exercise (Environmental improvement)

a. Situation

(Patients transferred from Futaba Hospital)
- It was unknown how long the patients had not received continence care. Although heating devices and blankets were used to protect them from the cold, ventilation was not maintained at a shelter where they

had stayed.

b. Responses (actual measures)
- Continence care and diaper exchange support were provided to the patients transferred from Futaba Hospital. The city strived to secure disposable diapers and other nursing-care items.
- The city made the arrangement for nursing-care staff members to assist patients transferred from Futaba Hospital.

c. Summary/measures in the future
- It is almost impossible to continue providing nursing care and medical support to residents requiring assistance at temporal emergency centers, due to a lack of necessary equipment.

3 Rest (mind, anxiety, suicide, etc.)

a. Situation
(Patients transferred from Futaba Hospital)
- Although most patients transferred from Futaba Hospital had communication problems, they managed to convey somehow their distress and pain to others.
- Patients with mental disabilities experienced a worsening of health conditions.

b. Responses (actual measures)
- After receiving continence care and assistance in taking water from nursing-care staff members, some patients transferred from Futaba Hospital gradually began talking again.
- The city officials provided frequent interviews with the patients and proceeded with necessary procedures for their consultation or hospitalization in medical institutions.

c. Summary/measures in the future
- To respond to the needs of patients having communication problems, it is essential to make sure that triage results and other critical information about the patients are shared among medical and nursing-care staff members. In addition to the development of such an information sharing system, it is also necessary for the city to assign medical workers and dedicated nursing-care stuff members at an early stage of evacuation to promptly respond to the urgent needs of persons requiring assistance.
- It is indispensable for the city to keep collaborative relationships with medical institutions in local communities.

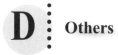

D Others

- The city gave priority to medical institutions for receiving a supply of gasoline, with the aim of securing emergency medical assistance for victim residents.
- The first issuance of the city's newsletter "Disaster Management," the decontamination promotion center's newsletter, and an information magazine on agriculture named "*kou*" were issued.
- The city conducted an explanatory meeting about the designation as a "specific spot recommended for evacuation" for the residents concerned. For households wishing to evacuate the designated area, the city helped them to find shelter.
- Summer camp programs were conducted for elementary school students.
- The city conducted measurements of residents' external exposure to radiation and internal exposure to

Chapter 3 | Situation of and Countermeasures by Each Individual Municipality

radiation, using personal dosimeter (glass badges) and Whole Body Counters, respectively.

- Decontamination work was implemented with the cooperation of volunteer members.
- The city held group meetings for parents and guardians of young children so that they can communicate and share information with each other.
- As part of post-disaster mental health care efforts, the city has conducted playing programs for mothers and young children, friendly gathering for new mothers, exercise classes for young children, lecture meetings on radiation for parents/guardians, and the distribution of glass badges. Moreover, they have been involved in support services for residents taking shelter in other municipalities such as announcements of medical examinations for young children. Having been fully occupied with regular duties and the heavy extra workload, the city officials have grown increasingly exhausted.

(Patients transferred from Futaba Hospital)

- At 23:00 on March 15, through Fukushima Prefecture, the city received a request for acceptance of patients that had come from medical staff members working in the Soso region. Those who were transferred to the city were inpatients at Futaba Hospital. It was already 02:00 on March 16 when the transfer of the inpatients was completed. Although Futaba Hospital staff members said that they would come to meet the inpatient at 10:00 on the day, no one came. The city officials, who were busily responding to the needs of residents at evacuation centers, did not receive any detailed information on the transfer; such as the number of patients to be transferred and their health condition. The lack of information caused a delay in preparing for the acceptance and the provision of necessary nursing care support for the patients. In such a situation, the city officials strived to prepare continence care items and drinking water. After the inpatients were transferred to evacuation centers, the city officials took a photograph of each individual patient and started his/her hospital chart so that the officials and other medical staff members can distinguish inpatients transferred from Futaba Hospital.
  - When changing a disposable diaper, the city officials confirmed each patient's name tag and filled in as much personal information as possible on individuals' hospital chart.
  - A record of nursing care for each individual patient was made.
  - When changing a disposable diaper, the city officials noticed there were some patients receiving intravenous hyper-alimentation. The patients were promptly referred to medical institutions.
  - Although triage cards were found under blankets, it was impossible to identify each card's owner.
  - For patients referred to medical institutions, the city officials made a copy of their medical charts. One copy was submitted to the medical institution and the other was sent to the city's emergency response headquarters.
  - Even in an extremely confused situation after a disaster, information transmission to emergency assistance staff members at evacuation centers is indispensable to promptly respond to the urgent needs of evacuees. Especially, personal information about patients with communication disabilities must be promptly transmitted to on-site care givers and shared among all staff members.
  - Photograph of patients was sent to the city's disaster response headquarters.

(Seiko Kanno, Kayoko Ito, Kanae Hata, Yoko Watanabe, Nobutaka Taniguchi)

27 Efforts of Fukushima City

1 Situation of the municipality

(1) Demographics (as of January 1 of each year)

	2011	2012	2013
Population	292,489	286,963	284,113
Number of households	113,187	112,646	113,374
Average number of people per household	2.6	2.5	2.5
Number of births	2,171	1,935	
Birth rate	7.5	6.8	
Number of deaths	2,942	2,921	
Mortality	10.2	10.3	
Ratio of the elderly aged 65 or older	23.7	24.56	

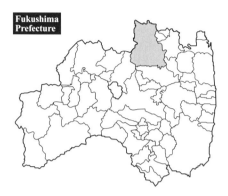

(2) Geographical features
Total area: 767.74 km² (approximately 30.2 km east-west; approximately 39.1 km north-south)
Distance from the Fukushima Daiichi Nuclear Power Station of the Tokyo Electric Power Company: approximately 63 km
Evacuation area: None
Transportation network: National Route 4; a starting point of the National Route 13; Tohoku Expressway; a junction of the JR Tohoku Line and the JR Ou Line; a junction of Tohoku *shinkansen* bullet trains and Yamagata *shinkansen* bullet trains

2 Situation of damage by the earthquake, tsunami and the nuclear disaster

(1) Damage by the Great East Japan Earthquake (as of the end of March 2012)

Property damage	Completely destroyed	Half destroyed	Partially destroyed
House	204	3,981	6,548
Public institution	0	0	325
Other	0	0	4,915

Human damage	Deaths by disaster	Disaster-related deaths	Missing persons	Injured persons
	6	7	0	19

(2) Situation of evacuation
① Evacuation centers within the municipality (as of the end of March 2012)

	Number of evacuation centers	Number of evacuees	Available period
Residents	0		
Evacuees received	0		

② Approximate number of evacuees in evacuation centers outside the municipality (as of the end of March 2012)

	End/March 2011	End/September 2011	End/March 2012	Latest period
First evacuation center	0	0	0	0
Second evacuation center	0	0	0	0
Temporary housing	0	0	0	0
Municipally-subsidized housing	0	0	0	0

③ Approximate number of voluntary evacuees (as of the end of March 2012)

Inside Fukushima Prefecture	74	Outside Fukushima Prefecture	6,804 persons

Chapter 3 | Situation of and Countermeasures by Each Individual Municipality

Outlook of damage related to the nuclear disaster

In the evening of March 15, sleet mixed with radioactive materials from the nuclear accident at the Fukushima Daiichi Nuclear Power Station fell in the northern part of Fukushima Prefecture, even 60 km away from the power station. The dispersion of radioactive materials caused environmental contamination in the entire prefecture. Initially, a maximum of 24.24 μSv/hour was observed. The nuclear accident brought about the following four major consequences in Fukushima City:

①A fearful feeling about radiation

Residents, including the city officials, had no knowledge of radiation and its effects on human health. The lack of knowledge caused a growing fear and anxieties about radiation among residents.

Moreover, because perceptions about the risk of exposure to radiation varied among people, there existed a sharp divergence of opinion about radiation not only among friends and acquaintances but also among family members, making residents feel uneasy in their daily lives. Some residents are still suffering from a conflict of opinion with their family members.

②Confusion caused by differing information and a distrust of the administration

Shortly after the disaster, the city asked expert advisors to help disseminate correct information on radiation to residents. However, residents were initially swayed by differing reports in the mass media, becoming sometimes optimistic and sometimes pessimistic. Information disseminated from the national government and Fukushima Prefecture was also contradictory, creating further confusion among residents. Inevitably, residents were obsessed with the idea that "The city may conceal critical information from us" and "The administration may provide false information to us on purpose," increasing their distrust of the administration.

③Baseless rumors and voluntary evacuation

An increasing anxiety about radiation and a growing distrust of information disseminated from the administration resulted in the spread of baseless rumors among residents, and voluntary evacuation of mothers and children. The baseless rumors have also seriously damaged the primary industries of Fukushima Prefecture. Moreover, during a prolonged period of voluntary evacuation, mothers and young children have faced a separation from other family members, financial difficulties and other problems in an unstable living environment in host municipalities. Offering physical and mental health care support to such young children is one of the urgent tasks for the city.

④A drastic change in lifestyles

During a certain period of time after the nuclear power station accident, residents had reframed from going outside because of relatively high radiation levels in the air observed in the city, and from eating local farm products such as vegetables and milk due to baseless rumors. Although most residents gradually returned to their normal daily lives over time, there are some residents whose lifestyle has drastically changed after the nuclear accident. Such residents have gained weight and developed lipid abnormalities. An increase in the number of prospective patients with lifestyle-related diseases is a great concern for the city.

3 Countermeasures against nuclear disaster (as of January 2013)

		Name of project	Division in charge	Number of targeted persons (households)	Expectant mothers	Nursing mothers	Babies	Young children	Elementary school students	Junior high school students	Senior high school students	People age 19 to 39	People age 40 or older	Remarks (major operations)
Countermeasures against external exposure	1	Personal dose measurements	Radiation and Health Management Office	All residents (approximately 292,000 persons)	○	○	○	○	○	○	○	○	○	Distribution of glass badges for three months to approximately 38,000 young children, elementary school and junior high school students. Distribution of electronic personal cumulative dosimeters to high school students and adults. Year-round lending, notification, acceptance of applications, distribution, collection, notification of measurement results, and analysis & announcements of measurement results
	2	Refreshment for expectant mothers (relaxation programs in a low-dose area)												Unavailable
	3	Monitoring and measurement of the air radiation levels (Ministry of Education, Culture, Sports, Science and Technology)	Radiation Monitoring Center of Environment Division	All residents (approximately 292,000 persons)	○	○	○	○	○	○	○	○	○	Installation of 392 monitoring posts within the city. A link to the website of the Ministry of Education, Culture, Sports, Science and Technology
	4	Measurement and mapping of the air radiation levels in the whole city	Radiation Monitoring Center of Environment Division	All residents (approximately 292,000 persons)	○	○	○	○	○	○	○	○	○	Measurement of air radiation levels, creation of maps, and distribution of the map to each household (distributed in June 2011 and May 2012)

264

	#	Item	Division in charge	Target	C1	C2	C3	C4	C5	C6	C7	C8	C9	Remarks
Countermeasures against internal exposure	5	Measurement of the air radiation levels at 30 fixed spots within the city	Radiation Monitoring Center of Environment Division	All residents (approximately 292,000 persons)	○	○	○	○	○	○	○	○	○	Air radiation level measurement one to three days per week. Announcements of the measurement results on the city's website
	6	Replacement of the surface soil on the grounds in childcare facilities, child education facilities and schools	Board of Education and Child Welfare Division				○	○	○	○				Survey, planning, selection of soil replacement companies, ordering, implementation, and assessment
	7	Decontamination of houses	Comprehensive Radiation Countermeasures Division	110,000 households	○	○	○	○	○	○	○	○	○	The "Hometown Decontamination Project" started for five years from October 2011. Each branch office of Fukushima City established a "Special Committee on Decontamination of the Local Community" for the planning, ordering, implementation, and assessment of the decontamination projects.
	8	Decontamination of public and medical institutions	Comprehensive Radiation Countermeasures Division	All residents (approximately 292,000 persons)	○	○	○	○	○	○	○	○	○	Survey, planning, selection of soil replacement companies, ordering, implementation, and assessment
	9	Improvement of indoor playing spaces	Child Welfare Division	All residents (approximately 292,000 persons)	○	○	○	○	○	○	○	○	○	Securing of indoor sandboxes and outdoor playing spaces in areas with a relatively low air radiation levels
	10	Inspection of breast milk and counseling	Health Promotion Division	For those wishing to have the services		○								Counseling services for mothers worried about the safety of breast milk, and information provision services about breast-feeding mother support projects conducted by Fukushima Prefecture
	11	Whole Body Counter measurements (conducted by the city)	Radiation and Health Management Office	Residents age 4 years and older	○	○	○	○	○	○	○	○	○	A Whole Body Counter mounted on a vehicle that circles around the premises of elementary schools and junior high schools was used. For the measurements of young children, expectant mothers and high school students, the city entrusted to three inspection agencies.
	12	Whole Body Counter measurements (conducted by Fukushima Prefecture for children aged 4 to 18)	Radiation and Health Management Office	Residents age 4 to 18 years old			○	○	○	○	○			Notification to the subject residents, acceptance of applications, and arrangement of venues
	13	Food and water quality inspection	Radiation Monitoring Center of Environment Division		○	○	○	○	○	○	○	○	○	Inspection of food products and water, which are brought in by residents, are conducted every day at 28 locations throughout the city. The quality inspection results are announced to the public.
	14	Thyroid gland examination (conducted by Fukushima Prefecture)	Radiation and Health Management Office	Residents age 18 years and younger when the earthquake occurred			○	○	○	○	○			Sampling of examinees, arrangement of venues, and answering inquiries
	15	Inspection of school meals at primary schools and junior high schools	Board of Education and Health and Physical Education Division (each school meal center and schools equipped with private facilities to prepare school meals)								○	○		Food ingredients of school meals or a serving of a school meal are inspected every day before serving. The inspection results are announced to the public.

Chapter 3 Situation of and Countermeasures by Each Individual Municipality

	No.	Item	Division	Target											Remarks
	16	Inspection of school meals at nursery schools	Child Welfare Division (each nursery school)				○	○							After cooking, a serving of a school meal is inspected every day at nursery schools. The inspection results are announced at each nursery school.
	17	Inspection of rice for school meals	Health and Physical Education Division and Child Welfare Division				○	○	○	○					Rice to be used for school meals is inspected several times to ensure the safety and security of young children.
	18	Debriefing sessions for measurement results of exposure dose													Unavailable
	19	Study sessions and symposiums on radiation	Health Promotion Division	All residents (approximately 292,000 persons)	○	○	○	○				○	○		Plans according to the target participants. A total of 12 study sessions/symposiums were conducted at four venues in FY2011 and a total of 63 study sessions/symposiums were held at 16 venues in FY2012.
	20	Cancer screening	Health Promotion Division	Residents age 20 years and older for uterine cancer screening Residents age 40 years and older for other cancer screening								△ (uterine cancer screening for residents age 20 years and older)	○		Cancer screening tests under the Health Promotion Law
	21	Replacement of the surface soil in rice paddies													Unavailable
	22	Measurement and mapping of the radiation dose in the soil within the whole city													Unavailable
Others	23	Lecture meetings on radiation	Health Promotion Division	All residents (approximately 292,000 persons)	○	○	○	○	○	○	○	○	○	○	Plans according to the target participants. A total of 20 lecture meetings were conducted at 19 venues in FY2011 and a total of 37 lecture meetings were held at 19 venues in FY2012.
	24	Sampling of respondents for a basic survey in the Fukushima Health Management Survey	Radiation and Health Management Office	All residents (approximately 292,000 persons)	○	○	○	○	○	○	○	○	○	○	Sampling of respondents, and the submission of survey results to Fukushima Prefecture
	25	Publication of disaster information magazines	Public Relations Division	All residents (approximately 292,000 persons)	○	○	○	○	○	○	○	○	○	○	Publicity through the city's newsletters
	26	Issuance of citizen health cards (containing a column for recording radiation exposure levels)													Unavailable
	27	Mental health counseling	Health Promotion Division	Parents with young children			○	○	○			Parents/ guardians with young children			Mental health counseling services by a psychologist, as needed, at medical examinations for young children
	28	Preparation and distribution of leaflets about radiation and its effects on human health	Health Promotion Division	All residents (approximately 292,000 persons)	○	○	○	○				○	○		Planning, preparation of leaflets (under the supervision of an advisor), and ordering to suppliers. Distribution of leaflets at the time of home visits, medical examinations for young children and lecture meetings, etc.

No.	Program	Division	Target										Description
29	Refreshment programs in *onsen* hot spring	Child Welfare Division	For those wishing to participate in the programs		○	○							A program for preschool children and their family members, aiming to encourage them to feel both physically and mentally refreshed at *onsen* accommodation facilities within the city
30	Summer refreshing programs for young children	Lifelong Learning Division	For those wishing to participate in the programs				○	○	○				The purpose of the project is to foster the sound development of young children, by helping them acquire hands-on experience with nature, friendly communication with each other, and restoration of youthful vigor and vitality in beautiful natural settings.
31	Measurement of the radiation levels at the poolside of schools	Educational General Affairs Division	All schools					○	○				Regular quality inspection of water taken from pools and poolside at schools to ensure the safety and security of students.
32	Education on radiation	School Education Division	All schools					○	○				Utilizing original instruction materials, each school has educated students about radiation in classes.
33	Projects to protect children from radiation damage	Health and Physical Education Division	For schools wishing to receive support					○	○				Doctors, sports trainers and sports instructors have been assigned to schools to help students develop healthy lifestyles and the habit of exercise.

Chapter 3 | Situation of and Countermeasures by Each Individual Municipality

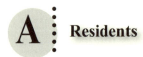 Residents

1 Nutrition (meals/water)

a. Situation

(Immediately after the earthquake)

- Although residents took shelter in evacuation centers due to the power failure, most of them returned home within two to three days because electricity came back on promptly. However, a cutoff of the water supply persisted for a maximum of almost two weeks, so residents had to walk or bicycle to an emergency water station every day and line up to receive water. There were also many residents who brought their young children with them to form a line in front of the emergency water station.
- Fresh food, gasoline and other daily commodities were in short supply for almost one month after the earthquake. There were many convenience stores that ran out of almost all goods, except tobacco and snacks.
- Because many stores suffered property damage from the earthquake or were at the risk of being damaged by aftershocks, they had to sell food and other goods in front of the store. Moreover, due to the overall short supply of commodities, stores had to limit their opening hours. Therefore, residents formed a line and had to wait a long time in front of stores, so as not to miss a chance to purchase a limited amount of daily commodities.
- There were many cases where residents, particularly residents working during the daytime, were not able to purchase fresh food due to the limited opening hours of stores.

(One to two years after the earthquake)

- Residents increasingly felt anxious about radioactive contamination of food and water.
- Due to concerns about possible contamination by radiation, an increasing number of residents avoided purchasing farm products produced in Fukushima Prefecture and Fukushima City.
- The city conducted a survey on the health conditions and lifestyle of residents in October 2011. The survey results revealed a tendency towards a decreased intake of vegetables and dairy products among residents.

(Two years after the earthquake)

- Residents increasingly accepted vegetables grown within Fukushima Prefecture.

b. Responses (actual measures)

(Immediately after to two years after the earthquake)

- The city issued its newsletter named "Prompt Report on the Off the Pacific Coast of Tohoku Earthquake" (from the 1st to the 23rd issues), in an effort to announce radiation and other necessary living information to the residents.
- After the resumption of regular duties, the Health Promotion Division strived to respond to the residents' urgent needs and concerns about radiation through home visits, health counseling services at each administrative ward, educational services, and medical examinations.
- The city conducted lecture meetings titled "Radiation, Health and Our Daily Lives" at several administrative wards, inviting Osamu SAITO (a doctor) as a lecturer.
- In collaboration with Nagasaki University and Kagawa Nutrition University, a lecture meeting on radiation was held as part of event programs at a health festival.

27 Efforts of Fukushima City

- The city has made strenuous efforts to establish an effective radiation inspection system for water and food. For example, the city embarked on water quality inspection immediately after the earthquake and incorporated a radiation screening system into a distribution process of farm products. In addition to these efforts, the city also set up a radiation measurement center for home-grown vegetables and other farm crops. Moreover, one year after the earthquake, the city has established a total of 28 radiation measurement centers for any food products that are brought in by residents.
- The city held a seminar on radiation effects on human health at the request of neighborhood associations, clubs for elderly people, and the Japan Agricultural Cooperative. At the seminar, an explanation about the radiation screening system that was incorporated into a distribution process of farm products was provided to the participants. The participating residents were also encouraged to have a radiation measurement done for their home-grown vegetables so that they could reduce the internal exposure dose as much as possible.
- Because many residents had nutritionally unbalanced meals due to anxiety about exposure to radiation, the city frequently conducted seminars on healthy and well-balanced diets.

2 Exercise (Environmental improvement)

a. Situation

(Immediately after the earthquake, at evacuation centers for both residents and evacuees from other municipalities)

- Because evacuation centers were densely crowded with evacuees, the city felt concerns about a decrease in activities of daily livings (ADLs) and the development of pulmonary deep vein thrombosis/thrombo-embolism (economy-class syndrome) among evacuees.

(Immediately after to two years after the earthquake)

- For fear of being exposed to radiation, an increasing number of residents reframed from going outdoors, leading to a decrease in their total exercise.
- Some of the public facilities were damaged by the earthquake. Although several learning centers and sports/exercise facilities were left undamaged, they were used as evacuation centers. Due to inaccessibility to these public facilities, residents lost an opportunity to go outside and add some physical activity to their daily lives.
- The city conducted a survey on the residents' health conditions and lifestyle in October 2011. The survey results revealed a tendency toward a decreased amount of exercise among an increasing number of residents.

b. Responses (actual measures)

(Immediately after the earthquake, at evacuation centers for both residents and evacuees from other municipalities)

- Evacuees were advised to drink a lot of water and take more exercise to prevent the development of the economy-class syndrome.
- To call evacuees' attention to the necessity of taking exercise, the city distributed pamphlets to each individual resident and posted them at evacuation centers.

(Residents)

- The city promptly repaired learning centers and sports/exercise facilities that had been damaged by the earthquake. Public facilities, which had been temporarily used as evacuation centers, also resumed normal services and programs.

Chapter 3 | Situation of and Countermeasures by Each Individual Municipality

- Welfare facilities strived to resume regular care services as early as possible.
- Various events were held to encourage residents to take exercise.

3 Rest (mind, anxiety, suicide, etc.)

a. Situation
(Immediately after the earthquake, at evacuation centers for both residents and evacuees from other municipalities)

- Residents were filled with extreme anxiety about their future due to a lack of information as to when they would be able to return home.
- An increasing number of residents felt completely exhausted, both physically and mentally, from their unstable life as evacuees. There were some residents who became unable to communicate with others and did not show any emotions to others.
- There were some cases in which residents, who were extremely possessed with an uneasy feeling, had no outlet but to take aggressive attitudes to others. This caused troubles between residents at evacuation centers.
- A conspicuous deterioration in the mental health conditions was observed both for families and for individual residents who had suffered from some mental health problems before the earthquake.

(Residents immediately after the earthquake)

- An increasing number of residents did not go outside and remained shut up at home for fear of being exposed to radiation.
- Public facilities such as learning centers and sports/exercise facilities became inaccessible because they were damaged by the earthquake or used as evacuation centers. The inaccessibility to these facilities resulted in lost opportunities for residents to communicate with each other.

(One to two years after the earthquake)

- Evacuees and residents remaining in their homes within the city had different concerns about radiation. As a result, it gradually became difficult for residents to easily understand and communicate each other. Such divergence of opinions was not limited to old friends and residents from the same area; even in a family, different members had different opinions, creating difficulties for their mutual understanding.
- Many elderly residents were forced to live separately from their children and grandchildren because the highest priority after the earthquake was to immediately evacuate young children to safer municipalities. The more the number of households of only the elderly increased, the more the city received complaints of loneliness from such elderly persons. Some elderly residents living apart from their family members complained, "No matter how tasty are the vegetables and other farm crops I grow, I cannot let my grandchildren eat them and see their happy face anymore. I completely lost my purpose in life."

b. Responses (actual measures)
(Immediately after the earthquake, at evacuation centers for both residents and evacuees from other municipalities)

- The city asked listening volunteers and event volunteers to visit evacuation centers to offer mental health support programs/services to evacuees.
- For evacuees who were in need of special counseling services, the city asked the staff members of the Fukushima Center for Disaster Mental Health and local psychiatrists to visit evacuation centers to offer necessary services for them.

(Residents immediately after to two years after the earthquake)

- The city issued its newsletter named "Prompt Report on the Off the Pacific Coast of Tohoku Earthquake" (from the 1st to the 23rd issues), in an effort to announce radiation and necessary living information to the residents.
- One month after the earthquake, the Health Promotion Division and the Longevity and Welfare Division resumed regular duties, striving to respond to the residents' urgent needs and concerns about radiation through home visits, health counseling services at each administrative ward, educational services, and medical examinations.
- With the aim of helping to reduce residents' anxiety about radiation, the city held a seminar on "radiation and health management."

c. Summary/measures in the future

- It can be said that a community's resilience to a disaster depends on the daily efforts to foster region-wide collaboration among various organizations and institutions. In light of this, daily health-care activities based on regional collaboration will not only accelerate regional development but also be indispensable to maintain disaster preparedness in each individual local community.
- Because Fukushima City accepted a large number of evacuees from other affected municipalities immediately after the earthquake, most public health nurses of the city had to be involved in emergency response activities at evacuation centers set up for area-wide evacuees. Inevitably, the city faced a lack of manpower to provide home visits and other personal public health services to residents. This was a totally different situation from the Great Hanshin-Awaji Earthquake and the Niigata Prefecture Chuetsu Earthquake. After these earthquakes, local public health nurses were able to focus on emergency response activities and attentive personal health-care support for local resident victims. It was also regrettable that only a few public health nurses from other municipalities came to Fukushima to assist local officials, for fear of exposure to radiation. As a lesson learned from the disaster, it is required for Fukushima City to estimate how many people will be forced to evacuate to other municipalities if a serious nuclear accident occurs again, and run a simulation of the worst scenario based on the estimation. Then, if Fukushima City is expected to serve as a host municipality in case of a nuclear disaster, the city should develop a local emergency response plan as a host municipality.
- The primary role of municipalities as an administrative body is to offer personal administrative services to each individual resident. To ensure that municipalities can fulfill this role even in times of disasters, it is important to take necessary measures to protect prefectural/city/town office buildings and other local tangible assets from disasters. As part of such disaster preparedness efforts, for example, Fukushima City had rebuilt the city office into an earthquake-proof building and started administrative operations at a new office on January 1, 2011. Because the earthquake-proof city office was not damaged by the earthquake, the city was able to continue to offer regular administrative services to residents even after the earthquake.
- A growing anxiety about radiation among residents is attributable to the fact that radiation is invisible and residents have almost no knowledge of its effects on human health. Residents' distrust of the administration has also been a factor that has increased concerns about exposure to radiation. After the nuclear power station accident, the national government has reviewed guidelines on the issuance of evacuation orders and the acceptable level of radioactive materials contained in food. To obtain the understanding and trust from residents (the general public), the guideline review process should be transparent. A top-down decision making process may create further distrust among residents.
- The city conducted a survey on the health conditions and lifestyle of residents after the earthquake. According to the survey results, residents' lifestyle drastically changed due to a growing fear of possible exposure to radiation. Although health improvement/promotion programs to minimize radiation effects

Chapter 3 | Situation of and Countermeasures by Each Individual Municipality

on human health are essential, the city believes that a clear distinction be made between "health effects of exposure to radiation" and "health effects of unregulated rhythms of daily lives (such as obesity caused by a lack of exercise and a worsening of lifestyle-related diseases)" in offering health promotion programs to residents. Otherwise, as can be seen from the city's experience, residents could think that "The city makes light of the health effects of exposure to radiation" and "The intention of the city is to shift our attention from the nuclear accident to a lack of exercise among us," leading to a growing distrust of the administrative efforts. In light of this, Fukushima City will intensify educational programs on how to reduce radiation exposure in daily life, while at the same time focusing on general health improvement initiatives based on its health promotion plans for residents.

- To help residents feel at ease without being worried about exposure to radiation, the city is required to repeatedly provide educational programs and counseling services that residents can voluntarily participate in. Easy-to-understand publicity service announcements and the establishment of a system enabling officials to promptly respond to the needs and problems of residents are also essential. Of course, the city had made strenuous efforts to provide attentive administrative services to residents. However, the situation has been completely changed after the earthquake and the nuclear accident, calling for a full-scale review of the services. "What are the resident-oriented health educational programs, publicity activities, and counseling services that can be accepted by residents and that will motivate them to pursue a more healthy lifestyle on their own?" is a new task under consideration by the city.

B: Expectant/nursing mothers and children

1 Nutrition (meals/water)

a. Situation
(Immediately after the earthquake, at evacuation centers for both residents and evacuees from other municipalities)

- At gymnasiums and other evacuation centers, a combination of "rice balls and Japanese tea" or "pastries and juice" constituted the majority of three meals at the time. Later, *bento*-style meals were distributed only once a day. In some areas, volunteer residents cooked *miso* soup with vegetables and other emergency foods for evacuees.
- Because most evacuees took shelter with the barest necessities, artificial milk (milk powder) and baby foods were in short supply at evacuation centers. It was difficult to secure these commodities within the city until emergency relief supplied reached the city.

(Residents immediately after the earthquake)

- Fresh food, milk powder, disposable diapers, gasoline, and other daily commodities were in short supply for almost one month after the earthquake.
- Most residents who took shelter at evacuation centers were able to return home within two to three days. However, because of a cutoff of the water supply that lasted for a maximum of almost two weeks, residents had to walk or bicycle to an emergency water station every day and line up to receive water. There were many residents who brought their young children with them to form a line in front of the emergency water station.

(One to two years after the earthquake)

- There was a growing anxiety among residents about contamination of food and water by radiation.
- Being worried about using tap water to prepare artificial milk and baby foods, many parents purchased

bottled water for young babies.

- Due to concerns about possible contamination by radiation, many parents increasingly reframed from using farm products produced in Fukushima Prefecture and Fukushima City to cook baby foods. There were some residents who decreased their intake of vegetables, irrespective of the origin of the vegetables.

(Two years after the earthquake)

- Parents increasingly used tap water and purchased vegetables grown in Fukushima Prefecture for young children's meals.

b. Responses (actual measures)

(Immediately after the earthquake, at evacuation centers for both residents and evacuees from other municipalities)

- The city distributed milk powder, baby foods and bottled water that were sent to the city as emergency relief supplies.

(Residents immediately after the earthquake)

- The city officials answered inquiries from households with young children about the safety of food and water as well as about the supply of milk powder, baby foods and disposable diapers.
- The city independently conducted water quality inspections. Although radioactive materials were not detected in tap water, the city instructed each branch office to prepare bottled water stocks so that households with young children could secure water in case radioactive materials are detected by the inspection.

(One month after to two years after the earthquake)

- After the resumption of regular duties, the Health Promotion Division strived to respond to the residents' concerns about possible exposure to radiation from food through home visits, child-rearing counseling services at each administrative ward, and medical examinations for young children.
- One year after the earthquake, the city established a total of 28 radiation measurement centers for food products that are brought in by residents.
- Information on radiation was disseminated to residents in the city's public relations magazine.
- Lecture meetings on "young children's health and radiation" were held in each administrative ward, in which pediatricians explained about the characteristics of radioactive materials contained in water and food as well as their possible effects on the health of young children.
- In collaboration with doctors and nationally certified senior nutritionists, health seminars on "babies' health and radiation" were conducted for expectant mothers and their family members. At the seminars, the nutritionists emphasized how the health of babies would be adversely affected if expectant mothers continue to take nutritionally-unbalanced diets for fear of radioactive materials contained in water and food products.
- To raise residents' awareness of the relationship between radiation and human health, the city prepared pamphlets titled "Radiation and Our Health" and "Let's Increase Physical Strength to Avoid Health Damages by Radiation!" and distributed them to residents.
- To conduct internal exposure dose measurements, the city procured a Whole Body Counter. The actual measurement was entrusted to an inspection agency.

c. Summary/measures in the future

- Each municipality is advised to include disposable diapers, milk powder and baby foods into stockpiles for emergencies. However, it is also advisable to pay attention to expiration dates of milk powder and baby foods that store safely for relatively shorter times than other emergency food supplies.

Chapter 3 | Situation of and Countermeasures by Each Individual Municipality

- If a nuclear disaster occurs, radioactive materials could be released into the natural environment, causing radioactive contamination of water and farm products. The city is urgently required to establish an effective quality inspection system that enables early detection of radioactive materials contained in water and food, thereby helping to reduce residents' anxiety about radiation.
- When a relatively high air radiation level is observed due to atmospheric dispersion of radioactive plumes, residents should tightly close windows and stay indoors. Ventilation of a room should be avoided. Because the period of high radiation levels in the air may extend to several days or longer, the city has to ensure that residents, particularly households with young children, store several days' or one week's worth of daily necessities such as bottled water, milk powder, baby foods and disposable diapers.
- An effective measure to reduce the intake of radioactive iodine (^{131}I) is to saturate the thyroid with enough non-radioactive iodine in advance. Because there are many kinds of iodine-rich food, the city must ensure that residents are fully aware of how important it is to increase a dietary intake of iodine by having nutritionally well-balanced diets every day.

2 Exercise (Environmental improvement)

a. Situation

(Immediately after the earthquake)

- Being worried about exposure to radiation, residents stayed indoors almost all day long. When going outside, many residents wore masks and long-sleeved clothes even in high temperatures.
- The city received a request for information on indoor playing spaces for young children such as learning facilities and children's halls.

(One to two years after the earthquake)

- Decontamination work at elementary schools, junior high schools, kindergartens, and nursery schools was completed by the end of summer vacation in 2011.
- Even after the completion of decontamination work in parks and public facilities, there was a divergence of opinion among residents and facility managers over when to allow young children to engage in outdoor physical activities.
- At elementary schools, junior high schools, kindergartens, and nursery schools, children/students were allowed to engage in outdoor activities for a restricted amount of time in 2011, at the facility manager's discretion. In 2012, city-owned nursery schools and the board of education removed the time restriction of outdoor physical activities at school grounds.
- It was often the case that when parents and children were playing in a decontaminated park, neighboring residents admonished the parents "Why do you allow your children play outdoors? Don't you think children should stay indoors?" Because different persons had different opinions on outdoor activities, many parents were confused as what to trust.

(Two years after the earthquake)

- The city set up an outdoor playing area in the Moniwa district, where a relatively low dose was observed. More indoor playing spaces were also established, totaling two facilities owned by the city and four facilities managed by the private sector. All these indoor and outdoor playing spaces gained great popularity with young children and their parents.
- Swimming classes were resumed at all elementary schools and junior high schools, except schools of which pools were inaccessible.
- An increasing number of young children were able to enjoy playing outdoors.

b. Responses (actual measures)

(One month after to two years after the earthquake)

- After the resumption of regular duties, the Health Promotion Division strived to help reduce parents' anxiety about their children's possible exposure to radiation from outdoor activities, through home visits, child-rearing counseling services in each administrative ward, and medical examinations for young children.

- At the lecture meetings on "young children's health and radiation—outdoor playing," pediatricians emphasized the significance of outdoor physical activities for the healthy development of young children.

- The city conducted health seminars for parents and young children, with the aim of supporting the health improvement of young children. To be specific, the participating young children were encouraged to "keep a regular rhythm of daily life" and "actively conduct physical activity."

- At the time of home visits and medical examinations for young children, the city officials provided information on facilities and places where young children can enjoy outdoor playing.

- In collaboration with doctors and nationally certified senior nutritionists, health seminars on "babies' health and radiation" were conducted for expectant mothers and their family members. At the seminars, effective ways to reduce an external exposure dose during outdoors playing were explained to participants.

- The city set up an outdoor playing area in the Moniwa district, where a relatively low dose was observed.

- The city also increased the number of indoor playing spaces and managed them.

  c. Summary/measures in the future

- When a relatively high air radiation level is observed due to atmospheric dispersion of radioactive plumes, residents should tightly close windows and stay indoors. Although the city has to ensure that residents are well aware of what they should do when the radiation level in the air is high, it is also a responsibility of the city to provide information on conditions, in terms of radiation levels in the air, when residents will be allowed to go outside.

- The city is required to conduct health-related educational programs so that residents can fully recognize the importance of physical activity for the healthy development of young children.

- From the perspective of parents, it is desirable if the city to make a comprehensive list of both indoor and outdoor playing spaces.

3   Rest (mind, anxiety, suicide, etc.)

a. Situation

(Immediately after the earthquake, at evacuation centers for both residents and evacuees from other municipalities)

- Evacuees increasingly felt anxious because there was no prospect of returning to the normal pace of life in their hometown. Increased anxiety made them irritable, causing troubles among evacuees at evacuation centers.

(Residents immediately after to one year after the earthquake)

- There was a growing anxiety among residents about exposure to radiation.

- Many residents regretted having taken their young children to line up for a long time in front of an outdoor emergency water station immediately after the earthquake.

- In April, an increasing number of mothers and young children began evacuating to municipalities outside Fukushima Prefecture. In most cases, fathers stayed within the prefecture for employment reasons.

- Of course, there were many mothers who wished to evacuate the city with children but were unable to do so for various reasons. The city officials increasingly received complaints from such mothers about

Chapter 3 Situation of and Countermeasures by Each Individual Municipality

unsatisfactory services, arising from anxiety about their children's exposure to radiation.
- A sharp divergence of opinion on radiation gradually became obvious among residents. Growing disagreement with friends and even family members made it difficult for residents to maintain favorable human relationships with others and to communicate with each other. As a result, cases in which residents were homebound or kept to their own rooms increased.

(One to two years after the earthquake)
- There was a difference in level of concern about children's exposure to radiation between parents who took shelter in other municipalities and those who remained within the city. Although parents staying within the city gradually began feeling at ease, parents taking shelter in host municipalities were still fearful of radiation, remaining almost as afraid as they were immediately after the earthquake. Such fears and anxiety might be attributed to the city's insufficient provision of necessary information.
- Two years after the earthquake, parents and children taking shelter in other municipalities gradually began returning to Fukushima City. However, not all such evacuees were willing to return to the city. There were some who had no other alternative but to reluctantly return for various reasons.

b. Responses (actual measures)
(Immediately after the earthquake, at evacuation centers for both residents and evacuees from other municipalities)
- The city asked midwives to go around to evacuation centers, where expectant mothers were accommodated, to offer mental health consultations for them.
- As needed, the city asked Fukushima Prefecture to dispatch a school counselor to offer mental health care support to students.
- Residents who were supposed to need special mental health care were referred to the Fukushima Center for Disaster Mental Health.

(Residents one to two years after the earthquake)
- A lot of lecture meetings and study sessions on radiation were held, for the purpose of helping to reduce residents' anxiety about exposure to radiation.
- In cooperation with pediatricians, lecture meetings on "young children's health and radiation" were held in each administrative ward.
- Health seminars on "babies' health and radiation" were conducted for expectant mothers.
- Friendly meetings for nursing mothers were conducted. The purpose of the meetings was to provide nursing mothers an opportunity to share information and communicate with each other, thereby reducing their anxiety and fear about radiation. The city assigned a psychologist as a facilitator of the meetings.
- At the time of medical examinations for young children, the city provided personal consultation services by a psychologist to mothers and young children as needed.
- Stretching exercise classes for fathers, mothers, and young children were provided, with the aim of helping parents feel mentally and physically relaxed.

c. Summary/measures in the future
- Fukushima City is located more than 70-km from the Fukushima Daiichi Nuclear Power Station of the Tokyo Electric Power Company. Due to the distance from the power station, residents in the city had almost no knowledge of radiation, causing confusion among residents after the accident. To avoid unnecessary confusion in times of disasters, the city is urgently required to offer various educational programs, thereby ensuring that both the officials and residents are well educated about radiation.
- After the nuclear power accident, the System for Prediction of Environmental Emergency Dose Infor-

mation (SPEEDI) did not work properly and vital information on radiation and emergency instructions were not disseminated to the city. Not knowing the risk of exposure to radiation, many pregnant women and mothers carrying babies on their backs formed a line outdoors to obtain water at an emergency water station during a period of high air levels of radiation. These expectant mothers and parents have remained worried about their children's possible exposure to radiation. As can be seen from this example, information dissemination through SPEEDI is indispensable in times of disaster.
- It is difficult for young children and expectant mothers to stay for a long period of time under inconvenient living conditions at a gymnasium and other evacuation centers. For such evacuees, it is necessary to partition off space or secure evacuation centers with private rooms/spaces.
- Against a backdrop of a rapidly changing child-rearing environment, Fukushima City had focused on support programs for nursing mothers as one of its urgent tasks. After the nuclear power station accident, however, "to reduce anxiety about children's exposure to radiation" was also added to the list of the city's child-rearing support initiatives. To attentively support nursing mothers, dissemination of information on child-rearing alone is insufficient; case-by-case assistance based on the sense of value and a family background of each individual mother is also indispensable. Particularly, post-disaster mental health care programs for mothers are one of the high priority tasks for the city. Although the severity and details of mothers' fear of radiation have gradually changed over the course of time, most mothers are still suffering from mental turmoil caused by the disaster. The city needs to have a long-term vision in taking measures to support their mental health needs.

People requiring assistance during a disaster (vulnerable people in case of a disaster)

1 Nutrition (meals/water)

a. Situation
(Immediately after the earthquake, at evacuation centers for both residents and evacuees from other municipalities)
- At gymnasiums and other evacuation centers, a combination of "rice balls and Japanese tea" or "pastries and juice" constituted the majority of three meals at first. Later, *bento*-style meals were distributed only once a day. In some areas, volunteer residents cooked *miso* soup with vegetables and other emergency foods for evacuees.
- Some residents tried to drink as little water as possible because they wanted to reduce the frequency of going to the toilet at evacuation centers. The development of economy-class syndrome among such residents was a great concern of the city.
- For residents who have chronic health problems and need therapeutic/restricted diets, it was almost impossible to accommodate their special dietary needs at evacuation centers.

(Residents immediately after the earthquake)
- Immediately after the earthquake, some persons requiring assistance took shelter in evacuation centers due to the cutoff of the water/electricity supply and a fear of aftershocks, while others stayed in their homes. After electricity came back on, most people requiring assistance returned home.
- Fresh food, gasoline and other daily commodities were in short supply for almost one month after the earthquake.
- Residents who took shelter in evacuation centers due to power failures were able to return home within two to three days. However, because of a cutoff of the water supply for as long as two weeks, residents had to walk or ride a bicycle to an emergency water station every day and line up to receive water.

Chapter 3 | Situation of and Countermeasures by Each Individual Municipality

Because it was difficult for persons requiring assistance and elderly residents to travel to the water stations and wait in line every day, their neighbors and other volunteer members strived to secure water for them.

- Some residents tried to drink as little water as possible because they wanted to reduce the frequency of going to the toilet during the cutoff of the water supply.

(One to two years after the earthquake)
- There was a growing anxiety among residents about contamination of food and water by radiation.
- Due to concerns about possible contamination by radiation, residents increasingly began to reframe from purchasing farm products produced in Fukushima Prefecture and Fukushima City. There were some residents who had a decreased intake of vegetables, irrespective of their origins.

b. Responses (actual measures)
(At evacuation centers immediately after the earthquake)
- The city strived to respond to the case-by-case needs of persons requiring assistance. For persons in need of some special support services, the city officials asked nearby medical institutions to visit evacuation centers to examine them, or referred them to nursing-care facilities.
- To prevent residents from getting dehydrated, the city officials encouraged them to make sure to take plenty of water.
- For residents needing therapeutic diets, the city provided relevant information to them and distributed therapeutic diets sent from the public health office of Fukushima Prefecture.

(Residents)
- The city called for help from neighborhood association members, commissioned welfare volunteers, and other volunteer staff members to take care of persons requiring assistance with their daily diets and all other aspects of daily living.
- The city has made strenuous efforts to establish an effective radiation inspection system for water and food. For example, the city embarked on water quality inspection immediately after the earthquake and incorporated a radiation screening system into the distribution process of farm products. In addition to these efforts, the city also set up a radiation measurement center for home-grown vegetables and farm products. Moreover, one year after the earthquake, the city established a total of 28 radiation measurement centers for any food products that are brought in by residents.
- Through its newsletters and the website, the city announced the radiation inspection results for food and water and disseminated other relevant information to residents.
- The city assigned dedicated personnel to offer consultation services for residents who were filled with concerns about radiation.
- Lecture meetings on health and radiation were held in each administrative ward, in which doctors explained in detail about the characteristics of radioactive materials contained in water and food as well as their possible effects on human health.

2 Exercise (Environmental improvement)

a. Situation
(At evacuation centers immediately after the earthquake)
- Because evacuation centers were densely crowded with evacuees, the city had concerns about a decrease in the activities of daily livings (ADLs) and the development of pulmonary deep vein thrombosis/thromboembolism (economy-class syndrome) among evacuees.

(Immediately after to two years after the earthquake)

- For fear of being exposed to radiation, many residents reframed from going outdoors, leading to a decrease in the amount of exercise they were getting and in their physical function.
- After the earthquake, elderly residents who had lived alone increasingly moved to their children's houses due to fear of aftershocks, resulting in a structural change in local communities. Inevitably, elderly residents remaining in their houses lost opportunities to go outside to communicate with neighbors, causing a decrease in their physical activity.
- Public facilities such as learning centers and sports/exercise facilities became inaccessible because they were damaged by the earthquake or used as evacuation centers. Due to the inaccessibility to these facilities, elderly residents and residents with disabilities experienced a decrease in their physical activity.
- Because some welfare facilities were also used as evacuation centers for evacuees from other municipalities, elderly residents and residents with disabilities were forced to receive only a limited frequency/duration of day-care services and short-term stay services. As a result of their decreased physical activity, the number of certified nursing-care recipients increased.

b. Responses (actual measures)

(Immediately after the earthquake, at evacuation centers for both residents and evacuees from other municipalities)

- For evacuees who were at risk of developing economy-class syndrome, all staff members at evacuation centers strived to share information on such evacuees and pay close attention to their health conditions, encouraging them to drink plenty of water and actively take exercise.
- To call evacuees' attention to the necessity of actively taking exercise, the city distributed pamphlets to each individual resident and posted them at evacuation centers.

(Residents)

- The city promptly repaired learning centers and sports/exercise facilities that were damaged by the earthquake. Public facilities, which were temporarily used as evacuation centers, also resumed normal services and programs.
- Welfare facilities strived to resume regular care services as early as possible.
- Information on elderly residents who were left stranded was shared among the city officials, local commissioned welfare volunteers, and other volunteer staff members.

3 Rest (mind, anxiety, suicide, etc.)

a. Situation

(Immediately after the earthquake, at evacuation centers for both residents and evacuees from other municipalities)

- Evacuees from other municipalities, who lost family members and houses to the tsunami, shared their overwhelming grief and consoled each other at evacuation centers.
- Evacuees were filled with extreme anxiety about their future due to a lack of information on when they would be able to return home.
- An increasing number of evacuees became completely exhausted, both physically and mentally, from their unstable life as evacuees. There were some evacuees who became reluctant to communicate with others and showed no emotions to others.
- There were some cases in which residents, who had an extreme feeling of uneasy, had no other way but to take an aggressive attitude toward others. This caused troubles between residents at evacuation centers.

Chapter 3 Situation of and Countermeasures by Each Individual Municipality

(Residents immediately after the earthquake)

- After the earthquake, most elderly residents who had lived alone moved to their children's houses due to fears of aftershocks. Therefore, elderly residents, who took shelter in local evacuation centers, felt isolated and helpless after returning from the shelters because of the absence of their old friends and neighbors in local communities.
- Public facilities such as learning centers and sports/exercise facilities became inaccessible because they were damaged by the earthquake or used as evacuation centers. Due to the inaccessibility to these facilities, residents with disabilities and elderly residents lost an opportunity to communicate with each other.
- Because some welfare facilities were also used as evacuation centers for evacuees from other municipalities, elderly residents and residents with disabilities were forced to receive only a limited frequency/duration of day-care services and short-term stay services. As a result, these residents lost an opportunity to regularly communicate with others.

(One to two years after the earthquake)

- Different residents had different opinions and concerns about radiation. Therefore, it gradually became difficult for residents to easily understand and communicate with each other. Such a divergence of opinion was not limited to old friends and residents from the same area; even within a family, different members had different opinions, creating a difficulty in their mutual understanding.
- Many elderly residents were forced to live separately from their children and grandchildren because the highest priority after the earthquake was to immediately evacuate young children to safer municipalities. The more the number of households with only elderly persons increased, the more the city received complaints of loneliness from them. Some elderly residents living apart from their family members complained, "No matter how tasty are the vegetables and other farm crops I grow, I cannot let my grandchildren eat them and see their happy face anymore. I completely lost my purpose in life."
- On the other hand, there were elderly residents who had at first evacuated to other municipalities with their grandchildren but eventually returned to their own homes to live separately from family members. Such elderly residents commented, "Even if I live with my children and grandchildren, I cannot feel at ease in an unfamiliar living environment."

b. Responses (actual measures)

(Immediately after the earthquake)

- The city officials went around to evacuation centers to respond to needs of residents and evacuees from other municipalities.

(One to two years after the earthquake)

- The city asked a regional comprehensive support center and livelihood support center to focus on counseling and consultation services for residents.

4 Summary/measures in the future

- As part of the city's disaster preparedness efforts, it is necessary to make a list of residents requiring assistance in times of disaster so that they can receive prompt and special emergency relief support during a disaster. It is also essential for the city to include in its disaster mitigation plan special response activities for residents requiring assistance and to ensure that all relevant parties fully understand the plan and know what to do in an emergency situation.
- With a prolonged period living as evacuees in an inconvenient environment at a gymnasium or other evacuation centers, persons requiring special assistance may face a worsening of their health condition.

To avoid such a scenario, the city has worked hard to establish an effective system to promptly offer special emergency assistance to vulnerable people in times of disaster. As part of such efforts, the city built a welfare shelter in March 2012.

- For national nursing-care service recipients, welfare officials are advised to decide in advance who will confirm the safety and living situation of each individual recipient, thereby avoiding overlaps in the safety confirmation process in an emergency situation.
- Municipalities with a wide land area, like Fukushima City, are advised to make sure to secure gasoline in times of disaster so that emergency relief activities can be promptly conducted.
- It can be said that community's resilience to a disaster depends on the daily efforts for region-wide collaborative relationships among various organizations and institutions of the public health, welfare, and medical fields. No matter how good is the disaster preparedness manual that the city develops, its resilience to a disaster will not be realized without such region-wide cooperative daily efforts.
- Local organizations (such as neighborhood associations), patient advisory groups, and associations of families with mentally disabled members played an important role in local-level emergency assistance activities during the disaster. To conduct effective emergency response activities in times of disaster, the city should build a close relationship with these organizations.
- Because Fukushima City accepted a large number of evacuees from other affected municipalities immediately after the earthquake, most public health nurses of the city had to be involved in emergency response activities at evacuation centers set up for area-wide evacuees. Inevitably, the city faced a lack of manpower to understand and accommodate the urgent needs of local young children, expectant mothers, persons requiring assistance during a disaster, and other residents. As a lesson learned from the disaster, it is required for Fukushima City to estimate how many people will be forced to evacuate to other municipalities if a serious nuclear accident occurs again, and run a simulation of the worst case scenario based on the estimation. Then, if Fukushima City is expected to serve as a host municipality in case of a nuclear disaster, the city should develop a local emergency response plan as a host municipality.

D Others

(Immediately after to one year after the earthquake)
- Emergency night clinics resumed regular consultations as early as on the day of the earthquake.
- The city established a contact section of comprehensive livelihood consultations (including health-related counseling) and assigned dedicated officials.
- The city officials answered inquiries about the short supply of daily commodities such as disposable diapers, milk powder, disinfectants, emergency medical supplies, and medical care items. Upon reaching the city, emergency relief supplies were distributed to residents.
- The city officials responded to inquiries from residents about radiation, while at the same time disseminating information on radiation exposure screening tests to the public.
- After the earthquake, the city established many evacuation centers within the city. Until the end of April 2011, the city officials visited a maximum of 61 evacuation centers per day. At each evacuation center, the officials strived to confirm the safety and health conditions of all evacuees, respond to the needs of persons requiring assistance, and encourage evacuees to maintain good hygiene in evacuation centers.
- Giving priority to medical institutions for receiving water, the city strived to secure water to be used for artificial dialysis and other medical treatment.
- Emergency response activities that the city conducted at evacuation centers for about three months were as follows:
  - There was an evacuation center where all inpatients from a mental hospital were transferred. Although

Chapter 3 — Situation of and Countermeasures by Each Individual Municipality

the city officials partitioned off the space at the evacuation center, it was almost impossible to accommodate both the evacuees with mental diseases and other evacuees within the evacuation center. Therefore, the city asked Fukushima Prefecture to refer the inpatient evacuees to a dedicated shelter within the prefecture.

- For persons requiring assistance, the city officials asked nearby medical institutions to visit evacuation centers to examine them. As needed, some persons requiring assistance were referred to nearby nursing-care facilities.
- Medical staff went to evacuation centers to examine persons requiring assistance. Because the staff made a medical/nursing-care record of each individual person in need of assistance at the time of the first examination, it was possible for all relevant staff members and the city officials to share the records to provide continued assistance to such persons.
- For persons needing therapeutic diets, the city distributed therapeutic diets sent from the public health office of Fukushima Prefecture. The city also provided information on medical care items to them.
- There were some bedridden elderly residents and persons requiring assistance who were forced to stay for a longer period of time at gymnasiums that served as evacuation centers. The city secured electric beds for such evacuees.
- The city provided information on medical institutions and pharmacy stores located near evacuation centers.
- The city officials answered inquiries about the short supply of daily commodities such as disposable diapers, milk powder, disinfectants, emergency medical supplies, and medical care items.
- The city provided information to evacuees on how to undergo radiation exposure screening tests.
- The city obtained cooperation from staff members of local medical institutions, schools of nursing, and other volunteer members to accommodate the needs of evacuees at each evacuation center.
- In collaboration with the Fukushima City Medical Association and the Japan Medical Association Team (JMAT), the city officials went around to evacuation centers to examine each individual evacuee.

(Four months to two years after the earthquake)
- The city established a health management committee consisting of five doctors.
- To measure an external exposure dose, personal dosimeters (glass badges) were distributed to residents.
- Internal exposure dose measurement was conducted, using a Whole Body Counter.
- The city provided information on its food inspection system, encouraging residents to utilize the system to reduce their personal dose to as low as possible.
- The city conducted health seminars for parents and young children, with the aim of supporting the health improvement of young children. To be specific, the participating young children were encouraged to "keep a regular rhythm of daily life" and "actively conduct physical activity."
- To raise residents' awareness of the relationship between radiation and human health, the city prepared pamphlets titled "Radiation and Our Health" and "Let's Increase Physical Strength to Avoid Health Damages by Radiation!" and distributed them to residents.

(Two years after the earthquake)
- As part of regional disaster preparedness efforts after the earthquake, the city has focused on the review/improvement of a regional disaster prevention plan, the preparation of the city's original "manual for regional support for persons requiring assistance in times of disaster," and the establishment of welfare evacuation centers and their management manual. As a result, a welfare evacuation center was built in March 2012. A conventional "disaster prevention guide for households" was also reviewed. Newly prepared guides were distributed to each household in April 2013.
- Living conditions of residents drastically changed after the earthquake. Therefore, based on the newly

developed "Fukushima City Health Promotion Plan," the city has been accelerating efforts to prevent the development and worsening of lifestyle-related diseases among residents.

(Junko Okubo)

28 Efforts of Nihonmatsu City

1 Situation of the municipality

(1) Demographics (as of January 1 of each year)

	2011	2012	2013
Population	61,192	59,901	58,810
Number of households	19,255	19,092	19,114
Average number of people per household	3.18	3.14	3.07
Number of births	418	382	
Birth rate	6.8	6.4	
Number of deaths	839	751	
Mortality	13.7	12.5	
Ratio of the elderly aged 65 or older	25.9	26.0	26.9

* The number shown in the "Population" column is the total of residents recorded in the city's basic register and includes foreign residents.

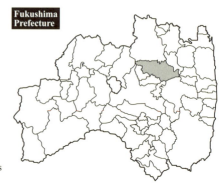

Fukushima Prefecture

(2) Geographical features
Total area: 344.65 km^2 (approximately 35 km east-west; approximately 17 km north-south)
Distance from the Fukushima Daiichi Nuclear Power Station of the Tokyo Electric Power Company: approximately 35–70 km
Evacuation area: None. But Namie Town and Kawamata Town, adjacent to the city, have a designated evacuation area.
Transportation network: One I.C of the Tohoku Expressway; three stations of the JR Tohoku Line; National Route 4

2 Situation of damage by the earthquake, tsunami and the nuclear disaster

(1) Damage by the Great East Japan Earthquake (as of March 31, 2013)

Property damage	Completely destroyed	Half destroyed	Partially destroyed
House	11	475	5,399
Public institution	0	0	93
Other	0	0	140

Human damage	Deaths by disaster	Disaster-related deaths	Missing persons	Injured persons
	0	0	0	0

* The number shown in the "Injured persons" column indicates severely injured persons. On March 11, 2011, the day of the occurrence of the earthquake, the city's head office building experienced a power failure. Because the Adachi Public Health and Welfare Center, where the Health Promotion Section was located, did not have any property damage and did not lose a water and power supply, the office building served as an evacuation center for the city residents and evacuees from neighboring municipalities affected by the tsunami and the nuclear power station accident.

(2) Situation of evacuation
① Evacuation centers within the municipality (The number of centers was the largest on March 16, 2011.)

	Number of evacuation centers	Number of evacuees	Available period
Residents of Nihonmatsu City + evacuees from other municipalities	17	902	March 12 to July 28
Evacuees from Namie Town	14	3,026	March 15 to September 1

* The city officials began visiting evacuation centers on March 12 (Sun.), the day after the earthquake.
On March 15 (Tue.), the city received evacuees from neighboring Namie Town and set up evacuation centers with an accommodation capacity of a total of 8,000 persons.

② Approximate number of evacuees in evacuation centers outside the municipality (as of April 1, 2013)

	End/March 2011	End/September 2011	End/March 2012	Latest period
First evacuation center	0	0	0	0
Second evacuation center	0	0	0	0
Temporary housing	0	0	0	0
Municipally-subsidized housing	0	0	0	0

28 Efforts of Nihonmatsu City

③ Approximate number of voluntary evacuees (as of September 1, 2012)

Inside Fukushima Prefecture	100	Outside Fukushima Prefecture (number of evacuees & prefectures)	665 persons in 33 prefectures

* Most residents who have been voluntarily taking shelter within Fukushima Prefecture are not registered in the evacuee management system of the city.

Outlook of damage related to the nuclear disaster

① With almost no people injured, Nihonmatsu City was not severely damaged by the earthquake. However, because the distribution of gasoline and food was stopped due to the release of radioactive materials, it was difficult for the city officials to commute to the office by car and visit evacuation centers using public vehicles.

② Without the experience of nuclear disaster drills, the city had no option but to follow a manual for radiation emergency medical responses provided from Fukushima Prefecture. Moreover, radiation-related information announced by the national government was the only available source of information for the city after the earthquake. Under these circumstances, it was announced that air radiation levels observed in some districts within the city were higher than those in areas within a 30-km distance from the Fukushima Daiichi Nuclear Power Station, where an evacuation order was issued. This announcement inevitably caused Nihonmatsu city residents to feel a growing fear of exposure to radiation. As of the end of 2012, residents were still worried about exposure to radiation.

③ Although having had no radiation specialist personnel, the city independently embarked on the measurement of air radiation levels in March 18, 2011.

④ During the first month after the earthquake, the city officials were busily occupied with the response to the needs of evacuees from Namie Town and other municipalities located in the severely damaged Hama-dori district. Therefore, the officials could not afford to address the local residents' various problems arising from the nuclear disaster.

⑤ Although a relatively high air radiation level was observed in some districts in Nihonmatsu City, an evacuation order was not issued to the city. Therefore, no emergency relief staff members were dispatched to the city from Fukushima Prefecture or from the national government. With no additional support, the administrative workload of the city officials almost doubled due to administrative procedures for local residents who voluntarily took shelter in other municipalities (such as a request to host municipalities for home-visiting services for babies and medical examinations for expectant mothers, young children and adults) as well as measures against radiation. As of the end of 2012, officials were still forced to manage an increased work load.

3 Countermeasures against nuclear disaster (as of January 2013)

		Name of project	Division in charge	Number of targeted persons (house-holds)	Expect-ant mothers	Nursing moth-ers	Babies	Young children	Elemen-tary school students	Junior high school students	Senior high school students	People age 19 to 39	People age 40 or older	Remarks (major operations)
Countermeasures against external exposure	1	Personal dose measurements (using glass badges)	Health Promotion Division	16,000	○	○	○	○	○	○	○	At their request	---	Distribution & collection, notification & analysis of measurement results, arrangement, and contracts
	2	Refreshments for pregnant women (relaxation in low-dose areas)	Health Promotion Division	400	○									Development of programs outline, meeting with suppliers, contracts, notification, and bill payment
	3	Refreshment for young children	Child-rearing Support Division	500			○	○						Planning, contracts, notification, acceptance of participating young children, and guiding support
	4	Refreshments for elementary school and junior high school students	School and Education Division	(500 students per school grade) × (9 school grades)					○	○				Planning, arrangement with school, contracts, notification, acceptance of participating students, and guiding support
	5	Monitoring and measurement of the air radiation levels (until April 2012)	Radiation Measurement and Decontamination Division	Measurement at 21 monitoring spots twice a day	○	○	○	○	○	○	○	○	○	Procurement of equipment, measurement, recording, and announcements of measurement results
		Real-time measurement of the radiation dose (Ministry of the Environment)		118 monitoring spots	○	○	○	○	○	○	○	○	○	Started in May 2012 by the Ministry of the Environment
	6	Measurement and mapping of the air radiation levels in the whole city			○	○	○	○	○	○	○	○	○	Arrangement, contracts, measurement, analysis & collection of measurement results, and the creation & distribution of maps

285

Countermeasures against internal exposure

No.	Item	Division	Target										Notes
7	Replacement of the surface soil on the grounds in childcare facilities, child education facilities and schools	Educational General Affairs Division				○	○	○	○				Arrangement and contracts
8	Decontamination of houses	Radiation Measurement and Decontamination Division	All households	○	○	○	○	○	○	○	○	○	Planning, contracts, collection & report of decontamination results, and arrangement of waste treatment
9	Decontamination of public and medical institutions	Facility Management Division		○	○	○	○	○	○	○	○	○	Planning, contracts, collection & report of decontamination results, and arrangement of waste treatment
10	Examination of breast milk	Health Promotion Division	400	---	○								Meeting with suppliers, contracts, notification, acceptance of breast milk samples, and bill payment
11	Whole Body Counter measurements (conducted by the city)	Health Promotion Division	All residents	○	○	○	○	○	○	○	○	○	Installation of equipment, calibration, schedule arrangement, request for analysis, notification of measurement results, aggregation & report of results, and clerical work
12	Whole Body Counter measurements (conducted by Fukushima Prefecture for children aged 4 to 18 years old)	Health Promotion Division	7,000	○	○		○	○	○	○			Arrangement of venues & schedules, notification of measurement results, and publicity
13	Food and water quality inspection	Radiation Measurement and Decontamination Division	All households	○	○	○	○	○	○	○	○	○	Meeting with suppliers, contracts, notification, acceptance of food and water samples, and bill payment
14	Thyroid gland examination (conducted by Fukushima Prefecture)	Health Promotion Division	Children age 18 or younger			○	○	○	○	○			Sampling of examinees, arrangement and announcements of venues & schedules
15	Inspection of school meals (Radiation dose in foodstuffs is measured at each school facility.)	Educational General Affairs Division	Public nursery schools, kindergartens, primary schools, and junior high schools			○	○	○	○				Consideration of measurement devices, contracts, carrying-in of devices, training, and announcements of measurement results to parents/guardians
16	Debriefing sessions for measurement results of exposure dose	Health Promotion Division	All households	○	○	○	○	○	○	○	○	○	Aggregation & analysis of measurement results, preparation of materials, publicity, announcements, and preparation of Q & A for debrief sessions
17	Study sessions on radiation (for young children and their parents/guardians)	Health Promotion Division	Parents/guardians			○	○	○	○				Planning, arrangement of lecturers & venues, publicity, and management
18	Medical examinations and cancer screening (for residents age 19 to 39*)	Health Promotion Division	Residents age 19 to 39								○		Sampling of examinees, arrangement of medical examinations, contracts, notification, and aggregation of examination results
19	Quality inspection of bagged rice	Agricultural Policy Planning Division	All rice produces	○	○	○	○	○	○	○	○	○	Schedule arrangement with relevant parties, publicity, announcements, measurements, and collection of measurement results
20	Measurement and mapping of the radiation dose in the soil within the whole city	Radiation Measurement and Decontamination Division	The entire city	○	○	○	○	○	○	○	○	○	Arrangement of measurement venues, measurements, collection & analysis of measurement results, and publicity
21	Lecture meetings on radiation	Radiation Measurement and Decontamination Division	All households	○	○	○	○	○	○	○	○	○	Arrangement of lecturers & venues, publicity, and reports

28 Efforts of Nihonmatsu City

22	Sampling of respondents for a basic survey in the Fukushima Health Management Survey	Health Promotion Division	All house-holds	○	○	○	○	○	○	○	○	○	The survey is conducted by Fukushima Prefecture. Publicity is conducted by Nihonmatsu City.
23	Publication of disaster information papers twice a month (a double-sided A-4 size paper)	Secretary and Public Relations Division	All house-holds	○	○	○	○	○	○	○	○	○	Collection of articles, proofreading, printing, sorting out, and distribution
24	Issuance of citizen health cards (containing a column for recording radiation exposure levels)	Health Promotion Division	All resi-dents	○	○	○	○	○	○	○	○	○	Preparation of health cards, contracts, proofreading, distribution preparation, and publicity

* For residents age 40 or older, medical examinations and cancer screenings are conducted separately.

Chapter 3 Situation of and Countermeasures by Each Individual Municipality

A Expectant/nursing mothers and children

1 Nutrition (meals/water)

a. Situation
- Immediately after the nuclear power station accident, it was reported that there was no need for Nihonmatsu City residents to be worried about their safety and security. However, as more details about air radiation levels within the city were announced, the more the residents become anxious about exposure to radiation.
- In response to a media report that told about water contamination by radioactive substances in the Tokyo metropolitan area, there was an increasing demand for bottled water from mothers with babies in the city. However, it was difficult for the city to secure enough bottled water to distribute to all babies within the city.
- Initially, artificial milk (milk powder) was in short supply because the distribution of commodities stopped after the earthquake. Although a large amount of milk powder arrived to the residents as emergency relief supplies after the resumption of a distribution system, the city officials had to pay close attention to the expiration date of the milk powder before distributing it to residents.
- Food contamination by radioactive substances was one of the great concerns among residents. Because the city failed to explain about the food quality inspection system and provide sufficient information on the inspection results to residents, opinions on consuming local rice, vegetables and water varied by person even within a family, resulting in disorganized family diets.

b. Responses (actual measures)
- As a measure to cope with the short supply of milk powder, the city provided baby foods to babies who had been weaned from milk powder. For mothers who had fed both breast milk and milk powder to their babies, the city asked them to feed as much breast milk as possible.
- The city officials made rules as to the provision of artificial milk and other emergency relief supplies to babies and young children.
- After the distribution of commodities was resumed, the city established an independent food radiation level inspection system.
- The food inspection results were announced to the residents through disaster information magazines.
- The city independently conducted breast milk examinations.
- The city purchased devices to measure radioactive substances contained in food. The measurement started in December, 2011 at each community center within the city.

c. Summary/measures in the future
- Although the city received no severe damage from the earthquake, the distribution of daily commodities stopped due to the nuclear power station accident. As a lesson from the nuclear disaster, the city needs to ensure that each individual household maintains enough stockpiles of commodities such as milk powder, disposable diapers, bottled water, and baby foods, thereby being well prepared for any emergencies.
- As one of the future tasks for the city, emergency food for young children with allergies should be stored. How to respond to the special needs of such young children should also be considered.
- The city is required to increase the number of devices to measure radioactive substances contained in food.
- When measuring radioactive substances contained in food, as much as 1kg of a foodstuff sample is

needed to be cut into tiny pieces in advance. Despite this laborious sample preparation for measurements, no severe food contamination was detected. Therefore, residents' interest in food quality inspection began declining about one year after the earthquake. However, radioactive substances have a tendency of migration, for example, from mountains through fields, rivers to ocean, or from higher to lower elevations above the sea level. To accurately understand food contamination by radiation, it is necessary to measure respective foodstuffs seasonally in the future.

2   Exercise (Environmental improvement)

a. Situation
- Immediately after the earthquake, accurate air radiation levels were unknown, and there were young children who played outdoors.
- Air radiation levels in some parts of Nihonmatsu City were higher than those in areas where an evacuation order was issued. Due to the results of the observation, residents were increasingly worried about the risk of exposure to radiation during outdoor activities.
- Even six months after the earthquake, there were some parents who did not allow their children to play outdoors. As a result, the number of obese young children increased.
- Although decontamination work at schools was completed, it was difficult for the city to make a decision on the resumption and length of safe outdoor activities at schools. This was attributed to a divergence of opinion among parents and the daily changing observed results of air radiation levels.
- As part of refreshment programs for expectant mothers, the city encouraged them to stay in other prefectures with a relatively low radiation levels in the air for their health. However, the longer the period of their stay became, the more they felt financially and mentally stressed.

b. Responses (actual measures)
- On March 18, 2011, the city independently started the measurements of air radiation levels at 21 monitoring spots within the city. (See Figure 28-1 for details.)
- The city replaced the surface soil on the grounds of all nursery schools, kindergartens, primary schools, and junior high schools located within the city.
- The city installed air conditioners at all nursery schools, kindergartens, primary schools, and junior high schools located within the city.
- The city distributed personal dosimeters (glass badges) to residents.
- The Ministry of Education, Culture, Sports, Science and Technology began installing real-time air radiation monitoring posts at 118 public facilities within the city in August 2012.
- The city lent to residents devices that measured radioactive substances contained in food.

c. Summary/measures in the future
- As an important point to remember, when a nuclear disaster occurs, the national government and Fukushima Prefecture will be fully occupied with emergency response activities in areas designated as evacuation zones. It is highly likely that municipalities to which no evacuation order is issued cannot count on any support from the government and prefecture.
- Although the city is required to judge a critical situation and address many issues at its own discretion, the absence of judgment criteria is a serious problem for the city.
- Radioactive substances do not necessarily expand in a circular pattern from the nuclear power station. Based on the assumption that radioactive substances might be observed anywhere within the prefecture, each municipality is strongly advised to be well prepared for a nuclear disaster.
- It is required for the city to prepare survey meters (scintillation counters) and ensure that officials have

Chapter 3 Situation of and Countermeasures by Each Individual Municipality

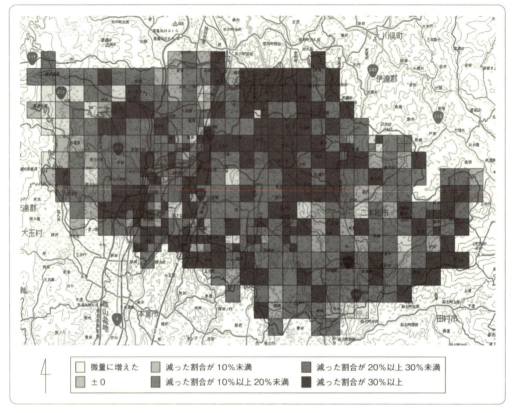

Figure 28-1 Observed changes in air radiation levels within Nihonmatsu City
Note: The figure shows a change in measurement results obtained from June 25 to July 11, 2012, compared to the baseline results from June 28 to July 1, 2011.

knowledge of how to use them to measure radioactive substances.
- Real-time air radiation monitoring posts installed by the Ministry of Education, Culture, Sports, Science and Technology are solar power-driven equipment. To accurately monitor radioactive substances, the city should install other monitoring equipment (not solar power-driven) that enables 24-hour monitoring of air radiation.

3 Rest (mind, anxiety, suicide, etc.)

a. Situation
- The more the details about the damage from the nuclear accident were brought to light, the more differing information was communicated through the media, which caused confusion among residents.
- In some cases, the city was also not sure what information/instructions to trust.
- Immediately after the nuclear accident, the mass media reported that there was no need for Nihonmatsu City residents to be worried about their safety and security. However, various controversial facts about the report were revealed, as a result of which residents became distrustful of the mass media.
- Due to differing information disseminated through the Internet and publications, residents became confused.
- Residents felt a growing anxiety about many aspects of daily living, including as to whether it is safe or

not to hang the laundry and *futon* bedclothes outdoors.

- For residents who evacuated to other prefectures, inaccessibility of necessary information announced by the city caused them to feel a growing sense of uneasiness.
- Disorganized daily diets within a family accelerated the uneasy feeling among family members.

b. Responses (actual measures)
- The city asked a radiation expert to serve as a radiological protection advisor and help the city to secure the safety and security of residents.
- The city held lecture meetings on radiation, in which an invited lecturer explained to the participants about the risks of low-dose exposure to radiation and how to avoid radioactive substances in daily lives.
- The city conducted study sessions on radiation for parents/guardians, under the themes of "basic knowledge of radiation," "daily diets," "outdoor playing" and "mental health care." (See Table 28-1 for details.)
- The city offered group work programs to residents, aiming to help participants feel at ease through friendly conversation with others.

c. Summary/measures in the future
- When a nuclear disaster occurs, an indoor evacuation will be issued and the distribution of papers, gasoline, and other daily commodities will stop. It is also highly likely that only a limited source of information will be available for the city and residents.
- The air radiation level and the situation surrounding the nuclear power station showed a rapid change every day. Nevertheless, the city was unable to announce the latest information to residents through its website and other information tools, failing to reduce a residents' growing fear of exposure to radiation.
- The city asked the radiological protection advisor to form a team with an internal exposure analyst, soil contamination analyst, and other specialists. Because radiation-related problems caused by the disaster are wide-ranging, collaboration with specialists from various fields is indispensable for a radiological protection advisor to provide effective advice to the city. The problem is that there are not many available radiation specialists in Japan.
- To help residents feel at ease, the city has to improve the networking system so that important information can be immediately updated on its website, as needed. The establishment of a prompt decision-making system is also a future task for the city.

4　Others

- Immediately after the earthquake, the city gave a priority for receiving gasoline to doctors, nurses, medical administrators, pharmacists, and the city officials (public vehicles), so that emergency response activities by the city officials and medical relief activities could be promptly conducted at evacuation centers.
- In June Nihonmatsu City became the first municipality, among municipalities not designated as an evacuation zone, to conduct a preliminary survey on exposure to radiation using a Whole Body Counter for 20 persons in municipalities other than Fukushima Prefecture.
- In May, the city asked for the cooperation of a radiological protection advisor. Because one advisor cannot provide effective advice on how to protect residents from exposure to radiation, the city asked the advisor to form a team of six radiation-related specialists.
- The city issued disaster information magazines twice a month and distributed them to each household.
- Nihonmatsu City became the first municipality, among municipalities not designated as an evacuation zone, to distribute personal dosimeters (glass badges) to residents. The city also conducted a survey on behavioral patterns of residents.

Chapter 3 Situation of and Countermeasures by Each Individual Municipality

Table 28-1 A poster for study sessions on radiation

Study sessions on radiation for parents and children

With the aim of helping residents to increase their knowledge of radiation and health management of young children, Nihonmatsu City will hold study sessions at local public health and welfare centers. At the study sessions, tips for protecting young children from exposure to radiation in daily living will be explained. Prior application should be made to participate in the study sessions.

Themes and schedules

	Nihonmatsu Public Health and Welfare Center	Adachi Public Health and Welfare Center	Iwashiro Public Health and Welfare Center	Towa Public Health and Welfare Center *Towa Cultural Center on November 20
Effects of Low-dose Exposure to Radiation on Human Health	October 2 (Sun.) 13:15 - 15:30	October 23 (Sun.) 13:15 - 15:30	October 24 (Mon.) 13:15 - 15:30	Scheduled on September 27 (Tue.)
Tips for Ensuring the Safety of Food	November 12 (Sat.) 13:15 - 15:30	November 27 (Sun.) 13:15 - 15:30	October 13 (Thur.) 13:15 - 15:30	October 4 (Tue.) 13:15 - 15:30
Physical Exercise for Parents and Children	November 21 (Mon.) 09:45 - 12:00 (For children under 3 years old)	November 20 (Sun.) 09:45 - 12:00 (For children under 3 years old)	November 21 (Mon.) 13:15 - 15:30 (For children age 3 years or older)	November 20 (Sun.) 13:15 - 15:30 (For children age 3 years or older)
Mental Health Care for Young Children	December 5 (Mon.) 13:15 - 15:30	December 4 (Sun.) 09:45 - 12:00	December 4 (Sun.) 13:15 - 15:30	November 28 (Mon.) 13:15 - 15:30

* Participation in all the four sessions is desirable. Different venues can be chosen according to theme.
* Participation in a single session is possible, depending on availability.

Details

Session on "Effects of Low-dose Exposure to Radiation on Human Health"

A doctor from Takagi School for Alternative Scientists, an NGO aiming to foster citizen scientists, will explain about radiation effects on human health and how to protect young children from low-dose exposure in their daily lives to radiation.

Session on "Tips for Ensuring the Safety of Food"

Keisuke AMAGASA, a free-lance journalist specializing in food safety problems, will offer daily diet tips for reducing internal exposure to radiation, and explain about the relationship between radiation problems and food safety problems, in an easy-to-understand format.

Session on "Physical Exercise for Parents and Children"

A collaborative program with Kodomo-no-Shiro, a national indoor play center.
Participating parents and young children can enjoy indoor exercise. Because there are many exercise programs adapted to the age of the children, both parents and young children can feel refreshed.

Session on "Mental Health Care for Young Children"

Taku IWAKURA, a clinical psychologist of Azamino Shinri Office (a psychological counseling office), will show examples of post-disaster mental health care support for both young children and adults.

Target residents

For each study session, a total of 30 parents/guardians of preschool children (on a first-come, first-served basis)
* Participants are asked to communicate information obtained at the study sessions to their friends and close acquaintances, so that correct information on radiation and health management can be disseminated to as many residents as possible.
* For participation of persons other than Nihonmatsu City residents, please contact the section below.

How to apply

Please apply to the contact section below by phone or fax. Information necessary to apply includes a name, date of birth, address and phone number of the applicant, as well as preferred dates of sessions, and the necessity of nursery services during a session.

Application deadline

No later than one week before each study session

Others

During a study session, free nursery services are available for about 10 young children at each venue. A prior reservation is required (on a first-come, first-served basis).
Contact/Application: Health Promotion Section　　　　Phone number: 55-xxxx　　　　Fax number: 23-xxxx

- The city established a registry system to manage each individual resident's exposure data obtained from a personal dosimeter, a Whole Body Counter, and from thyroid gland examinations.
- To evaluate measurement results from a Whole Body Counter, the city has not only conducted a software analysis but also asked for the re-analysis of measurement data from an internal exposure evaluation expert.

Summary/measures in the future

- Although the supply of water and electricity was secured, the city received complaints from mothers with babies about the short supply of disposable diapers and baby wipes. Of course, it is necessary to maintain full stockpiles for an emergency situation. However, it is also indispensable for the city to ensure that residents are aware of ways and means to cope with the lack of daily commodities; some of which have been passed down from generation to generation.
- The city received a wide variety of requests, inquiries and complaints from residents, most of which arose from a growing distrust of the national government, Fukushima Prefecture, and of the Tokyo Electric Power Company. Because the city officials had to attentively listen to residents and accommodate their needs, they were put under tremendous mental stress. The city needs to recognize the importance of mental health care programs for such "support providers" in times of disaster.

(Yoko Abe)

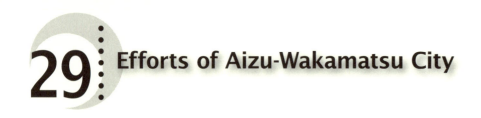

29 Efforts of Aizu-Wakamatsu City

1 Situation of the municipality

(1) Demographics (as of January 1 of each year)

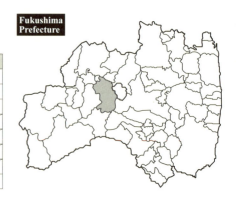

	2011	2012	2013
Population	126,114	125,472	124,515
Number of households	47,909	48,164	48,094
Average number of people per household	2.6	2.6	2.6
Number of births	993	971	
Birth rate			
Number of deaths	1,543	1,590	
Mortality			
Ratio of the elderly aged 65 or older	25.5	25.6	26.3

(2) Geographical features

Total area: 383 km² (approximately 20 km east-west; approximately 29 km north-south)
Distance from the Fukushima Daiichi Nuclear Power Station of the Tokyo Electric Power Company: approximately 97–115 km
Evacuation area: None
Transportation network: Banetsu Expressway; the JR Banetsu-sai Line; Aizu Railway; National Route 49

2 Situation of damage by the earthquake, tsunami and the nuclear disaster

(1) Damage by the Great East Japan Earthquake (as of February 20, 2013)

Property damage	Completely destroyed	Half destroyed	Partially destroyed
House	4	87	5,720
Public institution			
Other			

Human damage	Deaths by disaster	Disaster-related deaths	Missing persons	Injured persons
	1	3	0	6

(2) Situation of evacuation

① Evacuation centers within the municipality (as of December 28, 2011)

	Number of evacuation centers	Number of evacuees	Available period
Residents	8	221	March 11 to 13
Evacuees received	5	1,015	March 14 to December 28

② Approximate number of evacuees in evacuation centers outside the municipality (as of February 28, 2013)

	End/March 2011	End/September 2011	End/March 2012	Latest period
First evacuation center	0	0	0	0
Second evacuation center	0	0	0	0
Temporary housing	0	0	0	0
Municipally-subsidized housing	0	0	0	0

③ Approximate number of voluntary evacuees (as of February 28, 2013)

Inside Fukushima Prefecture	7	Outside Fukushima Prefecture (number of evacuees & prefectures)	168 persons in 24 prefectures

29 Efforts of Aizu-Wakamatsu City

Outlook of damage related to the nuclear disaster

① After the Great East Japan Earthquake, many people living in municipalities located near the Fukushima Daiichi Nuclear Power Station were evacuated to Aizu-Wakamatsu City. To receive as many evacuees as possible, the city set up a maximum of four evacuation centers within the city, including a general gymnasium with a large accommodation capacity.

② The city established a disaster response headquarters to promptly conduct emergency relief activities in collaboration with various organizations concerned. To be specific, the city strived to provide emergency assistance at evacuation centers, secure disaster emergency supplies for evacuees, and assess the damage the city received from the earthquake.

③ In providing emergency medical treatment and relief activities at evacuation centers, the city obtained cooperation from medical aid staff members of the city's medical association, the society of dentists, and the pharmacist association.

❸ Countermeasures against nuclear disaster (as of January 2013)

		Name of project	Division in charge	Number of targeted persons (households)	Expect-ant mothers	Nursing mothers	Babiesy	Young children	Elemen-tary school students	Junior high school students	Senior high school students	People age 19 to 39	People age 40 or older	Remarks (major operations)
Countermeasures against external exposure	1	Personal dose measurements (lending of cumu-lative dosimeters)	Health Promotion Division		○		○	○	○	○				Distribution & collection of cumulative dosimeters, and notification & analysis of measurement results
	2	Measurement of radiation dose (lending of air dosimeters)	Environ-ment and Living Division		○	○	○	○	○	○	○	○	○	Lending of air dosimeters, and analysis of measurement results
	3	Monitoring and measurement of the air radiation levels	Environ-ment and Living Division	9 posts										Installation of equipment, measurement, recording, and analysis & announcements of measurement results
	4	Real-time measurement of the radiation dose (Ministry of the Environment)	Environ-ment and Living Division	143 posts										Installation of equipment, measurement, recording, and analysis & announcements of measurement results
	5	Measurement of the radiation levels at sightseeing spots and public facilities	Tourism Division Greenery Division School Education Division		○	○	○	○	○	○	○	○	○	Installation of equipment, measurement, recording, and analysis & announcements of measurement results
	6	Playing programs for young childreny	Children's Affairs Division					Parents and children ○						A program by Fukushima Prefecture conducted at public nursery schools and child- rearing support centers. Planning, publicity and management of the program
	7	Decontamina-tion of public kindergartens and schools (cleaning of ditches and other work)	School Education Division	33 facili-ties				○	○	○				Procurement & installation of equipment, analysis & announcements of decontamination results, meetings with suppliers, contracts, notification, acceptance of samples, and bill payment
	8	Decontamination of nursery schools (cleaning of ditches and other work)	Children's Affairs Division				○	○						Procurement & installation of equipment, analysis & announcements of decontamination results, meetings with suppliers, contracts, notification, acceptance of samples, and bill payment
	9	Radiation level mitigation pro-gram (subsidized by Fukushima Prefecture)	Environ-ment and Living Division											Meeting with suppliers, contracts, notification, and bill payment
	10	Measures to sup-press the absorp-tion of radioactive materials into crops	Agricultural Policy Planning Division											Meeting with suppliers, contracts, notification, and bill payment

295

	#	Measure	Division	Target										Remarks
Countermeasures against internal exposure	11	Disposal of sediment dredged from a river, and sludge dredged from ditches, and sediment waste from water purification process	Waste Management Division Land Readjustment Division Road Maintenance Division Waterworks Section of the Water Utility Diviziony											Mechanical cleaning of streets, dredging work in ditches, and outsourcing of a temporary site for sludge/sediment disposal
	12	Measurement of the radiation dose in timber and forests and decontamination work	Agriculture and Forestry Division											Measurement and investigation of air levels
	13	Inspection of the radiation dose in food products	Health Promotion Diviziony	All households	○	○	○	○	○	○	○	○	○	Meeting with suppliers, contracts, acceptance of samples, and bill payment
	14	Whole Body Counter measurements (conducted by the city)	Health Promotion Division	Residents	○	○		○	○	○	○	○	○	Installation of devices, calibration, schedule arrangements, requests for analysis, and notification/ aggregation/ analysis of measurement results
	15	Water quality inspection	General Affairs Section of the Water Utility Division		○	○	○	○	○	○	○	○	○	Meeting with suppliers, contracts, notification, acceptance of samples, and bill payment
	16	Inspection of rice (independently conducted by the city)	Agricultural Policy Planning Division											Meeting with suppliers, contracts, notification, acceptance of samples, and bill payment
	17	Inspection of school meals	Children's Affairs Division School Education Division				○	○	○	○				Meeting with suppliers, contracts, notification, acceptance of samples, and bill payment
	18	Monitoring and measurement of the radiation dose in farm and forest products	Agricultural Policy Planning Division Agriculture and Forestry Diviziony											Procurement of equipment, measurement, recording, and analysis & announcements of measurement results
Others	19	Post-disaster mental health care program for young children and their family members	Health Promotion Division				○	○						Counseling services by a clinical psychologist for parents/guardians at medical examinations for young children (a program by Fukushima Prefecture)
	20	Sampling of respondents for a basic survey in the Fukushima Health Management Survey	Health Promotion Division	All households	○	○	○	○	○	○	○	○	○	Conducted by Fukushima Prefecture. The city conducts publicity.
	21	Sampling of respondents to a survey on the physical/mental development of young children in affected areas	Health Promotion Division				○	○						A survey by the Ministry of Health, Labour and Welfare. The city received a request from Fukushima Prefecture.
	22	Measurement of radiation levels in the soil	Agricultural Policy Planning Division											Measurement, and analysis & announcements of measurement results

A : Residents

1 Nutrition (meals/water)

a. Situation
- Residents were worried about radioactive contamination of their home-grown vegetables and other edible wild plants.

b. Responses (actual measures)
- In March 2012, the city started the measurement of radiation levels of food.

c. Summary/measures in the future
- For some food radiation level measurement devices, as many as 1,000cc of foodstuffs need to be cut into tiny pieces in advance. There were complaints from residents about the laborious preparation steps.

2 Exercise (Environmental improvement)

a. Situation
- Immediately after the earthquake, many residents reframed from going outdoors or wore a mask when going outside, due to anxiety about exposure to radiation.

b. Responses (actual measures)
- In October 2012, the city independently began internal exposure measurement using a Whole Body Counter, for residents age 4 years or older within the city.
- In April 2013, the city started the lending of electronic personal dosimeters to residents within the city.

c. Summary/measures in the future
- The city is required to make continuous efforts to understand the possible harmful effects of radiation on the health of the residents and take necessary measures to help residents feel at ease in their daily lives.

3 Rest (mind, anxiety, suicide, etc.)

a. Situation
- After the earthquake, there was no significant increase in the number of mental health-related counseling services that the city offered to residents.

b. Responses (actual measures)
- As part of its suicide prevention initiatives, the city held lecture meetings on measures to be taken against suicide. The city also prepared pamphlets containing information on its mental health care counseling services and contact information, and distributed them to all the households.

c. Summary/measures in the future
- Key points for successful suicide prevention programs as part of disaster preparedness initiatives are "to notice the distress of family members, friends and close acquaintances," "to encourage them to consult a medical institution" and "to always be considerate of them and mindful of their needs." The city intends

Chapter 3 — Situation of and Countermeasures by Each Individual Municipality

to ensure that residents fully recognize these key points, while at the same time focusing on the development of human resources who can contribute to the continued suicide prevention efforts of the city.

B Expectant/nursing mothers and children

1 Nutrition (meals/water)

a. Situation
- Because the distribution of daily commodities stopped immediately after the earthquake, the city received inquiries about the short supply of artificial milk (milk powder).
- The city received an increasing number of inquiries from parents with babies about radiation effects on breast milk and radioactive contamination of drinking water.
- There were many parents who purchased bottled water to prepare milk for babies.

b. Responses (actual measures)
- To address the short supply of milk powder, the city asked for cooperation from the local social welfare council to secure milk powder as emergency relief supplies.
- As to inquiries about the radiation effects on breast milk, the city officials initially introduced mothers to institutions within the prefecture that conducted breast milk examinations. After the start of food inspection programs, the city also embarked on breast milk inspection within the city.
- Aiming to share important information with residents, the city posted information and materials obtained from the national government and Fukushima Prefecture, at local public health centers.

c. Summary/measures in the future
- The city is required to ensure that each individual household maintains full stockpiles such as milk powder, disposable diapers, and baby foods for emergencies.
- The city reconfirmed how important it is to decide in advance how to and where to distribute emergency relief supplies in case the distribution of daily commodities stops in an emergency situation.

2 Exercise (Environmental improvement)

a. Situation
- The more the details about atmospheric contamination by radioactive substances were revealed, the more parents restricted their children from playing outdoors.
- Nursery schools, kindergartens, and primary schools also restricted outdoor activities. Young children and students were told to be sure to wear a mask when playing outdoors.

b. Responses (actual measures)
- The city independently conducted the measurement of air radiation levels.
- In November 2011, the city started the distribution of personal dosimeters (glass badges) only to expectant mothers and to young children under 16 years old at their or their parents' request. However, the city expanded the target to all the residents living within the city in April 2013.
- Based on "post-disaster mental health care initiatives for young children and their family members" by Fukushima Prefecture, the city provided physical activity classes at child-rearing support centers within the city.
- Because it was sometimes necessary to shut the windows, even in the hot summer, when an air radiation

level was high, the city installed electric fans at public schools within the city.

c. Summary/measures in the future

- The city is required to conduct timely announcements to the public of the measurement and analysis results of air radiation levels.
- Limited outdoor activities caused a lack of exercise among young children. To prevent them from becoming obese, it is necessary for the city to advise children (or their parents) to actively do indoor exercise as part of their daily lives.

3　Rest (mind, anxiety, suicide, etc.)

a. Situation

- The more the details about the damage from the nuclear power station accident were reported by the mass media, the more anxiety about the safety of young children was created among parents. The city's health consultation line also became increasingly deluged with inquiries from such parents. There were many parents who complained that they did not know what information to trust due to the flood of differing information. According to a questionnaire survey conducted by Fukushima Prefecture at medical examinations for young children as part of "post-disaster mental health care initiatives for young children and their family members", some parents suffered from sleeplessness and were seriously stressed after the earthquake and the nuclear power station accident.

b. Responses (actual measures)

- Based on "post-disaster mental health care initiative for young children and their family members" by Fukushima Prefecture, the city conducted a questionnaire survey for parents at the time of medical examinations for young children. At the respondent's request, counseling services by a clinical psychologist were also offered.

c. Summary/measures in the future

- The counseling services by a clinical psychologist for parents, offered at examinations for young children, were helpful for the city in reducing strong anxiety about radiation among parents and guardians.

C　Public health activities at evacuation centers

- For approximately four months after the earthquake, the city officials strived to provide physical/mental health management programs to residents at four evacuation centers set up within the city.
- The city officials made strenuous efforts to prevent the development of deep vein thrombosis/pulmonary embolism (economy-class syndrome), while at the same focusing on the understanding of the physical health conditions of residents. To be specific, the city officials confirmed whether each individual resident had a consultation with a doctor, and helped them acquire the prescribed medicines. As needed, they also encouraged residents to have an examination at a medical institution. Health-related counseling services were also offered to residents. In addition to these efforts, dedicated officials provided counseling services for residents as part of the city's post-disaster mental health care programs.
- When conducting public health activities, the city officials obtained cooperation from the local pharmacist associations, the medical associations, the societies of dentists, and medical volunteer staff members, as well as public health nurses dispatched from Kyoto Prefecture.

(Yoshino Muroi)

Chapter 4

Activities of Various Professional Organizations

30 Fukushima Medical Association

In the Great East Japan Earthquake, Fukushima Prefecture was seriously damaged by not only the earthquake and tsunami, but also by radioactive contamination caused by the nuclear accident at the Fukushima Daiichi Nuclear Power Station of the Tokyo Electric Power Company ("Fukushima Daiichi Station"). Consequently, the area within a 20km radius from the Fukushima Daiichi Station was designated as a restricted area, the area within a 20 to 30km radius as an emergency evacuation preparation area, and adjacent areas with high radiation levels as deliberate evacuation areas. Many residents were evacuated inside and outside the prefecture, and most of them were forced to live inconvenient lives in evacuation centers. These evacuees were mainly elderly people and those who require continuous therapy, and some people fell sick due to an unfavorable living environment. Accordingly, it became an urgent issue for administrative bodies and medical associations to ensure medical treatment in evacuation centers.

Immediately after the earthquake occurred, the Fukushima Medical Association ("the Association"), in collaboration with the Japan Medical Association, had become involved in diverse activities related to health assistance for disaster victims to protect the lives and health of residents in Fukushima Prefecture. This section introduces visiting clinic services in evacuation centers, which were provided with the assistance of Japan Medical Association Teams (JMATs). In addition, several issues related to nuclear disaster responses are described[1,2].

A Activities after the occurrence of the earthquake

1 Establishment of a disaster response headquarters and its initial activities

The Association established a disaster response headquarters at 15:30 on March 11, immediately after the occurrence of the earthquake, under the supervision of President Yuzo Takaya. However, due to a power failure, which was recovered on March 12, and a water cut-off, which lasted over a week, the activities of the disaster response headquarters remained sluggish. Since communication functions were recovered on March 12, the Association began to gather information from county and city medical associations in Fukushima Prefecture and respond to requests from its members. Although communication functions were recovered, phone connections remained bad. Consequently, clerical staff members sometimes had to visit the prefectural government. On March 13, the Association asked the Fukushima Prefecture Disaster Response Headquarters to secure water necessary to respond to dialysis patients. On March 14, it asked the headquarters to distribute iodine preparations, and dispatch medical examiners to county and city medical associations under the name of the Fukushima Prefectural Police Headquarters, Fukushima Medical Association, and Fukushima Prefecture Police Doctor Society. It also made a request for providing information on the summary of the situation of damage and responses of the individual county and city medical associations, and dispatching physicians to Minamisoma City Hospital. On March 15, it asked medical associations in Ibaraki, Tochigi, Gunma, Yamagata, and Niigata Prefectures to receive patients as well as asked the governor of Fukushima Prefecture to encourage these neighboring prefectures to receive patients.

Moreover, on March 15, the Japan Medical Association asked the Association to make arrangements for the dispatch of JMATs. On March 16, the Association asked county and city medical associations and hospitals to provide information on the lack of medical support in association with the dispatch of JMATs. On March 17, the Association asked the Japan Medical Association to dispatch JMATs to Fukushima Pre-

| Chapter 4 | **Activities of Various Professional Organizations** |

fecture. In addition, the governor of Fukushima Prefecture requested governors of individual prefectures to cooperate with the dispatch of JMATs.

2 Establishment of JMATs and their activities in Fukushima Prefecture

A JMAT is a group of medical personnel, which was designed by the Japan Medical Association to provide disaster medical care in case of large-scale disasters. On March 15, the Japan Medical Association decided to establish JMATs in the wake of this earthquake, and required medical associations in 43 prefectures, excluding affected prefectures, to dispatch JMATs to four affected prefectures (Iwate, Miyagi, Fukushima and Ibaraki Prefectures). Major activities of JMATs are as follows: 1) providing medical care in evacuation centers and aid stations; 2) offering support for daily medical care in hospitals and clinics in affected areas; 3) evaluating and improving the situation of evacuation centers (health and sanitary conditions of evacuees, trends in the occurrence of infection, dietary habits, etc.); and 4) providing medical care to home patients and managing their health.

The focus of the activities were: 1) responding to requests from medical associations in affected prefectures (prefectural medical associations and county and city medical associations in affected prefectures serve as the coordinator to grasp the situation of local medical care); 2) dispatching JMATs according to the "dispatch calendar" (continuing to dispatch JMATs so that there may be no time gap between the withdrawal of advance teams and the commencement of activities by subsequent teams; 3) ensuring a smooth handover of operations and withdrawal after medical institutions are rebuilt in affected areas; and 4) recruiting participants from member physicians based on professional autonomy. As an example of team formation, a team was required to consist of one physician, two nursing staff members and one clerical staff member at first. In fact, however, the formation changed depending on the situation of the medical association which dispatched JMATs. Moreover, staff members in other job categories, such as pharmacists and physical therapists, also participated in teams to provide support for rescue activities. The Japan Medical Association had dispatched a total of 1,395 JMATs by July 15, 2011, when its operations were completed.

In Fukushima Prefecture, the whole area of the Futaba District and Iitate Village and part of Minamisoma City, Kawamata Town and Tamura City were designated as a restricted area and a deliberate evacuation area, due to extensive damage from the tsunami and the nuclear power station accident. Accordingly, county and city medical associations in these areas were unable to offer visiting clinic services in evacuation centers. Under these circumstances, what was most needed was the dispatch of JMATs, which took over the operations of Disaster Medical Assistance Teams (DMATs) that assumed a major role in medical care at this very acute stage of the disaster.

The activities of JMATs continued until July 2011. A total of 274 teams were dispatched from Fukuoka Prefecture to Shinchi Town, from Ishikawa and Shizuoka Prefectures to Soma City, from Nagasaki Prefecture to Minamisoma City, from Aichi, Toyama, Fukuoka, Kyoto, Yamanashi Prefectures and the Metropolis of Tokyo to Iwaki City, from Shiga Prefecture to Fukushima, Date and Nihonmatsu Cities, and from Shiga and Kyoto Prefectures to Aizuwakamatsu City. I would like to take this opportunity to express my sincere gratitude to medical associations in these prefectures.

Since July 2011 the Japan Medical Association has continuously dispatched JMATs II, primarily aiming to prevent disaster-related deaths. In Fukushima Prefecture, Minamisoma City has received a total of 138 teams as of March 31, 2013.

30 Fukushima Medical Association

3 Activity situation of county and city medical associations after the occurrence of the earthquake

a. Futaba District Medical Association

Since the whole area of the Futaba District was designated as an evacuation area, the district faced a difficult situation where it had to offer support to disaster victims in evacuation destinations. Dr. Akira Isaka, President of the Futaba District Medical Association, as well as Dr. Akihito Horikawa and Dr. Masanori Sato, who were all evacuated to the Big Palette Fukushima in Koriyama City, set up a medical team with nurses, public health nurses and pharmacists and commenced to provide medical care in evacuation centers, while living together with 3,000 evacuees. After the DMAT of Toho University conducted support activities for a week, a JMAT began to provide support in April. Physicians from the Futaba District offered visiting clinic services in the evacuation center as a medical visiting team for 2.5 hours a day, and provided outpatient treatment with the JMAT on April 16. In addition, medical specialists were dispatched from the Koriyama Medical Association three times a week. Severely injured persons were transferred to hospitals in Koriyama City by fire engines from the Futaba District. There were no deaths in the evacuation center.

The Tsushima District in Namie Town received 6,400 evacuees from coastal districts, who were affected by the tsunami and the nuclear power station accident. The Tsushima Clinic, where Dr. Shunji Sekine, Vice President of the Futaba District Medical Association worked, struggled to respond to 300 patients a day. However, since an indoor evacuation order was issued on March 15, he was evacuated with residents to Towa Town, Nihonmatsu City, where he temporarily established the National Health Insurance Tsushima Clinic in the Towa Meaningful Life Center. Vice President Shunji Sekine, Dr. Shinya Imamura, Dr. Hiroaki Kanno, Dr. Kazumi Sato, Dr. Toru Tezuka, and Dr. Sadataka Nishi provided medical care to disaster victims by rotation. On April 18, they moved to Dake Hot Spring in Nihonmatsu City to offer medical treatment. Then, on October 1, they opened a clinic in the Tomioka Town Temporary Housing in Otama Village, where they continued to provide medical treatment. In evacuation destinations outside the prefecture, some physicians, including Dr. Akira Konno and Dr. Shuichi Ishida, continued to conduct medical activities at their evacuation destinations, such as Sanjo City in Niigata Prefecture and Saitama Prefecture.

b. Soma-gun Medical Association

In Minamisoma City, Odaka Ward was designated as a restricted area, Haramachi Ward and Iitate Village were designated as a deliberate evacuation area, and other areas were designated as emergency evacuation preparation areas. Since the government required children, expectant mothers and inpatients not to enter these areas, the city was unable to provide hospital treatment. As a result, two mental hospitals were closed and four general hospitals only provided outpatient care in Minamisoma City. Since many patients who required hospitalization were rushed to the Public Soma General Hospital and Soma Central Hospital, these hospitals faced difficulties in responding to these patients. To meet the medical needs of residents in Minamisoma City, Dr. Toshiyuki Higuchi, Vice President of the Soma-gun Medical Association, and the eight other member physicians in the local area opened a temporary clinic in Kashima Kosei Hospital to provide medical examinations. In addition, the Soma-gun Medical Association was required to identify hospitals which could receive patients in the departments of brain surgery and psychiatry and made arrangements to respond to the request. Consequently, Sendai Kosei Hospital proposed to prepare 70 beds, and other hospitals in Fukushima City and Koriyama City also provided help to receive patients.

Meanwhile, in Soma City, 15 evacuation centers were set up for 4,674 evacuees. On March 14, three to four medical teams, which consisted of member physicians in local areas, began to offer visiting clinic services in these evacuation centers. Since this function was taken over by a JMAT, which came to Soma

Chapter 4 | Activities of Various Professional Organizations

City on March 21, the local physicians became committed to conducting medical examinations at their own clinics. Dr. Katsutoshi Kashimura, President of the Soma-gun Medical Association, served as a coordinator for a JMAT. Although visiting clinic services in the evacuation centers ended on June 10, JMAT II continued to provide medical support to Minamisoma City, as stated before. There were no deaths in the evacuation centers.

c. Iwaki City Medical Association

Not only residents in coastal districts, which were heavily damaged by the tsunami, but also evacuees from Naraha and Hirono Towns, which were affected by the nuclear power station accident, rushed to Iwaki City. The city established 140 evacuation centers, where 19,574 evacuees moved. The Iwaki City Medical Association commenced visiting clinic services in evacuation centers on March 13, while sharing areas with Iwaki Kyoritsu General Hospital. These services were provided with support from the Tokyo DMAT and Dr. Takashi Nagata, a researcher at the Japan Medical Association Research Institute, who came to Iwaki City as requested by Dr. Masami Ishii, who was an Executive Board Member in charge of Emergency Medicine, Japan Medical Association and the former President of the Iwaki City Medical Association. However, no vehicles entered Iwaki City due to concerns about radioactive contamination. Moreover, there was a shortage of human resources, food, medical products and gasoline, and the water supply was also disrupted over long periods. It seemed to people in the city that they were forced to hold up in a castle and were deprived of supplies of food. Accordingly, support teams were asked to leave the city briefly, and only local medical teams continued to engage in smaller activities.

The radiation dose was soon found to be relatively low in Iwaki City. Although the radiation dose rose sharply to 23.72μSv on March 15, it then rapidly decreased and continued to diminish gradually. Serving as President of the Iwaki City Medical Association at the time, I visited Tokyo and asked the Japan Medical Association to provide support to Iwaki City to defuse the situation. Assistance was provided under the auspices of Dr. Masami Ishii, Executive Board Member of the Japan Medical Association. Upon a request from the Japan Medical Association, medical products began to be supplied again to medical institutions in the city. In addition, approximately 800kg of medical products were transported from the Aichi Medical Association to the Iwaki City Medical Association by air. Moreover, the first team of JMATs from the Aichi Medical Association entered Iwaki City on the evening of March 18, and full-fledged activities of JMATs began on March 19. Thereafter, the city was able to continuously receive support from JMATs that were dispatched from various prefectures. Although most hospitals in the city were facing various problems, such as property damage resulting from the earthquake, a water failure and absenteeism of employees due to a gasoline shortage, they managed to maintain their medical function, while transporting inpatients to hospitals outside the city. Accordingly, the city asked JMATs to offer visiting clinic services in evacuation centers, while sharing areas with medical teams from the city. Evacuees who required psychological care were introduced to mental health-care teams from Fukushima Medical University, which provided visiting care services in evacuation centers from the end of March.

When physical distribution service and water supply were recovered, evacuees began to move to municipally-subsidized housing in the middle of April and the number of evacuees in evacuation centers decreased. Approximately 80% and 96.2 % of medical institutions in local areas resumed providing medical care by the end of April and by the middle of May, respectively, and transportation service also began between evacuation centers and medical institutions. Accordingly, the activities of the JMATs ended on May 3. A total of 73 JMATs and 331 persons, including 127 physicians, had been dispatched to the city. There were no deaths in evacuation centers.

30 Fukushima Medical Association

d. Other county and city medical associations

Medical associations in the Central Region, such as the Fukushima City Medical Association and the Koriyama Medical Association, and the Aizuwakamatsu Medical Association formed local medical teams to offer visiting clinic services in evacuation centers. Services were offered in cooperation with support teams from other prefectures, such as JMATs and teams from the Japanese Red Cross Society. Thus, health assistance was smoothly provided to evacuees in individual areas.

B ⋮ Issues related to nuclear disaster responses

1 Participation in disaster administration of Fukushima Prefecture

Although the Association had concluded the Disaster Health Care Agreement with Fukushima Prefecture, it was not included in the Fukushima Prefecture Disaster Response Headquarters. As a result, the collaboration between Fukushima Prefecture and the Association did not work well for the acquisition of necessary information and overall medical support. This was a very regrettable response during this disaster. Fortunately, since the collaboration between Fukushima Prefecture, Fukushima Medical University and the Association was rebuilt thanks to the efforts of President Yuzo Takaya, who made full use of his personal network, everything proceeded without problems. Since the earthquake, the Japan Medical Association has been actively involved in the disaster prevention administration of the national government. Fukushima Prefecture also should make sure to incorporate the Association and JMATs into its basic disaster management plan and disaster medical system.

2 Countermeasures against exposure to radiation

Regarding countermeasures against exposure to radiation, the Act on Special Measures Concerning Nuclear Emergency Preparedness was established after the JCO criticality incident occurred at Tokai Village in 1999. The act required 19 prefectures where nuclear facilities are located and neighboring prefectures, to develop a radiation emergency medical system. Although large-scale nuclear disaster drills were conducted annually, these drills were of no help because severe accidents like this nuclear accident had not been assumed. In the future, practical and effective countermeasures should be taken based on a thorough investigation of this nuclear power station accident.

In addition, there were other major problems. Evacuation instructions based on scientific data obtained from the System for Prediction of Environmental Emergency Dose Information (SPEEDI) were not issued. Moreover, the Off-Site Center (OFC), which should transmit accurate information, did not work properly. During evacuation, huge traffic jams were caused because adequate escape routes had not been ensured. Consequently, many inpatients and residents in nursing facilities, who were transported for evacuation, died at evacuation destinations due to stress during transportation. There were 380 such disaster-related deaths. It is a big challenge to ensure escape routes and determine how to guide evacuation.

Furthermore, the national government and Fukushima Prefecture did not provide clear instructions concerning the administration of stable iodine preparations. This caused confusion in affected areas. The administration of stable iodine preparations is determined as follows: Measures for preventive administration should be taken when the projected thyroid equivalent dose for children of radioactive iodine (^{131}I) is judged to likely exceed 100 mSv (currently changed to 50 mSv) based on the data from SPEEDI and emergency monitoring. Instructions to administer stable iodine preparations were supposed to be issued by

Chapter 4 | Activities of Various Professional Organizations

a local nuclear emergency response headquarters of the national government (with the Prime Minister serving as Director-general) to relevant local governments via a local nuclear emergency response headquarters of Fukushima Prefecture (with the governor of the prefecture serving as Director-general). Given that this system failed to work well, it is necessary to conduct an extensive review of the system, including transferring the authority to determine the administration of stable iodine preparations to local governments.

3 Suggestions related to recovery and reconstruction from nuclear disaster

Here we introduce the summary of suggestions related to recovery and reconstruction from the nuclear disaster. These suggestions were provided to the national government and Fukushima Prefecture by the Project Committee on the Reconstruction from the Fukushima Nuclear Disaster, which was established by the Japan Medical Association in response to requests from the Association.

The national government, which has promoted a nuclear energy policy as a national policy, has a responsibility. The government should take responsibility for not only securing the safety of the Fukushima Daiichi and Daini Nuclear Power Stations until they are decommissioned, but also taking measures to remove radioactive materials from Fukushima Prefecture and ensure the return and resettlement of evacuated residents. Moreover, the government needs to secure the safety of nuclear power stations, disclose information and improve a second opinion system for nuclear power, which consists of nuclear experts who do not have a conflict of interest.

In addition, the national government is required to design flexible systems to revitalize local communities and establish them in law, as well as to create systems for disaster assessment with consideration of evacuation areas that are off limits.

Furthermore, an urgent issue for the national government is to build a system in which the government can continuously monitor the health damage of disaster victims in a responsible manner. The government is also required to mobilize experts in various fields, such as decontamination, impact of radioactive materials on soil and the ocean, waste disposal, food safety, and education and enlightenment of residents, and to establish an interdisciplinary and comprehensive national center beyond the boundaries of government offices[3].

It is no exaggeration to say that the recovery and reconstruction of Fukushima Prefecture depends on that from nuclear disaster. I hope that the issues mentioned here will be resolved and that health assistance for disaster victims will be promoted.

(Koichi Kida)

References
1) Masami Ishii: *Responses of the Japan Medical Association and Roles of JMATs*. The Journal of the Japan Medical Association. vol. 141, No. 1: 32–36, 2012
2) Koichi Kida: *Responses of the Fukushima Medical Association to the Great East Japan Earthquake and Future Issues*. The Bulletin of the Fukushima Medical Association, Vol. 73, No. 4/5: 4–10, 2011
3) Japan Medical Association Research Institute. *Research on Damage Compensation for the Fukushima Nuclear Disaster and Recovery and Reconstruction from the Disaster*:

31 Fukushima Dental Association

On March 11, 2011, the Great East Japan Earthquake occurred, and the tsunami following the earthquake caused tremendous damage mainly to the Pacific coast of the Tohoku region. The Fukushima Dental Association ("the Association") set up a disaster response headquarters on March 12. On the same day, the Association received a request for identity confirmation from the Fukushima Prefecture Police, and another request for dental relief activities from Fukushima Prefecture based on a cooperation agreement on disaster management. In response to these requests, the Association engaged in identity confirmation of unidentified bodies in collaboration with the Fukushima Prefecture Police and the Self-Defense Forces, and conducted dental relief activities for evacuees.

Here is reported the dental health support activities that the county and city dental associations in Fukushima Prefecture and other organizations provided to evacuees in various areas in Fukushima Prefecture from the occurrence of the earthquake until the end of June 2011.

A Report about dental health support activities

1 Survey method

The targets of a survey included county and city dental associations, dental hygienists' associations, dental technologists associations, Ohu University, Nagasaki University, dispatch teams from the Japan Dental Association and dental associations in other prefectures; dental associations in Hiroshima, Gifu, Miyazaki, Shimane and Wakayama Prefectures, and Tokyo Dental College. It also included volunteers; Dr. Koichi Nakakuki, Tokyo Medical and Dental University, volunteers from the Hokkaido Government and the Department of Dentistry, Ishikawa Medical Practitioners Association, and Yasushi Kunitomi, Kyodo Dental Clinic.

We asked these organizations and volunteers to submit reports about their support activities by the end of August 2011 to conduct a survey on the following items.

2 Frequency of going out for relief activities

We divided the number of times that they went out for relief activities in the months immediately following the earthquake into four time categories: March, April, May and June. Moreover, we divided areas where they visited into three areas (Coastal Region, Central Region and Aizu Region) in Fukushima Prefecture, and totaled the frequency of their going out to conduct relief activities. Survey results showed that they visited evacuation centers and other places a total of 525 times, with the greatest frequency being 278 times in April. The main areas of activities were the Coastal Region and the Central Region. The frequency of their going out for relief activities decreased in all areas in and after May (Figure 31-1).

3 Number of people engaged in support activities

We totaled the number of people who provided relief support, and classified them according to their job categories into dentists, dental hygienists, dental technicians, and others. According to the survey results, the total number of people who engaged in support activities was 1,504 persons. Dentists accounted for 68%, with 1,027 persons, followed by dental hygienists, who accounted for 21% with 312 persons (Figure 31-2).

Chapter 4 Activities of Various Professional Organizations

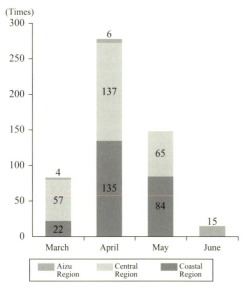

Figure 31-1 Frequency of going out for relief activities

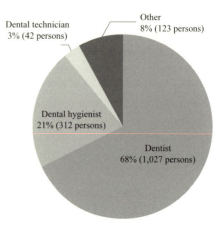

Figure 31-2 Composition of people engaged in support activities

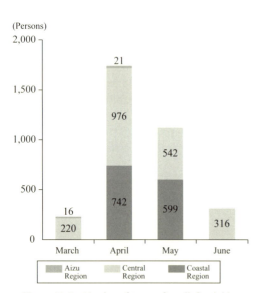

Figure 31-3 Number of targets for relief activities

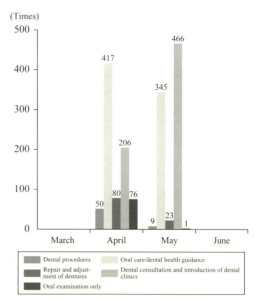

Figure 31-4 Contents of support activities by area (Coastal Region)

4 Number of targets for relief activities

With disaster victims who received dental relief defined as targets for relief activities, we sorted them by month from March to June, and further divided them into three areas according to their place of residence. The results showed that the total number of targets for relief activities was 3,414 persons. In terms of three areas in Fukushima Prefecture, the number of targets for relief activities reached the highest level in the Central Region in April with 976 targets for relief activities and in the Coastal Region in May with 599 (Figure 31-3).

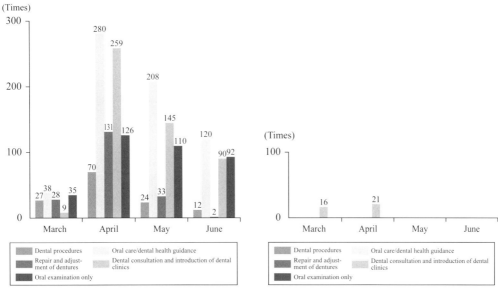

Figure 31-5 Contents of support activities by area (Central Region)

Figure 31-6 Contents of support activities by area (Aizu Region)

5 Contents of support activities

We broadly divided the contents of support activities into five categories; 1) dental procedures, 2) oral care and dental health guidance, 3) repair and adjustment of dentures, 4) dental consultation and introduction to dental clinics, and 5) oral examination. Moreover, we classified these activities into three groups according to areas where the activities were provided, and further divided them into four groups from March to June. According to the survey results, major support activities conducted in March and April were dental procedures, and repair and adjustment of dentures. In general, oral care and dental health guidance, and dental consultation and introduction to dental clinics were performed over the whole period and in all areas (Figure 31-4, 5 & 6).

 Consideration of dental health support activities

1 Situation at the time of support activities

In this earthquake disaster, all residents in Fukushima Prefecture, including members of dental associations, faced an unknown future due to the damage caused by the earthquake and tsunami, by the lack of information, shortages of fuel and food, and the nuclear power station accident.

On March 12, the Association received a request for dental relief activities from Fukushima Prefecture based on a cooperation agreement on disaster management that was concluded in December 2010. Although the Association took action in response to the request, Fukushima Prefecture did not provide information on evacuation centers and the number of evacuees to the Association, nor did it make necessary adjustments for municipalities. Accordingly, the Association independently began the procurement of goods, which was necessary at the initial stage of dental health relief activities, and gathered information. The Association was forced to conduct relief activities without prior arrangement by the prefecture. Moreover, the Associa-

Chapter 4 | Activities of Various Professional Organizations

tion did not reach an agreement with Fukushima Prefecture concerning who is responsible for a survey of necessary relief supplies and procurement and delivery of goods: The secretariat of the Association had to undertake these tasks instead of the prefecture. In Iwate Prefecture, a prefectural disaster response headquarters established a medical support network to share information, communicate and make adjustments with medical teams[1]. In Fukushima Prefecture, however, the disaster response headquarters was too confused to communicate due to responses to the unprecedented earthquake and the nuclear power station accidents. As a result, the Association was unable to provide systematic dental health support activities at the early stage of the disaster, and asked county and city medical associations in affected areas to conduct dental relief activities based on their independent judgment. Although members of individual county and city dental associations also faced various issues, they visited evacuation centers at an early stage after the earthquake. In addition, some county and city dental associations used holiday emergency clinics as fixed emergency clinics. Thus, dental personnel throughout Fukushima Prefecture worked to provide support to disaster victims.

2 Survey method and dental health support activities

The survey was conducted based on materials submitted by individual organizations that provided support to disaster victims. However, there were no reports about support activities in March when the earthquake occurred, although county and city dental associations did actually provided support. This was because the situation in the affected areas was very confusing. Accordingly, the detailed contents of the activities in March were unclear in some cases.

Since this earthquake caused widespread damage, county and city dental associations were required to play a central role in conducting dental health support activities in affected areas. At first, the support activities were left entirely to county and city dental associations and their members, and there were no uniform policies for support. This caused various problems as follows. Since gasoline was not secured due to a lack of logistic support, which was necessary for relief activities in affected areas, dental support teams and dental supplies were unable to be sent to evacuation centers. Relief supplies were not uniformly distributed to individual evacuation sites due to a lack of information. When dental support teams visited evacuees, the evacuees were sometimes absent from home. Even if dental support teams introduced dental clinics, evacuees did not know the way to the clinics. In addition, even if dental clinics were present, evacuees were unable to visit the clinics due to no means of transportation. Since medical coordinators for disaster management were not involved in dental relief activities in evacuation centers, people responsible for the operation of evacuation centers showed no understanding of dental support. Evacuees were unable to recognize who were dental support team members.

When medical support is provided at the time of a disaster, it is important to promptly collect information and analyze the demand for dental care and to establish support systems according to the results of analysis[2]. To this end, earthquake response manuals are indispensable, and support activities should be drawn up based on the manuals. In this earthquake, conventional manuals were inadequate to respond to the unprecedented nuclear power station accident. At first, the Association was unable to grasp the changing circumstances after the accident, and had difficulty forming support plans in line with the "responses immediately after the occurrence of disaster" included in the Dental Relief Manual for Large-scale Earthquake Management[3]. This led to confusion of support activities. Moreover, regarding the support activities in affected areas and their issues at the early stage after the earthquake, there was no feedback from the affected areas to the Association, and therefore, the Association was unable to respond as needed. This was also one of the factors that prevented information sharing and made support activities difficult.

Fukushima Dental Association

3 Results of the survey

a. Frequency of going out for relief activities

On March 11, individual dental professionals and local dental associations began to provide dental health support without a central plan. However, the situation after the nuclear power station accident was so confused that they were unable to conduct organized activities. In particular, they faced extreme difficulties conducting support activities in the Coastal Region at the early stage after the earthquake. This was due to a loss of essential utilities, a lack of supplies and information, and the risk of exposure to radiation. Consequently, the frequency of going out to conduct relief activities in March, immediately after the earthquake, was forced to be low.

From the end of March through April, dental health support activities, which were conducted mainly by the Association, went into full swing. Relief supplies began to be delivered to disaster victims. In addition, many organizations from other prefectures came to Fukushima Prefecture to provide dental health support. As the situation after the earthquake improved, support activities in evacuation centers were conducted more smoothly. Moreover, various areas in Fukushima Prefecture received evacuees from the nuclear power station accident and actively offered them support. For these reasons, the frequency of going out to conduct relief activities in this period was the highest during the entire survey period. In and after May, the frequency decreased, because dental health support activities were mainly conducted in dental clinics in a recipients' neighborhood, not evacuation centers.

b. Number of people engaged in support activities

Since 68% of the people engaged in support activities were dentists and 21% were dental hygienists, not only dental procedures but also dental health guidance was provided to disaster victims. According to reports, disaster victims were more comfortable with dental hygienists than with dentists on site. Accordingly, it was confirmed that the cooperation between dentists and dental hygienists was essential for smooth implementation of support activities.

c. Number of targets for relief activities

The number of targets for relief activities in individual areas tended to decrease in and after May. However, this did not mean that the number of disaster victims who needed assistance decreased over time, as seen with other large-scale earthquakes. The reason why the number of targets relief activities decreased was that the focus of support policies shifted from dental care support to dental health guidance.

d. Contents of support activities

At the early stage after the earthquake, the ratio of emergency dental procedures was high in evacuation centers. Among these procedures, the ratio of repair and adjustment of dentures was highest. This was because many elderly people moved to evacuation centers and needed to recover from masticatory disturbance. Mr. Yoichi Iijima indicated that people with problematic dentures had difficulty maintaining a healthy diet in evacuation centers in association with changes in food quality[4]. At this time, oral care and dental health guidance were often provided to disaster victims through visits to individual evacuation centers. These activities were conducted with the aim of preventing respiratory infection in disaster victims, especially elderly people, who were forced to live in evacuation centers for a long time. To raise awareness of the importance of oral care, posters about oral care were put up in evacuation centers.

The range of dental health support activities differed depending on areas. In areas with relatively little damage from the earthquake, dental clinics in the neighborhood of evacuation centers were judged to be able to receive disaster victims. Accordingly, the focus on support activities was placed on the introduction of nearby dental clinics from the early stage after the earthquake. This included provision of only dental consultation in evacuation centers and distribution of maps showing dental clinics in the neighborhood of evacuation centers.

C Dental care support activities in the future

In FY 2013, the Association revised its disaster response manual based on the experience and reflections from this earthquake. However, the Association needs to continue to make the manual more practical and ensure the high effectiveness of the manual in anticipation of responding to unpredictable disasters in the future. It is an important issue to clarify the position of dentistry in the medical system for disaster management in prefectural medical programs, partly to enhance cooperation with relevant organizations. In addition, it is necessary to reaffirm the significance of medical coordinators for disaster management and work to develop human resources in a systematic manner in cooperation with Fukushima Prefecture.

Although the Association encountered the unprecedented earthquake and the nuclear power station accident following the earthquake, and faced various unexpected issues, it worked to provide as much dental care support as possible. However, the reconstruction of affected areas has not yet been achieved, and it is still unclear when the problems caused by the nuclear power station accident will come to an end. Additionally, ultimate solutions to radioactive contamination issues have not been implemented. Accordingly, the Association is required to continue to offer dental care support to disaster victims.

> We would like to extend our heartfelt gratitude to relevant organizations for their support for the dental health support activities of the Fukushima Dental Association, and also express our sincere appreciation to all people involved in dental care support.

(Joji Ikeyama, Yutaka Tanaka, Masahiro Ando, Osamu Kaneko)

References
1) Toshiki Moriya, Keietsu Saigo, Hidenori Maekawa, Hideki Daikoku, Morio Hakozaki: *Recovery and Reconstruction of Dental Care Provision Function in the Coastal Region of Iwate Prefecture*. Program for the 60th General Meeting of Japanese Society of Oral Health, 83, 2011.
2) Akira Tanaka: *Dental Health Support Activities in Large-scale Disaster*. The Journal of the Japan Dental Association, vol. 62, No. 4: 2009–2007.
3) Fukushima Dental Association: *Dental Relief Manual for Large-scale Earthquake Management*, Fukushima Dental Association, 12–13, 1999.
4) Yoichi Iijima: *Dental Care Activities and Oral Care at Home (Visits) and Evacuation Centers in Affected Areas of the Great East Japan Earthquake*. Dental Diamond, 36, 149–151, 2011.

32 Fukushima Nursing Association

Two years have passed since the Great East Japan Earthquake and the accident at the Fukushima Daiichi Nuclear Power Station of the Tokyo Electric Power Company that occurred on March 11, 2011. However, many disaster victims are still unable to return to their homes. Although efforts have been made in affected areas toward the recovery from the earthquake disaster, the recovery has not gone smoothly. The earthquake and the nuclear power station accident have caused tremendous damage throughout Fukushima Prefecture, especially in terms of the social economy and assurance of medical care.

A Outline of the Fukushima Nursing Association

The Fukushima Nursing Association ("the Association") is a professional organization consisting of nursing personnel. The Association has a total of 11,487 members as of the end of March 2013, comprising 385 public health nurses, 324 midwives, 9,269 nurses, and 1,509 practical nurses. In July 24, 2012, the Nursing Hall and Nursing Training Center was established in Koriyama City. Based in the center, the Association runs training programs for its members and engages in operations related to the health and welfare of residents in Fukushima Prefecture.

On April 1, 2013, the Association commenced new activities as the Fukushima Nursing Association, Public Interest Incorporated Association.

B Contents and progress of support activities related to the earthquake

1 Survey of the damage situation

- First survey (from March 13, 2011)
  The Association conducted a survey of 114 facilities by fax to assess their damage situation, and received responses from 70 facilities. Nine facilities requested the dispatch of disaster relief nurses.
- Second survey (from March 25, 2011)
  The Association conducted a survey of 114 facilities by fax to assess their damage situation, and received responses from 48 facilities. Thirty-seven hospitals had received people from affected facilities (a total of 1,073 persons). Three facilities requested the dispatch of disaster relief nurses.
- Third survey (from May 19, 2011)
  The Association assessed the situation of affected facilities and members. As of the end of February 2012, of 846 affected members, two members had died, the homes of 97 members were entirely destroyed by fire or damaged and unlivable, those of 349 members were partially destroyed by fire or seriously damaged, those of 131 members leaned to one side, those of 10 members were inundated above the floor level, those of 16 members flowed out, and some members were forced to evacuate their homes by the evacuation order. As a result, the Association provided a total of 9.54 million yen of disaster relief money to its members. In addition, the Japanese Nursing Association offered a total of 56.3 million yen in disaster assistance grants to 58 facilities in the Soso branch and the Iwaki branch, which suffered damage due to the earthquake, the tsunami and from radiation, to support affected members.
  Moreover, many donations and relief supplies from around the country were delivered to affected mem-

Chapter 4 | Activities of Various Professional Organizations

bers and facilities.

2 Request for the dispatch of disaster relief nurses

- On March 18, in response to requests made in the survey, the Association asked the Japanese Nursing Association, a nationwide organization, to dispatch nurses to four facilities. However, the Japanese Nursing Association replied that it was unable to dispatch nurses to Fukushima Prefecture. Although the Association repeatedly asked it to dispatch nurses, it declined all requests from the Association. Later, it was revealed that the Japanese Nursing Association declined to dispatch nurses due to the nuclear power station accident.
- On March 22 and 23, the Association asked nurses to register as disaster relief nurses of the Association to commence the support activities of its disaster relief nurses.
- On March 29, Ms. Setsuko Hisatsune, President at the Japan Nursing Association, came to the Association. After visiting affected areas, she began disaster support activities for Fukushima Prefecture.

3 Situation of the dispatch of disaster relief nurses

- A total of 400 nursing staff members from 24 prefectures, who were dispatched by the Japanese Nursing Association, conducted support activities in the following places.

March 29 to April 1	Hirata Central Hospital
April 6 to 29	Big Palette Fukushima
April 10 to 16	Eight evacuation centers in Otama Village
April 10 to 29	Nasukashi National Children's Center

- A total of 64 nursing staff members mainly dispatched from neighboring prefectures (Tochigi and Chiba Prefectures)

  | May 1 to 13 | Big Palette Fukushima |

- A total of 56 nurses registered as disaster relief nurses of the Association

April 1 to 4 & 7 to 10	Tamura City General Gymnasium
April 1 to 10	Hirata Central Hospital
April 9 to 12 & 14 to 17	Iwaki Municipal Chuodai Minami Elementary School

- Research on the needs for support by public health nurses of the Japanese Nursing Association (a total of eight public health nurses)

  | From April 4 | Hara Town Public Health Center in Minamisoma City |

Based on the review of a series of support activities, the following situations were clarified.

- Since part of the information networks between the Association and individual hospitals were blocked immediately after the earthquake, the Association had difficulty collecting information on affected facilities.
- In the ever-changing circumstances of medical institutions and evacuation centers, adjustments for dispatching nurses were carried out between the Fukushima Prefecture Disaster Response Headquarters, the department in charge of dispatch of disaster relief nurses and the Japanese Nursing Association. However, it took a significant amount of time to ensure cooperation and share information between them.
- Disaster relief nurses from other prefectures took over operations in evacuation centers as nursing professionals, and provided appropriate assistance for infection control. Since norovirus infection was found in the Big Palette Fukushima, which was a large-scale evacuation center, nursing care was provided in three shifts in an infection observation room.

32 Fukushima Nursing Association

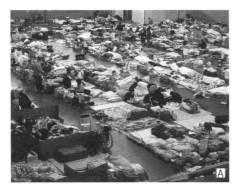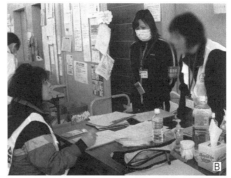

Figure 32-1 Activities of disaster relief nurses
A: Situation of an evacuation center   B: Conference for health care at a temporary shelter

The disaster relief nurses of the Association were involved in support activities from April 1 to April 17. A total of 56 nurses participated in the activities in hospitals and evacuation centers. Although the entire Fukushima Prefecture was affected by the earthquake, some facilities escaped damage from the disaster. The association asked these facilities to cooperate in dispatching nurses, while receiving patients transported from affected areas. Thus, the Association was able to achieve support activities as a professional nursing organization, through cooperation by directors of individual facilities and nursing administrators (Figure 32-1).

Here is introduced an e-mail from a disaster relief nurse from the Japanese Nursing Association (Shiga Prefecture), just for reference.

"I found that Fukushima Prefecture was hit hard by unpleasant rumors. Actually, when I was required to visit Fukushima Prefecture, I was immediately asked, "Has the situation of the nuclear power station already been controlled?" Since it was hard to distinguish between facts and rumors at the early stage of support activities, in particular, the Japanese Nursing Association might not be sure whether nurses should be dispatched to Fukushima Prefecture. However, when I saw the website of the Fukushima Nursing Association, I was very surprised and moved because residents in Fukushima Prefecture worked to support and protect their areas although they had to evacuate the areas. Although more than one month has passed since the disaster occurred, there seem to be many urgent issues, including improvement of a hygienic environment and provision of mental health care mainly in evacuation centers. I would be grateful if I can provide psychological and material support to people living as evacuees."

Meanwhile, the activities of disaster relief nurses organized by the Japanese Nursing Association were conducted by volunteer nursing professionals. Since they were required to show identification before participating in support activities, this delayed the start of their activities for victims of the nuclear power station accident, compared with disaster nurses from other prefectures. This highlighted the limits and issues in the scope of volunteer activities.

In addition, the Association felt the need to implement public relations concerning the activities of disaster relief nurses to gain the understanding of relevant organizations and persons, such as Fukushima Prefecture, municipalities, and other administrative bodies as well as social welfare councils.

Chapter 4 | Activities of Various Professional Organizations

C : Disaster support activities conducted as a general operation by the Fukushima Nursing Association

- On September 30, 2011, the Association held a discussion session with nursing administrators, in which group works were carried out to talk about how nursing administrators took action when the earthquake occurred, what the present situation was, and what were the future issues and requirements.

  In the session, various activities that nursing personnel conducted during the six months after the earthquake were reported. Some nursing personnel lived in hospitals due to a lack of gasoline for transportation. Other personnel evacuated patients from affected hospitals to safer places by using sheets instead of stretchers. All nursing personnel worked to protect the lives of evacuees. Moreover, the Association held a discussion session with nursing personnel from five local branches to have them report what activities they conducted at individual medical facilities after the earthquake. In these sessions, the following issues were clarified.
  - Some nursing personnel were evacuated due to concerns about the effects of radiation. Their absence from work led to a lack of nursing staff.
  - The stress of staff members should be considered and treated.
  - Disaster response manuals in facilities should be reviewed.
  - It is necessary to collaborate with administrative bodies in municipalities where facilities are located.
- On November 19, 2011, the Association held a joint meeting of public health nurses, midwives, and nurses. In the meeting, they reported on their activities and participated in group work to share information on activities for disaster management and establish networks between medical professionals. They reconfirmed the importance of information sharing and networks between professionals in individual areas.
- The Association conducted training workshops on radiation to support its members, and held lecture meetings to provide mental health care to nursing personnel.
- Training workshops on disaster nursing
  - At first, a training workshop on disaster nursing was planned to be conducted once in FY 2011, with prospective participants being 200. However, since numerous people applied for the workshop, the Association conducted two workshops in FY 2011, in which 452 people participated. Workshops were also conducted in FY 2012.
  - Social gatherings of disaster relief nurses

    On September 29, 2011, the Association held a social gathering for disaster relief nurses, in which a nursing staff member, who served as a disaster relief member of the Association, reported on her experience at the time of the disaster. In a situation where conflicting information was presented after the nuclear power station accident, she worked feverishly to help disaster victims; including responding to those who had bruises, became hypothermic, and drank muddy water due to the tsunami.

    Moreover, activities of disaster relief nurses, who worked in medical institutions and evacuation centers, were reported. Although they engaged in support activities separately from other disaster relief nurses, they were able to provide professional support as nursing personnel, including taking preventive measures against infectious disease.

    In FY 2012, the Association also held a lecture meeting on the theme of "What is required of nurses at the time of disaster – through the experience of evacuation activities in hospitals –." In the lecture meeting, participants learned lessons about ongoing disaster experience, such as response to disaster stress of patients and staff members and provision of mental health care, from the harrowing experience of evacuation activities in hospitals affected by the nuclear power plant accidents.

- PR magazine "*Nursing Fukushima*"

Since the occurrence of the earthquake, the Association has continuously published the "Activity Report about the Great East Japan Earthquake" in its PR magazine, which is published five times annually. The report has already been published ten times. The Association plans to report on its ongoing activities with a new theme "A Path toward Recovery."

D Outsourcing business from Fukushima Prefecture to promote measures to secure nursing staff

Under a situation where the nuclear power plant accident remains unresolved, one of the most urgent and important issues is to take measures to secure nursing personnel and prevent them from leaving their jobs, not only in the Soso and Iwaki Districts but throughout Fukushima Prefecture, to maintain the quality of health, medical and welfare services. The Association has been entrusted by Fukushima Prefecture to provide employment counseling for nursing personnel through visits to evacuation centers.

In June 2011, the Association began to hold employment counseling conferences, where nursing personnel served as advisers, while visiting various places in Fukushima Prefecture as well as Niigata and Yamagata Prefectures, where disaster victims were evacuated. As of the end of March 2012, a total of 61 conferences had been held, with a total of 110 participants. Consequently, 18 persons commenced work as nursing personnel.

In FY 2012, the Association looked for sources of employment for nurses, performed the matching of employment supply and demand, and held employment counseling conferences in three public employment security offices (Hello Work Offices) and other public institutions in Fukushima Prefecture. The Association visited 30 facilities to look for job offers, and held 46 employment counseling conferences. A total of 65 persons participated in the counseling conferences and 32 persons commenced work. In the Soso Public Employment Security Office in affected areas, 10 counseling conferences were held, with 31 persons participating and 17 persons starting work.

In FY 2013, expanding the range of activities to six districts in Fukushima Prefecture, the Association held employment counseling conferences in public employment security offices in the Fukushima, Koriyama, Shirakawa, Aizuwakamatsu, Soso and Iwaki Districts. Moreover, the Association plans to strengthen support activities in conjunction with nurse bank operations by conducting a model project for cooperation between nursing centers and public employment security offices in Fukushima, Toyama and Hyogo Prefectures.

E Health assistance projects in municipalities using health-care professionals

Like outsourcing business mentioned in the preceding section D), since January 2012 the Association has also been entrusted by Fukushima Prefecture to conduct a health assistance project for disaster victims. In this project, the Association employs public health nurses, nurses, senior nutritionists, nutritionists and dental hygienists to provide support to affected municipalities and public health and welfare offices ("health offices").

Chapter 4 — Activities of Various Professional Organizations

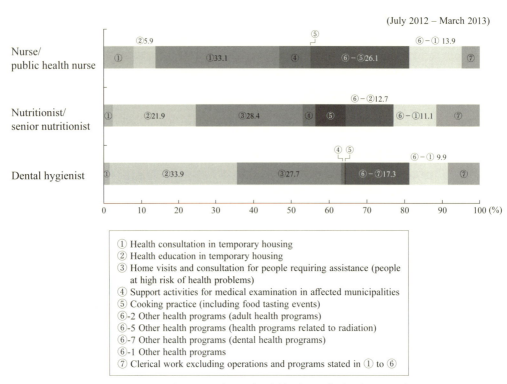

Figure 32-2 Summary of annual activities by professional personnel

In FY 2012, the Association provided assistance for health-care activities of staff members of affected prefectures (health offices) and municipalities. To this end, the Association received support from public health nurses from other prefectures (one from Hokkaido, one from Chiba Prefecture and two from Hyogo Prefecture) and employed a total 37 persons from Fukushima Prefecture, including 35 professional personnel; two public health nurses, 12 nurses, four senior nutritionists, seven nutritionists, six dental hygienists, as well as one coordinator and one clerical person. The Association conducted support activities in four cities, six towns and one village and provided assistance to four health offices and one local office. The major activities of these professional personnel were provision of health consultations and education and consultation services for people requiring assistance (people at high risk) in temporary housing. Meanwhile, public health nurses and nurses were more involved in health-care projects related to radiation (Figure 32-2).

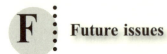

F Future issues

The Association concluded a cooperation agreement on disaster management with Fukushima Prefecture in March 2009, and created the "Disaster Relief Manual." Based on this agreement, the Association set up a disaster response headquarters and began support activities. In this disaster associated with the tsunami and the nuclear power station accident, it is necessary to take measures that take into account long-term evacuation and health-care management. These measures should continue to be examined on a national and prefectural level. Meanwhile, a review of the activities of the Association showed the following issues.

- It is necessary to improve and enhance training programs related to disaster nursing for the members of the Association and continuously cultivate disaster relief nurses.

Training programs concerning disaster nursing have already been offered. However, the contents of the training programs should be further improved and enforced, including improvement of hierarchical training programs, promotion of the members' understanding of radiation, and enhancement of nursing activities and health-care management during long-term evacuation. In addition, stress of the nursing staff should be more intensively treated.

- In long-term evacuation, it is important to establish networks between municipal health nurses and nursing administrators in individual facilities within divisional organizations in each district, aiming to promote health-care management for residents in Fukushima Prefecture.
- It is necessary to facilitate a smooth cooperation between the Association, the Fukushima Prefecture Disaster Response Headquarters, and the Japan Nursing Association. Moreover, it is also important to expand awareness of the activities and the organization/administration of the Fukushima Nursing Association after the disaster and ask for the understanding of relevant municipalities, relevant institutions such as fire and police departments, relevant organizations such as social welfare councils, and professional organizations such as medical associations and pharmacists associations. In particular, regular discussions should be conducted between medical, dental, pharmacists and nursing associations to share information and provide support.
- Since the disaster response headquarters of the Association failed to conduct organized activities, the Association should improve the organization of the headquarters, including clarifying the roles of staff members, to enable systematic activities.

Lastly, an issue that should be addressed immediately is to secure nursing staff to ensure medical treatment. However, there is not always one solution to the issue due to the seriousness of the situation, in which more young nurses and mid-career nurses with children left their jobs due to the nuclear power station accident. This was in addition to a long-term and chronic shortage of nursing staff.

The Association has consistently focused on various projects over many years as follows: 1) actively approaching high school students who want to be nursing personnel, 2) providing employment consultation for nursing staff, 3) taking measures to improve a working environment and prevent nursing staff from leaving their jobs, and 4) identifying potential nursing personnel using nurse banks. However, the Association has not yet succeeded in solving the chronic shortage of nurses.

Regarding securing nursing staff, there are limitations to improvement of the working environment and working conditions in medical institutions. Accordingly, the Association earnestly hopes that reform measures will be taken through discussions with the national government, Fukushima Prefecture and relevant organizations. Moreover, the Association intends to exert further efforts to be involved in cooperative activities as a nursing professional organization.

(Midori Suzuki)

33 Fukushimaken Association of Radiological Technologist

A : Initial response of the Fukushimaken Association of Radiological Technologist

The Fukushimaken Association of Radiological Technologist ("the Association") is designated as a protection program institution for residents in Fukushima Prefecture. The Association had its branch members participate in the Radiation Emergency Medicine Training Course, which is hosted annually by the Nuclear Safety Research Association. In the training course the members develop expertise as well as learn how to handle equipment, how to perform screening at aid stations in case of nuclear accidents and how to offer first-stage medical services for radiation exposure. Moreover, in response to a request from Fukushima Prefecture, the Association dispatched its members to the Fukushima Nuclear Disaster Drill, which was held annually by the prefecture. In the drill, the members belonged to screening teams, and their role as radiological technologists was determined by training manuals. Accordingly, when the Association learned about the accident at Fukushima Daiichi Nuclear Power Station of the Tokyo Electric Power Company ("Fukushima Daiichi Station") on March 11, it understood the urgency of the situation and the necessity of an immediate response to the accident.

In this accident, however, the Off-Site Center (OFC), a hub for emergency response in case of a nuclear disaster, was damaged by the earthquake and lost its function due to disrupted communication lines. Consequently, it was on March 13 that the Association received a call for service from the Fukushima Prefecture Disaster Response Headquarters.

Around noon of March 13, staff members of the Association were finally able to contact Mr. Kenji Suzuki, President of the Association, by phone. He asked the members to secure human resources so that three radiological technologists could be dispatched to each of the Fukushima Gender Equal Centre in Nihonmatsu City and the Koriyama General Gymnasium. The members faced difficulties in securing human resources under a situation where mobile phones and fixed-line phones were not easily connected. However, I (then Vice President) asked the Ken-nan branch to dispatch radiological technologists to the Koriyama General Gymnasium and the Fukushima Gender Equal Centre. Mr. Ikuo Watanabe, Assistant Branch Chief of the Aizu branch, asked individual facilities in Aizuwakamatsu City to secure human resources. President Kenji Suzuki made arrangements and adjustments of radiological technologists who should be dispatched to radiation screening venues mainly in Ken-poku District.

On March 13, staff members of health offices began to perform screening at the Koriyama General Gymnasium and the Fukushima Gender Equal Centre in Nihonmatsu City. In these two venues, decontamination buildings were also set up by the Self-Defense Forces. On the previous day, the Japan Association of Radiological Technologists, a higher body of the Association, had established a disaster response headquarters and had designated President Kenji Suzuki as a local director of the disaster response headquarters. Accordingly, President Kenji Suzuki visited the Fukushima Prefecture Disaster Response Headquarters in the morning and evening of March 14 to collect information and make arrangements for persons in charge of screening activities, for which individuals would be dispatched from individual organizations and relevant institutions, and classified destinations where radiological technologists should be dispatched.

Gasoline and other fuels began to run short around March 12. This made it more difficult to secure human resources. While asking various facilities to dispatch radiological technologists, the Association obtained information that some radiological technologists stood by at home because they were unable to go to work due to suspension of train services, no supply of gasoline, and damage of facilities. The Association asked these radiological technologists to work at radiation screening venues near their homes. However, the Fukushima Prefecture Disaster Response Headquarters did not function smoothly at first, and there was confusion concerning the dispatch of radiological technologists to screening venues.

For the dispatch of radiological technologists in Fukushima Prefecture, a system was established in which President Kenji Suzuki attended meetings at the Radiation Emergency Medicine Management Office at the Fukushima Prefecture Disaster Response Headquarters in the morning and evening every day and gave instructions to the Association after exchanging information and arranging schedules for personnel assignment at the meetings.

On March 16, the Japan Association of Radiological Technologists commenced to dispatch its personnel to provide support.

B : Screening activities for emergency radiation exposure

Table 33-1 shows 13 permanent screening venues in Fukushima Prefecture that were set up on March 13. The Radiation Emergency Medicine Management Office made adjustments and arrangements for personnel in charge of individual venues who were dispatched from associations of radiological technologists as well as associations of electric power companies and national universities across the country, from municipalities, the Fukushima prefectural government, local finance bureaus of the Ministry of Finance, and health offices in Fukushima Prefecture and its municipalities.

The basic principle of screening is to ensure the safety and security of residents. Until March 13, the standard for decontamination had been 13,000 cpm or higher levels according to the manuals, at which level decontamination of the whole body was required. However, the standard value was raised on March 14 due to emergency circumstances, where those exposed to less than 13,000 cpm of radiation required no decontamination, those exposed to 13,000 cpm to 100,000 cpm of radiation required decontamination by removing clothes and partial decontamination of the body, and those exposed to 100,000 cpm or higher of radiation required decontamination of the whole body. In addition, since the radiation levels of water discharged during the decontamination process were expected to have no impact on the environment, the water was handled as general wastewater.

Table 33-1 Permanent screening venues established on March 13

Ken-poku	Fukushima City: Azuma General Gymnasium Nihonmatsu City: Fukushima Gender Equal Centre (decontamination facility) Kawamata Town: Kawamata Town Health Center
Ken-chu	Koriyama City: Koriyama General Gymnasium (decontamination facility), Big Palette Fukushima Sukagawa City: Ken-chu Public Health and Welfare Office Tamura City: Tamura City General Gymnasium
Ken-nan	Shirakawa City: Ken-nan Public Health and Welfare Office
Aizu	Aizuwakamatsu City: Aizu Dome in the Aizu Athletic Park, University of Aizu
Soso	Minamisoma City: Soso Public Health and Welfare Office
Iwaki	Iwaki City: Iwaki City Public Health Center, Nakoso High School

Chapter 4 | Activities of Various Professional Organizations

At first, screening was performed only for persons, clothes and goods that were always close at hand, such as hand luggage. However, as the necessity for screening of residents decreased, residents brought pets and various goods that were not normally regarded as a target for screening. Accordingly, the Radiation Emergency Medicine Management Office set the following standards, because it would be unable to respond to all requests for screening unless a certain screening standard was established.

1. Screening is performed for private cars that have been left within a 20-km radius from the Fukushima Daiichi Station, because their counts are high.
2. Screening is performed for pets accompanying family members.
3. Screening is not necessary for vegetables, because (GM counter-type) survey meters can measure only radiation on their surface, and accurate assessment cannot be made.
4. Screening of industrial products is performed in the Fukushima Technology Centre, Koriyama City.

Moreover, the Nuclear Emergency Response Headquarters of the national government tightened the screening standard for goods that evacuated residents took out of homes in evacuation areas, which were within a 20-km radius from the Fukushima Daiichi Station, when they temporarily returned home for the second time. The standard value for decontamination was restored from 100,000 cpm to 13,000 cpm on September 16.

The Association started full-fledged operations in individual screening venues on March 14. Table 33-2 shows the number of personnel who were dispatched by the Association and the number of people who received screening in March.

Table 33-2 Breakdown of the number of radiological technologists dispatched by the Fukushimaken Association of Radiological Technologists and screening

Date	No. of screening venues	No. of dispatched personnel	No. of people who received screening	13,000 to 100,000 cpm	100,000 cpm or higher	100,000 cpm or higher in all venues
March 13	1	4	27	0	0	0
March 14	4	14	1,517	0	0	2
March 15	6	20	4,711	41	0	5
March 16	5	17	3,535	137	4	6
March 17	9	22	3,314	22	0	43
March 18	7	27	2,620	40	1	39
March 19	9	28	2,196	25	1	1
March 20	5	22	1,519	7	0	0
March 21	4	22	1,124	2	0	1
March 22	4	18	1,584	33	0	1
March 23	3	9	718	3	0	0
March 24	3	7	765	2	0	0
March 25	3	8	767	1	0	0
March 26	2	4	510	2	0	0
March 27	2	5	512	0	0	1
March 28	2	3	425	0	0	2
March 29	2	3	404	4	0	1
March 30	2	3	431	0	0	0
March 31	2	3	465	3	0	0
Total	75	239	27,144	322	6	102

Screening was performed in a total of 75 venues, where a total of 239 radiological technologists were dispatched. A total of 27,144 persons received screening, among whom there were 322 persons whose radiation level was 13,000 cpm to 100,000 cpm and six persons whose radiation level was 100,000 cpm or higher.

From March 14 through 16, a very high number of evacuees visited screening venues and that made for long waiting lines from opening to closing. In the screening venue at the University of Aizu, where many evacuees visited, screening did not end until 3:00 am of March 15. In April, a total of 34 radiological technologists were dispatched to a total of 17 venues, where 1,560 persons received screening. There was nobody whose radiation level was 13,000 cpm or higher.

Although certificates of screening were issued to those who received screening, their specifications were not unified and were handled differently among venues at first. In the Koriyama General Gymnasium, although certificates were not issued on March 14, those with the seal of the director of the Koriyama City Public Health Center were issued from March 15 to the morning of March 17, and those with the seal of Fukushima Prefecture were issued from the afternoon of March 17. In the Fukushima Gender Equal Centre, only slips, where a screening date was rubber-stamped, were delivered and no certificates were issued on March 14 and 15. Then, certificates with the stamp of Fukushima Prefecture were issued from March 16. Meanwhile, in another venue, certificates with the signature of the person who performed screening were issued by the Fukushima Prefecture Disaster Response Headquarters. The national government issued a notice that the issuance of a certificate of screening was not recommended because it might lead to discrimination against those who did not receive screening. In fact, however, those who came from evacuation order areas were not allowed to live in temporary housing, nor did they receive medical care in medical facilities, if they were unable to provide evidence that they were not contaminated. Taking into account these disadvantages, Fukushima Prefecture continued to issue certificates of screening.

In the screening that the Association preformed for two months, there was no case where radiation had an impact on health. The radiation level of all people that received screening fell below the standard value when their radiation level was measured after they took off their clothes or were decontaminated. The Association was involved in screening in a total of 35 permanent venues and evacuation centers in Fukushima Prefecture, in cooperation with associations of electric power companies and staff members of Fukushima Prefecture and municipalities. Then, based on a policy that encouraged the decrease of the number of venues, screening venues where less than 100 persons had visited were closed and integrated into other sites. By the end of October, screening was performed only in health offices in individual areas.

Although the Association was located in Fukushima Prefecture, where the nuclear power station accident occurred, it had difficulty securing personnel for screening over a long period, because local personnel were also affected by the earthquake. Accordingly, the Association recruited volunteers from across the country to dispatch them to affected areas, in cooperation with the earthquake disaster response headquarters of the Japan Association of Radiological Technologists.

Table 33-3 is the outline of screening personnel dispatched by the Japan Association of Radiological Technologists. The Japan Association of Radiological Technologists set up an earthquake disaster response headquarters on March 12 immediately after the nuclear power station accident, with President Yasuo Nakazawa serving as a director. On March 13, it urgently recruited screening personnel and secured survey meters (GM counter-type) as requested by the Japan Atomic Energy Commission, Cabinet Office, and the Guidance of Medical Service Division, Ministry of Health, Labour and Welfare. On March 16, in response

Chapter 4 | Activities of Various Professional Organizations

Table 33-3 Breakdown of radiological technologists dispatched by the Japan Association of Radiological Technologists

Name of crew	Period of dispatch (2011)	No. of dispatched personnel	Prefecture
1st crew	March 16 – 21	12	Hokkaido, Akita: 2; Tokyo, Saitama: 2; Kanagawa 5; Kagawa
2nd crew	March 21 – 25	5	Chiba: 5
3rd crew	March 22 – 27	4	Tokyo, Okayama, Tokushima: 2
4th crew	March 25 – 29	4	Saitama, Tokyo, Oita: 2
5th crew	March 26 – 31	5	Gifu: 5
6th crew	March 28 – April 1	4	Fukui: 4
7th crew	March 31 – April 4	4	Kyoto: 4
8th crew	April 2 – 7	4	Hyogo: 4
9th crew	April 6 – 10	5	Yamaguchi: 5
10th crew	April 9 – 14	4	Niigata: 2; Kanagawa: 2
11th crew	April 13 – 17	4	Kagawa: 4
Total	60 days	55	17 prefectures

to a request for cooperation from the Radiation Emergency Medicine Management Office, it dispatched the first crew, which consisted of 12 radiological technologists with President Tetsuo Tosa of the Akita Association of Radiological Technologists serving as a leader. It dispatched 55 radiological technologists from 17 prefectures, ranging from Hokkaido in the north to Oita Prefecture in the south. The dispatch lasted a total of 60 days from the first crew dispatched on March 16 to the 11th crew dispatched on April 17. These crew members of the Japan Association of Radiological Technologists performed screening in a total of 10 permanent screening venues and evacuation centers. The number of people who received screening was 15,600, among whom there were 82 persons whose radiation level was 13,000 cpm to 100,000 cpm and two persons whose radiation level was 100,000 cpm or higher. On and after April 18, the Japan Association of Radiological Technologists temporarily stopped the dispatch of screening personnel, because its original goal was achieved. It planned to resume the dispatch according to the situation of temporary home visits and secondary evacuation of residents, while making adjustments with associations of electric power companies throughout the country and the Ministry of Education, Culture, Sports, Science and Technology, which also dispatched radiological technologists.

C Screening before a postmortem examination of bodies

On April 7, the search for dead bodies was commenced within a 20-km radius from the Fukushima Daiichi Station, which was designated as an evacuation area after the accident. On April 8, the Fukushima Prefectural Police Headquarters requested the Japan Association of Radiological Technologists to perform screening before a postmortem examination of bodies. The screening of dead bodies began on April 11 in Soma City, Minamisoma City and Namie Town. From April 11 to 14, chief technologist Shunji Shimada, technologist Tatsuo Hanai and technologist Yuki Kumemoto were dispatched as the first crew members from Minamisoma City General Hospital in Fukushima Prefecture. The second and later crew members comprised volunteers who were recruited from across the country. A total screening period, from the first crew to the 14th crew, which was dispatched on June 14, was 69 days, and a total of 28 radiological technologists from 15 prefectures were dispatched during the period.

Table 33-4 shows the situation of screening activities before a postmortem examination of bodies, which

Table 33-4 Screening before a postmortem examination

Name of crew	Dispatch period	No. of dispatched personnel & prefecture	Venue of a postmortem examination	No. of dead bodies
1st crew	April 11 – 14	Fukushima: 3	Namie Town (Tsushima Junior High School), Minamisoma City General Sports Center, old factory site of Alps Electric Co., Ltd.	62
2nd crew	April 15 – 19	Okayama: 2; Toyama:1	Minamisoma City General Sports Center, old factory site of Alps Electric Co., Ltd.	118
3rd crew	April 20 – 24	Tokushima: 3		30
4th crew	April 25 – 29	Chiba: 2		32
5th crew	April 30 – May 4	Nagano: 2		34
6th crew	May 5 – 9	Kagoshima: 2		26
7th crew	May 10 – 14	Mie: 2		22
8th crew	May 15 – 17	Fukuoka: 2		8
9th crew	May 20 – 24	Shizuoka: 3		12
10th crew	May 25 – 29	Kumamoto: 2		0
11th crew	May 30 – June 3	Yamagata: 3		0
12th crew	June 4 – 8	Fukushima: 1; Saga: 1		
13th crew	June 9 – 13	Nara: 2		
14th crew	June 14 – 18	Fukui: 2		
Total	69 days	15 prefectures: 28 persons		344

was commenced on April 11. Dose measurement of bodies before a postmortem examination was carried out in Namie Town (Tsushima Junior High School), Minamisoma City (Minamisoma City General Sports Center), and Soma City (the old factory site of Alps Electric Co., Ltd.). The dose of a total of 344 dead bodies was measured as of June 3. Although dose measurements were carried out for a maximum of 30 dead bodies per day, the screening was distressing because some bodies had lost body parts or had decomposed and the bodies were decaying over time.

D : Future activities and expected roles

Since the occurrence of the earthquake, radiological technologists have been involved in radiation emergency medicine in response to various requests. However, what is introduced here is only the summary of the activities of the Fukushimaken Association of Radiological Technologist ("the Association") and a part of all the activities that its members have been committed to. The response of radiological technologists to the nuclear power station accident caused by the earthquake was not limited to screening. They were required to respond to the accident as experts on radiation in their individual workplace, and played a central role in addressing concerns of residents and securing their safety.

In individual areas, they conducted various activities related to radiation protection, including communicating knowledge on radiation, delivering lectures, providing consultations and performing decontamination, while making use of their expertise about radiation. They will be required to take such action in the future and must respond to the requests.

Nuclear reactors where the accident occurred are getting cool, and the situation after the accident is gradually returning to normal. Accordingly, the role of radiological technologists will change in the future. Radiological technologists have been involved in radiation emergency medicine, including providing support for smooth evacuation, and addressing concerns of residents. However, their next challenge will be to secure the safety and security of residents in a situation where they have to coexist with radiation over a

| Chapter 4 | Activities of Various Professional Organizations |

long period. Under these circumstances, what can they do? Although decontamination is given top priority as an emergency measure at the moment, too much focus seems to be placed on numerical values of dose. In addition to decontamination, what is needed in the future is for accurate information to be provided to make a correct assessment of the situation regarding radiation, and see that appropriate measures are taken depending on the situation.

When radiation exposure is monitored on a continuous basis, measurement of not only external exposure, but also internal exposure is required. In Fukushima Prefecture, there are many whole- body counters, most of which are operated and managed by radiological technologists. If they are also involved in quality control of the whole-body counters, they will be able to provide data, while ensuring consistency between facilities.

The nuclear power station accident caused by the earthquake was an unprecedented event. Although the Association has provided support by making full use of its organizational strength and human resources, it frequently operated under confusing conditions. The improvement of emergency contact and collaboration systems is also a challenge for the future.

By responding to this nuclear accident as an expert on radiation, I became keenly aware of the seriousness of the responsibility of radiological technologists, who have a national qualification. The Association intends to pursue its studies to carry out its mission as an expert group on radiation and respond to the mandate of residents in Fukushima Prefecture.

(Yasuo Saito)

References
1) Yasuo Saito: *Summary of Screening Activities for Emergency Radiation Exposure*. Fukushima Prefecture Health and Hygiene Magazine, vol. 21, No. 2: 24–28, Fukushima branch of the Japan Public Health Association, 2012
2) Japan Association of Radiological Technologists: *Response to the Great East Japan Earthquake – Efforts for the Fukushima Daiichi Nuclear Power Station Accident – Interim Report*. 2012

34 Fukushima Pharmacists Association

 Summary of the nuclear power station accident

The Great East Japan Earthquake, which occurred on March 11, 2011, caused an unprecedented catastrophe to coastal areas in Iwate, Miyagi and Fukushima Prefectures. The earthquake and tsunami destroyed and washed away many houses, killed approximately 30,000 people and affected approximately 0.35 million residents. On March 12, a hydrogen explosion occurred at the Fukushima Daiichi Nuclear Power Station of the Tokyo Electric Power Company ("Fukushima Daiichi Station"), which was located in the Coastal Region. The explosion destroyed a nuclear reactor building and caused meltdown in a nuclear reactor. The Nuclear Power Station office performed ventilation of the nuclear reactor to reduce the pressure inside. This led to release of a large amount of radioactive contaminants into the air. Consequently, radioactive contaminants were widely scattered. On the same day, 70,000 to 80,000 residents in Futaba County (Hirono Town, Naraha Town, Tomioka Town, Kawauchi Village, Okuma Town, Futaba Town, Namie Town, and Katsurao Village), Soma County (Shinchi Town and Iitate Village) and their surrounding municipalities were forced to urgently evacuate the areas and moved to municipalities in the Central Region. Radioactive materials formed plumes; a cloud of air including gaseous and particulate substances. The plumes diffused, moving downwind, and scattered radioactive materials in various areas in Japan because of strong winds. Soon, many hot spots (places with high radiation levels) were found in fields, mountains and residential areas in other prefectures.

After the accident, even experts on nuclear studies offered different views about released radiation levels. Moreover, the national government did not seem to present correct information. Accordingly, residents in Fukushima Prefecture, who did not receive accurate information, lived with fear and had concerns about radioactive contaminants without gaining knowledge and understanding of them. Fear about radioactive materials, which contaminated fields, mountains and, residential areas in Fukushima Prefecture, gradually grew stronger. This led to deep anxiety of residents, harmful rumors, and economic problems.

Residents in Fukushima Prefecture, especially expectant mothers, babies and little children, and younger-generation parents with children, who were afraid of exposure to radioactive contaminants and health damage, gradually moved out of the prefecture. According to the survey conducted by Fukushima Prefecture, 53,277 residents were reported to be evacuated outside the prefecture as of July 4, 2013. Although two years have passed since the earthquake occurred, the total population of Fukushima Prefecture continues decreasing. This reduces residents' motivation for economic activities and production. Meanwhile, as residents live as evacuees for a longer period of time, more people feel distressed in an unfamiliar environment and require psychological care. In addition, there are an increasing number of disaster-related deaths due to physical deconditioning and emotional distress. Although residents in Fukushima Prefecture have made efforts to recover from the earthquake, they will still have to face radiation issues over many generations in an environment contaminated by radioactive materials.

 Initial responses at the occurrence of the earthquake

The Fukushima Pharmacists Association ("the Association") offered the following responses at the early

Chapter 4 — Activities of Various Professional Organizations

stage of the nuclear accident.

- Establishing a disaster response headquarters of the Association
- Building a collaborative system with the Fukushima Prefecture Disaster Response Headquarters
- Concluding a cooperation agreement for disaster management with Fukushima Prefecture
- Instructing the secretariat of the Association to serve as a supervising center and take the leadership role
- Issuing instructions to prepare for distribution and arrangement of stable iodine preparations (in response to a request for arranging stable iodine preparations)
- Confirming the safety of its member pharmacies and their information and engaging in other operations (checking evacuation destinations)
- Conducting a conference with Fukushima Medical University and regional hospitals to talk about medical cooperation
- Asking for permission to give special treatment to emergency medical transport vehicles and issuance of permits
- Asking for issuance of certificates for refueling priority vehicles (from the Fukushima Prefecture Disaster Response Headquarters)
- Building a system to communicate and work together with pharmaceutical wholesalers
- Granting permission to prepare drugs based on prescription records and drug information lists without prescriptions (also allowing pharmacists to choose original drugs or generic drugs with the same indications with the agreement of clinics and hospitals)
- Asking medical institutions to issue prescriptions after prescribing drugs to patients
- Selecting core pharmacies and asking them to prescribe drugs (pharmacies where several pharmacists work)
- Compiling the number of evacuees and the name of facilities and municipalities where they were evacuated
- Requesting the Japan Pharmaceutical Association to dispatch pharmacists in association with medical relief operations in a disaster (attaching an agreement with the Governor of Fukushima Prefecture)
- Requesting the Japan Pharmaceutical Association to dispatch directors in charge of disaster management
- Securing accommodations for pharmacists dispatched from other prefectures (by the secretariat of the Association at the expense of the Association)
- Organizing pharmacies that provide logistic support (pharmacies where several pharmacists work)
- Visiting affected areas and having discussion with administrative bodies by the president of the Association (what is required of pharmacists associations)
- Summarizing requests to the national government and submitting formal requests for issuance of reconstruction bonds at the national budget level and establishment of a welfare tax through a Diet member elected from Fukushima Prefecture (Liberal Democratic Party), who served as a special adviser to the Association
- Discussing medical cooperation with public health and welfare offices ("health offices") in local areas, county and city medical associations and nursing associations in local areas
- Discussing requests for the dispatch of pharmacists associated with medical relief operations with the Japan Pharmaceutical Association
- Recruiting and dispatching volunteer pharmacists who would engage in sorting drugs and goods which were sent for support purposes at storage depots for drugs (logistics)
- Asking for stocking of relief supplies and drugs and delivering them (facilities of the Fukushima Prefectural Board of Education)
- Responding to requests for ordering take-along drugs in cooperation with pharmacist teams
- Using drugs, which were stocked at pharmacies operated by the Association, to compensate for the lack of drugs in evacuation facilities in the Ken-poku medical district (providing drugs to medical association

teams in individual public health centers)

- Providing support for purchasing and delivering drugs to be used by individual medical teams
- Responding to requests for securing pharmacists who would accompany individual medical teams
- Responding to requests for dispatching pharmacists from health offices in individual areas in Fukushima Prefecture
- Sending drugs and goods to health offices after they were sorted
- Attending meetings of medical teams, which were held at individual health offices every morning

These are the time-series responses that the secretariat and the disaster response headquarters of the Association offered cooperatively after the occurrence of the disaster. The following are issues to be addressed urgently in the future.

(Activities toward the future)

- Training radiation pharmacists and establishing a committee of them
- Recruiting and registering pharmacists who can accompany medical teams in case of disaster, and organizing teams
- Conducting programs that promote residents' understanding and awareness of the necessity of prescription records and drug information lists
- Training pharmacists who understand all about ethical drugs, herbal drugs and over-the-counter drugs, and can give an explanation of them
- Preparing stable iodine preparations

C ⋮ Radiation pharmacists

① Purpose of the activities of radiation pharmacists

The members of the Association aim to contribute to public health by actively and continuously pursuing their studies of radioactive materials in an academic and systematic manner and accurately conveying information to residents in Fukushima Prefecture, while making use of their academic skills and qualities as pharmacists, concerning various issues that residents face after the nuclear power station accident.

② Significance of the establishment of a committee

Pharmacists have (academic) qualifications to explain a radiation disaster.

- It is necessary to understand physics, chemistry, biology, epidemiology and clinical sciences to some extent to talk about the biological effect of radiation.
- Organic chemistry and biochemistry are necessary to explain the impact of the physical energy of radiation.
- The movement of radioactive materials, such as cesium, can be grasped by using inorganic chemistry and pharmacodynamics.
- The public can easily understand the biological effect of radiation, when the impact of radiation on food ingredients is contrasted based on the knowledge of environmental hygienics and food hygienics.

Only pharmacy training covers all these academic disciplines (physics, chemistry, biology, epidemiology, clinical sciences, organic chemistry, biochemistry, inorganic chemistry, pharmacodynamics, environmental hygienics, and food chemistry).

③ Vocational aptitudes

- Pharmacists have a shallow but wide knowledge in various areas.
- Pharmacists implement a practical science.

- Pharmacists have a habit of scrutinizing information.
- Pharmacists understand the stochastic effects on an empirical basis.
- Pharmacists are experts on chemical substances and living bodies.
- Pharmacists are medical scientists with a background of a scientific mind.

(Based on the lecture by Dr. Ishihara, National Institute of Radiological Sciences)

For the reasons ① to ③ mentioned above, pharmacists should and/or can be involved in environmental issues and food safety in terms of medical and health care. In particular, since pharmacists are engaged in health management and environmental issues for students through their operations as school pharmacists, they can support healthy lives of children. From these perspectives, the Association established a sub-committee within the Pharmaceutical Care Committee to hold frequent training workshops, with the aim of fostering pharmacists, for the first time in Japan, who have detailed knowledge of radioactive materials and their adverse effects.

The Association will address this challenge on a priority basis to eliminate the anxiety of residents in Fukushima Prefecture.

D Stock and distribution of stable iodine preparations

1 Medication of stable iodine preparations

When the nuclear accident occurred at the Fukushima Daiichi Station, gaseous radioactive materials were released into the air. These materials included rare gases, such as krypton and xenon, and volatile radioactive iodine (^{131}I), which might have an impact on the human body. As released radioactive plumes (radioactive clouds) were moving and spreading, their concentration of radioisotopes was deceasing. Given the weather conditions at the time, however, there was a possibility of external exposure, in which people might directly receive radiation from these plumes, and internal exposure, in which people might take in radioactive materials by breathing and from eating contaminated food. This threatened to have an adverse impact on the health of residents over wide areas. In particular, thyroid exposure to radioactive iodine was regarded as being most risky. Accordingly, appropriate measures were required to be immediately taken. Although the national government should have urgently taken measures for residents who might be exposed to radiation when the nuclear accident occurred on March 12, it did not even give instructions to take stable iodine preparations.

Physicians at Fukushima Medical University Hospital, a director of the pharmaceutical department at the hospital and the Association worried about thyroid cancer based on a report on the incidence rate of thyroid cancer after the Chernobyl nuclear power plant accident. Learning from the past case where Poland, which is adjacent to Belarus, took swift action to administer iodine, they were communicating with each other while waiting for the national government and Fukushima Prefecture to give instructions to administer stable iodine preparations to residents in Fukushima Prefecture. However, no instructions were provided, and all that they could do was to dispense stable iodine preparations, prepare for their distribution and wait for instructions. On March 12 and 13 in Kawamata Town, Miharu Town and part of Iwaki City, stable iodine preparations were administered to thousands of residents and evacuees coming from towns where the nuclear power station was located; as is described in the Fukushima Prefecture Radiation Emergency Medical Care Manual. It was not until much later that Fukushima Prefecture gave instructions not to administer stable iodine preparations and to collect them. During the few days after the nuclear accident, some evacuees obtained information on iodine preparations from the Internet, bought Isodine gargle solution, Isodine solution for external use, and Potassium Iodide tablets from the Internet market and at drugstores and pharmacies, and took them, while sometimes diluting them. Preventive administration of stable iodine preparations, by which stable iodine is taken into the body in advance, is effective in preventing accumulation of radioactive iodine inhaled from the outside air in the thyroid gland and it reduces exposure to radiation in the thyroid area. Quite a few people seemed to know this fact after obtaining information from the Internet.

However, stable iodine preparations have no effect on internal organs other than the thyroid gland, or on internal and external exposure to any type of radioactive material. It is important to publicize the fact that stable iodine preparations are not a panacea for protection against radiation. The national government and Fukushima Prefecture should prepare countermeasures against nuclear disaster, while assuming every possible situation.

2　Storing of stable iodine preparations

It is necessary to oblige prefectures and municipalities where nuclear power stations are located to store stable iodine preparations that are sufficient for the number of residents under the age of 40 living within approximately a 5- to 10-km radius from the power stations. In addition, three days' worth of stable iodine preparations should be reserved for residents within a 30-km radius from the power stations.

At the same time, powdered stable iodine preparations, purified water and simply syrup (flavoring agents) should also be stored for babies and little children and those who cannot swallow pills. Health insurance pharmacies and drug wholesalers are suitable for storing these medical goods. This is because pharmacies have grinders for tablets and pills and dispensing equipment. Moreover, pharmacists capable of dispensing drugs work at pharmacies. Since they have received nuclear disaster drills and training programs, they can act calmly.

3　Prescription records

When the nuclear accident occurred on March 11, 2011, residents who lived in towns where the nuclear power station was located and in neighboring municipalities urgently evacuated the areas on the same day and moved to facilities in municipalities in the Central Region in Fukushima Prefecture. As soon as they were placed in facilities, patients with chronic disease and parents with pediatric patients began to visit several hospitals and clinics in search of drugs that they had taken or used. After the earthquake, however, the water supply was shut off due to broken water pipes, and the power supply was also cut off. The supply of gasoline was stopped, and the damage to essential utilities and transportation persisted. In addition, many hospitals and clinics were unable to provide medical care due to the evacuation of staff members. In such a chaotic situation, a great number of affected patients, as well as general patients, who did not have their prescriptions became very anxious and rushed to dispensing pharmacies in search of drugs. The number of patients who came to dispensing pharmacies was five times as many as during ordinary times, and the waiting rooms were full of these patients. This made them more anxious. To respond to this situation, the disaster response headquarters of the Fukushima Pharmacists Association held a council on March 13 with the president, physicians and staff members at the Medical Affairs Department of Fukushima Medical University Hospital as well as medical institutions that dealt with the issuance of prescriptions. Consequently, they reached a consensus that dispensing pharmacies were able to prepare a week's worth of drugs based on electronic drug history lists, handwritten drug history lists, prescription records and drug

Chapter 4 | Activities of Various Professional Organizations

information lists, even if outpatients did not have prescriptions. Although dispensing pharmacies were then allowed to prepare two to four weeks' worth of drugs to eliminate congestion, the situation continued to be confusing until April.

In this disaster, prescription records and drug information lists that patients brought with them were of much help for identifying a patient's disease, and for preparing drugs and dispensing drugs at medical institutions and dispensing pharmacies. This was attributed to the guidance of pharmacists throughout the country. They had repeatedly introduced case examples on a daily basis, in which prescription records played a major role in protecting the lives of disaster victims in the Great Hanshin-Awaji Earthquake and the Mid Niigata Prefecture Earthquake, and had promoted public understanding of the importance of prescription records. It may be no exaggeration to say that prescription records supported patients and their family members as well as dispensing and medical services in local areas, prevented the breakdown of medical care, saved the lives of affected patients and relieved their family members.

Accordingly, I proposed that the Association should utilize television spots to promote the understanding of all residents in Fukushima Prefecture of the necessity of keeping prescription records. The Association was determined to continue this project for two years and asked all TV stations in Fukushima Prefecture for cooperation. It is six months since our message was broadcast in television spots. This has enhanced understanding of residents and patients in Fukushima Prefecture, and they have come to present their prescription records together with prescriptions to receptionists. The TV spot broadcast was realized thanks to the understanding and support of medical and dental associations. Health insurance pharmacies have long desired that all patients actively utilize prescription records, as described here. I expect that prescription records will be of help to patients not only at the time of a disaster but also during ordinary times and serve as a bridge between patients and medical institutions.

Researchers and experts are now issuing a warning that a Tonankai earthquake will occur in the near future. The Ministry of Health, Labour and Welfare should immediately publicize the necessity of prescription records to ensure the lives, safety and security of the public.

(Hideo Sakurai)

35 Fukushima Physical Therapy Association

Not only the large-scale earthquake and tsunami but also the unprecedented nuclear power station accident made a significant impact on the health of residents in Fukushima Prefecture. Residents who lived near the Fukushima Daiichi Nuclear Power Station of the Tokyo Electric Power Company ("Fukushima Daiichi Station"), were forced to evacuate their homes and live as evacuees. Inconvenient lives as evacuees undermined the physical and mental health of residents and gradually decreased their activity. Physical therapists placed special emphasis on support for preventing impairment of their motor ability and secondary complications associated with this in limited settings, such as evacuation centers and temporary housing.

A Disaster support activities immediately after the earthquake

Immediately after the earthquake occurred, it was imperative to collect information to understand the current conditions. The Fukushima Physical Therapy Association set up a disaster response headquarters to gather information on how many evacuees were there and where they were distributed in Fukushima Prefecture, and to know the actual circumstances of evacuees. There were 344 evacuation centers in Fukushima Prefecture, of which 87 evacuation centers received more than 100 evacuees. According to surveys conducted in evacuation centers, it was revealed that there were many elderly people with internal complaints and motor system diseases and many frail elderly people in the evacuation centers. An inconvenient living environment and poor nutrition and hygiene in evacuation centers gradually deprived evacuees of opportunities to take exercise and encouraged them to lead inactive lives. This involved a great risk of increasing the incidence of disuse syndrome, and was regarded as a major issue.

B Disaster support activities at the intermediate stage

Based on the survey results, the Fukushima Physical Therapy Association began to perform individual screening in evacuation centers. Members of the association identified what elements were actually disturbing the lives of people in evacuation centers, and worked to eliminate these elements in cooperation with local staff members, while responding to individual abilities and obstacles. The members considered a wide variety of people, ranging from people who suffered the aftereffects of strokes and those who became inactive due to dementia to those at high risk for secondary complications from impaired motor function and inactivity. The members focused on maintaining and increasing their motor function and ability, including suggesting the use of sticks and walking aids, and creating an environment that enabled people to move more easily. Through these activities, an environment that caused a decline in people's motor ability was found to be one of the major problems in evacuation centers.

C Disaster support activities at the later stage

As evacuees' living places shifted from evacuation centers to temporary housing, new problems arose. Since temporary housing had limited space and equipment, this caused damage to the motor ability of evacuees. Limited living conditions, such as a difference in levels of the floors and small bathrooms, definitely narrowed the range of daily activities of evacuees. Physical therapists continuously provided support as a member of the Fukushima Professional Team for Counseling and Support (Fukushima Care Manager Association, Fukushima Association of Certified Social Workers, Fukushima Society of Medical Social Workers, Fukushima Association of Psychiatric Social Workers, Fukushima Physical Therapy Association, and Fukushima Association of Occupational Therapists). They focused on promoting regional assistance, while responding to individual needs and providing general and comprehensive assistance, such as installation of railings, adjustment of a living environment, and support for a transition to local nursing-care insurance services. People need to maintain their goals and role in life. Moreover, healthy bodies and high motivation are essential for them to lead lives according to individual's motor ability, activity and purpose in life. For evacuees living in temporary housing and municipally-subsidized housing, it is necessary to continue to consider how to provide support to them from the perspectives of not only motor function but also maintenance and expansion of activity, so that they can live more independent lives in their own fashion.

D Rehabilitation continuing into the future

There are four stages in disaster countermeasures; initial responses, emergency measures, restoration, and revival. What is important is whether we can resolve issues at hand and promptly start action toward the future, and whether we can present visions for the future. Although individual rehabilitation in the area of medical and nursing care was required immediately after the earthquake, the focus of the rehabilitation will shift to regional development. The process toward revival can be said to be rehabilitation itself, in which it is crucial for physical therapists to play their respective roles. In particular, it is extremely important to rebuild health-care and nursing systems (revitalize regions) with a focus on regional residents. The Fukushima Physical Therapy Association intends to make the utmost effort for restoration and revival from the disaster and throw its energy into realizing a secure and safe society.

(Kazuyuki Yamaguchi, Hidenori Oriuchi)

36 Fukushima Association of Occupational Therapists

A Initial responses (confirmation of the safety of members)

The disaster response manual of the Fukushima Association of Occupational Therapists ("the Association") states that the Association shall promptly establish a disaster response headquarters in case of a disaster, with the President of the Association serving as Director-general, and respond to the disaster. However, President Koji Okamoto worked at a hospital located in the Central Region, and the hospital suffered serious damage from the earthquake. Since Mr. Takayuki Kimura, Chief of the Secretariat of the Association, and I worked in the Aizu Region which suffered relatively little damage, we took the initiative in setting up a disaster response headquarters and began to confirm the safety of members. Since phone and e-mail connections became bad immediately after the earthquake and many members were evacuated to inland areas, such as Fukushima City, Koriyama City, and outside Fukushima Prefecture, we had great difficulty making contact with members. In particular, we were scarcely able to grasp the situation of members in the Futaba District, which was designated as an evacuation area. In fact, we confirmed the safety of members using a check list, mainly based on secondhand information from other members saying "Mr. A said that he had seen Ms. B at an evacuation center." This was necessary because there were few members who were able to be directly contacted by phone and e-mail. With the fear of radiation, the chief of the Iwaki branch continued to send detailed information to us on a daily basis. Thanks to cooperation with him and with other members, we were able to confirm the safety of all members of the Association on March 31. We spent three weeks to confirm the safety of approximately 700 members: it seemed to us that it took too long.

B A period when members took action not as an organization but as an individual

The nuclear power station accident caused great concern among residents in Fukushima Prefecture. Deeply shocked by the fact that the nuclear power station exploded, most residents faced an unknown future and were tremendously anxious. All residents considered whether they should be evacuated further away or stay there. Occupational therapists also struggled to live their daily lives and carry out their tasks while in a mental state of anxiety and confusion. In the period immediately after the earthquake, the Association was not ready to decide how to provide support as an organization, nor did its members know how to take action as occupational therapists. Many occupational therapists seemed to just work as hard as possible almost on an individual basis. For instance, Mr. Takayuki Kimura, who served as Chief of the Secretariat of the Association, left the Aizu Region for facilities for the physically handicapped in Iwaki City, along with relief supplies being loaded onto a vehicle. At that time, many truck drivers hesitated to enter Fukushima Prefecture due to concerns about the nuclear power station accident. Residents in Fukushima Prefecture were asked to go to Tochigi Prefecture if they needed relief supplies. Since nobody tried to go to Iwaki City, for example, the city was completely cut off. Under these circumstances, Mr. Kimura worked hard along with social workers with whom he was acquainted. Due to a serious shortage of gasoline, they had to strive to procure gasoline to return from Iwaki City. In addition, they might have encountered a dangerous situation on the way because the earthquake might cause tremendous damage to roads to and from Iwaki City. However, many occupational therapists, including Mr. Kimura, worked furiously on an individual basis during this period when the Association found itself in a situation where it was unable to

Chapter 4 — Activities of Various Professional Organizations

provide organized support activities.

C. A period when the Fukushima Association of Occupational Therapists commenced activities as an organization

In April, the supply of gasoline was resumed almost to normal distribution levels. On April 16, the Association held an executive meeting, which had been postponed. The Association determined, as a basic policy, that disaster support activities should be conducted on a branch basis, because damage caused by the earthquake varied widely between areas. Since many residents in the Coastal Region were evacuated to inland areas in Fukushima Prefecture due to the nuclear power station accident, these areas were required to take individual action for evacuees. The Association asked each branch to provide support that would meet the needs of individual areas without placing a heavy burden on its members.

D. Support activities of the Aizu branch commenced

Although many members provided support on an individual basis, the Aizu branch with relatively little damage from the earthquake commenced support activities as an organization for the first time in memory.

On holidays in April, Ms. Chikako Ozaki, Chief of the Aizu branch, visited temporary evacuation centers, such as gymnasiums, to ask evacuees whether or not they faced any problems. Contrary to her expectation, many evacuees in most evacuation centers answered positively, saying, "Public health nurses perform radio gymnastic exercises with us every morning and evening," "Dance and yoga instructors come to teach exercises," and "I have no problem because I can walk." Accordingly, Ms. Ozaki left evacuation centers, asking evacuees to make contact with her if they faced any problems. As a result she did not immediately intervene. It seemed to her that many public health nurses, staff members of social welfare councils and volunteers were aware of the importance of prevention of disuse syndrome and deep vein thrombosis/pulmonary thromboembolism (economy class syndrome) from the experience in the Great Hanshin-Awaji Earthquake and the Mid Niigata Prefecture Earthquake and took preventive measures. Later, however, she realized that she had made a big mistake.

The members of the Aizu branch did nothing for some time because they heard that there were no problems with evacuees. However, some members gradually became motivated to provide support to evacuees as occupational therapists and do something recreational for evacuees. Therefore, they changed their purposes from support to entertainment, and decided to begin activities in evacuation centers. On May 1, they visited an evacuation center with materials for creating beanbags, origami paper and coloring books. Only a small number of evacuees participated in their activities, because it was the first time. However, as they became relaxed with the members, while creating beanbags together, they began to talk about the situation of their family members and their past lives. Then, they talked about their more immediate problems: For example, "Since I suffered a mini-stroke five years ago, I have had trouble with hand motion. As I don't do housework or any tasks at an evacuation center, my hands have become more stiff," "Since I wear slippers at the evacuation center, I have difficulty walking and easily stumble. Yesterday I fell down in the toilet and felt pain," and "Although I slept on a bed at home, I sleep on a futon here. I have difficulty standing up from a mattress laid on the floor." Soon the members provided a simple assessment of hand function and balance ability for the evacuees and found that most evacuees had some problems. The members were very surprised to realize that the situation of the evacuees was severe. The evacuees who said not long before that they had no problem began to express their true opinions as they became

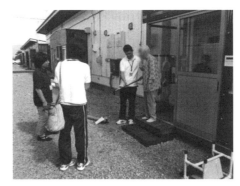

Figure 36-1 Guidance at a temporary housing
Telling an evacuee the position of a handrail at the entrance

physically and mentally relaxed through activities with the members. When the members talked with the evacuees, public health nurses came to tell what they worried about: For example, "I am concerned about the way Mr. C walks," and "The hands of Ms. D are shaky when she eats meals." The public health nurses seemed to have recognized the members as experts in rehabilitation. This provided a good opportunity for the members to learn the importance and potential of their activities. The members learned the lesson that they were unable to know what evacuees really felt only by a quick visit to the evacuation centers and asking evacuees whether or not they needed assistance.

From that day, the members of the Aizu branch hurriedly changed their schedule and visited evacuation centers every day during early-May holiday season in Japan, taking welfare equipment such as sticks and shoes with them. They asked for the cooperation of the Fukushima Physical Therapy Association and for prosthetists from the Association (Figure 36-1).

Thus, the Aizu branch began to provide support in evacuation centers. Probably, other branches also conducted support activities in a similar way. There were no coordinators in any branch of the Association with a clear intention of commencing support activities. During this earthquake, various people started unilateral support activities in their area within Fukushima Prefecture, while puzzling over and seeking what to do for evacuees.

E Activities of the Fukushima Counseling and Support Professional Team

The Fukushima Care Manager Association and five other organizations of counseling and support professionals formed the Fukushima Counseling and Support Professional Team, and built up a system in which they made collaborative efforts to provide support. The Association participated in the team and offered its cooperation. I remember that the team first provided support at the Big Palette Fukushima on June 26. Members of the Koriyama branch of the Association participated in the support activities. Team members continued to provide support, while collaborating with each other in individual areas. As evacuees began to move from temporary evacuation centers, such as gymnasiums, to secondary evacuation centers, such as hotels and inns, and temporary housing, the team gradually promoted cooperation with care managers and social workers to provide support in individual areas.

Chapter 4 — Activities of Various Professional Organizations

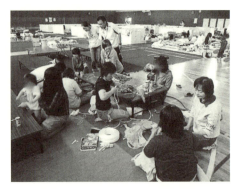

Figure 36-2 Support activities for disaster victims at Fureai Gymnasium
Creating cloth sandals

F. Support activities in temporary housing

For support activities in temporary housing, the Association started by providing advice about equipment and materials, such as installation of railings and elimination of differences in the levels of the floors. There were many points to be improved, such as big steps at the entrance and useless railings in a bathroom. The Association provided guidance in cooperation with the Fukushima Physical Therapy Association (Figure 36-2).

The Association cooperated in programs aimed at care prevention and preventing evacuees from being homebound all the time. These programs were conducted at support centers in temporary housing sites. The Association provided guidance concerning physical exercises and training as well as recreation and activities for fun. Given the number of temporary housing sites in Fukushima Prefecture, the activities of the Association were conducted in limited areas. However, the Association was able to offer occupational therapy, with the great assistance of the Ibaraki Association of Occupational Therapists and the Niigata Association of Occupational Therapists, which were located in adjacent prefectures.

These support programs have been continuously conducted at support centers in temporary housing sites from the beginning of evacuation up to the present date.

G. People become healthy through activities

The Japanese Association of Occupational Therapists promotes support activities with a focus on activities meaningful to individuals, under the slogan "People become healthy through activities." Most evacuees in Fukushima Prefecture were forced to be evacuated due to the nuclear power station accident. They were not only separated from their beloved homes, but also were robbed of an opportunity to engage in activities that were meaningful to them. When people become unable to engage in their daily activities, which were conducted in their hometowns, including going to work, working in the fields, going shopping at their favorite stores, and doing housework, they become gradually unhealthy both physically and mentally. I have seen such people in evacuation centers in various areas. As the flip-side of the slogan "People become healthy through activities," they proved that people became unhealthy without activities. They had been able to live active lives by working in the fields, cleaning large houses, cooking, and doing the laundry until the earthquake occurred. I realized that a daily routine, including weeding gardens, taking the dog for a walk and chatting with neighbors, made people healthy mentally and physically.

Although daily exercise is recommended to prevent disuse syndrome, only physical exercises and training are probably of no help. What is really important to health is to conduct activities meaningful to individuals and engage in a daily routine.

Evacuation after the nuclear power station accident surely robbed residents of many activities meaningful to them. Since I am an occupational therapist, I do not know the impact of low-dose exposure to radiation on health. However, it is apparent that living as evacuees has an adverse impact on health.

H Support activities in Minamisoma City

As stated before, the Association adopted a policy that support activities should be conducted on a branch basis. In the Soso branch in Minamisoma City, however, many members were evacuated to other areas inside and outside of Fukushima Prefecture, and only two members were left. Although members of other branches should have visited the Soso branch to provide assistance, they could not do so because support activities were conducted throughout Fukushima Prefecture. In addition, members of the Association were also wondering whether to evacuate their areas while engaging in support activities, as well as having to pour their energy into the operation of their own branches. Accordingly, the Association requested the Japan Association of Operational Therapists, a parent organization, to offer full support for the Soso branch. In a situation where other organizations announced that they would not conduct support activities in the Soso District due to the impact of radiation, the Japan Association of Operational Therapists provided support from November 2011 through March 2012. Moreover, it was actively involved in recruiting occupational therapists for Minamisoma City General Hospital. As a result, two occupational therapists were employed and worked at the hospital.

I Support activities in the future

Although I described the support activities of the Fukushima Association of Occupational Therapists in this section, what is introduced here is only part of the various support activities conducted throughout Fukushima Prefecture.

In Fukushima Prefecture, it is still unclear when the problems caused by the nuclear power station accident will come to an end. Probably the problems will remain unresolved for a while. While often feeling impatient at the slow progress toward the solution of the problems, the Association will continue to spend a great deal of time providing support.

(Keiichi Hasegawa)

37 Fukushima Dietetic Association

A Overall activities of the Fukushima Dietetic Association at the time of the earthquake

On March 11, 2011, the Great East Japan Earthquake and the following nuclear accident at the Fukushima Daiichi Nuclear Power Station of the Tokyo Electric Power Company ("Fukushima Daiichi Station") caused tremendous damage and sadness to Fukushima Prefecture. This earthquake and accident made me fully realize the obvious fact that people cannot live without water and food.

Due to the nuclear disaster, nine towns and villages were forced to relocate their administrative functions to other areas inside and outside of Fukushima Prefecture. In addition, harmful rumors about radiation spread throughout Fukushima Prefecture, including the Aizu Region, 100 km away from the Fukushima Daiichi Station. This inflicted significant damage on every industry in Fukushima Prefecture, including the agriculture, forestry and fisheries industry and the manufacturing industry. Thus, the nuclear disaster shook Fukushima Prefecture to its foundations.

Immediately after the earthquake, Fukushima Prefecture in particular was put into abnormal circumstances, where food and relief supplies were not delivered to the prefecture for nearly a month due to damage to transportation networks, a shortage of gasoline, and concerns about radiation.

Under these circumstances, the Fukushima Dietetic Association ("the Association") recruited volunteers to provide nutritional and dietary support for disaster victims, in collaboration and cooperation with administrative bodies, the Self-Defense Forces, and other institutions and organizations concerned. The Association delivered 139 senior nutritionists and nutritionists, who applied for support activities, including its members who were also living as evacuees after losing everything due to the earthquake, to evacuation centers and temporary housing. A total of 400 nutritionists were dispatched to provide support (Table 37-1).

Through this disaster, I fully realized that food was fundamental for living and that nutritional and dietary support at a time of a disaster was necessary immediately after the disaster.

Here is reported the volunteer support activities that the Association conducted over approximately a

Table 37-1 Situation of food support activities

Area	Group support & guidance			Individual support & guidance			No. of staff members (volunteers)			
	Frequency	No. of facilities & homes	No. of people	Frequency	No. of facilities & homes	No. of people	Nutritionists of health offices	Dietetic associations/volunteers	Temporary nutritionists employed urgently and through job-creation programs	Local governments & others
Fukushima Prefecture	523	940	36,879	1,134	2,098	3,724	693	400	380	379

(Surveyed by the Health Promotion Division, Fukushima Prefecture; "Situation of nutritional and dietary support of public health and welfare offices"; as of April 1, 2012)

year soon after the earthquake.

B. Outline of major support activities in collaboration with administrative bodies and relevant institutions/organizations

① From March 23 in collaboration with Fukushima Prefecture, the Association provided relief supplies more promptly to those who were unable to eat ordinary food
② On March 29, the Association accepted a request for dispatching volunteers to the Fukushima Nutrition Support Team
③ The Association cooperated with the first diet survey (from April 19) and the second diet survey (from June 3) at temporary evacuation centers in Fukushima Prefecture
④ Conducting activities for improving the dietary environment in evacuation centers in collaboration with Fukushima Prefecture, its municipalities and the Self-Defense Forces
  Ensuring necessary food and nutrition; preventing the outbreak of infectious diseases and food poisoning; providing support for nutritional assessment; smoothly providing warm meal service; and preventing secondary damage, such as aggravation of chronic disease
⑤ Conducting support activities for disaster victims living in temporary housing and municipally- subsidized housing and for affected municipalities
  • Providing group and individual nutritional guidance and implementing cooking practice programs at assembly rooms in temporary housing sites
  • Providing individual nutritional guidance by visiting temporary housing and municipally- subsidized housing

C. Concrete support activities

1 Providing relief supplies more promptly to those who cannot eat ordinary food

Since food distribution was stopped due to a shortage of gasoline, public health and welfare offices ("health offices") received many consultations from municipalities immediately after the earthquake concerning the lack of artificial milk (milk powder), thick liquid diets, baby food, and food allergy friendly foods. In cooperation with the Health Promotion Division of the Fukushima Prefectural Government and senior nutritionists of health offices, the Association promptly procured special nutritive foods and other foods from the Japan Dietetic Association and supporting member companies of the Association. The Association distributed them to disaster victims and municipalities, as well as stored them in three hubs of the Association in Fukushima Prefecture (Figure 37-1).

2 Improving a dietary environment in evacuation centers

a. Situation in evacuation centers

The situation in evacuation centers differed from site to site even in the same local community. In an evacuation center where the action for nutritional and dietary support was taken late, only bread, rice balls and water were distributed for more than two weeks (Figure 37-2). Accordingly, health offices and municipal nutritionists set priority tasks for each evacuation center, and provided nutritional and dietary support, in collaboration with relevant institutions and organizations, senior nutritionists dispatched from across the country, and other professionals (Figure 37-3).

Chapter 4 Activities of Various Professional Organizations

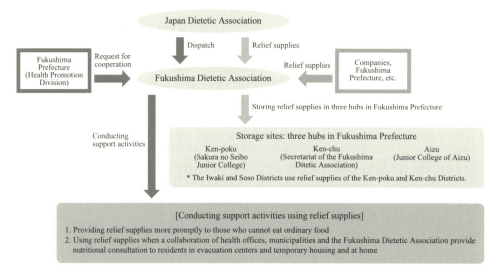

Figure 37-1 Emergency responses in a situation where there is no timely delivery of relief supplies
(Notification document of the Health Promotion Division, Fukushima Prefecture, 2011)

Figure 37-2 Situation of an evacuation center at the beginning of April

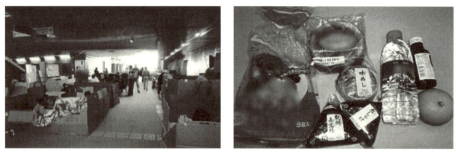

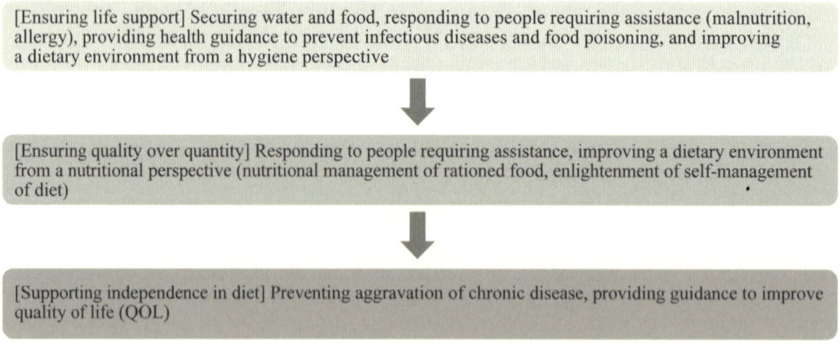

Figure 37-3 Nutritional and dietary support

b. Actual case examples

① Case example 1 (Figure 37-4)

The Association was involved in improving the dietary environment in evacuation centers in cooperation with the Self-Defense Forces and promotion members for diet modification, by request from local govern-

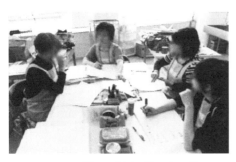
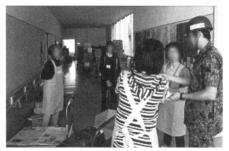

Figure 37-4   Situation of an evacuation center in April and May, 2011

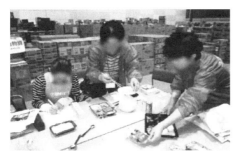
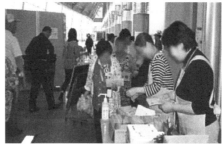

Figure 37-5   Situation of an evacuation center in April to July, 2011

ments that managed evacuation centers. Its efforts included management of foodstuffs, menu planning, procurement of foodstuff, cooking guidance, and health guidance.

② Case example 2 (Figure 37-5)

The Association conducted dietary surveys and engaged in educational activities for self-management of diet, in cooperation with health offices and senior nutritionists dispatched from across the country, by request from Fukushima Prefecture.

c. Reporting the situation at evacuation centers and addressing a request for improvement of the situation to the disaster response headquarters

The Fukushima Prefecture Disaster Response Headquarters was very busy and struggled to respond to requests from evacuation centers in individual municipalities. Accordingly, staff members of health offices and municipal senior nutritionists visited evacuation centers, and then, based on the results of visits, made requests for improving the diet at evacuation centers to local disaster response headquarters via directors of health offices. Moreover, the Health Promotion Division, Fukushima Prefecture, required the Fukushima Prefecture Disaster Response Headquarters to improve the dietary environment, based on the results of dietary surveys conducted throughout the prefecture. Hyogo Prefecture, which dispatched support members to Miyagi Prefecture, also made requests for the improvement of diet to the national government. Consequently, the food budget per person increased from 1,010 yen to 1,500 yen on May 2 in Miyagi Prefecture (on May 4 in Fukushima Prefecture).

Chapter 4 — Activities of Various Professional Organizations

3 Activities for supporting the health preservation and promotion and independence of disaster victims by request from Fukushima Prefecture and affected municipalities

- Providing group and individual nutritional guidance and implementing cooking practice programs at assembly rooms in temporary housing sites
- Providing individual nutritional guidance at temporary housing

D Issues and future activities

1 Present situation and issues

In Fukushima Prefecture, there seems to be the following nutritional issues due to the impact of the nuclear power station accident and prolonged living as evacuees.

- After the earthquake, there are growing concerns about an increase in the number of those tending to obesity and those suffering from hypertension.
- The amount of physical activity has decreased in residents of all generations.
- Salt intake of residents in the Tohoku Region originally tended to be higher. However, it is feared that salt intake may increase in association with changes in the cooking environment after the earthquake.
- There are fears about the decrease of vegetable intake and the increase of unbalanced nutrition.
- Residents' motivation for cooking and their will to live are decreasing due to small kitchens in temporary housing, a family environment in which family members have to live separately, and difficulty in procuring food.

2 Future activities

Since FY 2012, the Association has undertaken a project for nutritional and dietary support for disaster victims, which was sponsored by Fukushima Prefecture, and has continued to conduct support activities for affected municipalities and disaster victims to date.

Although the Association worked hard to do all that was possible after this earthquake, there remained many issues in need of reconsideration. The Association confirmed the necessity to conduct trainings and drills during ordinary times, to practice collaboration and cooperation with administrative bodies and relevant institutions and organizations during a disaster. The Association also needs to improve skills to provide nutritional and dietary support from the perspective of disaster victims.

The Association intends to make continuous efforts to be able to contribute to society in an emergency, although nobody wants to experience disasters like this.

> I would like to take this opportunity to extend my heartfelt gratitude to people in various professions and relevant institutions and organizations for their support and cooperation with our support activities.

(Keiko Nakamura)

38 Fukushima Society of Certified Clinical Psychologists

In the Great East Japan Earthquake, Fukushima Prefecture suffered from an unprecedented earthquake and tsunami, the nuclear power station accident and harmful rumors associated with radiation. Furthermore, dispersal and deposition of radioactive materials will continue to threaten the health of residents over decades. Under these conditions, the Fukushima Society of Certified Clinical Psychologists ("the Society") launched the Great East Japan Earthquake Response Project to provide psychological support throughout Fukushima Prefecture. This section reports mainly on how the Society grasped the situation after the disaster and exerted its ingenuity to provide support.

A Psychosocial situation of residents in Fukushima Prefecture

1 Psychologically traumatic experience

In disaster relief assistance, it is important to provide support to residents who suffered a psychologically traumatic experience, when their safety and security are ensured after disasters. This psychological support includes care for acute stress response and posttraumatic stress disorder (PTSD), and grief care for object-loss reaction. In this disaster, however, the crisis caused by the nuclear accident at the Fukushima Daiichi Nuclear Power Station of the Tokyo Electric Power Company was expected to last over a prolonged period of time. Residents in Fukushima Prefecture would be unable to ensure their safety and security and will continue to experience psychological trauma. Accordingly, the Society needed to exert its ingenuity to provide psychological support.

2 A vague sense of anxiety

Immediately after the earthquake, members of the Society visited emergency evacuation centers to provide support based on disaster relief support manuals, such as the Psychological First Aid (PFA). However, due to prolonged exposure to low-dose radiation, the safety and security of residents was not ensured either physically or psychologically. Accordingly, the Society was required to consider how to respond to their vague sense of anxiety.

3 A vague sense of loss

Residents, who were evacuated by the evacuation order, lost their homes and hometowns, although these homes and hometowns existed seemingly undamaged. Residents' expectations that they might return to their homes and hometowns caused a vague sense of loss for them. Moreover, residents in low-dose contaminated areas, who were not forced to evacuate the areas, also felt a vague sense of loss. Although they lived in a rich natural environment with an abundant crop, they were restricted from shipping agricultural and livestock products and their children were restricted from playing outside. The sense of loss that they faced seemed difficult to overcome due to its vagueness.

4 Self-determination

Residents were pressed to make a judgment and decision about the following matters.
- Whether they should stay and raise their children there, or evacuate outside Fukushima Prefecture for

Chapter 4 | Activities of Various Professional Organizations

the sake of their children's health

- On which should they be more focused; the merit of evacuation for protecting the health of their children, or the risk of feeling stressed due to adapting to new living environments and separation from what they are attached
- Whether they should believe inspection data showing that radiation dose in the areas has no immediate effect on health, and whether it is safe to breastfeed babies and to allow children to play outside, drink tap water and eat food grown in the area

5 Prolonged living as evacuees with no promise of the future

By living as evacuees, residents were forced to sever their ties with local communities, interrupt the continuity of their lives and lose their careers, thereby facing the crisis of losing their identity. They were anxious about when they would be able to return to their homes, and where and how they would live in the future. Some children suffered from separation anxiety and were unable to separate from their parents. They showed a tendency toward depression and behaved restlessly and wildly, while keeping a fixed expression. Moreover, when only mothers and children were evacuated, separation from the husband or the father imposed an enormous economic burden on them because they needed double living expenses. In addition, they might face the crisis of divorce. Thus, living lives as evacuees involved the risk of threatening mental health of residents and their family ties. Most evacuees living in temporary housing were middle-aged and elderly people. In particular, elderly men living alone were reluctant to talk with others, even if members of the Association visited their rooms, and did not participate in any events. The members were concerned seeing these elderly men sitting alone in their rooms.

6 Compensation issues

The indemnity and compensation for the nuclear power station accident were paid to disaster victims. This contributed to ensuring the livelihood of disaster victims. On the other hand, the compensation caused a feeling of unfairness among disaster victims and hurt the bonds of local communities. Some local residents were unable to understand how deeply evacuees were hurt by the loss of what they cherished, and criticized them for living rich lives thanks to receiving an indemnity and compensation. Some evacuees said that they tried to say nothing about the fact that they were evacuees, because they would not want anyone to ask about indemnities.

7 Restrictions on topics of daily conversation

Unwritten agreement is being made about restrictions on topics of daily conversation. As stated before, some residents try not to say that they are evacuees. Moreover, employees at Tokyo Electric Power Company (TEPCO) try to conceal their identity, because they find it absurd that residents turn their rage against TEPCO on them.

At first, the health hazards of exposure to low-dose radiation were said to be unclear. Concerns about radiation caused a kind of panic among residents and became a popular topic of conversation. However, due to the ambiguity of the impact of radiation, residents are gradually more likely to avoid talking about radiation. This is because topics related to radiation may make conversation uncomfortable due to the differences in the degree of anxiety among residents. This raises additional concerns that residents' anxiety may be hidden and prolonged.

Table 38-1 Comparison of disaster-related death and death directly associated to the disaster

Prefecture	A: No. of disaster-related deaths* (persons)	B: No. of deaths directly associated to the disaster** (persons)	A/(A+B) (%)
Fukushima	1,383	1,606	46.2
Miyagi	862	9,536	8.3
Iwate	389	4,673	7.7

Note) The percentage of 46.2% in Fukushima Prefecture is prominent.
(* Reconstruction Agency, as of the end of March 2013; ** Statistics Bureau, Ministry of Internal Affairs and Communications, as of March 11, 2013)

8 An extremely large number of disaster-related deaths

The situation of the psychosocial crisis in Fukushima Prefecture, which was created by the earthquake followed by the nuclear disaster, was different from that in Iwate and Miyagi Prefectures, as stated above. The uniqueness and seriousness of the situation in Fukushima Prefecture shows up in the large number of disaster-related deaths, including suicides.

The number of deaths resulting directly from the earthquake and tsunami in the Great East Japan Earthquake and disaster-related deaths caused by stress from living as evacuees was compared between Fukushima, Miyagi and Iwate Prefectures (Table 38-1).

In Fukushima Prefecture, the nuclear disaster prolonged the crisis, and caused a vague sense of anxiety and loss among residents. Moreover, issues mentioned in 1) to 6) were unlikely to be resolved. Accordingly, the Society was required to provide support that responded to individual cases.

B Devising ways to provide support

To respond to the unprecedented disaster in Fukushima Prefecture through the project, the Society devised ways to provide support that could respond to individual needs, based on the skills and experience of certified clinical psychologists. The Society developed the Parent-and-child Play and Parent Meeting program, which aimed to provide support to younger children and their parents, and the Class Meeting program, which was a Fukushima version of school support.

1 Parent-and-child Play and Parent Meeting

Due to concerns about prolonged lives as evacuees and low-dose exposure, parents with younger children were subject to greater stress and required mental health care. The mental stability of parents is essential for good mental health of children. To provide mental health care to parents and children, community support systems are indispensable. Accordingly, the Society planned the Parent-and-child Play and Parent Meeting program together with health offices, and regularly implemented the program (approximately once a month) in various areas, through collaboration between local professionals, such as certified clinical psychologists, childcare workers, public health nurses, midwives, nutritionists and child-support staff members.

a. Advance preparations
① Target people: Preschool children (0 to 6 years old) and their parents Municipal health nurses call for participation.

Chapter 4 Activities of Various Professional Organizations

② Venue: Local health centers, child-support centers, community centers, etc.
③ Date and time: Time zones when children and parents can easily gather together Morning hours are recommended.

b. Implementing procedures

① Reception: Confirm the name and age of participants and distribute name tags.
② Preparatory meeting: Staff members confirm the support schedule of the day, and share prior information on participants, if any. Participants play freely until all participants come.
③ Opening (5 min): Public health nurses introduce support staff members, and childcare workers introduce children and parents.
④ Parent-and-child play (approx. 30 min): Childcare workers contrive ways to play so that parents and children can relieve their stress, regain their smiles and share affection and a basic sense of trust (Figure 38-1). Other staff members support the progress of the program.
⑤ Parent meeting (approx. 60 min): Certified clinical psychologists serve as facilitators to form small groups. After relaxation, individual groups hold peer meetings (Figure 38-2). Other staff members participate in the meetings, where individual participants talk about what they worry about and are embarrassed about, and how they cope with issues. Participants listen to each other sympathetically, share information and offer advice to each other. Childcare workers take care of children at places where parents can see what their children are doing. Accordingly, parents and children can be separated with no worry.

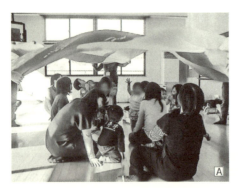 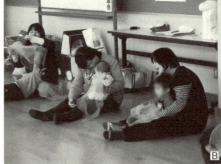

Figure 38-1   Parent-and-child Play
A: Wrapping cloth balloon   B: Scarf

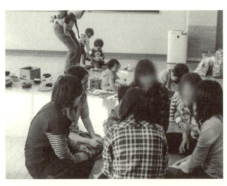 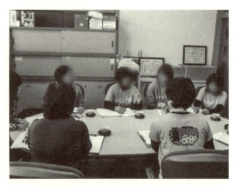

Figure 38-2   Parent meeting   **Figure 38-3**   Staff meeting after the program

⑥ Closing (5 min): Local health nurses close the program.

⑦ Staff meeting after the program (approx. 30 min): All staff members gather to review and examine their role in the program (Figure 38-3). Points to be checked include whether games were appropriate and effective, what was talked about in parent meetings, whether there were children and parents whom staff members felt anxious about, and what consideration they need to give in the future. In the case where staff members need to respond to children and parents on a continuous and individual basis by introducing them to consulting services and medical institutions, they request local health nurses to deal with such children and parents, while paying attention to ensure the continuity of support.

c. Effects of support

① The Parent-and-child Play program contributed to restoring a loving relationship between parents and children. Children with separation anxiety and stress reaction regained their smiles, and were able to separate from their parents and play with friends cheerfully. Their mental state also became stable.

② In parent meetings, which provided a receptive environment, parents were able to honestly talk on subjects – almost all issues mentioned in 1) to 7) of the paragraph A), which they were reluctant to discuss at other times. This helped to alleviate their vague sense of anxiety and loss. Their faces softened, and they were able to recover their confidence to raise children there. This program provided an opportunity to activate the capacity for peer support by encouraging ties between parents, while empowering participants and enhancing their resilience.

③ The Society regularly implemented the program to encourage parents and children to change and grow. Community support systems, where parents and children can continue to receive support from many sides, are being established, through the collaboration between various professionals involved in support activities in local areas.

d. Implementation status (two outsourcing projects)

① Project entrusted by the Japan Committee for UNICEF (FY 2011 – 2012)

The program was implemented at 25 sites in Futaba Town (Listel Inawashiro), Fukushima City, Miharu Town, Motomiya City, Koriyama City, Tamura City, the Ken-chu Public Health and Welfare Office, the Ken-nan Public Health and Welfare Office, Shirakawa City, temporary housing in Katsurao Village, Kitakata City, Ishikawa Town, Samegawa Village, Tamakawa Village, Asakawa Town, Nishigo Village, Date City, Yabuki Town, Nihonmatsu City, Kunimi Town, Kagamiishi Town, Hanawa Town, Namie Town, Otama Village, and Nakajima Village (Table 38-2).

② Parent-and-child Play Plaza and Counseling Workshop in the Mental Health Care Project for Affected Young Children and Their Family Members (November 2011 – March 2012)

The program was implemented at 13 sites in Shirakawa City, Motomiya City, Fukushima City, Kitakata City, Date City, Kunimi Town, Kagamiishi Town, Namie Town, Yabuki Town, Hanawa Town, Nishigo Village, Nakajima Village and Samegawa Village. The program was implemented a total of 65 times. A total of 114 certified clinical psychologists and 141 childcare workers were dispatched. A total of 1,309

Table 38-2 Frequency of the Parent-and-child Play and Parent Meeting program and number of participants

	Frequency of the program	No. of certified clinical psychologists	No. of childcare workers	No. of participants (Children)	No. of participants (Parents)	No. of participants (Children & Parents)	No. of volunteers
2011	78	149	149	555	902	1,457	37
2012	168	330	385	1,809	1,924	3,733	62
Total	246	479	534	2,364	2,826	5,190	99

Chapter 4 | Activities of Various Professional Organizations

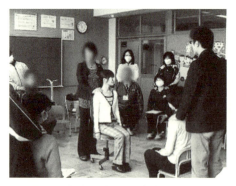

Figure 38-4 Bringing a feeling of relaxation to a teacher

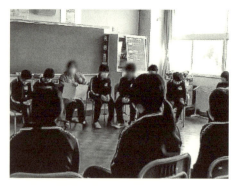

Figure 38-5 Class meeting

persons, comprised of 633 young children and 676 parents, received support.

2 Fukushima version of Class Meeting

The Society made strenuous efforts to provide support in a school setting, as mentioned below.
- Encouraging evacuated students and local students to make friends with each other and overcome the difficult situation through mutual peer support to lead relaxed school lives
- Providing mental health care to teachers, who work hard for students although they are also victims of the earthquake, so that they do not burn out (Figure 38-4)
- Identifying children with suspected PTSD and respond to them through individual counseling

The Fukushima version of the Class Meeting program is not performed in an invasive way, unlike debriefing sessions where disaster victims are required to talk about a painful experience to overcome the experience. The program includes a questionnaire on health and relaxation. In the program, participants freely talk about what they think at the moment, how they use their ingenuity in responding to issues, and what they can do in the future. The program is a class for mental health care with a focus on mutual support of group members (Figure 38-5, 6). Staff members teach teachers how to conduct the Class Meeting program after school hours on the day previous to the program. Then, they have teachers actually experience the program to provide mental health care for the teachers. On the following day, the teachers carry out the program for their students. Subsequently, individual interviews and consultations (suggestions and advice) with school counselors are provided to students who seem to require care.

The program was implemented at 35 schools; to the best of the Society's knowledge. These schools gave favorable feedback to the Society as follows: "The entire school has been restored to a relaxed atmosphere," "The program inspired a feeling of fellowship," "I was able to be honest about my own feelings," "I refreshed myself by talking about my concerns," and "The program filled me with courage and vigor."

(Kanae Narui, Keiko Omori, Takashi Tomimori: *Report of Support Activities, Report of Support during the Great East Japan Earthquake by the Fukushima Society of Certified Clinical Psychologists*. Great East Japan Earthquake Response Project of the Fukushima Society of Certified Clinical Psychologists, 2013)

Class Meeting (questionnaire on health)				(mm/dd/yy)
Name of school:	1. Elementary School 2. Junior High School 3. High School	grade		class
Your name:	Male/Female	Student No.		

Please tell us your physical and mental health conditions.

1) How often have you felt like as follows <u>during the past week (from the last week to today)</u>? Circle the number that applies to you.	Never (0)	Occasion ally (1)	Fre-quently (2)	Almost always (3)
1. I have difficulty falling asleep.				
2. I feel frustrated and irritated, and flare up in anger.				
	I become startled by the slightest sound and trivial				
3. things.				
4. I dream about my bitter experience and dream a horrible dream.				
5. I am reminded of unwanted memories by small events.				
6. I sometimes remember my bitter and shocking experiences, and become frightened and uncomfortable.				
7 I do not find my shocking experience real and true.				
8. I wonder why I cannot shed tears although I have had a sad experience.				
9. I try not to talk about my bitter and shocking experiences.				
10. I sometimes blame myself of doing (having done) wrong.				
11. I cannot enjoy what seems to be fun.				
12. I feel alone.				
13. I have a headache or a stomachache, and feel ill.				
14. I cannot enjoy my meals and do not want to eat them.				
15. I feel like doing nothing.				
16. I find it difficult to go to school.				
17. I can concentrate on studies.				
18. I have lots of fun at school.				
19. I enjoy talking with my friends.				
20. I am concerned about going out.				
21. I am worried about whether food is safe.				
22. I am concerned about my health in the future.				
				Total of items 1 to 16

2) How are you feeling now? What are you thinking now?

3) How do you manage to deal with your feeling?

4) What do you want to do in the future? What can you do in the future?

5) Please give us your feedback about the Class Meeting program.

Great East Japan Earthquake Psychological Support Center (Japanese Society of Certified Clinical Psychologists, Association of Japanese Clinical Psychology: Logistic Support WG, Psychological Assessment Team): Fukushima Society of Certified Clinical Psychologists

Figure 38-6 Class meeting (questionnaire on health)

Chapter 4 Activities of Various Professional Organizations

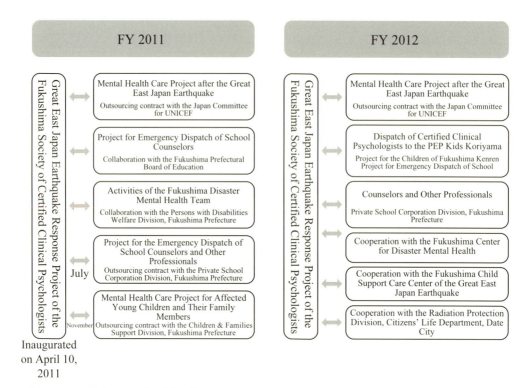

Figure 38-7 Projects conducted for disaster response support by the Fukushima Society of Certified Clinical Psychologists

C Summary of support activities

Since June 2011, the Society has been entrusted by the Japan Committee for UNICEF to conduct the Mental Health Care Project after the Great East Japan Earthquake. In addition, it has also conducted the Project for Emergency Dispatch of School Counselors and Other Professionals, which has been outsourced by the Private School Corporation Division, Fukushima Prefecture. From November 2011 through March 2012, the Society was entrusted by the Children & Families Support Division, Fukushima Prefecture to conduct the Mental Health Care Project for Affected Young Children and Their Family Members. Figure 38-7 shows the support activities in which the Society has been involved for the past two years.

D Toward the future

Although the number of children age 18 or younger who were evacuated to other areas inside and outside of Fukushima Prefecture temporarily exceeded 30,000, it had decreased to 27,617 as of October 1, 2013. Evacuees returned to their homes with children when the children started school and entered higher schools. In municipalities in Futaba County, restricted areas have been reorganized. Kawauchi Village has relocated its village office and is waiting for residents to return to the village, while decontaminating the local environment and improving infrastructure. More evacuees will gradually return home in the future. However, their homes, to which they felt attached, have remained untouched and are falling into decay after two and a half years have passed since the earthquake. Most homes have changed too much for resident to live in them. Moreover, the safety of residents has not been ensured, and infrastructure has not been completely repaired. Accordingly, there are still many residents who hesitate to return home with children.

Residents in Fukushima Prefecture will be continuously required to make decisions and judgments by themselves under increasingly difficult situations. Municipal health nurses, childcare workers and certified clinical psychologists need to provide ongoing support for families who struggle to live their daily lives in a fluid situation, while worrying about various issues. Accordingly, the Parent-and-child Play and Parent Meeting program, in which these professionals talk together with parents about the issues faced by families, while laughing and enjoying games with children, will be useful in the future. The program is also helpful when families who return home from evacuation destinations meet local residents again and fit in with them.

Meanwhile, some young children have not yet walked in bare feet on the ground and do not know how to play outdoors. There are actually children who have become obese and have experienced a loss of motor function. Moreover, it seems that an increasing number of children have recently shown PTSD signs and stress response. After the Chernobyl nuclear power plant accident, health care management and mental health care are still necessary 27 years after the accident. Therefore, we have the responsibility of doing our best, using our ingenuity, for residents in Fukushima Prefecture, in particular, so that children may grow up healthy and happy both physically and mentally. To this end, we have to further promote the establishment of a system in which parents and children can receive support through cooperation of local professionals involved in child rearing, continuously receive care from various sources, and be supported by local communities. We need to draw up comprehensive projects, in which more professionals (such as physicians, public health nurses, midwives, nurses, certified clinical psychologists, childcare workers, physical therapists, occupational therapists, certified social welfare workers, specialists on exercises and plays, radiation scientists, nutrition instructors, nurse-teachers, and teachers) work cooperatively. Furthermore, administrative bodies should implement these projects as part of their support measures.

(Kanae Narui)

References

1) National Child Traumatic Stress Network, National Center for PTSD, translated by the Hyogo Institute for Traumatic Stress: *Psychological First Aid. Field Operations Guide 2nd Edition.* htttp://www.j-hits.org/ 2009.

2) Kanae Narui: *Class Meeting Using Stress Management*, jointly edited by Koji Takenaka and Yoshiki Tominaga, *Stress Management Education for Daily Life and Disaster*, Sunlife Co., Ltd., pp. 26–29, 2011.

3) Kanae Narui, Keiko Omori, Takashi Tomimori: *Principles and Approaches in the Fukushima Version of Class Meeting. Mother and Child Well-being around the World*, vol. 73, 2012–10: pp. 69–76, Shiseido Social Welfare Foundation, 2012.

4) P. Boss (translated by Koji Minamiyama): *Leaving without Goodbye, Goodbye without Leaving*, Gakubunsha Co., Ltd., 2005.

5) Yoshiki Tominaga: *Basic Principles in Support for Disaster Victims. Clinical Psychology*, vol. 24, Kongo Shuppan, pp. 710–715, 2004.

6) Yoshiki Tominaga, Kanae Narui, etc.: *Fukushima Mental Health Care Manual ⟨Child Version⟩.* Fukushima Mental Health and Welfare Centre, 2013.

7) Kanae Narui, Keiko Omori, Takashi Tomimori: *Report of Support Activities, Report of Support during the Great East Japan Earthquake by the Fukushima Society of Certified Clinical Psychologists.* Great East Japan Earthquake Response Project of the Fukushima Society of Certified Clinical Psychologists, 2013.

8) *Mother and Child Well-being around the World*, vol. 73, Shiseido Social Welfare Foundation, 2012.

9) Edited by Yoshiki Tominaga, Kanae Narui, Keiko Omori, and Takashi Tomimori: *Fukushima Mental Health Care Manual ⟨Child Version⟩.*

39 Fukushima Ward Council on Social Welfare

A : Issues in support

In the Great East Japan Earthquake, which occurred on March 11, 2011, Fukushima Prefecture suffered from an earthquake and subsequent tsunami as well as the nuclear power station accident. Consequently, many residents from over a wide area were forced to be evacuated. The recovery of Fukushima Prefecture is expected to be delayed compared to other prefectures. Living as evacuees is also expected to be prolonged. Although it is two years since the earthquake occurred, more than 140,000 residents are still evacuated to areas inside and outside of the prefecture.

At the initial stage after the earthquake occurred, the Fukushima Ward Council on Social Welfare ("Fukushima Council") supported the operation of disaster volunteer centers, which were managed by the Municipal Councils on Social Welfare ("Municipal Councils"). The disaster volunteer centers matched volunteers, who came to provide support from inside and outside of the prefecture, and disaster victims, who asked for their support. Moreover, the Fukushima Council offered special financing of welfare loans to disaster victims, who could not cover the cost of living at the moment. A common issue for every social welfare council was how to provide livelihood support for temporary housing.

B : Activities of disaster volunteer centers

On March 11, when the earthquake occurred, the Fukushima Council contacted individual Municipal Councils by phone to confirm the damage situation in each area. As a result, the Fukushima Council determined to establish disaster volunteer centers of Municipal Councils ("Municipal VCs") and support their operation. On the same day, the Fukushima Council established its own disaster volunteer center.

On March 12, staff members of the Fukushima Council conducted an on-site survey to assess the damage situation of buildings of individual Municipal Councils, which would become bases for the establishment and operation of disaster volunteer centers. As a result of the survey, the Fukushima Council immediately determined that there was a need to receive many volunteers from inside and outside of the prefecture for the operation of disaster volunteer centers.

On March 14, the Fukushima Council held the Fukushima Disaster Volunteer Liaison Council, which was comprised of relevant organizations in Fukushima Prefecture. On the same day, the Fukushima Council established the Fukushima Disaster Volunteer Center ("the Fukushima VC") in the lobby on the first floor of the Fukushima General Social Welfare Center, where the Fukushima Council had its office, based on the Reception Policy for Disaster Volunteers of the liaison council.

Municipal VCs, which began to be set up on the very day when the earthquake occurred, increased in number and were established in a maximum of 34 out of 59 municipalities in the prefecture.

Since before the earthquake, Municipal Councils had prepared for the establishment and operation of disaster volunteer centers, which would handle matching between volunteers and victims requiring their

356

support in case of a disaster. However, they had no experience of actually establishing and operating disaster volunteer centers, because a large-scale disaster like this had never occurred in Fukushima Prefecture.

Due to the wide-reaching impact of the nuclear power station accident, recovery work was delayed, and the time people spent living as evacuees was expected to be prolonged. Accordingly, more supporters were required to conduct disaster volunteer activities and operate Municipal VCs over a long period of time.

The Japan National Council of Social Welfare made arrangements to increase the number of supporters in charge of operation of disaster volunteer centers, and received a total of 7,895 supporters from other prefectures, ordinance-designated cities, and Municipal Councils outside of the prefecture from March 17 through August 31. Fukushima Prefecture received support from the Kanto bloc A (Tokyo Metropolis, Chiba, Saitama, Gunma, Tochigi, and Ibaraki Prefectures and Saitama City), the Kyushu bloc (Okinawa, Fukuoka, Saga, Nagasaki, Kumamoto, Oita, Miyazaki and Kagoshima Prefectures, and Fukuoka and Kitakyushu Cities) and the Hokkaido/Tohoku bloc (Hokkaido and Yamagata Prefectures, and Sapporo City). Their support enabled a smooth operation of the Fukushima VC and 14 Municipal VCs (Shinchi Town, Soma City, Minamisoma City, Iwaki City, Kawauchi Village, Tomioka Town, Namie Town, Okuma Town, Kunimi Town, Fukushima City, Nihonmatsu City, Sukagawa City, Shirakawa City, and Aizuwakamatsu City).

From September 1 up to December 3, the Fukushima VC made arrangements for and received a total of 1,145 supporters in charge of the operation of disaster volunteer centers from eight social welfare councils (Tokyo Metropolis, Ibaraki, Gunma, Hokkaido, Tochigi, Fukuoka and Saitama Prefectures, and Chiba City). These supporters were dispatched to seven Municipal VCs (Iwaki City, Soma City, Minamisoma City, Kawauchi Village, Tomioka Town, Okuma Town, and Namie Town), which needed support for operating disaster volunteer centers.

In Fukushima Prefecture, the Cooperation Agreement on Disaster Management between the Fukushima and Municipal Councils on Social Welfare had been concluded before the occurrence of the earthquake. Based on the agreement, a total of 114 staff members of Municipal Councils in the Central and Aizu Regions and the Fukushima Council supported the operation of the Municipal VCs.

From June 2011, temporary housing was gradually built in Fukushima Prefecture. Many disaster victims moved from temporary evacuation centers and secondary evacuation centers to temporary housing from August. In association with this, Municipal VCs, mainly on the Pacific Coast, changed their names to life recovery volunteer centers (specific names were given individually), and began to engage in efforts at the next phase. The Fukushima Council provided support for the activities of welfare counselors who were assigned to Municipal Councils in 30 out of 59 municipalities. It also worked to watch over disaster victims and support their livelihood as they moved toward recovery, under the slogan of victim-centered recovery and prevention of isolation and loneliness of disaster victims.

C ⋮ Activities of welfare counselors

The Fukushima Council assigned 171 welfare counselors (196 welfare counselors as of the end of FY 2012) to 30 out of 59 Municipal Councils in the prefecture. In cooperation with Municipal Councils it aimed to watch over disaster victims living in temporary housing through visiting activities, and to conduct support activities to maintain and restore communities of disaster victims.

Chapter 4 — Activities of Various Professional Organizations

The main purpose of assigning welfare counselors to Municipal Councils was to prevent the loneliness and isolation of evacuees. The importance of prevention of loneliness and isolation had been indicated from case examples in other large-scale disasters, and a wide variety of approaches were taken. Welfare counselors regularly visited individual households to confirm the safety of evacuees, watch over them and to understand what they were worried about and were bothered by. In some cases, they provided consultation and information to individual evacuees. In other cases, they offered assistance for evacuees in group settings, including providing opportunities to promote friendship between evacuees in temporary housing. Moreover, they provided regional support to build relationships between residents in temporary housing and local residents and organizations around the temporary housing.

While regularly visiting temporary housing and watching over evacuees, welfare counselors heard about a number of problems from the evacuees. The most common problems were about their daily lives, followed by the health of and medical care for evacuees themselves and their family members, and then by the worries about their family members. Many evacuees coming from areas around the Fukushima Daiichi Station were worried that they did not know when they could return to their hometowns and had no idea what their future lives would be.

In addition, there was a big difference between the situation of evacuees living in temporary housing and that of those living in municipally-subsidized housing, such as apartment houses. In temporary housing, evacuees tended to reduce their independence due to being accustomed to support, while good relationships were maintained in communities. Meanwhile, in municipally- subsidized housing, it became obvious that evacuees suffered from a feeling of loneliness and a lack of information.

D Importance of support activities

In Fukushima Prefecture, many evacuees are still unable to return to their homes due to the nuclear power station accident, and are forced to live in unfamiliar areas away from their familiar surroundings over a long period of time. They also feel various stresses due to significant changes in human relationships as well as from a new living environment and different communities. Although two years have passed since the earthquake occurred, they live with anxiety while facing an unknown future.

Under these conditions, the Fukushima Council realizes that support activities of welfare counselors will become increasingly important. They watch over evacuees, listen to them and provide consultation, while building close relationships with the evacuees. They also provide opportunities for evacuees to communicate with each other, and hold events, so that the evacuees can have something to live for. It is two years since evacuees moved to temporary housing. The Fukushima Council intends to continue to provide support for evacuees in collaboration and cooperation with administrative bodies, commissioned welfare volunteers, and medical and welfare professionals, so that they can return to their old lives as soon as possible.

(Seiichi Watanabe)

40 Fukushima Acupuncture and Moxibustion Association

Two years have passed since the Great East Japan Earthquake occurred on March 11, 2011. Since the occurrence of the earthquake, I have asked myself whether I played my full part as a health-care professional in Fukushima Prefecture after it was hit by the earthquake. When disaster medical care systems are built up in Japan based on the experiences from past large-scale earthquakes, I hope that practitioners of acupuncture and moxibustion will be effectively used as medical resources. I also hope that practitioners of acupuncture and moxibustion will be of some help to community health care in Fukushima Prefecture, where local communities are on the brink of collapse after the earthquake. The following is my report on support activities of the Fukushima Acupuncture and Moxibustion Association at the time of the disaster.

A Acupuncture and moxibustion

Acupuncture and moxibustion are traditional therapies, in which a noxious stimulus and a thermal stimulus are applied to skin by acupuncture needles and by moxa, respectively, to adjust bodily functions. To become practitioners of acupuncture and moxibustion, people must complete a three- or four-year specialized course for acupuncture and moxibustion at universities or professional schools, and pass national examinations to acquire licenses as acupuncturists and moxibustionists. Practitioners with these licenses are permitted by law to practice medicine to a limited extent.

B Support activities

The Fukushima Acupuncture and Moxibustion Association ("the Association") commenced support activities on March 19, a few days after the nuclear power station accident occurred. Initially, the Association gave acupuncture and moxibustion therapies and massage mainly to evacuees from the nuclear power plant accident in the Central Region and the Aizu Region located in internal regions which had a low impact from the earthquake. At that time, due to a lack of gasoline, there were long waiting lines at gas stations. At supermarkets that were damaged by the earthquake, goods remained scattered, and only a few undamaged goods were sold at temporary cash desks. The situation in the Coastal Region, which was tremendously affected by the earthquake, the tsunami, and the nuclear power station accident, was more confusing than inland regions. Accordingly, in Iwaki City, which was located in the southern part of the Coastal Region, volunteer activities for medical care were started as late as at the end of March. In the northern area of the Coastal Region, which was close to the nuclear power station, support was not provided at the initial stage of the disaster. This was because there were fewer practitioners from the Association in the area because the area was geographically separate from other areas and because of the impact of the nuclear power station accident. It was in June that members of the Association eventually began support activities in the area. A total of 289 practitioners, including those dispatched from other prefectures, gave acupuncture and moxibustion therapies and massage to approximately 1,000 disaster victims. Support was also provided by other types of professionals, such as nurses, judo healing therapists, certified health and athletic trainers, as well as students at professional schools for acupuncture and moxibustion. Medical care was provided not only to evacuated residents but also to staff members of local governments who operated evacuation centers.

Chapter 4 — Activities of Various Professional Organizations

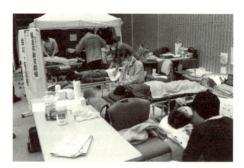

Figure 40-1 Providing medical care at evacuation centers

When providing support in evacuation centers, members of the Association found that many people complained of motor system symptoms, which are generally known as indications for acupuncture and moxibustion. Meanwhile, there were also many people who exhibited various other symptoms, such as insomnia, loss of appetite and constipation, due to stress caused by living as evacuees. One of the features of acupuncture and moxibustion therapies is that practitioners of acupuncture and moxibustion can provide comprehensive medical care for various symptoms of the body, not limited to the motor system. In evacuation centers, practitioners of acupuncture and moxibustion provided medical care to people who complained of several symptoms, and were able to relieve pain in the whole body (Figure 40-1).

In acupuncture and moxibustion therapies, it takes nearly one hour to provide medical care to one patient. Since acupuncture and moxibustion therapies stabilize the autonomic nervous system, patients can be relaxed mentally and physically through the therapies. In evacuation centers, many evacuees spoke of their distress, while receiving medical care. Acupuncture and moxibustion therapies seemed to provide opportunities for evacuees, who had significant stress in evacuation centers, to regain their mental and physical calmness and temporarily release their emotional baggage.

Many patients come to receive the therapies due to fatigue, including stiffness in the shoulders, cramps in the back and the lower back, and weariness in the legs, which are not medically regarded as a disease. In evacuation centers, many evacuees complained of these symptoms. Even if they were not medically sick, provision of medical care contributed to healing their tiredness and maintaining their bodily functions. I believe that acupuncture and moxibustion therapies helped evacuees live their lives in evacuation centers in a slightly more positive manner, helping them cope with the stress by healing their tired bodies. I also believe that acupuncture and moxibustion therapies were able to help evacuees in evacuation centers, who could not be medically treated, by using a different approach from general medical care.

In some evacuation centers, members who had received a license as instructors in preventive health care for the elderly from the Tokyo Metropolitan Geriatric Hospital and Institute of Gerontology (Tokyo Metropolitan Institute of Gerontology), visited evacuees to teach exercises. At first, exercise guidance was provided to evacuees to prevent deep vein thrombosis/pulmonary thromboembolism (economy class syndrome). New programs which focused on improving strength were then added to the usual exercise programs to prevent muscle weakness of the elderly due to a lack of activity in evacuation centers. Although information on the effects of the new programs was not collected, not only elderly people but also younger people seemed to enjoy doing the exercise. When hearing evacuees say, "We are waiting for you to come," and "Come visit us again," members of the Association believed that they were able to help evacuees refresh themselves, even if only temporarily.

C : Issues

We had some trouble in conducting support activities in evacuation centers. Since acupuncture and moxibustion therapies were virtually unknown among evacuees, not many evacuees wanted to receive the therapies. Some practitioners of the Association had a license as practitioners of Japanese traditional massage, massage and finger pressure, and were allowed to provide medical care with massage techniques. When many evacuees wanted to receive not acupuncture and moxibustion therapies but massage therapy, only members who had a license as practitioners of Japanese traditional massage, massage and finger pressure were asked to provide care and became overworked. In some cases, the Association was reluctantly compelled to restrict the number of people who could receive a massage therapy. Less recognition for acupuncture and moxibustion therapies also became an obstacle in situations other than medical necessity. Evacuation centers, where members of the Association conducted support activities, were operated by administrative bodies, and staff members of these administrative bodies were responsible for securing places for support activities at evacuation centers. Since these staff members had little knowledge about acupuncture and moxibustion therapies and practitioners, members of the Association were very careful about asking the staff members to secure places for conducting the therapies. As members of the Association continued to provide medical care, fewer evacuees hesitated to receive acupuncture and moxibustion therapies, and more evacuees came to receive therapies after they had undergone therapy and found it effective. If acupuncture and moxibustion therapies had been more widely recognized, the Association could have provided medical care to more evacuees. The Association realizes that it will confront this issue whenever it tries to conduct similar activities in the future.

D : To contribute to support activities with acupuncture and moxibustion therapies in case of a disaster

Through its support activities in this earthquake, the Association realized that practitioners of acupuncture and moxibustion were able to provide medical care even in a chaotic situation immediately after the earthquake, because they needed only simple medical tools. The Association also confirmed that acupuncture and moxibustion therapies were effective in easing the suffering of people living in evacuation centers. Although acupuncture and moxibustion therapies are unsuitable for people who are in mortal danger, they can help people restore their energy.

Ideally, practitioners of acupuncture and moxibustion should be included in disaster medical support teams to provide support in collaboration with other medical professionals. I heard that some practitioners of acupuncture and moxibustion actually worked that way in this earthquake. Although collaboration between acupuncture and moxibustion therapies and general medical treatment is ideal, there are various obstacles, such as less recognition of acupuncture and moxibustion therapies, in the present environment. These obstacles should be cleared away one at a time to realize a collaboration.

Acupuncture and moxibustion therapies can heal tiredness and maintain bodily functions. Making use of these features, practitioners of acupuncture and moxibustion can assist administrative and medical staff members who provide support to disaster victims, like conditioning trainers do for sport teams. I heard that a group of practitioners of acupuncture and moxibustion in another prefecture provided medical care mainly to staff members who conducted support activities.

Chapter 4 | Activities of Various Professional Organizations

Acupuncture and moxibustion therapies are traditional medicine that has been handed down from ancient times. However, they are not yet widely prevalent in contemporary Japan, and therefore can be said to be an unknown and new medicine. With features completely different from conventional medical treatment, acupuncture and moxibustion therapies have the potential of opening a new phase of medical support in case of a disaster. The Association intends to find ways to have acupuncture and moxibustion therapies effectively used as new medical resources, while building collaborative relationships with general medical professionals.

(Yohei Imaizumi)

41 Fukushima Association of Medical Social Workers

Two years have passed since the Great East Japan Earthquake occurred. In Fukushima Prefecture, the nuclear power station accident has made the recovery from the disaster more difficult than it already was. The evacuation order due to the nuclear power station accident was issued to eight municipalities in Futaba County and surrounding four municipalities. It is said that 96,000 residents were evacuated to other areas inside of the prefecture, and 56,000 residents to areas outside of the prefecture.

Since the occurrence of the earthquake, the Fukushima Professional Team for Counseling and Support, which comprised six professional organizations, has been involved in diverse support activities for disaster victims in various areas in the prefecture. Here is stated the issues of support activities for people whose human rights were infringed by the nuclear power plant accident, from the perspective of social workers.

A Immediately after the disaster (activities as hospital personnel)

Ohta Atami Hospital, where I worked at the time of the earthquake, is a secondary-level emergency hospital with 420 beds. The hospital was not significantly damaged by the earthquake. However, since large aftershocks continued, the hospital had inpatients in the old ward evacuated to the new wards. The halls and corridors of the new wards were filled with beds. Due to instability of the supply of food, fuel oil and medical products, it took three weeks for the hospital to return to a normal medical schedule.

The Koriyama Yulux Atami, a convention hall, is located near the hospital. After the earthquake, 1,000 residents were evacuated to this hall after their reception was refused by three to four other facilities designated as evacuation centers that were already filled with other evacuees. The residents evacuated to the hall included 70 residents and 40 staff members of special nursing homes for the elderly in Futaba County. The staff members evacuated these residents, who required intensive nursing care with an average nursing care level of 4.7, by bus without causing any deaths. With only the barest necessities, and with no personal information or drugs for the residents having been brought, the staff members provided round-the-clock care to the residents in a situation where they were unable to confirm the safety of their own family members. The residents were forced to lie down on blankets spread directly on the floor. Both the residents and the staff members, who carried out nursing care for such residents, were exhausted. The director of the Ohta Atami Hospital, who rushed to the hall in response to a request, found that the residents and the staff members had reached the limits of their physical strength and that they required an environment where beds were prepared to make nursing care more comfort and easy. Accordingly, he offered one of the hospital wards as an evacuation center (Figure 41-1). They moved to the hospital on March 14 (Figure 41-2). As the environment for nursing care was improved and even bathing was made possible, the staff members seemed to be somewhat refreshed.

In Koriyama City, some hospitals were completely destroyed or seriously damaged by the earthquake, and asked other facilities to receive their patients. The city faced an urgent need to restore the function of the hospitals. Social workers were required to promptly search for facilities where residents requiring intensive nursing care could receive comfortable care. They coordinated the reception of residents with special nursing care facilities for the elderly and geriatric health service facilities in neighboring municipalities. Consequently, all residents who were in stable condition were able to move to 12 other facilities between March 15 and 18.

Chapter 4 — Activities of Various Professional Organizations

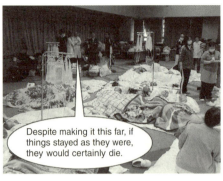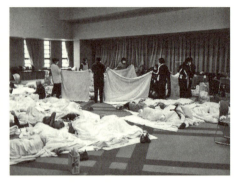

Figure 41-1 Environment for evacuees at the Koriyama Yulux Atami

Approx. 1,000 evacuees, including residents in special nursing care facilities for the elderly with an average nursing care level of 4.7

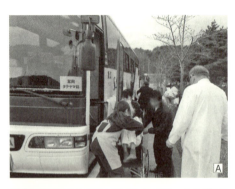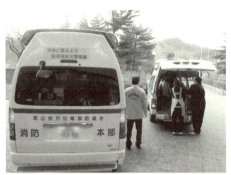
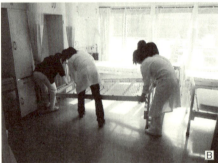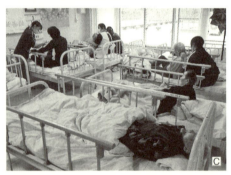

Figure 41-2 Moving to Ohta Atami Hospital

A: The director of the hospital determined to offer his hospital as an evacuation center, while consulting with Fukushima Prefecture and making arrangements to be covered by the Disaster Relief Act.
B: Preparing beds with the concerted efforts of all staff members
C: Staff members are also disaster victims. They continue to provide round-the-clock care in a situation where they are unable to confirm the safety of their own family members. They need to be free from work.
   It is imperative to restore hospital functions.
   Social workers having coordinated the secondary evacuation with neighboring special nursing care facilities for the elderly, while using their networks.
   (It is important to obtain confirmation from administrative bodies and keep records.)

B: What was learned through support activities for special nursing care facilities for the elderly

① Understanding the Disaster Relief Act
- In evacuation centers, disposal diapers and commodities can be procured from relief supplies. Meanwhile, when evacuees are hospitalized, they have to bear the cost of these items.
- Although the expenses required for emergency evacuation can be covered by the Disaster Relief Act, those needed when evacuees return home must be borne by the individuals. For instance, a patient on a ventilator, who was transferred to a hospital in an adjacent prefecture, had to pay the transportation cost of 200,000 yen when he returned home. The amount is too high and unreasonable for individual evacuees to bear.

② Keeping basic information about patients and residents, such as medical history, medication profile and family information, with the individuals.

This time, names of evacuated residents were clear because they were accompanied by staff members. However, they had no other information, such as medical history and medication profiles. Immediately after the nuclear power station accident, it was said that if another explosion occurred at the nuclear power station, residents in Koriyama City would also have to evacuate the area. Accordingly, basic information about individual patients was compiled in an A4-sized form and all patients were to keep them at hand in case of evacuation. Since personal computers may be unavailable in case of a disaster, paper-based patient information should be prepared and kept with individual patients.

③ Teamwork and networks required on a routine basis

Each facility that received residents requiring intensive nursing care responded to requests from social workers in a cooperative manner, although they were also affected by the earthquake. After the disaster social workers were able to defuse the situation through their networks with acquaintances. However, it is crucial to create organizational networks, including preparing evacuation centers for those requiring special care, on a routine basis.

C: Activities of the Fukushima Professional Team for Counseling and Support

The Great East Japan Earthquake is said to be different from the Great Hanshin-Awaji Earthquake and the Mid Niigata Prefecture Earthquake, in that disaster victims either died from the tsunami or they suffered no or slight injuries, and that there were no seriously-injured people. As a result, even bedridden elderly people and disabled people were evacuated to temporary evacuation centers, where sufficient nursing care was not provided to them due to the chaotic situation. Although many professionals and volunteers were involved in support activities in evacuation centers, their activities were not conducted in an effective manner due to poor management. Under these conditions, the Fukushima Professional Team for Counseling and Support was organized in response to the demand by the President of the Fukushima Care Manager Association that every association should work together, as a single association was unable to do everything. The Fukushima Association of Medical Social Workers ("the Association"), the Fukushima Association of Certified Social Workers, the Fukushima Physical Therapy Association, the Fukushima Association of Occupational Therapists, and the Fukushima Association of Psychiatric Social Workers formed the team. Working with Fukushima Prefecture, the Fukushima Professional Team for Counseling and Support devised a provisional plan in which only the first assessment was necessary for evacuees to be eligible for nursing care insurance services. Consequently, nursing care insurance services were able to be provided to all people that needed them. The Fukushima Professional Team for Counseling and Support mainly engaged in coordination of these nursing care insurance services at temporary and secondary evacuation centers. This led to the establishment of the Fukushima Dispatch Project of Professional Teams for Counseling and Support for Livelihood Support for Affected Elderly People in Temporary Housing." The Fukushima Professional Team for Counseling and Support conducted unique support activities in various areas in Fukushima Prefecture to meet welfare needs. In Koriyama City, the team opened social workers' rooms in temporary housing to provide consultation once a week. The team introduced medical institutions near evacuation centers to evacuees, cared for lonely elderly people, and addressed the needs for evacuees to live in ways they like in evacuation centers. However, over time the team members faced greater difficulties in providing support. This was because the unknown future created increasing anxiety and frustration among evacuees, and different backgrounds of individual evacuees caused disputes between them. Some evacuees were hurt by biased views and harsh words of residents at evacuation destinations.

After the earthquake, the Association participated in the Fukushima Professional Team for Counseling and Support, and conducted diverse activities in various areas in Fukushima Prefecture. The following is a review of these activities from three phases.

① Support activities in temporary and secondary evacuation centers under a crisis situation

Social workers puzzled over what they could do for evacuees, while providing support. However, as times went by, obstacles in the lives of evacuees became obvious, and social workers gradually recognized that they needed to make adjustments to regional resources systems.

② Support activities when evacuees moved from secondary evacuation centers to temporary housing and municipally-subsidized housing

Social workers provided information on temporary housing to evacuees, so that the evacuees could select the best temporary housing where they would live over the following few years. Moreover, they provided support for a smooth transition from lives in evacuation centers, where food, clothing and shelter were secured, to lives in temporary housing.

③ Livelihood support in temporary and municipally-subsidized housing

Social workers conducted unique activities in various areas, including offering health classes. In Koriyama City, they opened social workers' rooms, partly thanks to the efforts of the Fukushima Ward Council on Social Welfare. Some evacuees masochistically tormented themselves over the fact that they had to depend on relief supplies, while others became addicted to gambling and drinking. Evacuees also suffered from a sense of isolation due to their prolonged lives as evacuees. Social workers regularly visited evacuees to provide support. Meanwhile, some evacuees enjoyed growing vegetables, although they were leading inconvenient lives in unfamiliar areas. When social workers asked local residents to lend part of their fields to these evacuees, the residents willingly accepted the request. The evacuees saw their vegetables transplanted to the fields with great joy.

D Toward the reconstruction of lives

The nuclear power station accident destroyed people's lives, hurt people, and broke ties between people. Administrative bodies intend to solve issues caused by the accident with money. However, the recovery of Fukushima Prefecture depends not on money, but on how disaster victims can regain their own lives. Issues related to human dignity and health may not be solved with money. I intend to keep this in mind as a social worker.

Even in such a situation, some people find joy in connecting with others, and send messages that they should keep their hopes up for the sake of the next generation. People living as evacuees patiently endure hardship. Fukushima Prefecture will not recover unless individual residents can reconstruct their lives. Having experienced the earthquake on March 11, the Association is filled with a sense of their mission to provide support to disaster victims until they require no more support.

(Junko Okawara)

42. Universities and other educational research institutions (1)
— Guidelines for childcare support in areas around evacuation zones

The nuclear accident at the Fukushima Daiichi Nuclear Power Station of the Tokyo Electric Power Company drastically changed daily lives of parents and children in Fukushima City. Immediately after the accident, I tried to investigate what measures had been effective for maternal and child health in the previous overseas cases: This for my own reference. Unfortunately, there were few available practical materials concerning maternal and child health. The following is a paper that summarized the process of how a university and a local government worked together to consider childcare support measures after the earthquake. The contents of the paper were partially altered and were translated into Japanese[1]. I hope that publication in several languages of regional activities at the time of the nuclear accident will serve as a useful reference in cases of unexpected accidents and for preparedness for unexpected disasters.

A Changes in lives

Among areas located around evacuation zones in Fukushima Prefecture, Fukushima City had relatively higher levels of air radiation. A significant feature of the situation in the city was that there was a large migration of the population after the earthquake; although the city was not designated as an evacuation area. In particular, the number of children under the age of five rapidly decreased by approximately 17% during the two years after the earthquake.

Under these conditions, medical students at Fukushima Medical University conducted a survey to compare childcare concerns before and after the earthquake in Fukushima City, in cooperation with public health nurses in the city. They summarized the records of health checkups for children age 3 to 4 months, using 82 cases in 2010 and 88 cases in 2011. As a result, they classified the contents of childcare concerns into six major categories (child development, child nutrition, child diseases, child physical shape, daily lives, and radiation). A new category "radiation," which did not exist a year before, appeared after the earthquake, and accounted for 30% of the childcare concerns. Moreover, the ratio of "child diseases" increased from 14% in 2010 to 27% in 2011.

This kind of parental anxiety, which does not reach a pathological level, is considered to be a natural reaction of parents to uncertain risks and new regulation, which have come into their daily lives. It is reported that the Chernobyl nuclear accident had a long-term impact on the mental health of parents and children[2]. After the earthquake, parents and children carried personal dosimeters (glass badges) with them whenever they went outside, and large radiation monitoring equipment was set out in public places in the city. Although decontamination was gradually performed in nursery schools, kindergartens, schools, and parks, most parents restricted children's outdoor activities, depending on radiation levels. Schools distributed leaflets to parents through students, which explained radiation levels, decontamination and food monitoring.

The following is a case example of how a children's educational facility called "Comcom (a facility to foster children's dreams)," which was located in the central part of the city, addressed the anxiety of parents and children in the post-quake period. With science and computer laboratories, art and music rooms, a library, a rock climbing wall, a playroom for younger children, a planetarium and a science exhibition room, the facility held workshops and events for children and families. A characteristic feature of the facility was that residents participated in a construction project at the facility, and therefore it reflected the needs of users. Although the building was severely damaged by the earthquake, the facility was re-opened in July 2011. Thereafter, residents used the facility as a safe indoor play space with little exposure to radiation. The facility also conducted classes to teach parents and children about radiation, and held many science events in collaboration with academic institutions inside and outside of the prefecture. Moreover, at the end of 2011, a large- scale indoor facility was opened in Koriyama City, which had a relatively high radiation level, as did Fukushima City.

B　Collaboration between a university and a local government

Immediately after the earthquake, public health nurses in Fukushima City worked ceaselessly, in particular, to provide support to disaster victims in evacuation centers. Despite engaging in extra duties, public health nurses resumed their regular activities, including child health checkups that restarted one month after the earthquake. Around that time, the city requested me to provide advice to support parents who faced anxiety about radiation exposure of their children.

This request from Fukushima City to Fukushima Medical University was made based on the collaboration between the university and local governments. The Department of Public Health, Fukushima Medical University School of Medicine had conducted joint projects with several local governments in the prefecture since before the earthquake. In the field of maternal and child health, the university and the local governments worked together to collect childcare data, and conduct and assess childcare support programs in various areas in the prefecture. The long trial-and-error efforts of researchers in the university and public health nurses in the local governments contributed to support activities after the earthquake.

C　Short-term measures

After the initial request from the city in April 2011, three meetings were held with public health nurses in the city in May, September, and November 2011. Table 42-1 presents recommendations from each meeting, which were summarized by consulting experts in disaster mental health and psychology as needed. To prepare for the first meeting, I asked public health nurses in the city to list items about which parents with small children frequently asked advice. The items were mainly about the safety of going out, opening windows, using ventilation fans, drying laundry outside, and water. Items specific to parents engaging in

Table 42-1　Summary of meetings between the university and the city

	Time of meeting	Major recommendations
1st meeting	May 2011 (2 months after the earthquake)	Aim: To respond to parents' anxiety at the initial stage 1) Providing consistent information 2) Setting up indoor play spaces and watching over children and parents 3) Increasing mental health awareness of public health nurses
2nd meeting	September 2011 (6 months after the earthquake)	Aim: To respond to parents' continued anxiety 1) Continuing to provide consistent information 2) Improving individual consultations and group meetings 3) Introducing screening to identify parents with anxiety 4) Responding to separated families
3rd meeting	November 2011 (8 months after the earthquake)	Aim: To build a long-term care system 1) Improving early childcare support 2) Promoting cooperation with residents and collaboration between different sections in the city office 3) Improving training programs for public health nurses

child rearing included the safety of breast milk, the necessity of evacuation and other preventive measures to reduce children's exposure to radiation. In addition, a sense of distrust of information provided by the national government was also listed.

In the first meeting, three specific proposals were presented as countermeasures against parents' anxiety at the initial stage, with the aim of reducing the provision of inconsistent information that fuel parents' anxiety and showing a receptive attitude toward parents' anxiety.

① Providing comprehensive and consistent information: creating leaflets for distribution and consultation materials based on close consideration and consensus so that public health nurses will not make inconsistent statements that could confuse residents and can share a common view about information to be provided

② Setting up indoor play spaces where children can play without fear of radiation and mothers can communicate with each other under the benevolent watch of public health nurses

③ Sharing the recognition among public health nurses that parents' anxiety immediately after the earthquake is a natural response and that receptive attitudes toward parents' anxiety and efforts to protect the health of family members are important

An earlier study on residents' risk awareness and behavior after the Three Mile Island accident indicated that voluntary evacuation of residents in wide areas beyond the governor's evacuation advisory resulted not only from providing confusing information, but also from residents' unique risk awareness of a carcinogenic and genetic influence[3]. Accordingly, the first proposal alone was insufficient to address parents' anxiety. The national government explained that exposure to radiation due to the nuclear accident at the Fukushima Daiichi Station had little impact on an increased cancer risk. However, parents' concerns about the appearance of invisible and dangerous environmental factors cannot be easily resolved, regardless of the degree of risk. Health behavior is formed through complicated processes, and good compliance can be obtained only if information is considered credible. The second and third proposals were designed to help public health nurses build a trusting relationship with residents by showing their receptive attitudes toward parents' anxiety.

In September 2011, I received another request for providing advice. I asked public health nurses to report their activities during the past three months to confirm that my initial advice was of help to their activities. According to a report, they discussed and created leaflets on radiation, its health effects and daily preventive measures against radiation exposure, and widely distributed them to residents. They also used the leaflets at childcare consultations. Moreover, they regularly held lecture meetings concerning radiation with support from local medical associations, and provided support to parents in group settings with assistance from societies of certified clinical psychologists. In addition, they conducted a questionnaire survey about changes in the lives of parents and children as part of their independent epidemiological study, at the time of child health checkups in July.

Major issues in the second meeting were how to respond to parents' continued anxiety and how to give attention to separated families. In most of these families, fathers stayed at home to work in the city, and mothers and children voluntarily evacuated the city. Meanwhile, some parents were worried and complained about their inability to move out of the city due to economic reasons. Public health nurses were concerned about these parents as well. In these cases, careful responses should be offered, depending on the situation of individual families.

Based on assessment of these conditions, four measures were proposed.

① Continuing to provide consistent information.

② Increasing opportunities for individual childcare consultations and parents' group meetings.

In particular, I proposed to include parent-and-child play programs and learning activities into group meetings to attract more participants; for example, classes on radiation were conducted at Comcom for parents and children. Science lab activities for children and consultation sessions for parents were combined in classes in which parents were able to ask experts questions about radiation, while their children were carrying out experiments.

③ Introducing systematic screening for identifying high-risk families.

Maternal and child health services should not be provided uniformly to everyone. Systematic screening should be performed to grasp the situation of individual parents and children and identify those in need of support.

④ Reaching out to fathers.

There were many cases where family members were forced to be separated. One of the ways to address problems caused by this situation might be to listen to fathers' views through questionnaires used in child health checkups.

Since the second meeting was brief with participation of a few public health nurses, the third meeting was immediately scheduled to discuss in detail about longer-term measures.

D : Long-term prospects

In November 2011, the third meeting was held as a larger-scale training workshop, which was attended by 27 public health nurses. In the meeting, lectures were delivered by two lecturers invited by the university, and public health nurses were provided with an opportunity for an exchange of views. Topics of the lectures were about mental health in case of a disaster, long-term benefits of early childcare support and practical childcare support methods. Subsequently, public health nurses and lecturers in groups exchanged opinions concerning the needs of residents, current public health responses and future prospects.

Based on their discussions, three major guidelines were suggested concerning long-term prospects.
① Improving early childcare support.

At the time of a disaster, top priority should be placed on support for parents and children so that they can return to their daily lives. It is apparent that the earlier childcare support is provided, the higher cost-effectiveness can be achieved to promote the sound growth of children[4]. Healthy development of young people leads to an increase of social productivity and a decrease of social burden imposed by negative outcomes, such as crimes.

② Effectively providing information in cooperation with resident organizations.

Residents may make proactive decisions and ease their sense of distrust of local governments by more voluntarily obtaining information that responds to individual needs. At the 60th Annual Meeting of the Tohoku Public Health Association, which was hosted immediately after the earthquake by the Department of Public Health, School of Medicine, Fukushima Medical University, Professor Michael Reich of the Harvard School of Public Health delivered a lecture, and proposed six public health guidelines for post-disaster recovery. As one of the guidelines, he suggested enhancing social capital in local communities[5]. Social capital refers to features of social organization, such as trust, norms, and networks that can improve the efficiency of society by facilitating coordinated actions. Interestingly, residents in areas with high social capital returned from their evacuation destinations to their hometowns much earlier after both the Great Kanto Earthquake and the Great Hanshin-Awaji Earthquake.

Chapter 4 | Activities of Various Professional Organizations

③ Improving training programs for public health nurses

The improvement of training programs can increase the skills and knowledge of public health nurses, who make first contact with residents, and can provide an opportunity for public health nurses to independently determine their course of action. Moreover, participation of public health nurses from different sections of the city office and different local governments can provide a valuable opportunity to strengthen the formation of networks. The workshop held in 2011 was evaluated by participants, and more than 90% of the participants answered that the workshop was useful and that they wanted to attend another workshop.

E   Residents and scientists

In cases of unintended pregnancy or a first pregnancy, mothers tend to lose their confidence in child rearing. Thus, unexpected and first-time events, even though they are pregnancies that are generally considered as a happy event, may have an adverse impact on mental health. This corresponds to the features of the nuclear accident. Scientific data on the mental health effects of the nuclear accident has been established. The carcinogenic effects of prolonged exposure to low-dose radiation are still under debate. The Fukushima Health Management Survey, an epidemiological investigation, is being conducted targeting residents in Fukushima Prefecture. However, it is extremely difficult to identify a small increase in cancer risk caused by low-dose exposure, while taking into account many carcinogenic risks, such as biological factors, socio-economic factors, and health behavior[6]. In addition to these complex confounding associations, there is a tendency for mothers to make exaggerated reports on physical symptoms of their children after a nuclear accident. Studies by medical students showed that this tendency was observed in Fukushima City. This information bias will make epidemiological assessments of carcinogenic risk of low-dose exposure more difficult.

The nuclear accident has created a large gap between residents and scientists. Under a situation where scientific evidence on health effects of low-dose exposure has not been clarified, if scientists state that current exposure levels present no risk to daily lives, residents may consider that the scientists reject their anxiety and infringe upon their right to protect their lives. Similar conflicts were reported from the Love Canal incident in the U.S. Although many residents in an area where chemical waste had been dumped complained of health problems, scientists did not reach a consensus view on a causal relationship between chemical waste and health problems, thereby creating further confusion. Meanwhile, the media effectively turned this into a social issue, and the government was forced to respond.

The occupational philosophy of public health nurses, who support the health of residents, is to identify the needs of residents, offer appropriate and prompt responses, and establish a trusting relationship with residents. Meanwhile, epidemiologists disclose scientific evidence, but the results are inaccessible and incomprehensible to residents. To narrow the gap between residents and scientists, it is necessary to develop human resources who can accurately convey information between the two groups. Our example of collaboration between researchers at the university and public health nurses can serve as a stepping-stone to reducing the gap. A major overseas example is the Council on Linkages between Academia and Public Health Practice, in which 20 member organizations work to strengthen partnerships between relevant organizations, foster experts in public health and promote joint research, aiming to pursue public health activities based on scientific evidence.

F Conclusion

In Fukushima City, low-dose exposure is expected to persist in the future. Amid parents' continuing concerns about radiation, children will continue to grow. Experts in the field of public health should have long-term prospects and make constructive responses by taking this earthquake as an opportunity to improve maternal and child health systems. To this end, the details of the collaboration between the university and the local government were introduced in this section as one of the effective measures. Although more than two years have passed since the earthquake, the university is conducting workshops for public health nurses on an increasing scale.

(Aya Goto)

References

1) Goto A, Reich MR, Yuriko S, Tsutomi H, Watanabe E, Yasumura S: Parenting in Fukushima City in the post-disaster period: Short-term strategies and long-term perspectives. Disasters, 2014.

2) Bromet EJ: Mental health consequences of the Chernobyl disaster. Journal of Radiological Protection, 32 (1), N71–N75, 2012.

3) Lindell MK, Barnes VE: Protective response to technological emergency: Risk perception and behavioral intention. Nuclear Safety, 27 (4), 457–467, 1986.

4) Heckman JJ: Skill formation and the economics of investing in disadvantaged children. Science, 312 (5782), 1900–1902, 2006.

5) Michael Reich: *A Public Health Perspective on Reconstructing Post-disaster Japan*. The Journal of the Japan Medical Association, 140 (7), 1480–1485, 2011.

6) Boice, JD Jr.: Radiation epidemiology: a perspective on Fukushima. Journal of Radiological Protection, 32 (1), N33–N40, 2012.

43 Universities and other educational research institutions (2) — Overview of the Fukushima Health Management Survey

More than two years have passed since the Great East Japan Earthquake occurred at 2:46 p.m. on Friday, March 11, 2011. Currently, street scenes and facial expressions of residents in Fukushima Prefecture seem perfectly ordinary. People who visit Fukushima Prefecture now may not feel the direct impact of the massive earthquake and subsequent tsunami. However, they will find that there still remains temporary housing in suburb areas, about a 10-minute drive from the city center, and that there are few vegetables grown in the prefecture and no fish caught off the coast of the prefecture to be found on shelves at supermarkets.

In Fukushima Prefecture, the nuclear accident at the Fukushima Daiichi Nuclear Power Station of the Tokyo Electric Power Company ("Fukushima Daiichi Station") caused many issues, such as evacuation due to the accident, concerns about the health effects of radiation, delay of decontamination, contaminated water treatment, and harmful rumors. Unfortunately, it seems that we are a long way from the restoration and recovery of Fukushima Prefecture. Not only the approximately 210,000 residents who were forced to be evacuated, but also other residents in the prefecture must make a living there, while feeling a vague anxiety.

The national government, the prefectural and municipal governments, and other administrative bodies have acted responsibly and taken diverse measures to alleviate the sufferings of residents who lost jobs or the foundations of their livelihood, or were forced to live separately from their families. Moreover, specified non-profit corporations (NPO corporations), public-service corporations, incorporated foundations, academic societies and volunteers as well as universities and other educational research institutions also have played a large role in dealing with various issues that have not been adequately or fully addressed by administrative bodies.

According to the Ministry of Education, Culture, Sports, Science and Technology, there were 771 universities (86 national universities, 82 public universities and 603 private universities), 373 junior colleges (22 public junior colleges and 351 private junior colleges) in Japan in 2012. In addition, there are approximately 840,000 scientists in Japan, in the fields of arts, social science, life science, physical science and engineering (Science Council of Japan). In the post-quake situation, it is worthy of note that universities and other educational research institutions, such as Hiroshima University, Nagasaki University and the National Institute of Radiological Sciences, were very active in taking measures against the nuclear disaster while working as organizations. Meanwhile, many educational researchers throughout Japan also undertook various efforts on an individual basis after the Great East Japan Earthquake.

A   Major activities of universities in Fukushima Prefecture

1   University of Aizu

The University of Aizu established the Reconstruction Support Center on March 4, 2013, aiming to contribute to the recovery of Fukushima Prefecture from the Great East Japan Earthquake by making use of its expertise in Information and Communication Technology (ICT). According to the website of the university, "through the establishment of the Reconstruction Support Center, the University of Aizu and the Junior College of Aizu intend to promote university-wide efforts to support reconstruction of Fukushima Prefecture." Moreover, "One of the aims of the establishment of the center is to offer technical assistance to the Fukushima Health Management Survey conducted by Fukushima Medical University. The university will work cooperatively to manage a large amount of data in a safe and secure manner by taking full advantage of its ICT expertise. Moreover, it will contribute to overcoming the nuclear disaster and harmful rumors from an aspect of ICT." Director Jiro Iwase is involved in creating a database as a member of a database committee established within the Radiation Medical Science Center for the Fukushima Health Management Survey, Fukushima Medical University.

2 Iwaki Meisei University and Higashi Nippon International University

Iwaki Meisei University and Higashi Nippon International University established the Iwaki Community Reconstruction Center, in cooperation with Fukushima Prefecture and Iwaki City. Aiming for early reconstruction of Fukushima Prefecture, they are involved in four projects: 1) a research project measuring radiation and radioactivity and their reduction, 2) an earthquake record maintenance project, 3) a tourism and regional development project through provision of information on affected areas, and 4) an independence support promotion project for affected disabled people.

3 Ohu University

In response to a request for postmortem examination of unidentified bodies in the Soma area in Fukushima Prefecture, postmortem teams were formed at the School of Dentistry, and a total of over 50 dentists were dispatched to the area. Moreover, faculties of the university are engaged in research, which has been adopted in the Revitalization Promotion Program conducted by the Japan Science and Technology Agency (JST).

4 College of Engineering, Nihon University

To assist in the recovery from the Great East Japan Earthquake, the College of Engineering, Nihon University has conducted diverse projects, making use of the features of the College of Engineering, as follows.
1. Conducting a sports festival support project and other unique projects as part of the efforts of the Nichidai Sustainable Platform, which supports activities for the restoration and recovery from the earthquake
2. Planning various symposiums as part of the efforts for the recovery from the earthquake by making full use of research and technologies in its specialized field

5 Fukushima University

Fukushima University established the Fukushima Future Center for Regional Revitalization on April 13, 2011, immediately after the earthquake. The university aims to "scientifically conduct survey research on facts concerning damage resulting from the Great East Japan Earthquake and the nuclear accident at the Fukushima Daiichi Nuclear Power Station of the Tokyo Electric Power Company. Moreover, it intends to provide support for the restoration and recovery from the earthquake by forecasting developments in affected areas based on the facts." Currently, a total of 55 experts in the fields of the environment, regional policies, industry, education and psychology, as well as industrial recovery, radiation, and energy are working energetically.

6 Fukushima Medical University

Since Fukushima Medical University Hospital was designated as a secondary-level hospital for radia-

Chapter 4 | Activities of Various Professional Organizations

tion exposure, immediately after the earthquake it was preoccupied with responses to patients who were exposed to radiation and were radioactively contaminated. Since it also served as the only tertiary-level emergency hospital in Fukushima Prefecture, it was expected to play a larger role in providing medical care after the earthquake, and was very busy responding to patients. Regarding the overview of university-wide efforts, please refer to the website: http://www.fmu.ac.jp/univ/chiiki/dbook.html (in Japanese) and http://www.fmu.ac.jp/univ/en/about/e_dbook.html (in English).

B : Efforts of Fukushima Medical University (Fukushima Health Management Survey)

In light of the health effects of radiation resulting from the nuclear power station accident, Fukushima Prefecture decided to conduct the Fukushima Health Management Survey, aiming to care for the health of residents for many years to come. Fukushima Medical University received a commission to conduct the survey.

1 Roles of the university

Fukushima Medical University was founded with the aim of training and fostering medical professionals who contribute to health, medical and welfare services for residents in Fukushima Prefecture. The Fukushima Health Management Survey is regarded as part of support activities for health management of residents, and was requested by the residents. Fukushima Medical University took the lead in planning and implementing the survey. On June 1, 2011, less than three months after the earthquake, the university established the Radiation Medical Science Center for the Fukushima Health Management Survey as an internal organization to prepare a draft of the survey. The Review Committee for the Fukushima Health Management Survey, which was set up by Fukushima Prefecture, is responsible for examination of survey methods, and progress management and assessment of the survey.

2 Overview of the Fukushima Health Management Survey

The details of the Fukushima Health Management Survey were stated previously. Here is introduced the overview of the survey. The survey comprises a basic survey and four detailed surveys; 1) thyroid ultrasound examination, 2) comprehensive health check, 3) mental health and lifestyle survey, and 4) pregnancy and birth survey (Figure 43-1).

a. Basic survey

The release of radioactive materials after the nuclear power station accident disturbed not only residents living in the evacuation area within a 20-km radius of the Fukushima Daiichi Station, but also all residents in Fukushima Prefecture. Accordingly, the basic survey was conducted to estimate external exposure levels among all of approximately 2.05 million residents in the prefecture. In the survey, questionnaires were distributed to the residents to ask about their movements and locations (movement record) during the four months after the occurrence of the nuclear power station accident until July 11, when air radiation levels were the highest. Based on the concept that accurately knowing external exposure levels that may pose a health risk is the basis for health management, this survey was named as a basic survey. Estimated external exposure levels (effective dose levels) were calculated using an external exposure dose assessment system, which was developed by the National Institute of Radiological Sciences.

By the end of July 31, 2013, a total of 445,015 residents had responded. The results for 435,788 resi-

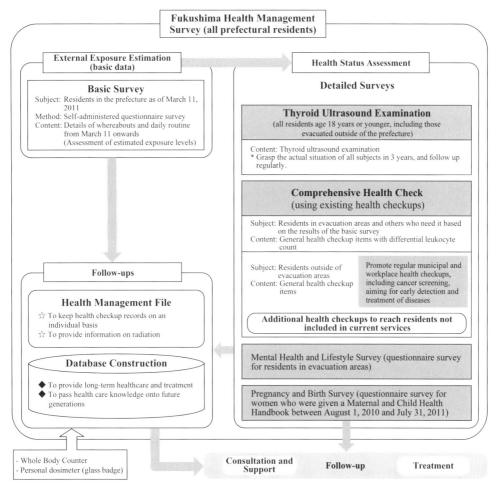

Figure 43-1 Overall picture of the Fukushima Health Management Survey at an initial stage

dents, excluding radiation workers, showed that the estimated external exposure levels for 99.8% of the respondents were less than 5 mSv. On the whole, it is determined that released radiation is unlikely to cause damage to human health.

However, the response rate to the questionnaires was only 23.5% as of July 31, 2013. The purposes of the survey did not seem to be fully understood by residents. Accordingly, various efforts are implemented, including providing face-to-face support for completing the questionnaires, to increase public awareness of the survey.

b. Detailed surveys

In principle, detailed surveys were conducted targeting all of approximately 210,000 residents who lived in the evacuation area within a 20-km radius of the Fukushima Daiichi Station and evacuated the area at the direction of the national government (residents in Hirono Town, Naraha Town, Tomioka Town, Kawauchi Village, Okuma Town, Futaba Town, Namie Town, Katsurao Village, Iitate Village, Minamisoma City, Tamura City, Kawamata Town, and part of Date City 〈areas related to Specific Spots for Recommended Evacuation〉). This was based on the idea that appropriate health care should be provided to evacuees

Chapter 4 | **Activities of Various Professional Organizations**

since health effects caused by evacuation were known to be significant.

① Thyroid ultrasound examination

Considering that parents throughout Fukushima Prefecture were concerned about pediatric thyroid cancer, thyroid ultrasound examinations were conducted targeting all residents age 18 years or younger at the time of the earthquake. The examinations were commenced in October, 2011. At first, preliminary examinations were conducted until March 2014 to confirm the actual situation during the period when radiation was unlikely to have an effect on the thyroid. After April 2014, formal examinations are held every two years for residents age 20 years or younger. For those who become 20 or older, examinations are undertaken every five years to watch over the health of residents throughout life.

Initially, thyroid ultrasound examinations are conducted. If nodules and cysts are detected, secondary examinations, such as detailed thyroid ultrasound examinations, blood collection, urine testing, and cytodiagnosis as needed, are conducted. A system in which approximately 20,000 evacuees living outside of the prefecture can also undergo the examinations at medical institutions at their evacuation destinations, has been improved.

Of 289,960 target residents living in the prefecture as of August 23, 2013, 238,785 residents underwent the examinations. Consequently, 225,537 residents who obtained the results of the examinations needed no secondary examinations, and 99.31% of them obtained Level-A assessments (A1 and A2), which needed only follow-up care until the next examination after 2014. Meanwhile, secondary examinations were required for 0.69% of the residents (1,558 persons) who had a Level-B assessment with nodular lesions of over 5.1 mm and cysts of over 20.1 mm being detected, and one resident who had a Level-C assessment. Of 897 residents who completed secondary examinations, 59 residents were found to have lesions and cysts that were malignant and were suspected of malignancy. However, these lesions and cysts were considered to have already existed before the earthquake and they were detected early by the examinations.

② Comprehensive health check

Residents in restricted areas were forced to be evacuated and lost opportunities to receive health checkups, thereby facing issues of health care. Moreover, they were also forced to drastically change their lifestyles, such as dietary habits and physical exercise habits. Accordingly, comprehensive health checkups were conducted to assess their health conditions, with the aim of prevention of lifestyle-related diseases and early detection and early treatment of such diseases.

Checkup methods and items are as follows: 1) For residents age 16 years or older living in the prefecture, additional checkup items, such as blood count (red cell count, hematocrit, hemoglobin, platelet count, white cell count, and differential leukocyte count) serum creatinine, eGFR, and uric acid are included in specific health checkups provided by municipal governments. Those who cannot receive health checkups including these additional items can undergo comprehensive health checkups in other areas in the prefecture. Comprehensive health checkups for residents age 15 years or younger are provided in medical institutions where designated pediatricians work; 2) Comprehensive health checkups for target residents evacuated outside of the prefectures are provided in medical institutions that belong to the Japan Municipal Hospital Association, the Japan National Health Insurance Clinics and Hospitals Association, and the Association of National Social Insurance Society, with the assistance of the Japan Anti-Tuberculosis Association.

The results of general health checkups before the earthquake and comprehensive health checkups after the earthquake were compared upon request from Iitate Village. Target residents for comparison were 1,503

Table 43-1 Comparison of the results of health checkups

	Before the earthquake	After the earthquake
Obesity (BMI)	36%	48% ↑
Hypertension	57%	65% ↑
Diabetes	9%	11% ↑
Dyslipidemia	40%	52% ↑

men and women age 40 years or older living in Iitate Village (714 men and 789 women with an average age of 65 years old) who underwent one or more specific health checkups, and health checkups for the elderly (age 75 years or older) between 2008 and 2010. The study included 1,032 of these residents (489 men and 543 women; follow-up rate of 69% and an average follow-up period of 1.8 years) who underwent comprehensive health checkups after the earthquake between 2011 and 2012. The comparison results revealed that checkup scores declined as shown in Table 43-1. Iitate Village publicized the comparison results to residents through its public relations magazines, in order to increase public awareness about health conditions after the earthquake. Furthermore, the village held health classes designed to increase the amount of physical activity, in collaboration with medical institutions.

③ Mental health and lifestyle survey

Since physical and mental health problems were identified as part of long-term health effects of the Chernobyl nuclear accident, a mental health and lifestyle survey was conducted targeting the same people who received the comprehensive health checks. From January 18, 2012, questionnaires were sent by mail to residents who were eligible for comprehensive health checks in FY 2011. Four different types of questionnaires were prepared according to age groups, and survey items were set for each age group. Major survey items included current mental and physical health conditions, lifestyles (dietary habits, sleep, smoking, drinking, and exercise), activities in the past six months, and experience in the Great East Japan Earthquake.

If respondents were determined to be in need of consultation and support after filing the survey, clinical psychologists, public health nurses and nurses provided telephone consultations. If needed, and with the consent of the respondents, they offered their information to the Fukushima Center for Disaster Mental Health and municipal governments to provide further support. If respondents were determined to need medical advice, physicians who were registered with medical institutions in the prefecture were introduced to them. Of 210,189 target people, 18,745 children and 73,569 adults responded to the survey. According to the survey results, 1,363 children (7.3%) and 5,359 adults (7.3%) were found to require assistance. Regarding lifestyles, 3,351 persons (4.6%) of 73,569 respondents were found to need support.

The survey was conducted in FY 2012 as well, when a major change was made to questionnaires for children age 0 to 6 years old. Since the Strengths and Difficulties Questionnaire (SDQ), which was used as an index for assessing mental health status of children, was designed for children age 4 years or older, the questionnaires for children age 0 to 6 years were divided into two types: those for children age 0 to 3 years and those for children age 4 to 6 years. Although the final results have not yet been obtained, psychological effects in children and adults seem to be slightly less.

④ Pregnancy and birth survey

To respond to the anxiety of expectant and nursing mothers in the prefecture, a pregnancy and birth survey was conducted targeting all women who were pregnant at the time of the Great East Japan Earthquake. The survey aimed not only to provide support to expectant and nursing mothers, but also to improve

Chapter 4 | Activities of Various Professional Organizations

medical services in the field of obstetrics and perinatal medicine in the prefecture.

Questionnaires were distributed to 16,001 women in the prefecture who were given a Maternal and Child Health Handbook between August 1, 2010 and July 31, 2011. Survey items included the situation of receiving pregnancy checkups after the earthquake, health conditions during the progress of pregnancy, the situation of giving birth, and mental health status. The survey for expectant and nursing mothers evacuated outside of the prefecture was provided in cooperation with the Japan Society of Obstetrics and Gynecology and the Japan Association of Obstetricians and Gynecologists.

After the survey, call centers were established to respond to concerns about health care and child rearing, and midwives and public health nurses provided telephone consultations. Consultations were also provided by e-mail. Those who were determined to be in need of assistance based on the survey results were given telephone consultations by midwives and nurses. Those who were determined to need medical advice received care from their regular obstetricians and gynecologists, and if needed, from physicians at universities. In FY 2011, 9,316 women (58.2%) responded to the survey. Of the respondents, 1,401 women (1,224 women who checked items of depression, and 177 women chosen based on their free comments) were determined to require assistance, and were given telephone consultations. The consultations were provided concerning radiation (409 cases), mothers themselves (283 cases), child rearing (196 cases), and children (147 cases).

Almost the same survey was conducted in FY 2012. The proportion with a tendency toward depression (25.6%) fell below the level of the previous year (27.1%). The survey was conducted in FY 2013 as well. The survey should be continued to watch over expectant and nursing mothers in the future.

(Seiji Yasumura)

References

1) Website of Fukushima Medical University: http://fukushima-mimamori.jp/outline/
2) Yasumura S, Hosoya M, Yamashita S, Kamiya K, Abe M, Akashi M, Kadoma K, Ozasa K, for the Fukushima Health Management Survey Group: Study Protocol for the Fukushima Health Management Survey. J Epidemiol, Vol. 22 (2012) No. 5: 375–383, http://dx.doi.org/10.2188/jea.JE20120105.
3) Tanigawa K, et al: Loss of life after evacuation: lessons learned from the Fukushima accident. The Lancet, Volume 379, Issue 9819, 889–891, 10 March 2012, doi: 10.1016/S0140-6736 (12) 60384-60385
4) Yasumura S, Goto A, Yamazaki S, Reich MR: Excess mortality among relocated institutionalized elderly after Fukushima nuclear disaster. Public Health, Volume 127, Issue 2, February 2013, 186–188.
5) Reconstruction Agency. *Report on Consideration of Prevention of Disaster-related Death in Fukushima Prefecture* (March 29, 2013): http://www.reconstruction.go.jp/topics/20130329kanrenshi.pdf

44 Expectations for public health from medical perspectives

I served as a diagnostic radiologist at the Department of Radiology of Fukushima Medical University before the Great East Japan Earthquake occurred. After the earthquake, however, I moved to the Department of Radiation Health Management of Fukushima Medical University. The reason was as follows. Since Fukushima Medical University Hospital was designated as the only secondary-level hospital for radiation exposure in the prefecture, I was deeply involved in radiation emergency medicine after the earthquake. Consequently, I was required to provide support for internal exposure testing, mainly using Whole Body Counters to address the post-quake situation in the prefecture.

In addition, I was required to respond to residents who lived surrounded by radioactive materials, which were widely dispersed from the Fukushima Daiichi Nuclear Power Station of the Tokyo Electric Power Company ("Fukushima Daiichi Station"). While increasingly engaged in providing diverse information on radiation exposure to residents and administrative bodies, I realized that public health nurses in municipalities were forced to play a central role in responding to residents on behalf of administrative bodies. They faced entirely new issues of residents' concerns about radiation exposure, and even had to prepare personal dosimeters (glass badges) and Whole Body Counters. Although they took a greatest deal of care in carrying out their work after the earthquake, they received only a little support and training, and no extensive human support was provided to them.

To reduce the burden of public health nurses, I was mainly involved in providing information on radiation exposure over a year after the earthquake. However, I heard in FY 2012 that public health nurses in the eight towns and villages in Futaba County, where residents were evacuated from restricted areas, were forced to shoulder an increasingly heavy burden, while facing new problems other than radiation exposure. Thus, health consultation Yorozu was commenced.

A Health consultation Yorozu

In FY 2012, I often heard from public health nurses in evacuation areas that prolonged evacuation was aggravating the health problems of residents. As many intellectuals had warned, evacuation actually caused changes in the living environment and lifestyles and increased stress of residents. This led not only to weight gain and a lack of exercise, but also to an increase in lifestyle-related diseases and disuse syndrome. Accordingly, active and prompt approaches to primary prevention of diseases were required before medical care became necessary.

It is difficult to say how medical professionals should address this situation. However, we reached a conclusion that medical professionals should try to respond to on-site needs by listening to worries of individual residents, checking their health conditions, and providing human support for health services from medical aspects, even though only a small number of personnel could be involved. We decided to provide consultations concerning all matters, including health issues, radiation issues, and even trivial problems. At the end of May 2012, the health consultation Yorozu was commenced in parallel with health checkups in Iitate Village[1]. Subsequently, the health consultation Yorozu and health checkups were provided in a similar way in other municipalities where residents were evacuated. By the end of FY 2012, the health consultation Yorozu was also provided in parallel with debriefing sessions on health checkup results. In the health consultation of Yorozu, physicians at the National Hospital Organization Disaster Medical Center, which collaborated with Fukushima Medical University, directly visited individual municipalities to carefully identify the needs of public health nurses and meet their needs as a liaison between public health

Chapter 4 Activities of Various Professional Organizations

nurses and residents.

 B **What was learned through the health consultation Yorozu**

Only approximately 10% of residents who received health checkups came to the booth for the health consultation Yorozu. However, this inefficiency was anticipated from the beginning. Nevertheless, we carried out the health consultation Yorozu to listen to concerns of individual residents about health and radiation and respond to the needs of public health nurses in local areas. Moreover, we believed that it was significant to build a face-to-face relationship between medical professionals and public health nurses.

Medicine aims to treat diseases and restore health to patients. Meanwhile, primary prevention of diseases, which requires individual responses (self-care), is promoted on a daily basis by municipal staff members in charge of health welfare. However, I realized through the health consultation Yorozu that a more close relationship between existing medical professionals and staff members in charge of health welfare was necessary in the difficult situation after the earthquake, in which a large-scale and prolonged evacuation was required. In the following, the negative impact that this situation had on primary prevention of diseases is discussed from four aspects, mainly based on what was learned from the situation in Iitate Village.

1 Aging of the population

Before the earthquake, Iitate Village had a population of 6,187 people as of November 1, 2010. Of these people, 1,859 were the elderly, age 65 years or older, with the population aging rate being 30.0%. As of April 1, 2013, the overall population and the elderly population of the village were 5,931 and 1,838, respectively, with the population aging rate being 31.0%[2]. In the entire Fukushima Prefecture, the population aging rate also increased by approximately 1% from 2011 to 2012. However, this was not because the actual number of the elderly increased, but because of a decrease in the younger population that accelerated the increase of the population aging rate. In addition, the population aging rate in areas where residents continued to stay around the 20-km zone of the Fukushima Daiichi Station, might be higher than statistical figures show. An increase in the population aging rate after the nuclear power station accident was a common tendency throughout Fukushima Prefecture.

2 Decentralization of population

Table 44-1 shows the situation of evacuees, which was published by Iitate Village. The information is updated as needed, and is posted on the official website of Iitate Village at all times[3]. According to the table, the number of residents who lived in temporary housing was 1,177. On the other hand, the number of residents who lived in their acquaintances' houses and municipally-subsidized housing was 4,909, which was nearly five times as many as those living in temporary housing. When compared with other data that were published, the situation in Iitate Village was found to be completely different from that of Minamisoma City in terms of the distribution of population in the various housing sites[4] (Table 44-2). Meanwhile, detailed information on evacuation in other municipalities has not yet been clarified. To obtain accurate information on evacuation in other municipalities, it is essential to continuously make contact with staff members on site.

In Iitate Village, public health nurses faced great difficulties in completing their daily tasks, including visiting individual homes and providing information on health guidance, although they were able to deal

Table 44-1   Current situation of evacuation in Iitate Village

Residents in the village	Their own homes in the village	13
	Iitate Home	5
	Total	18
Evacuees outside of the village	Acquaintances' houses or municipally-subsidized housing in Fukushima Prefecture	4,909
	Temporary housing in Fukushima Prefecture	1,177
	Outside of Fukushima Prefecture	502
	Whereabouts unknown	2
	Total	6,590

(As of April 1, 2013; surveyed by Iitate Village and altered by the author) Figure 44-2 Current situation of evacuation in Minamisoma City

Figure 44-2   Current situation of evacuation in Minamisoma City

Residents in the city	Their own homes	34,995
	Acquaintances' houses or municipally-subsidized housing in the city	5,470
	Temporary housing in the city	5,612
	Total	46,077
Evacuees outside of the city	Acquaintances' houses or municipally-subsidized housing outside of the city	17,002
	(of the above, outside of Fukushima Prefecture)	(10,295)
	Total	17,002
Others	Death (including death not from the earthquake)	2,270
	Move-out	6,090
	Whereabouts unknown	122
	Total	8,482

(As of March 28, 2013; surveyed by Minamisoma City)

with these tasks before the earthquake. In temporary housing, where many residents lived on the same site, public health nurses were able to effectively provide support. However, municipally-subsidized houses were scattered over a wide area, and this made their support activities more difficult. In addition, evacuation had broken up large families in which several generations lived together, and the family trends were shifted from large families to nuclear families. This led to an increase in the number of households, including those with elderly people living alone. Consequently, staff members of administrative bodies, as well as family members and neighbors, had difficulty watching over the health of individuals.

3   Changes in lifestyles

Many residents complained of the loss of purpose in life because they had fewer opportunities to enjoy nature and engage in agricultural work in temporary housing and municipally-subsidized housing. Even though encouraged to take exercise due to weight gain, most residents were reluctant to just take a walk. In addition, there were changes in ways of procuring food. Although many residents had used home-grown foods before, they were forced to procure foodstuffs at supermarkets after the earthquake. This promoted modernization and urbanization of dietary habits.

Meanwhile, some residents realized how convenient it was to live near supermarkets and hospitals, after they left the village. Other residents who had chronic diseases were able to receive more constant care than before the evacuation. However, another issue was that if residents suffered new health problems, they had difficulty choosing appropriate medical institutions in unfamiliar areas.

Chapter 4 | **Activities of Various Professional Organizations**

4 Collapse of communities

Various issues mentioned here, such as the aging of the population, population decline, decentralization of the population, separation of family members and urbanization of lifestyles, were considered to be the appearance of existing structural vulnerability that was faced by many underpopulated areas in Japan. A large-scale evacuation rapidly increased this vulnerability. Moreover, prolonged living as evacuees with an unknown future not only caused these issues, but also enormously increased fatigue of residents and decreased the capacity of local communities. The collapse of communities was expected to have an adverse impact on residents' health. Elderly people who had been watched over by family members and neighbors in their communities and those whose medical condition was between healthy and unhealthy could not be prevented from falling sick. Furthermore, the difficulty in choosing personal physicians might increase lifestyle-related diseases and promote their progress.

C : How can medical professionals work together?

How can medical professionals address the actual situation of disaster victims? Although I was not an expert in community medicine and health welfare, I happened to be involved in the efforts to respond to the post-quake situation. While providing support, I found that an unprecedentedly large- scale evacuation involving all residents in towns or villages and living as evacuees with an unknown future had a far greater impact on residents' lives than I might imagine. Moreover, I realized through case examples in Iitate Village that the post-quake situation and needs in individual municipalities were completely different.

The only common feature was that many people were unable to find motivation for self-care, while worrying about whether they were able to maintain good health. If existing primary prevention systems did not work well to prevent diseases, this might eventually lead to an increase in the number of people requiring medical care and shorting of their lives. In the following, I will offer my opinions as to whether health deterioration can be prevented.

1 Time-oriented collaboration between public health nurses and medical professionals

It is more than two years since the earthquake occurred. However, the post-disaster situation still continues and shows no sign of improvement. An immediate and urgent challenge is to stem the increase of disaster-related deaths. The Reconstruction Agency has already offered a direction to take countermeasures[5]. In the short term, focus should be placed on identifying people at high risk of soon developing health-related problems. In the medium term, measures should be taken to curb the increase in the number of people requiring medical care. In the long term, self-care should be promoted to deal with a variety of existing health risks. Furthermore, a final goal in the long term is to extend the lives of residents, while keeping them healthy, through collaboration between public health nurses and medical professionals. To this end, it is necessary to promptly draw up time- oriented road maps according to each term. The road maps should always be revised based on on- site needs.

2 Listening to residents, arranging personnel serving as a liaison and identifying on-site needs

To take short-term measures based on collaboration between public health nurses and medical profes-

Expectations for public health
from medical perspectives

44

sionals it is essential to know the actual on-site situation. Some people may think that staff members who listen to views of individual residents through the health consultation Yorozu may feel burdened, and that views of only a small number of residents cannot lead to resolution of problems. However, I believe that it is crucial to build a trusting relationship between staff members and residents through direct communication. Even if the individual views of residents are not very influential, staff members can identify on-site needs by regularly listening to residents as a liaison. Furthermore, they can summarize the needs and share them between all members involved. I believe that this can broaden the perspectives of individual staff members.

Insufficient information sharing has been a critical and unexamined issue since the initial stage of the disaster, and has frequently caused a delay in determination of further responses. To avoid making the same mistakes, it is important to involve as many people as possible and share information with each other. I believe that this provides wisdom that can respond to new challenges. One of purposes of the health consultation Yorozu is to have many people, including those from other prefectures, share and remember important information. From the initial stage, many people have been dispatched from other prefectures to join the health consultation Yorozu as staff members. I believe that it is crucial to continue to receive supporters from other prefectures to have them share and remember important information.

3 Toward the establishment of a sustainable medical care system

Living as evacuees is expected to be prolonged. However, most of the issues that should be urgently addressed in this situation may not be immediately resolved. Although medical professionals can provide support from only from a health aspect, they should not end support activities too soon, as long as there are on-site needs. To continue to provide support, not only efforts and funds but also human support are indispensable. One of the problems is that medical professionals have little training to be actively involved in primary prevention of diseases. The other problem is whether the results of primary prevention of diseases can be confirmed when medical professionals are involved. However, these problems cannot prevent medical professionals from implementing short-term efforts. If they judge that there is no need for them to provide support after grasping the situation, then this is one of their conclusions. However, they should make efforts to gain information before making a final decision. Furthermore, information should be shared among those involved so that continuous support can be provided even if personnel are replaced.

I believe that sharing information and enabling free access to information lead to more appropriate decisions and more choices to provide support. Currently, individual municipalities in Fukushima Prefecture are not sure what efforts are being made and what kind of support are being provided in other municipalities. If information is shared, cooperative structures may be able to be built on site. I propose that communications should be improved in all directions before planning the establishment of any one medical care system.

D How to respond to the appearance of structural vulnerability

As mentioned before, a large-scale evacuation revealed existing structural vulnerability that was faced by many underpopulated areas in Japan, and the vulnerability was rapidly increased. Are there any means to respond to this structural vulnerability? The following two examples in island medicine and community medicine may provide clues on collaboration between medicine and primary prevention of diseases.

One example is the efforts at Okidozen Hospital, Shimane Prefecture[6]. The hospital regularly held meet-

Chapter 4 | Activities of Various Professional Organizations

ings, where care managers, home-care helpers, staff members at day care centers, and business operators who lease welfare products as well as physicians, floor nurses, home-visiting nurses, office-based nurses, and occupational therapists from the hospitals participated. All participants discussed 10 to 20 cases for approximately two hours. The purpose of the meetings was to share information and to prevent staff members and institutions from facing future difficulties individually. One of the most important features of the meetings was that the meetings were run without placing a high value on only the physicians' point of view.

The other example is the efforts at National Health Insurance Fujisawa Municipal Hospital, Iwate Prefecture[7]. When the hospital had faced difficulty surviving immediately after its founding, it had overcome the crisis by adopting a new policy, "Hospitals can be raised by communities." Based on the policy, the hospital continuously held night school courses as well as open seminars and workshops in which residents were able to participate.

In both cases, residents and staff members involved worked together to increase public interest in primary prevention of diseases, aiming to raise awareness that they should and/or can support community medicine. I believe that these approaches are necessary for most underpopulated areas in Japan. I do not think that improvement of medical care systems and functions is the only good answer.

To address common issues between island and community medicine and medicine for disaster victims, it is important for physicians, nurses, public health nurses and administrative officers in charge of welfare to support and complement each other by sharing information, as stated above. What is learned from these efforts will help formulate suggestions of how to provide support to disaster victims in the future. We need to have the vision that hospital personnel should respond to the needs of public health nurses and involve local volunteers and residents in health-maintenance activities, while taking primary prevention of diseases as a basis for medical care and making use of limited human resources.

I also believe that these efforts will be helpful not only to improve medical care for disaster victims, but also to provide clues for the revival of community medicine for local residents. Improvement of current community medicine is another major issue to be tackled on a long-term basis. Based in Fukushima Prefecture, I aim to offer a range of ways to effectively provide support through collaboration between medicine, health welfare, and public health.

> I would like to extend my sincere gratitude to staff members at the National Hospital Organization Disaster Medical Center, who were committed to planning and operation of the health consultation Yorozu. I am also deeply grateful to staff members at the municipal government in Iitate Village, who provided information to us, while engaged in support activities on site.

(Makoto Miyazaki)

References

1) Makoto Miyazaki: *What Is Learned through the Health Consultation Yorozu – Lessons from Medical Care in Remote Islands and Remote Rural Areas.* Japan Medical Weekly Journal, No. 4625: 27–31, Japan Medical Journal, 2012.

2) Website of Fukushima Prefecture, *Estimated Population of Fukushima Prefecture (results of a survey of resident population of Fukushima Prefecture).* http://wwwcms.pref.fukushima.jp/pcp_portal/PortalServlet?DISPLAY_ID=DIRECT&NEXT_DI SPLAY_ID=U000004&CONTENTS_ID=15846

3) Website of Iitate Village, *Evacuation Situation of Residents as of March 1, 2013.* http://www.vill.iitate.fukushima.jp/saigai/?p=8445

4) Website of Minamisoma City, *Situation of the City and State of Residence Evacuation*. http://www.city.minamisoma.lg.jp/index.cfm/10,853,58,html

5) Website of the Reconstruction Agency, *Report of Examination for Prevention of Disaster-related Death in Fukushima Prefecture (as of March 29, 2013)*. http://www.reconstruction.go.jp/topics/20130329kanrenshi.pdf

6) Yoshihiko Shiraishi: *Support for Medical Care in Remote Islands and Remote Rural Areas – Multisystems by Comprehensive Physicians and Comprehensive Nursing Care*, Hospital, vol. 70- 3: 190–193, Igaku-Shoin Ltd., 2011.

7) Motomi Sato: *What Municipal Hospitals Should Be to Support Community Medicine – Establishing Medical Services with the Efforts of Everyone*, Hospital, vol. 70–3: 186–189, Igaku- Shoin Ltd., 2011.

Chapter 5

**Measures taken by
Hiroshima University**

Hiroshima University (HU) plays the role of "Tertiary Radiation Medical Institution" for the western-Japan block, and functioned as a base for radiation emergency medicine (REM) during the accident at the Fukushima Daiichi nuclear power plant (FDNPP). Thus far, more than 1,300 people, including doctors, radiological technologists, nurses, office personnel, and others have been dispatched as members of HU Radiation Emergency Medical Assistance Teams (REMATs). This involvement has allowed for the development of a comprehensive and systematic emergency support program. However, even with this program in place, during the course of both the emergency response activities and post-response reflection, a number of challenges were identified. By identifying these challenges we were able to accelerate and build on the progress of HU's previously established radiation disaster medicine program with regards to the development of well-trained, interdisciplinary human resources (Ministry of Education, Culture, Sports, Science and Technology (MEXT) 21st Century Center of Excellence (COE) Program "Radiation Casualty Medical Research Center"). This experience and knowledge ultimately led to the creation of a new graduate education program. This chapter describes the background of and philosophy behind the establishment of the "Phoenix Leader Education Program (Hiroshima Initiative) for Renaissance from Radiation Disaster" as well as an overview of its structure. Furthermore, I discuss the various measures taken by HU following the FDNPP accident.

45 : Recovery Support and Carrying out Radiation Emergency Medicine at the Main Site — As a Tertiary Radiation Medical Institution —

In 2004 HU was designated as Tertiary Radiation Emergency Medical Institution by MEXT and subsequently implemented a number of projects with the intention of developing a protocol for providing REM. With these collaborative projects, a broad, interconnected "human network" was established throughout the "western block of Japan" which connects municipal governments representing areas with nuclear facilities, the secondary radiation emergency medical care facilities in the immediate vicinity, and Hiroshima University. HU has contributed to the establishment of an effective Radiation Emergency Medicine System designed to provide training for REM, decontamination, and screening for radioactive substances, and to the development of pre-determined patient transport routes. Therefore, following the FDNPP accident, the HU REMAT was dispatched immediately to Fukushima. The REMAT utilized its accumulated knowledge and specialized skills for the security and safety of the affected population of Fukushima prefecture. Additionally, following the accident, REM specialists currently working throughout Japan, but who had been trained in the "western block" network, were able to rush expeditiously to Fukushima. Due to their high level of professionalism and expertise, the HU REMAT and the REM specialists were able to work together in a mutually supportive and trusting relationship, and keep disorder, confusion, and mishaps within the locally compromised Fukushima REM system to a minimum. This section outlines the support services in place to respond after an accident.

Chapter 5   Measures taken by Hiroshima University

 Radiation Emergency Medical Assistance

The Great East Japan Earthquake occurred on March 11th, and the Declaration of a Nuclear Emergency Situation was made that evening by former Prime Minister Kan. However, despite the passing of a full day's worth of valuable time, no updated information about the state of the nuclear reactor at the FDNPP or levels of radioactive environmental contamination reached Hiroshima University, the Tertiary Radiation Medical Institution. Although no new information from the national government had been released well into the morning of March 12th, Hiroshima University made the proactive decision to establish the Radiation Emergency Medicine Committee with Professor Kenji Kamiya being installed as chair. Thus, substantive preparations for an accident possibly involving radiation exposure were begun. This committee became the focal point for determining and carrying out countermeasures involving REM. The first REMAT group was dispatched to Fukushima on the afternoon of March 12th. Following this initial team, more than one thousand three hundred HU faculty and administrative staff, 37 groups in total, have been dispatched thus far to the various evacuation points for residents. These locations include the Fukushima Medical University, J-Village (where a temporary emergency medical room has been installed), school facilities, local community assembly halls, and the emergency medical room in the FDNPP. These groups took proactive measures to prepare for possible instances of injury or sickness due to radiation exposure, and to ensure the safety and security of local residents.

In the offsite center that had previously been moved to the Fukushima Prefectural Governmental Hall (Fukushima Prefectural Jichi-Kaikan) and then to the Fukushima Prefectural Office after March 13th, 2011, doctors, nurses, and radiation technologists remained on standby in preparation for possible incidents of radiation exposure from the nuclear power plant accident.

When the case of an injured worker with a suspected "beta ray burn" occurred at the FDNPP on March 16th, the HU Emergency Medical doctors departed Fukushima Medical University by Japan Self-Defense Force helicopter and flew to the grounds of the plant in order to transport the patient to Fukushima Medical University for treatment. Furthermore, in their role as medical support members of the Offsite Center, HU emergency physicians were involved in establishing the triage protocols and the patient transportation system for instances of injury or illness due to possible radiation exposure from the contamination of the nuclear accident. However, in order to offer emergency medical treatment to the sick or injured residents suspected of having been contaminated by radiation, a better option needed to be established. Thus, with the support of HU REMAT, J-Village, located 20 km south of the FDNPP, was designated and equipped as a triage site to be used as an alternative to the closed medical institutions located within the 20km exclusion zone. Additionally, it was an urgent necessity to also develop a system for providing medical care to the thousands of workers who were involved in the restoration of the crippled nuclear power plant and may have been exposed to radiation. For that reason, on July 1st an onsite "Emergency Room" (ER) was established in the FDNPP to allow for immediate response to radiation exposure or other emergencies that might occur during the course of the restoration work. After establishing the *Fukushima Daiichi Nuclear Power Plant Emergency Medical Service System Network*, Koichi Tanigawa, the deputy director of the HU Radiation Emergency Medicine Promotion Center, was appointed director in charge of managing the onsite ER. The secretariat overseeing this network was installed at Hiroshima University with the mandate to coordinate emergency medical staff dispatched to Fukushima from all over Japan. This support work remains ongoing.

Following the evacuation order, perhaps the most significant of the initial challenges was to develop an effective radiation screening system for potentially externally-contaminated evacuated residents. In order to properly carry out this task, HU worked with specialists from the National Institute of Radiological Sciences (NIRS), in conjunction with the Fukushima Prefectural Government to convene a Radiation Emergency Medicine Coordination expert's council. This emergency council formalized a coordinated contamination screening and decontamination system for evacuated residents as well as grouping procedures for volunteers arriving from throughout Japan into contamination screening teams. It was now March 14th while the emergency response systems and procedures were being finalized, the evacuation of all remaining hospital patients as well as the residents of assisted living facilities found within the 20km radius emergency zone was taking place. Moreover, radiological contamination screening and healthcare management were taking place at the "So-So" health office in Minamisoma. At the same time, in order to reflect more accurately the scientific data and to employ a more pragmatic screening approach, the HU medical team made the suggestion that the radiological contamination screening level should be raised from 13,000 cpm to 100,000 cpm. This revised criterion was subsequently adopted as the standard by the Fukushima Prefectural Government. As a result of this revised screening level the number of individuals requiring whole body cold water decontamination was reduced dramatically, and the physical burden placed on evacuees was significantly lessened. Of important note, during the emergency evacuation of vulnerable groups such as hospital patients and the elderly, many precious lives were lost. As people with intimate knowledge of the actual situation, the faculty and staff members of Hiroshima University chose to disseminate this information in an effort to improve the nuclear power plant disaster prevention system. In collaboration with the NIRS, HU REMAT was also responsible for measuring for internal contamination levels and carrying out thyroid examinations for children living in areas of Fukushima such as Iitate Village in the Soma District where airborne levels of radiation were relatively high. This data was used to develop reference materials and a database of internal exposure levels of children's thyroid glands.

Given the urgency of the evacuation, residents were forced to leave without even the most basic of necessities. Due to this, evacuated residents were given supervised opportunities to enter the 20 km exclusion zone and retrieve certain belongings beginning on the 22nd of April, 2011. In order to carry out these return visits safely, specific health care precautions were taken and radioactive contamination screening of these residents was performed. HU doctors, radiological technologists, nurses, and administrative staff members were dispatched continuously on Fukushima rotations in order to properly conduct the previously mentioned responsibilities, as well as to support the residents' who were entering the exclusion zone for their temporary return visits.

The assessment of internal exposure doses was carried out with a whole body counter for the people of Fukushima prefecture who had been evacuated and who had entered the restricted area designated by the national government. In total, the assessment of 142 people had been carried as of summer, 2013.

B : Support services at Fukushima Medical University

Of particular significance is the role played by Fukushima Medical University (FMU) as a base for medical services and health care administration, as well as its efforts to investigate the health effects of the FDNPP accident on the people of the prefecture. Due to this HU pursued and reached an *Inclusive and Comprehensive Research Cooperation Agreement* with FMU on April 2nd, 2011, which covered health research and health management in Fukushima Prefecture. This framework also laid the foundation for long term cooperation with a specific eye towards Human Resource Development.

The Fukushima Health Management Survey was conducted by the Fukushima Prefectural Government with FMU as the executing agency, and targeted the 2.05 million people living in the prefecture. In order to fully support FMU in its endeavors, highly-skilled individuals such as university vice-presidents, professors, and researchers have been dispatched from Hiroshima University to offer assistance as specialists, and to ensure the smooth implementation of the Fukushima Health Management Survey. Implementation of this specific survey represented a unique challenge for FMU not only because of insufficient experience dealing with REM, but more specifically due to the uncommon characteristics of the circumstances surrounding a nuclear accident. With this in mind, the support of HU, a specialized institution for REM, became indispensable.

Furthermore, in terms of support for REM, beginning in May of 2011 doctors and radiological technologists with expertise using whole body counters were dispatched weekly from HU. As of June 29th, in cooperation with doctors from FMU and Nagasaki University, these medical specialists had measured the internal radiation dose of approximately 60 firefighters. Additionally, in order to develop a low dose radiation exposure assessment system for REM applications, a joint project was carried out by HU and FMU entitled "Development of a low dose radiation exposure monitor", and funded by the MEXT. This project was used to successfully establish a biological dose assessment system at FMU.

C Risk Communication

Following the FDNPP accident a wide range of conflicting information regarding the health risks associated with radiation exposure was disseminated throughout the country by media outlets. This contributed to increased anxiety and confusion among both the local population in Fukushima Prefecture and the general Japanese population at large. Furthermore, at both a domestic and international level unsubstantiated rumors proliferated in the business community and led to substantial economic damage. Given such a confusing situation, both scientists and radiation specialists were required to repeatedly explain the health effects of radiation exposure in simple, clear language, as reassuringly as possible. The fact that many of the specialists involved in the risk communication for the FDNPP accident came from Hiroshima University (located in the only city to have ever experienced an atomic bomb) helped to reassure residents, reduce their anxiety levels, and counteract the abundant negative rumors. Kenji Kamiya, senior professor at the Research Institute for Radiation Biology and Medicine was appointed to the post of Prefectural Radiation Health Risk Management Advisor by the governor of Fukushima Prefecture. On April 12th, 2011, he began his duties which included advising the prefectural government on health management and giving lectures on the health risks associated with radiation exposure. Providing 83 lectures in total, both within and outside of Fukushima Prefecture as of August 2012, professor Kamiya strove to disseminate clear and accurate knowledge about both health management and radiation exposure. He was genuine in his sincere efforts to contribute to easing resident's worries about health hazards and helped to prevent further damage from harmful rumors. Beyond the efforts in Fukushima, on April 19th Hiroshima University established the 'Radiation Protection Fundamental Information Portal Site' in order to provide clear and accurate information about radioactivity and surrounding issues.

D Monitoring Environmental Radiation

Importantly, HU researchers drawn from a variety of academic fields beyond medicine have carried out support activities for the recovery from the radiation disaster. At the request of the MEXT Radio Isotope

Division of Natural Science, Center for Basic Research and Development, from September, 2011, HU began environmental radioactivity monitoring in the specified evacuation areas. Using HU supplied analysis instruments experts measured for the presence of radioactive nuclides in water sources (well water, river water, etc.) and reported the results. Furthermore, in order to prepare for the lifting of the evacuation order, beginning in May, 2012, environmental monitoring for radioactive substances in the restricted areas was instituted and is ongoing to this day. Building on the environmental monitoring efforts, between September and December, 2012, on three separate occasions, faculty members and students from the HU Graduate Schools of Engineering and Biosphere Science were dispatched to Minamisoma City to take samples of soil and atmospheric dust.

While supporting the recovery from the disaster caused by the FDNPP accident, the acute need for highly-skilled and adaptable people able to cope with the challenges faced during a radiation accident situation became clearly apparent. It was this understanding that lead to the launching of a unique, inter-disciplinary graduate program. It was designed to foster the education and training of leaders equipped with a wide range of knowledge drawn from across academic disciplines who are able to effectively and confidently lead disaster recovery efforts. It was this range of specific tasks, some mentioned above, that were carried out by HU staff in their efforts to support the recovery from the nuclear accident that would come to form the educational basis of the new graduate program, and act as an inspiration for them to work collectively towards establishing it.

46 Initiation of Measures for Human Resource Development
— Establishment of the Phoenix Leader Education Program (Hiroshima Initiative) for Renaissance from Radiation Disaster —

This chapter describes the establishment of the Phoenix Leader Education Program (Hiroshima Initiative) for Renaissance from Radiation Disaster. Due to the FDNPP accident a large amount of radioactive materials were released into the environment. This lead to serious concerns about not only the health issues of the residents but also other critical consequences such as potential environmental radiological contamination and the possible collapse of local communities. To put it another way, the effects of a radiation disaster influence all aspects of society. This includes, among other things, human health – both physical and mental, societal well-being, the environment, agriculture and forestry, commerce and industry, the general economy at large, and local communities. In order to effectively promote a revival from such a broad-ranging disaster, we need to enlist talented people with knowledge and technological know-how who come from many scientific disciplines. Virtually all areas of academic enquiry including the medical sciences, radiation and nuclear science, environmental science, the physical sciences, engineering, sociology, pedagogy, psychology, etc. are essential. However, as things currently stand such an interdisciplinary education, integrated research program to foster the talented individuals mentioned above does not presently exist at any university, either domestically within Japan or abroad. Having identified this gap in available graduate education, using its academic resources HU was ideally positioned to assume this mission to develop just such a graduate education and research program. One that integrates a wide range of academic fields based on the university's experiences and achievements accumulated during its intimate involvement with the recovery process that followed the destruction caused by the atomic bombing. HU's expertise, coupled with the recent experience gained from its efforts with *Radiation Emergency Medical Assistance* in the regions affected by the accident at the FDNPP, has helped to clearly identify the specific human resources needed to work as specialists in the field of radiation disaster recovery.

HU specialists involved with REM, radiation health risk management, and environmental radiation measurement clearly saw the limitations of their own educational backgrounds, and those of other experts involved in the emergency response and subsequent recovery. The HU Research Institute of Radiation Biology and Medicine which has investigated the radiation specific damages caused by the 1945 atomic bombing is one of top academic radiation research institutes in the world. Despite this, these researchers also recognized the limits of their ability when they left the laboratories to engage the actual radiation disaster on the ground, at a personal level. The worries and the sufferings of the people were made clear, as well as the extent of the tragedy of their destroyed livelihoods. For example, although 1 millisievert literally has a risk value of 1 millisievert of radiation in a textbook, the meaning of this numerical value varies depending on the person who is exposed, and in turn its seriousness can be interpreted at a wide level of disparity. HU members involved in the recovery efforts recognized this knowledge disconnect between the lab and the people with whom they were interacting. This interaction was one of the catalysts that lead to the realization that an all-round approach to solving the problems of a radiation disaster should be one of the missions of their university. Despite the tremendous efforts usually associated with establishing a new graduate program, the groundwork to educate and train specialists with expertise in radiation disaster recovery already existed at HU. As a research intensive university located in one of only two cities to have suffered an atomic bombing, and the ability to build on this historical foundation of radiation recovery expertise, made developing this new program with limited preparation time possible. Specialist researchers in the sciences and humanities from a number of institutes and graduate schools, including the Research Institute for Radiation Biology and Medicine, HU Hospital, Graduate School of Biomedical and Health Sciences, joined in this collaborative effort to establish, in this extremely compressed time-frame, a unique and targeted graduate program. The fruits of their efforts became the Phoenix Leader Education Program (Hiroshima Initiative) for Renaissance from Radiation Disaster. It was selected and formally recognized in FY 2011 as a new graduate program within a government educational initiative sponsored by the Ministry of Education, Culture, Sports, Science and Technology (MEXT) known as the Leading Graduate Schools. The first 8 students were welcomed into the program in October, 2012, after a detailed and comprehensive arrangement was made with 8 of HU's graduate schools including among others the Graduate School of Letters, Social Sciences, and Biomedical and Health Sciences.

Although the historical and empirical background behind the establishment of the program made it unique, the academic structure was also distinctly unlike traditional graduate education programs whose focus lay in training researchers. It was founded on the philosophy of utilizing extensive cross-disciplinary, educational resources. Through comprehensive four and five year doctoral courses, this program aims to develop specialists in the area of radiation disaster recovery who possess academic expertise, and a broad range of practical skills and competencies. The program is composed of three unique, yet synergistic training courses. The first is designed to nurture personnel capable of protecting human lives from radioactivity in the four year *Radiation Disaster Medicine Course*. The second is focused on protecting the environment from radioactivity in the five year *Radioactivity Environmental Protection Course*. Finally, the third course aims to protect society in the five year *Radioactive Social Recovery Course*. These three courses consist of neither a narrow educational focus nor a concentrated research activity in any one specialized academic field. For example, the curriculum in the *Radiation Disaster Medicine Course* is designed to enable students to gain knowledge and skills for the proper diagnosis and treatment of pathological conditions affected by radiation, the evaluation of the mechanism, the possible risks of carcinogenesis and genetic damage due to radioactivity, the assessment of the psychological effects of stress caused by the radiation contamination, and the delivery of adequate mental health care.

Furthermore, the three courses have foundational common core course requirements that must be completed by the end of the fourth semester which embody a radical, hands-on, practice-focused approach to graduate education. A typical, required subject is the "short-term fieldwork" for students in their second semester, which involves a one week, on-site learning experience about the influences and effects of the FDNPP accident. This Fukushima, on-site learning experience, takes place at cooperating institutions such as FMU and Fukushima University, temporary evacuation housing facilities, a hospital in Minamisoma city, and a temporary elementary school for children from three different schools from within the evacuation zone. While participating, the graduate students are expected to actively understand the region's circumstances, consider the challenges it's facing, and to reflect on the diverse perspectives they encounter. It is also expected that they will recognize that resolving the problems in Fukushima will require much more than a singular focus on a specialized field of study. Based on the feedback and opinions of the first cohort of graduate students, the initial short-term fieldwork was a rewarding experience that both motivated and inspired them. Considering this, an additional two day, on-site learning opportunity was instituted as a first semester component for all incoming students in order to give them early exposure to the actual situation on the ground in affected areas such as Minamisoma City.

HU faculty involved in this program sincerely appreciate the understanding and support of the onsite partners, without which certain fundamental components such as the short-term fieldwork and the early exposure to the reality of Fukushima would not be possible. All stakeholders share a strong commitment to achieving similar goals which has allowed for such successful cooperation. With this appreciation foremost in their minds, the faculty recognizes that engaging personally with the recovery efforts offers them the opportunity to utilize their research achievements to accomplish the program mission and give

Chapter 5 | Measures taken by Hiroshima University

back to the community. Although research outcomes are vital, the program's primary purposes remain the establishment of Radiation Disaster Recovery Studies (RDRS) as a new academic field and the development of human resources able to respond to and cope with a radiation disaster. Researchers, coming from a variety of academic backgrounds, are setting up, revising and finalizing the new academic framework as well as working together to successfully implement, promote and expand the program. The graduates of the Phoenix Leader Education Program will embody its goals and diligently carry out their roles as researchers and specialists within this new academic field. They will be able to draw upon their practical experiences and inter-disciplinary skills to confidently lead the recovery from a radiation disaster. One of the historic missions of HU, built in a city that experienced an atomic bombing, is to establish and foster the academic field of radiation disaster recovery studies, and demonstrate a genuine commitment to this mission through educating and training specialists.

As developing human resources to lead the recovery from possible radiation disasters is recognized as an urgent need both in Japan and around the world, expectations for the success of the program, among both domestic and international stakeholders, are immense. Researchers from institutions including FMU, Fukushima University, Nagasaki University, Tohoku University, the Radiation Effects Research Foundation, and the National Institute of Radiological Sciences have joined those from Hiroshima University as faculty members who teach classes and conduct research under the auspices of the program. Furthermore, the program receives substantial assistance from partners outside Japan such as the International Atomic Energy Agency (IAEA) and the International Commission on Radiological Protection (ICRP). These organizations actively welcome students as interns and dispatch experts who act as seminar instructors and symposium speakers. Education beyond any one organization or country plays a fundamental role in the program, and functions to extend a student's worldview, spur enthusiasm, and cultivate their academic and professional growth into the multitalented personnel, with both the knowledge and skills required, able to navigate the challenges of radiation disaster recovery.

As of October, 2015, twenty-nine students, representing ten different nations, were enrolled in the program and striving towards their PhD. With a genuine effort, these students are maximizing their experience to become specialists in the field of radiation disaster recovery. A noteworthy example of this can be seen in the eight students who have participated in both short and long-term internships at the IAEA. With a view towards the future, the program works continuously to build upon its foundation and develop the most well-prepared, human resources possible. It aims to further its role as the focal point for the human network involved in the recovery from the accident at the FDNPP, as well as supporting all aspects of radiation security and safety around the world.

Chapter 6

Suggestions
— Toward the Future —

47 Measures to be Taken

In this chapter, I will suggest measures to be taken in the field of public health in case of a nuclear disaster from the position of a researcher at the Department of Public Health, School of Medicine, Fukushima Medical University, which is located in Fukushima Prefecture and was affected by the Great East Japan Earthquake. Although making suggestions in a systematic and comprehensive manner is far beyond my capacity, I hope that my suggestions will be of some help for those involved in public health to develop their future activities according to their positions and roles.

A Features of the nuclear disaster (its position in disasters)

In Japan, disaster is defined as any abnormal natural phenomenon, including any storm, tornado, torrential rain, heavy snow, flood, rock slide, debris flow, tidal wave, earthquake, tsunami, volcanic eruption, and landslide. It includes any large-scale fire and explosion, as well as any damage caused by the reasons that are stated in government orders to be similar to these phenomena in terms of the degree of damage (Item 1, Article 2, Chapter 1 of the Basic Act on Disaster Control Measures). Nuclear disaster is a type of disaster. According to the Act on Special Measures Concerning Nuclear Emergency Preparedness ("Nuclear Emergency Preparedness Act"), a nuclear disaster is defined as damage caused to the lives, bodies or properties of citizens due to a nuclear emergency situation (Item 1, Article 2, Chapter 1 of the Nuclear Emergency Preparedness Act). Moreover, the act prescribes that a nuclear emergency situation means a situation in which radioactive materials or radiation at an abnormal level has been released outside the nuclear site of a nuclear operator (in the case of the transport of radioactive materials outside the nuclear site, outside a vessel which is used for said transport), due to the operation of the reactor, etc. by said nuclear operator (omitted) (Item 2, Article 2, Chapter 1 of the said Act). In Japan, the JCO criticality accident that occurred at Tokai Village on September 30, 1999 is often cited as an example of nuclear accidents. This accident triggered the establishment of the Nuclear Emergency Preparedness Act. The act stipulates that when the Prime Minister has issued a declaration of a nuclear emergency, he/she shall be given full authority. This is a major difference between the Nuclear Emergency Preparedness Act and the Disaster Countermeasures Basic Act, which states that affected municipalities should assume primary responsibility to settle the situation in case of disaster. This is based on the recognition that a nuclear disaster has the potential to cause a national crisis, unlike other disasters.

As mentioned in "Chapter 1 – What Nuclear Disaster Means" (P. 1), nuclear disaster has taken on a very different aspect from other disasters in past cases, because it reminds us of the health effects of radioactive materials and radiation, which are invisible to the eye. In the Great East Japan Earthquake, Fukushima Prefecture was affected by not only the earthquake and tsunami but also a nuclear disaster. In addition, the prefecture was also damaged by harmful rumors. Accordingly, the situation caused by the damage to the nuclear reactors as well as necessary support in Fukushima Prefecture was significantly different from that in Iwate and Miyagi Prefectures. To cite an example, the Japanese Nursing Association rejected a request to dispatch nurses to Fukushima Prefecture due to the nuclear power station being in a critical state. This was very regrettable because nurses were not asked to be dispatched to areas with high radiation levels but to areas where local nurses and public health nurses engaged in their activities. This symbolizes how great the concern was caused by invisible radiation. In particular, concerns about the medium- and long-term impact of radiation on the health of local residents have become a major issue in Fukushima Prefecture.

Chapter 6 | Suggestions — Toward the Future —

Although some books deal with efforts in public health in case of general disaster[1], there is no book concerning public health efforts in the case of a nuclear disaster; at least in Japanese. This is because a nuclear disaster and radiation associated with the nuclear disaster are difficult to handle. According to the Nuclear Emergency Preparedness Act, the national government should take on the responsibility to implement efforts in public health to protect people's health in Fukushima Prefecture, where the nuclear power station accident occurred, and to create manuals that serve as guidelines for these efforts. Unfortunately, the manuals have not been created yet. Although public health is expected to play an important role in coping with a nuclear disaster, the response in Fukushima Prefecture and its municipalities seem to represent one trial and error after another and they are still seeking ways to respond to the disaster.

B ⋮ Attitudes of the national government, prefectures and municipalities toward responses in public health in case of a nuclear disaster

I have discussed with members of the Fukushima Prefecture Community Health Association, which mainly comprises public health nurses, about how to organize a public health response, while reviewing what we should communicate to the public from a perspective of public health. Public health covers a very wide range of areas. When it is broadly defined as an area related to human life and health, almost all administrative operations are included in public health when it is closely examined. With such an interpretation, some local governments took radiation measurement of potable water and food to be part of the services of public health nurses.

1 Responses of the national government

Regarding responses of the national government, page 27 and the "*Record of the 3.11 Great Earthquake*"[2] issued by the Executive Committee for Earthquake Response Seminars can be referenced. However, it is a little known fact that the national government faces the challenge that there is not a clear distinction between the roles of individual government offices concerning disaster responses, especially responses to radiation exposure. Table 45-1, which I created, shows the roles of major government offices that are heavily involved in support of disaster victims and the health effects of radiation in association with the nuclear disaster following the Great East Japan Earthquake. It does not provide a comprehensive overall picture as there are other government offices, which are not included, whose function and responsibility are related to the disaster response.

The issue of environmental contamination by radioactive materials associated with the nuclear power station accident was thought at first to be within the jurisdiction of the Ministry of the Environment. However, when I asked the Ministry of the Environment via web conference about responses to environmental contamination, including responses of the Japan Environment and Children's Study Fukushima Unit Center, which conducts the Eco & Child Study, it answered as follows: "Environmental contamination by radioactive materials is exempt from the Basic Environment Act, and should be handled by the Nuclear Safety Commission (currently the Nuclear Regulation Authority) defined in the Atomic Energy Basic Act. The Ministry of the Environment only has charge of the disposal of radiation-contaminated waste as part of the disposal operations of disaster waste." In August 2011, however, the Act on Special Measures concerning the Handling of Pollution by Radioactive Materials was promulgated (enforced in January 2012). The act aims "to quickly mitigate the impact of environmental contamination on human health and the living environment by stipulating measures to be taken by the national government, local public bodies, relevant nuclear operators, etc. concerning handling of environmental contamination caused by the diffusion of radioactive materials associated with the Fukushima Daiichi Nuclear Power Station accident." Therefore,

Table 45-1 Major government offices involved in support for disaster victims and monitoring health effects of radiation in association with nuclear accident

Cabinet Office:	Core agency for disaster-prevention measures (Office for Nuclear Disaster Countermeasures), promotion of nuclear regulation on a fair basis (former Nuclear Safety Commission, Nuclear Regulation Authority)
Ministry of Economy, Trade and Industry:	Regulation and disaster-prevention measures related to nuclear facilities (Nuclear and Industrial Safety Agency)
Ministry of Education, Culture, Sports, Science and Technology:	Environmental radiological monitoring, prevention from radiation hazards (Science and Technology Promotion Bureau)
Ministry of Health, Labour and Welfare:	Responses to radioactive materials in food (Department of Food Safety, Pharmaceutical and Food Safety Bureau), health crisis management (Health Sciences Division)
Ministry of the Environment:	Clerical work related to radiation, such as were related to the Fukushima Health Management Survey (Radiation Health Management Office, Environmental Health Department), Eco & Child Study (Environmental Risk Assessment Office, Environmental Health and Safety Division, Environmental Health Department)
Ministry of Agriculture, Forestry and Fisheries:	Measurement of radioactive materials contained in food and agricultural products (Pharmaceutical and Food Safety Bureau, Agricultural Production Bureau)
Ministry of Land, Infrastructure, Transport and Tourism:	Restoration of transportation including roads
National Police Agency:	Evacuation guidance for disaster victims, search of missing people, identity confirmation of dead bodies
Fire and Disaster Management Agency:	Fire companies: evacuation guidance, search of dead bodies
Ministry of Defense:	Rescue, search, transportation of goods and personnel
Reconstruction Agency:	Infrastructure development, industrial promotion, employment, decontamination, health management

The names in parentheses refer to divisions and departments in charge.

the Ministry of the Environment now plays a central role in measures taken against contamination by radioactive materials.

Although the Ministry of Health, Labour and Welfare tends to be considered as a core agency to respond to environmental contamination from the perspective of human health, many other government offices are also associated with the health effects of radiation. A distinction between their roles is very complicated. Accordingly, **integration of various authorities handling radiation-related matters** was required by, in particular, prefectures and municipalities.

2 Responses of prefectures (Fukushima Prefecture) and public health and welfare offices

Regarding responses of prefectures, it is necessary to distinguish between the roles of prefectural governments and public health and welfare offices ("health offices").

The prefectural governments serve as a headquarters and a liaison with the national government. In the case of Fukushima Prefecture, the policies and attitudes of the prefectural government have determined the course of action of municipalities. Since the prefectural government has to consider a wide range of issues related to public health as well as continue to face new problems even two years after the earthquake, it is still busy with disaster-related work, and this shows no sign of decreasing. Accordingly, **it is essential that every prefecture should take measures to prepare for a nuclear disaster on a routine basis.**

Health offices have always had significant duties and roles to engage in public health activities for residents and to support municipalities under their jurisdiction. In Fukushima Prefecture, there are eight health

Chapter 6 | **Suggestions — Toward the Future —**

offices, two of which are located in central cities (Iwaki City and Koriyama City). The Fukushima Daiichi Nuclear Power Station of the Tokyo Electric Power Company is located in Okuma and Futaba Towns and is under the jurisdiction of the Soso Public Health and Welfare Office. This book describes the responses offered by all health offices, including the Soso Public Health and Welfare Office. However, what I most want to emphasize is that **not only municipalities where nuclear power stations are located but also surrounding municipalities will be forced to take some measures in case of a nuclear disaster, and that all public health centers that hold jurisdiction over municipalities which receive evacuees must also take some measures**. Actually, not only health offices throughout Fukushima Prefecture, including the public health centers whose jurisdiction covered the area where the nuclear power station was located, but also those in adjacent prefectures had to take various measures in this disaster. This shows that if nuclear power station accidents occur, even prefectures where nuclear power stations are not located may be forced to respond to the accidents[3]. Accordingly, every prefecture in Japan should prepare for a nuclear disaster on a routine basis.

3 Responses of municipalities

Responses of municipalities are exactly the same as those of prefectures and health offices in that **even municipalities where nuclear power stations are not located have to take some measures**. As stated in this book, responses of municipalities in Fukushima Prefecture varied between the 13 affected municipalities, which were designated as evacuation areas, and the other 46 municipalities. However, since almost all municipalities received evacuees, they had to provide support services for the evacuees including various operations related to radiation exposure; for example, responding to local residents' concerns about health. While municipalities where the nuclear power station is located conducted emergency drills in preparation for a nuclear disaster before the earthquake, administrative staff in the other municipalities lacked crisis awareness and knowledge of nuclear disasters. Therefore, they had trouble responding to the diversity of demands following the power station accident. I believe that their experience can serve as a reference point for, not only prefectures where nuclear power stations are located, but also municipalities geographically apart from nuclear power stations.

With the prospect that municipalities throughout Japan will use it as a reference, I set a framework for their response in matters of public health. To organize health issues, or simplify them, I divided them into **three categories: nutrition, exercise and rest**, which are three elements of good health. Although these categories seem to be classified rather roughly, this is based on the following reasons:

- In theory, these elements have been generally established as three elements of good health, and have been accepted in the field of public health as well as other fields.
- These elements are prevalent among health experts and the public, and are easily accepted as important factors in determining health.
- It is not always practical to subdivide health issues to grasp their actual situation and devise specific measures according to an individual situation. In many cases, measures for health issues have much in common and are related to each other. Accordingly, measures become more feasible when considered in a larger context.

Although there seems to be various views of how targeted people should be categorized, they are classified in this book into **three groups: independent residents; people requiring assistance during a disaster (vulnerable people in case of a disaster), especially elderly people, disabled people, those who living alone, inpatients, and residents in nursing facilities; and expectant and nursing mothers,**

47 Measures to be Taken

Example ①From the occurrence of the disaster on March 11, 2011 to April 30 (up to 1 month)

Figure 45-1 Municipalities' perspective to examine disaster responses and their actual efforts

and children. Ideally, specific support should be provided to these targeted people to respond to their special needs, and such support is recommended when feasible. However, although detailed responses can be planned during ordinary times, such responses are difficult to provide in the actual situation of an earthquake disaster and may even cause confusion. Accordingly, I believe it important to broadly classify targeted people first, and then consider more detailed responses for them.

As stated above, it is effective to consider disaster responses from two perspectives; categorization of health issues and categorization of attributes of targeted people. In addition, it is recommended to divide the stages of the response after the disaster into an acute stage, an intermediate stage and a later stage for classification, as follows. (Figure 45-1)

(1) From the occurrence of the disaster on March 11, 2011 to April 30 (up to 1 month)
(2) From May 1 to September 30, 2011 (2 to 6 months)
(3) From October 1, 2011 to March 31, 2012 (7 months to 1 year)
(4) April 1, 2012 to March 31, 2013 (1 year and 1 month to 2 years)

C Major issues in public health at the time of a nuclear disaster

In this nuclear disaster, several issues of public health have been pointed out concerning screening, preventive medication with stable iodine preparations, support for people requiring assistance during a disaster, and handling of dead bodies contaminated by radioactive materials[3].

1 Radioactive contamination & screening

On March 15, instructions to perform screening were issued to heads of Fukushima Prefecture, Okuma

Town, Futaba Town, Tomioka Town, Namie Town, Naraha Town, Hirono Town, Katsurao Village, Minamisoma City, Kawauchi Village, and Tamura City based on the Nuclear Emergency Preparedness Act. A report "*How to provide radiation emergency medicine*" (2011; Nuclear Safety Commission) states that local public bodies should designate places for relief to provide screening as needed, in cooperation with relevant institutions. In this disaster, there were so many targeted people that even all staff members in Fukushima Prefecture could not respond to them. Thanks to the many people dispatched from public health centers throughout Japan and the Japan Association of Radiological Technologists, screening was provided to all targeted people. However, there was confusion concerning the establishment of standards for decontamination. These issues should be examined for the future.

Even municipalities where nuclear power stations are not located should make arrangements to promptly implement screening by having radiologists participate in training courses, such as the Radiation Emergency Medicine Course hosted by the Nuclear Safety Research Association. Staff members can then acquire expertise and master how to handle medical equipment used for screening.

2   Preventive medication of stable iodine preparations

To prevent thyroid cancer caused by radioactive iodine (^{131}I), it is effective to take stable iodine preparations with no radioactive iodine before radiation exposure.

On March 16, 2011, written instructions were issued to the heads of Fukushima Prefecture and 12 relevant municipalities to require administration of stable iodine preparations to residents when they leave evacuation areas (within a 20km radius). However, Fukushima Prefecture did not give instructions to take iodine preparation as it had already confirmed that there were no targeted people in areas within a 20-km radius from the nuclear power station. Meanwhile, Miharu Town, which was not designated as an evacuation area, determined on March 15 to distribute stable iodine preparations to residents and instruct them to take it. Although the prefecture required Miharu Town to withdraw its instructions, the town did not obey the prefecture. There are still many discussions about the propriety of the instructions to take stable iodine preparations.

On June 5, 2013, the Nuclear Disaster Response Guidelines were revised, in which basic principles for distribution and medication with stable iodine preparations, including distribution in advance, were newly offered[4]. Moreover, The Secretariat of the Nuclear Regulatory Authority created practical guidelines based on these principles to clarify specific measures related to distribution and medication with stable iodine preparations. Prefectures and municipalities are required to be familiar with the information in these guidelines as well.

3   Support for people requiring assistance during a disaster

People requiring assistance during a disaster refer to those who need help to take necessary actions in case of disaster. This includes acquiring accurate and necessary information in a prompt manner and getting evacuated to safer places to protect them against the disaster. Generally, they include elderly people, disabled people, foreigners, expectant mothers, and younger children. Since people requiring assistance may lack adaptability to new circumstances, they often face difficulties adapting to changes in the living environment caused by the disaster, evacuating to safer places, and living in evacuation centers. However, if they can receive necessary support when needed, they can live independent lives[5].

Table 45-2 Number of disaster-related deaths resulting from the Great East Japan Earthquake (as of March 29, 2013)

Prefecture	Total	Age bracket		
		20 years old or younger	21 to 65 years old	66 years old or older
All prefectures in Japan	2,688	5	287	2,396
Iwate Prefecture	389	1	48	340
Miyagi Prefecture	862	1	109	752
Fukushima Prefecture	1,383	0	121	1,262
Others	54	3	9	42

In this section, elderly people (including those living alone), disabled people, inpatients, and residents in nursing facilities are defined as vulnerable people in case of a disaster. This definition covers a wider range of people than those generally defined as people requiring assistance during a disaster.

One of the major features of the Great East Japan Earthquake is that the number of deaths from the disaster in Fukushima Prefecture was smaller than in Miyagi and Iwate Prefectures. Specifically, the number of deaths in Fukushima Prefecture was 1,606 (as of September 11, 2013; National Police Agency) compared to 9,537 in Miyagi Prefecture and 4,637 in Iwate Prefecture. On the other hand, the number of disaster-related deaths (defined as those who died from deterioration of wounds suffered in the Great East Japan Earthquake, and who became eligible for disaster condolence grants based on the Act on Payment for Solatia for Disaster) in Fukushima Prefecture was larger than in the other two prefectures, with an absolute majority of more than a thousand (Table 45-2). In particular, the number of elderly people suffering disaster-related deaths is significantly larger, with the ratio of approximately 90%. This is common to any prefecture. This shows that elderly people are vulnerable people in case of a disaster and need support as people requiring assistance during a disaster.

In association with the nuclear power station accident, all residents, including inpatients and residents in nursing facilities, who lived within a 20-km radius were forced to be evacuated by the evacuation order issued on March 12. Although the evacuation of ordinary residents was nearly completed on March 13, approximately 840 inpatients were left behind. To take these patients out of hospitals, rescue efforts were conducted. However, it was reported that 12 patients died during transportation, and 50 patients died at evacuation destinations immediately after they were transported[6]. Moreover, it was revealed that many of the elderly people who lived in 34 geriatric facilities within a 20-km radius (special nursing care facilities for the elderly, geriatric health care facilities, group shared residences, etc.) died in association with the evacuation. Excess mortality, the number of deaths is significantly larger than in the previous year, was observed not only immediately after the earthquake but also for approximately one year after the event. Unfortunately, evacuation, which was conducted to avoid the health effects of radioactive materials, resulted in the death of elderly people. It is no exaggeration to say that excess mortality at this time was closely related to the earthquake (Figure 45-2).

Learning from this experience we have to prepare for disaster on a routine basis, including setting guidelines for evacuation, establishing appropriate procedures for evacuation, ensuring evacuation destinations and securing means of communicating and cooperating with the evacuation destinations, securing routes to procure necessary medical products and goods, and training staff to give evacuation guidance. Furthermore, we need to share our conclusion that determination of whether evacuation is necessary or not is very important, because evacuation may be harmful or life threatening if we make no provision for it.

Chapter 6 Suggestions — Toward the Future —

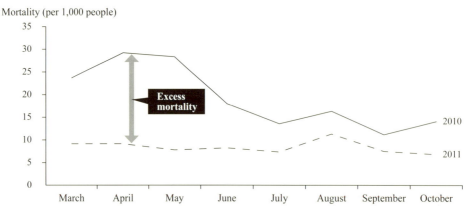

Figure 45-2 Comparison of the number of deaths in geriatric facilities in 2010 and 2011 (Yasumura S, Goto A, Yamazaki S, Reich MR. Excess mortality among relocated institutionalized elderly after the Fukushima nuclear disaster. Public Health, 127: 186-188, 2013)

Some physicians say that families with elementary school children should be evacuated in a group for a certain period of time, and some people involved in public health empathize with them. This is regrettable because they take no thought of what a large impact is made on health by evacuation, as stated above. If experts in public health argue for evacuation, they should make a comprehensive assessment, in advance, of what specific measures should be taken to avoid and reduce risk concerning physical, psychological and economic problems, which are expected to arise in association with evacuation. Considering what a great influence their remarks have, they cannot avoid blame for their irresponsible comments if they express their opinions with no regard to the risk of evacuation.

4 Handling of dead bodies contaminated by radioactive materials

There had been no specific rules concerning handling of dead bodies contaminated by radioactive materials in case of a nuclear disaster. In this earthquake disaster, decontamination procedures for dead bodies were set so that those who would conduct a postmortem examination of dead bodies would not be exposed to radiation[3].

5 Preparations during ordinary times

a. Stockpile for emergency

Basically, individual households should prepare a minimum amount of preserved food and emergency provisions in anticipation of disaster. Individual family members need to prepare emergency sets or evacuation sets packed in backpacks by themselves. Regarding vulnerable people in case of a disaster, however, administrative bodies need to provide support and public help for their preparations.

Municipalities are also required to have a minimum stock of supplies, such as preserved food, emergency provisions, medical products, artificial milk (milk powder), bottled water, blankets, cold weather protection gear, and makeshift beds. However, this is no simple task because they have to bear a considerable burden of the cost and management of these stocks, regardless of the size of the population. In particular, emergency provisions, such as food, medical products, milk powder and bottled water, have limited shelf lives, it takes a lot of money to keep them in stock, while regularly replacing them with new supplies. In addition, when residents are forced to be evacuated, municipalities are required to ensure transportation means for goods, distribute them according to the needs in individual evacuation destinations, and devise appropriate ways to store them.

Many public health nurses in municipalities where residents were forced to evacuate due to the Great East Japan Earthquake stated their views as below: "If necessary goods can be fully stored, this leaves nothing to be desired. However, it is a hard work for us to manage stocks while busily engaged in daily operations even during ordinary times. **It is effective to make preparations for physical and material support concerning various emergency recovery services in case of disaster by concluding a mutual support agreement in disaster between local governments or with private businesses**."

b. Preparation for physical support & human resources development

As one of the means to provide physical support at the time of a nuclear disaster, experts in radiation need to be dispatched. However, those most required by municipalities are public health nurses and clerical staff members. In the Great East Japan Earthquake, only a few nursing staff members were dispatched to Fukushima Prefecture at first. This comprised a major obstacle to health-care activities. Moreover, it was extremely regrettable that the Japanese Society of Public Health, which aims to contribute to the improvement of public health in Japan, was unable to offer direct and specific support to Fukushima Prefecture as well as to Iwate and Miyagi Prefectures. Since I serve as Director of the Japanese Society of Public Health, I feel partly to blame for this inconvenience. It is necessary to review the roles and tasks of professional organizations and academic societies in terms of physical support.

A Mutual Support Agreement in Disaster is very important, in particular, as a means to enhance a physical support system. At the time of disaster, not only expert personnel involved in public health but also clerical personnel become very busy with emergency responses. This leads to a significant delay of office work, and effective activities related to public health may become impossible. Accordingly, the assistance of clerical personnel from other prefectures and municipalities are indispensable. Although a Municipal Support Agreement in Disaster has already been concluded between many municipalities that have established sister city relationships, those which have not yet concluded the agreement are encouraged to sign it as soon as possible.

In Fukushima Prefecture, the national government, the prefecture and municipalities were required to take unprecedented measures in the aftermath of the accident in all aspects since the earthquake. Although human resources capable of responding to a disaster are required, there are not many people who have any experience with disaster response and can share their experiences. Accordingly, to develop human resources that can respond to a radiation disaster, which is different from other disasters, **it is most efficient to dispatch people to prefectures and municipalities which require an enormous amount of time for earthquake disaster recovery and reconstruction, aiming to promote personnel exchange, and to have them involved in reconstruction activities with local people**. In particular, it is very effective to dispatch not only expert personnel, such as public health nurses and nutritionists, but also clerical personnel. Even two years after the earthquake in the Radiation Medical Science Center for the Fukushima Health Management Survey of Fukushima Medical University, where I work, ten people dispatched from other prefectures are continuously involved in operations along with other staff members. This serves as on-the-job training (OJT), or in-house education and training. When returning to their municipalities after their term of service, dispatched staff members can share the knowledge and experience that they have acquired through the activities in affected areas. Consequently, this leads to human resource development. Meanwhile, local governments that receive staff members from other municipalities can reduce the burden of operations due to the increase of personnel, as well as gain empirical knowledge derived from the other

Chapter 6　Suggestions — Toward the Future —

municipalities. Thus, physical support is the most helpful for affected areas, aside from monetary support.

D Aiming to provide appropriate information (Toward better risk communication)

In this nuclear power station accident, residents in Fukushima Prefecture seemed to have been confounded by information obtained through the mass media. The explanation about the nuclear power station accident by the national government and Tokyo Electric Power Company (TEPCO) was inappropriate, was hard to understand and was offered too late. This incurred the distrust of residents in Fukushima Prefecture, and has led to an atmosphere in which they do not believe information from the national government and TEPCO concerning their questions, as is shown in Table 45-3. Accordingly, even though the national government shows scientific evidence that the impact of radiation is minimal for the residents, that only reinforces the suspicion that the government intends to underestimate the impact of the accident and damage. On the other hand, they rather tend to believe the government's views when it suggests the possible greatest risk (overestimates the risk) of the accident. The national government and TEPCO have raised doubts among not only residents but also experts, and have not gained their confidence yet.

Risk communication is defined as a communication where positive information on targeted activities and scientific technologies as well as negative information, such as risk to targets, are fairly passed on between individuals, groups and organizations, and where those involved exchange their opinions about it to communicate and interact with each other. The important thing is that those concerned, such as administrative bodies, experts, residents, and stakeholders, should share accurate information about the risk of radiation and enhance their mutual communication. A one-sided communication from administrative bodies and experts to residents never works effectively.

Table 45-4 shows the issues and ideal pathways of risk communication concerning radiation. Although this does not cover everything, I hope that it will be helpful.

Table 45-3　Examples of questions that residents have

- What happened in the nuclear power station? Did core meltdowns occur in nuclear reactors?
- When did radioactive materials begin to be dispersed, and how much and where were they dispersed?
- To avoid exposure to radiation, to where should we evacuate, and what should and shouldn't we do?
- Are crops, seafood and other food of Fukushima Prefecture origin safe to eat?
- Are adults, who were exposed to more or less radiation, likely to develop cancer?
- Are children, who were exposed to more or less radiation, likely to develop thyroid cancer?
- What is the safety level of exposure to radiation?

Table 45-4　Better risk communication concerning radiation

- Direct communication in smaller groups is an effective means for mutual understanding.
- Some materials should be prepared when explanations are given. Materials should be the same for each theme. In addition, individual speakers should give the same explanation for each theme. This is effective to increase residents' confidence in the information.
- Regarding risk management information (ways to respond to risk), several ways should be presented so that individual residents can make a voluntary choice.
- Information that is not abstract but specific, direct and experiential is more easily accepted by residents.
- Information on not only conclusions but also processes leading to the conclusions should be provided.
- On the assumption that participants have some questions, adequate time for question-and-answer sessions should be given.
- Opportunities to provide consultation to individual residents should be offered as much as possible, even if it is difficult to do so.

In addition to comprehensive medical examinations conducted by affected local governments, the Radiation Medical Science Center for the Fukushima Health Management Survey, Fukushima Medical University has provided health consultation "*Yorozu Kenko Sodan*" to residents who are concerned about the health effects of radiation. By so doing, it aims to ensure and enhance the safety and security of affected residents. The health consultation, in which faculties and physicians at the university communicate directly with residents, has earned high satisfaction ratings from residents and has received a good evaluation from local governments. Thus, it is very important to establish systems that enable face-to-face communication.

Furthermore, public health centers in Fukushima Prefecture have offered to deliver lectures on radiation based on the philosophy that information should not be presented in a one-sided manner and that interactive communication is needed. These lectures have been helpful in conveying information on radiation to residents. According to questionnaire surveys of participants in the lectures, the following points received a favorable reception: (1) Participants were able to determine the themes of lectures; (2) Lectures included hands-on learning, such as practical trainings for radiation measurement. Interactive communication and hands-on experience were effective for providing information.

E : Importance of accumulating experience and transmitting information

In Fukushima Prefecture, all residents were not only affected by the earthquake and tsunami, but also were forced to face radiation issues caused by the nuclear power station accident. Roughly more than two hundred thousand residents, who were forced to be evacuated, had an extremely problematic experience and are still forced to live inconvenient lives. Other residents, who were not evacuated, also had a highly painful and bitter experience. It will take a good amount of time to heal the emotional wounds inflicted by their unhappy experience. Meanwhile, there are concerns that peoples' memories might fade with time, and that even the tragedy caused by the disaster might be gradually forgotten. Accidents, such as leakage of contaminated water, may remind people that the nuclear power station accident has not been settled yet. However, those involved in public health in Fukushima Prefecture should have the responsibility to preserve peoples' memories of the accident and make use of the experience gained during the accident to prepare for similar disasters in the future.

(Seiji Yasumura)

References

1) Editor: Osamu Kunii: *Public Health in Case of Disaster – What We Can Do.* Nanzando Co., Ltd.: Tokyo, P. 1–437, 2012.

2) Executive Committee for Earthquake Response Seminars: *Record of the 3.11 Great Earthquake – Responses by national government offices, affected local governments and various professionals.* Civil Law Study Group Co., Ltd.: Tokyo, P. 1–788, July 11, 2012.

3) Yasuhiro Kanatani: *Public health response to the nuclear accident.* Journal of the National Institute of Public Health, Vol. 62, No. 2: P. 125–131, 2013.

4) Nuclear Regulation Authority website: http://www.nsr.go.jp/public_comment/bosyu130130/130130-01.pdf

5) *Guidelines for Evacuation Support for People Requiring Assistance during a Disaster.* Committee Support for Vulnerable People in Disasters, March 2006.

6) Tanigawa K, Hosoi Y, Hirohashi N, et al: Loss of life after evacuation: lessons learned from the Fukushima accident. Lancet, 379: 889–891, 2012.

7) Radiation Medical Group, Fukushima Medical University Hospital: *Facing Nuclear Disaster — Messages from medical professionals living in Fukushima.* Life Science Co., Ltd.: Tokyo, P. 1–273, May 1, 2013.

Materials

List of the Situation and Measures of Other Municipalities

Name of municipality				Aizubange Town	Aizumisato Town	Asakawa Town	Ishikawa Town
1 Situation of the municipality							
Population (persons) (upper part: as of January 1, 2011; lower part: as of January 1, 2013)				17,837 17,413	23,524 22,812	7,094 6,965	17,526 17,110
Ratio of the elderly aged 65 or older (%) (upper part: as of January 1, 2011; lower part: as of January 1, 2013)				28.8 29.3	30.7 31.4	25.3 26.1	27.72 28.70
Total area (km²)				91.65	276.37	37.43	115.71
Distance from Fukushima Daiichi Nuclear Power Station of the Tokyo Electric Power Company (km)				Approximately 108	106	67	60
2 Situation of damage by the earthquake, tsunami and the nuclear power station accident							
Property damage	House	Completely destroyed		2 (as of February 28, 2013)	0 (as of January 1, 2013)	0 (as of October 2013)	1 (as of October 11, 2013)
		Half destroyed		7 (″)	2 (″)	1 (″)	32 (″)
		Partially destroyed		32 (″)	325 (″)	586 (″)	2,602 (″)
	Public institution	Completely destroyed		0 (″)	0 (″)	0 (″)	0 (″)
		Half destroyed		0 (″)	0 (″)	0 (″)	0 (″)
		Partially destroyed		2 (″)	0 (″)	17 (″)	27 (″)
	Other	Completely destroyed		6 (″)	1 (″)	0 (″)	0 (″)
		Half destroyed		70 (″)	7 (″)	0 (″)	0 (″)
		Partially destroyed		233 (″)	114 (″)	134 (″)	207 (″)
Human damage	Deaths by disaster			0 (as of February 28, 2013)	0 (as of January 1, 2013)	0 (as of April 2011)	0 (as of October 11, 2013)
	Disaster-related deaths			0 (″)	0 (″)	0 (″)	1 (″)
	Missing persons			0 (″)	0 (″)	0 (″)	0 (″)
	Injured persons			1 (″)	1 (″)	3 (″)	4 (″)
Establishment of evacuation centers (total number)				2 (as of February 28, 2013)	9 (as of January 1, 2013)	1 (as of April 2011)	2 (as of October 15, 2013)
Evacuees received (total number)				1,095 (as of February 28, 2013)	36,762 (as of September 6, 2012)	170 (as of April 2011)	Approximately 730 (as of July 11, 2013)
Establishment of temporary housing for residents and evacuees received (total number)				0 (as of February 28, 2013)	259 (as of January 1, 2013)	0 (as of October 2013)	0 (as of October 11, 2013)
Approximate number of voluntary evacuees	Inside Fukushima Prefecture (number of people)			0 (as of February 28, 2013)	0 (as of January 1, 2013)		0 (as of October 1, 2013)
	Outside Fukushima Prefecture (number of people/ prefectures where people are evacuated)			0 (″)	14/7 (″)		56/14 (″)
3 Whole efforts							
Countermeasures against external exposure	Personal dose measurement			○	○	○	○
	Refreshment for expectant mothers (relaxation in low-dose areas)						
	Refreshment for young children						
	Refreshment for elementary school and junior high school students						
	Monitoring of air levels			○	○	○	○
	Real-time measurement of radiation dose (Ministry of the Environment)			○	○ (Ministry of Education, Culture, Sports, Science and Technology)	○	○ (Ministry of Education, Culture, Sports, Science and Technology)
	Measurement of air levels in the whole jurisdiction & creation of maps			○	○		○
	Replacement of the surface soil on the grounds in childcare facilities, child education facilities and schools			○	○ (disposal of surface soil)	○	○
	Decontamination of houses				○ (in preparation/planned to be conducted)		○
	Decontamination of public and medical institutions				○ (in preparation/planned to be conducted)		○
Countermeasures against internal exposure	Examination of breast milk						
	Whole Body Counter measurements (conducted by municipalities)					○	
	Whole Body Counter measurements (conducted by Fukushima Prefecture, targeting those age 4 to 18)			○		○	○
	Food and water quality inspection			○	○	○	○
	Thyroid gland examination (conducted by Fukushima Prefecture)					○	○
	Inspection of school meals			○	○	○	○
Others	Debriefing sessions for measurement results of exposure dose						○
	Study sessions on radiation			○		○	
	Cancer screening				○ (in accordance with the Health Promotion Act)	○	○
	Replacement of the surface soil in rice paddies				Measures to inhibit the absorption of cesium taken		
	Measurement of radiation dose in soil in the whole jurisdiction & creation of maps			○	Only measurement in farmland conducted; maps not created	○	
	Lecture meetings on radiation			○	○	○	○
	Sampling of respondents for a basic survey in the Fukushima Health Management Survey			○	○	○	○
	Publication of disaster information magazines			○	○		
	Issuance of citizen health cards (containing a column for recording radiation exposure levels)						
	Other measures						

Name of municipality			Izumizaki Village	Inawashiro Town	Otama Village	Ono Town
1 Situation of the municipality						
Population (persons) (upper part: as of January 1, 2011; lower part: as of January 1, 2013)			6,892 6,806	15,776 15,435	8,640 8,539	11,597 11,144
Ratio of the elderly aged 65 or older (%) (upper part: as of January 1, 2011; lower part: as of January 1, 2013)			22.7 23.4	30.8 31.5	22.81 23.41	27.8 28.7
Total area (km²)			35.4	395.0	79.46	125.11
Distance from Fukushima Daiichi Nuclear Power Station of the Tokyo Electric Power Company (km)			70	Approximately 80	60	35
2 Situation of damage by the earthquake, tsunami and the nuclear power station accident						
Property damage	House	Completely destroyed	59 (as of April 1, 2013)	17 (as of February 7, 2013)	29 (as of November 8, 2013)	4 (as of February 14, 2013)
		Half destroyed	331 (〃)	76 (〃)	41 (〃)	45 (〃)
		Partially destroyed	630 (〃)	704 (〃)	916 (〃)	1,397 (〃)
	Public institution	Completely destroyed		0 (〃)	0 (〃)	0 (〃)
		Half destroyed		0 (〃)	0 (〃)	
		Partially destroyed		9 (〃)	0 (〃)	39 (〃)
	Other	Completely destroyed	12 (〃)	80 (〃)		44 (〃)
		Half destroyed	32 (〃)	116 (〃)		116 (〃)
		Partially destroyed	43 (〃)	548 (〃)		175 (〃)
Human damage	Deaths by disaster		0 (as of April 1, 2013)	0 (as of February 7, 2013)	0 (as of November 14, 2013)	0 (as of February 14, 2013)
	Disaster-related deaths		0 (〃)	0 (〃)	1 (〃)	0 (〃)
	Missing persons		0 (〃)	0 (〃)	0 (〃)	0 (〃)
	Injured persons		0 (〃)	1 (〃)	0 (〃)	
Establishment of evacuation centers (total number)			2 (as of April 1, 2013)	10 (as of February 7, 2013)	9 (as of November 14, 2013)	3 (as of May 2, 2012)
Evacuees received (total number)			115 (maximum actual number) (as of March 11, 2011)	8,428 7, 2013)	533 (as of February 5, 2013)	13,235 (as of May 2, 2012)
Establishment of temporary housing for residents and evacuees received (total number)			0 (as of April 1, 2013)	10 (as of February 7, 2013)	630 (as of February 5, 2013)	
Approximate number of voluntary evacuees	Inside Fukushima Prefecture (number of people)		1 (as of April 1, 2013)	0 (as of February 7, 2013)	4 (as of August 1, 2013)	3 (as of October 1, 2012)
	Outside Fukushima Prefecture (number of people/ prefectures where people are evacuated)		30/9 (〃)	37/12 (〃)	48/Unknown (〃)	23/Unknown (〃)
3 Whole efforts						
Countermeasures against external exposure	Personal dose measurement		○	○	○	○
	Refreshment for expectant mothers (relaxation in low-dose areas)					
	Refreshment for young children					
	Refreshment for elementary school and junior high school students				○	
	Monitoring of air levels		○	○	○	○
	Real-time measurement of radiation dose (Ministry of the Environment)		○	○	○	○
	Measurement of air levels in the whole jurisdiction & creation of maps		○	○	○	○
	Replacement of the surface soil on the grounds in childcare facilities, child education facilities and schools		○	○	○	○
	Decontamination of houses		○	○	○	
	Decontamination of public and medical institutions		○	○	○	△ (partially conducted 〈schools, child education facilities, etc.〉)
Countermeasures against internal exposure	Examination of breast milk					
	Whole Body Counter measurements (conducted by municipalities)			○	○	○
	Whole Body Counter measurements (conducted by Fukushima Prefecture, targeting those age 4 to 18)		○		○	○
	Food and water quality inspection		○	○	○	○
	Thyroid gland examination (conducted by Fukushima Prefecture)		○		○	
	Inspection of school meals		○	○	○	○
Others	Debriefing sessions for measurement results of exposure dose		○			
	Study sessions on radiation				○	○
	Cancer screening			○	○	○
	Replacement of the surface soil in rice paddies			○	△ (reversal tillage)	
	Measurement of radiation dose in soil in the whole jurisdiction & creation of maps				○	
	Lecture meetings on radiation		○	○	○	○
	Sampling of respondents for a basic survey in the Fukushima Health Management Survey		○	○	○	○
	Publication of disaster information magazines					○ (through public relations magazines, etc.)
	Issuance of citizen health cards (containing a column for recording radiation exposure levels)					
	Other measures					Health checkups with an additional test item (a blood test corresponding to one for ionizing radiation workers) ; regeneration project for self- supplied feed producing farms (reversal of the surface soil of grassland) ; Lending of air dosimeters

416

Name of municipality			Kagamiishi Town	Kaneyama Town	Kitakata City	Kitashiobara Village
1 Situation of the municipality						
Population (persons) (upper part: as of January 1, 2011; lower part: as of January 1, 2013)			13,056 / 12,842	2,579 / 2,412	52,267 / 50,953	3,294 / 3,166
Ratio of the elderly aged 65 or older (%) (upper part: as of January 1, 2011; lower part: as of January 1, 2013)			20.90 / 22.13	53.70 / 55.43	31.4 / 32.0	17.27 / 16.89
Total area (km²)			31.25	293.97	554.67	233.94
Distance from Fukushima Daiichi Nuclear Power Station of the Tokyo Electric Power Company (km)			64	133	106.4	100
2 Situation of damage by the earthquake, tsunami and the nuclear power station accident						
Property damage	House	Completely destroyed	173 (as of May 31, 2012)	0 (as of October 1, 2013)	0 (as of February 15, 2013)	
		Half destroyed	768 (″)	0 (″)	0 (″)	
		Partially destroyed	1,623 (″)	0 (″)	0 (″)	
	Public institution	Completely destroyed		0 (″)	0 (″)	
		Half destroyed	983 (″)	0 (″)	0 (″)	
		Partially destroyed		0 (″)	19 (″)	
	Other	Completely destroyed		0 (″)	0 (″)	
		Half destroyed	450 (″)	0 (″)	0 (″)	
		Partially destroyed		0 (″)	16 (″)	
Human damage	Deaths by disaster			0 (as of October 1, 2013)	0 (as of February 15, 2013)	
	Disaster-related deaths		2 (as of May 31, 2012)	0 (″)	0 (″)	
	Missing persons		0 (″)	0 (″)	0 (″)	
	Injured persons		2 (″)	0 (″)	0 (″)	
Establishment of evacuation centers (total number)			20 (as of May 31, 2012)	0 (as of October 1, 2013)	1 (as of February 15, 2013)	1 (as of April 13, 2011)
Evacuees received (total number)			317 (as of October 17, 2013)	13 (as of October 1, 2013)	10,174 (as of February 15, 2013)	360 (as of April 13, 2011)
Establishment of temporary housing for residents and evacuees received (total number)			100 (as of October 17, 2013)	0 (as of October 1, 2013)	0 (as of February 15, 2013)	
Approximate number of voluntary evacuees	Inside Fukushima Prefecture (number of people)		3 (as of July 10, 2013)	0 (as of April 1, 2012)	0 (as of October 1, 2012)	
	Outside Fukushima Prefecture (number of people/ prefectures where people are evacuated)		112/20 (″)	3/1 (″)	25/7 (″)	
3 Whole efforts						
Countermeasures against external exposure	Personal dose measurement		○	○	○	○
	Refreshment for expectant mothers (relaxation in low-dose areas)		Refreshment projects are conducted by relevant business operators.			
	Refreshment for young children					
	Refreshment for elementary school and junior high school students					
	Monitoring of air levels		○	○	○	○
	Real-time measurement of radiation dose (Ministry of the Environment)		○	○	○	○
	Measurement of air levels in the whole jurisdiction & creation of maps		○			○ (only dose measurement)
	Replacement of the surface soil on the grounds in childcare facilities, child education facilities and schools		○			
	Decontamination of houses		○			
	Decontamination of public and medical institutions		○	○		
Countermeasures against internal exposure	Examination of breast milk					
	Whole Body Counter measurements (conducted by municipalities)		○			
	Whole Body Counter measurements (conducted by Fukushima Prefecture, targeting those age 4 to 18)		○	○		
	Food and water quality inspection		○	○	○	○
	Thyroid gland examination (conducted by Fukushima Prefecture)		○	○		
	Inspection of school meals		○	○	○	○
Others	Debriefing sessions for measurement results of exposure dose		○		○ (combined with lecture meetings and study sessions)	
	Study sessions on radiation		○		○ (combined with lecture meetings and study sessions)	○
	Cancer screening		○	○	Only usual cancer screening	
	Replacement of the surface soil in rice paddies		○			
	Measurement of radiation dose in soil in the whole jurisdiction & creation of maps		○			
	Lecture meetings on radiation		○	○	○	○
	Sampling of respondents for a basic survey in the Fukushima Health Management Survey		○		○	○
	Publication of disaster information magazines		○		○	○
	Issuance of citizen health cards (containing a column for recording radiation exposure levels)		Not issued independently by the town			
	Other measures					

Name of municipality				Kunimi Town	Koori Town	Samegawa Village	Shimogo Town
1 Situation of the municipality							
Population (persons) (upper part: as of January 1, 2011; lower part: as of January 1, 2013)				10,340 10,123	13,154 12,651	4,151 3,985	6,661 6,445
Ratio of the elderly aged 65 or older (%) (upper part: as of January 1, 2011; lower part: as of January 1, 2013)				30.0 31.0	28.01 28.20	29.8 30.49	36.1 36.5
Total area (km²)				37.90	42.97	131.3	317.09
Distance from Fukushima Daiichi Nuclear Power Station of the Tokyo Electric Power Company (km)				Approximately 66	65	63	104
2 Situation of damage by the earthquake, tsunami and the nuclear power station accident							
Property damage	House		Completely destroyed	191 (as of March 15, 2013)	55 (as of October 1, 2013)	7 (as of February 12, 2013)	0 (as of October 1, 2013)
			Half destroyed	565 (″)	187 (″)		0 (″)
			Partially destroyed	508 (″)	1,883 (″)	112 (″)	0 (″)
	Public institution		Completely destroyed		0 (″)		0 (″)
			Half destroyed		1 (″)		0 (″)
			Partially destroyed		4 (″)	11 (″)	0 (″)
	Other		Completely destroyed	306 (″)	223 (″)		0 (″)
			Half destroyed	177 (″)	178 (″)		0 (″)
			Partially destroyed	153 (″)	539 (″)	39 (″)	0 (″)
Human damage	Deaths by disaster			1 (as of March 15, 2013)	0 (as of October 1, 2013)		0 (as of October 1, 2013)
	Disaster-related deaths			0 (″)	0 (″)		0 (″)
	Missing persons			0 (″)	0 (″)		0 (″)
	Injured persons			20 (″)	1 (″)		0 (″)
Establishment of evacuation centers (total number)				17 (as of March 15, 2013)	2 (as of October 1, 2013)	1 (as of February 12, 2013)	2 (as of April 28, 2011)
Evacuees received (total number)				11,641 (as of March 15, 2013)	140 (as of October 1, 2013)	272 (as of February 12, 2013)	503 (as of March 25, 2011)
Establishment of temporary housing for residents and evacuees received (total number)				135 (as of March 15, 2013)			0 (as of October 1, 2013)
Approximate number of voluntary evacuees	Inside Fukushima Prefecture (number of people)			Unknown (as of March 15, 2013)	Unknown (as of October 1, 2013)		0 (as of October 1, 2013)
	Outside Fukushima Prefecture (number of people/ prefectures where people are evacuated)			179/12 (″)	102/Unknown		0 (″)
3 Whole efforts							
Countermeasures against external exposure	Personal dose measurement			○	○	○	○
	Refreshment for expectant mothers (relaxation in low-dose areas)					○	
	Refreshment for young children					○	
	Refreshment for elementary school and junior high school students			○		○	
	Monitoring of air levels			○	○	○	○
	Real-time measurement of radiation dose (Ministry of the Environment)			○	○	○	○
	Measurement of air levels in the whole jurisdiction & creation of maps			○	○	○	
	Replacement of the surface soil on the grounds in childcare facilities, child education facilities and schools			○		○	○
	Decontamination of houses				○		
	Decontamination of public and medical institutions			○	○	○	
Countermeasures against internal exposure	Examination of breast milk						
	Whole Body Counter measurements (conducted by municipalities)			○	○		○
	Whole Body Counter measurements (conducted by Fukushima Prefecture, targeting those age 4 to 18)			○		○	○
	Food and water quality inspection			○	○	○	○
	Thyroid gland examination (conducted by Fukushima Prefecture)			○	○		○
	Inspection of school meals			○	○	○	○
Others	Debriefing sessions for measurement results of exposure dose						
	Study sessions on radiation					○	
	Cancer screening			○ (only usual cancer screening)		○	
	Replacement of the surface soil in rice paddies			○			
	Measurement of radiation dose in soil in the whole jurisdiction & creation of maps			○		○	
	Lecture meetings on radiation			○	○	○	○
	Sampling of respondents for a basic survey in the Fukushima Health Management Survey			○		○	○
	Publication of disaster information magazines			○			
	Issuance of citizen health cards (containing a column for recording radiation exposure levels)						
	Other measures						Project for lending air dose measuring instruments

418

Name of municipality			Showa Village	Shirakawa City	Shinchi Town	Sukagawa City
1 Situation of the municipality						
Population (persons) (upper part: as of January 1, 2011; lower part: as of January 1, 2013)			1,559 1,499	64,651 63,261	8,429 8,024	79,202 77,508
Ratio of the elderly aged 65 or older (%) (upper part: as of January 1, 2011; lower part: as of January 1, 2013)			52.2 53.2	22.5 23.3	27.5 27.6	21.8 22.9
Total area (km²)			209	305.30	46.4	279.55
Distance from Fukushima Daiichi Nuclear Power Station of the Tokyo Electric Power Company (km)			126	Approximately 80	62.6	59
2 Situation of damage by the earthquake, tsunami and the nuclear power station accident						
Property damage	House	Completely destroyed	0 (as of March 31, 2013)	240 (as of December 14, 2012)	474 (as of November 18, 2013)	1,249 (as of December 1, 2012)
		Half destroyed	0 (″)	1,818 (″)	156 (″)	3,503 (″)
		Partially destroyed	0 (″)	6,748 (″)		10,563 (″)
	Public institution	Completely destroyed	0 (″)	Unknown (″)		Unknown (″)
		Half destroyed	0 (″)	Unknown (″)		Unknown (″)
		Partially destroyed	0 (″)	Unknown (″)		Unknown (″)
	Other	Completely destroyed	0 (″)	420 (″)		Unknown (″)
		Half destroyed	0 (″)	603 (″)		Unknown (″)
		Partially destroyed	1 (″)	1,026 (″)		Unknown (″)
Human damage	Deaths by disaster		0 (as of March 31, 2011)	12 (as of April 1, 2011)	110 (as of November 18, 2013)	0 (as of December 1, 2012)
	Disaster-related deaths		0 (″)		8 (″)	10 (″)
	Missing persons		0 (″)		0 (″)	0 (″)
	Injured persons		0 (″)		3 (″)	Unknown (″)
Establishment of evacuation centers (total number)			1 (as of March 31, 2011)	22 (as of May 6, 2011)	8 (as of November 18, 2013)	48 (as of December 1, 2012)
Evacuees received (total number)			4 (as of March 31, 2013)	65 (as of October 25, 2012)	50,076 (as of November 18, 2013)	612 (as of March 1, 2013)
Establishment of temporary housing for residents and evacuees received (total number)			0 (as of March 31, 2013)	140 (as of October 25, 2012)	573 (as of November 18, 2013)	177 (as of February 8, 2013)
Approximate number of voluntary evacuees	Inside Fukushima Prefecture (number of people)		0 (as of March 31, 2013)	4 (as of February 22, 2013)	126 (as of November 18, 2013)	3 (as of March 1, 2013)
	Outside Fukushima Prefecture (number of people/ prefectures where people are evacuated)		0 (″)	467/34 (″)	6/Unknown (″)	674/33 (″)
3 Whole efforts						
Countermeasures against external exposure	Personal dose measurement			○	○	○
	Refreshment for expectant mothers (relaxation in low-dose areas)					
	Refreshment for young children					○
	Refreshment for elementary school and junior high school students					
	Monitoring of air levels		○	○	○	○
	Real-time measurement of radiation dose (Ministry of the Environment)		○	○	○	○
	Measurement of air levels in the whole jurisdiction & creation of maps			○	○	○
	Replacement of the surface soil on the grounds in childcare facilities, child education facilities and schools		○	○	○	○
	Decontamination of houses			○		○
	Decontamination of public and medical institutions		○	○	○ (only public institutions)	○
Countermeasures against internal exposure	Examination of breast milk				○ (Prefecture)	
	Whole Body Counter measurements (conducted by municipalities)				○	○
	Whole Body Counter measurements (conducted by Fukushima Prefecture, targeting those age 4 to 18)			○	○	○
	Food and water quality inspection		○	○	○	○
	Thyroid gland examination (conducted by Fukushima Prefecture)			○	○	○
	Inspection of school meals		○	○	○	○
Others	Debriefing sessions for measurement results of exposure dose			○		○
	Study sessions on radiation		○	○	○	○
	Cancer screening		○ (provided as a usual health checkup)	○	○	○
	Replacement of the surface soil in rice paddies					
	Measurement of radiation dose in soil in the whole jurisdiction & creation of maps				○	
	Lecture meetings on radiation			○	○	○
	Sampling of respondents for a basic survey in the Fukushima Health Management Survey			○	○	○
	Publication of disaster information magazines			○		○
	Issuance of citizen health cards (containing a column for recording radiation exposure levels)					
	Other measures					

Name of municipality				Soma City	Tadami Town	Tanagura Town	Tamakawa Village
1 Situation of the municipality							
Population (persons) (upper part: as of January 1, 2011; lower part: as of January 1, 2013)				38,085 36,507	5,054 4,906	15,346 15,060	7,307 7,159
Ratio of the elderly aged 65 or older (%) (upper part: as of January 1, 2011; lower part: as of January 1, 2013)				25.05 26.12	40.48 41.72	24.8 Unknown	23.2 23.9
Total area (km²)				197.67	747.53	159.82	46.56
Distance from Fukushima Daiichi Nuclear Power Station of the Tokyo Electric Power Company (km)				42.94	151.9	73	Approximately 60
2 Situation of damage by the earthquake, tsunami and the nuclear power station accident							
Property damage	House	Completely destroyed		1,087 (as of February 29, 2012)		1 (as of February 12, 2013)	0 (as of October 31, 2013)
		Half destroyed		941 (″)		24 (″)	45 (″)
		Partially destroyed		3,556 (″)		594 (″)	654 (″)
	Public institution	Completely destroyed				1 (″)	0 (″)
		Half destroyed				1 (″)	0 (″)
		Partially destroyed					20 (″)
	Other	Completely destroyed					
		Half destroyed					
		Partially destroyed					
Human damage	Deaths by disaster			458 (as of February 12, 2013)			0 (as of October 31, 2013)
	Disaster-related deaths			21 (″)			0 (″)
	Missing persons						0 (″)
	Injured persons						3 (″)
Establishment of evacuation centers (total number)				23 (as of June 17, 2011)	2 (as of April 1, 2011)	2 (as of February 12, 2013)	3 (as of April 20, 2011)
Evacuees received (total number)				144,229 (as of June 17, 2011)	1,932 (as of August 1, 2011)	1,126 (as of February 12, 2013)	1,897 (as of April 20, 2011)
Establishment of temporary housing for residents and evacuees received (total number)				1,420 (as of January 31, 2013)			20 (as of October 31, 2013)
Approximate number of voluntary evacuees	Inside Fukushima Prefecture (number of people)			69 (as of October 12, 2011)		4 (as of February 12, 2013)	0 (as of October 31, 2013)
	Outside Fukushima Prefecture (number of people/ prefectures where people are evacuated)			929/34 (″)		19/7 (″)	27/5 (″)
3 Whole efforts							
Countermeasures against external exposure	Personal dose measurement			○	○	○	○
	Refreshment for expectant mothers (relaxation in low-dose areas)						
	Refreshment for young children						
	Refreshment for elementary school and junior high school students						
	Monitoring of air levels			○	○	○	○
	Real-time measurement of radiation dose (Ministry of the Environment)						○
	Measurement of air levels in the whole jurisdiction & creation of maps			○		○	○
	Replacement of the surface soil on the grounds in childcare facilities, child education facilities and schools			○		○	○
	Decontamination of houses			○			○
	Decontamination of public and medical institutions			○			○
Countermeasures against internal exposure	Examination of breast milk				○ (by institutions commissioned by the prefecture)		
	Whole Body Counter measurements (conducted by municipalities)			○			○
	Whole Body Counter measurements (conducted by Fukushima Prefecture, targeting those age 4 to 18)				○	○	○
	Food and water quality inspection			○	○	○	○
	Thyroid gland examination (conducted by Fukushima Prefecture)					Planned to be conducted in FY 2013	○
	Inspection of school meals			○	○		○
Others	Debriefing sessions for measurement results of exposure dose						
	Study sessions on radiation			○ (inviting lecturers; targeting children)			○
	Cancer screening			○	○		Screening for general residents
	Replacement of the surface soil in rice paddies						
	Measurement of radiation dose in soil in the whole jurisdiction & creation of maps						○
	Lecture meetings on radiation			○	○	○	○
	Sampling of respondents for a basic survey in the Fukushima Health Management Survey				○	○	○
	Publication of disaster information magazines						
	Issuance of citizen health cards (containing a column for recording radiation exposure levels)						
	Other measures			Individual consultation based on measurement results by personal dosimeters; special committee for health measures; city's public relations magazines (containing Q&A on radiation)			

420

Name of municipality			Tenei Village	Nakajima Village	Nishiaizu Town	Nishigo Village
1 Situation of the municipality						
Population (persons) (upper part: as of January 1, 2011; lower part: as of January 1, 2013)			6,480 6,265	5,257 5,216	7,764 7,464	19,791 19,949
Ratio of the elderly aged 65 or older (%) (upper part: as of January 1, 2011; lower part: as of January 1, 2013)			25.77 26.52	21.8 22.7	39.86 40.38	18.3 19.3
Total area (km²)			225.56	18.91	298.13	192.32
Distance from Fukushima Daiichi Nuclear Power Station of the Tokyo Electric Power Company (km)			70	68	Approximately 120	83.57
2 Situation of damage by the earthquake, tsunami and the nuclear power station accident						
Property damage	House	Completely destroyed	74 (as of March 13, 2013)	3 (as of October 15, 2013)		43 (as of January 31, 2013)
		Half destroyed	138 (″)	9 (″)		305 (″)
		Partially destroyed	1,560 (″)	954 (″)		1,975 (″)
	Public institution	Completely destroyed		0 (″)		8 (″)
		Half destroyed		0 (″)		3 (″)
		Partially destroyed	16 (″)	3 (″)		36 (″)
	Other	Completely destroyed		0 (″)		75 (″)
		Half destroyed		0 (″)		50 (″)
		Partially destroyed		3 (″)		143 (″)
Human damage	Deaths by disaster			0 (as of October 15, 2013)		3 (as of March 1, 2013)
	Disaster-related deaths			0 (″)		0 (″)
	Missing persons			0 (″)		0 (″)
	Injured persons		3 (as of March 13, 2013)	0 (″)		4 (″)
Establishment of evacuation centers (total number)			1 (as of July 31, 2011)	2 (as of October 15, 2013)	1 (as of May 12, 2011)	3 (as of March 1, 2013)
Evacuees received (total number)			2,364 (as of July 31, 2011)	132 (as of October 15, 2013)	2,408 (as of May 12, 2011)	31,349 (as of March 1, 2013)
Establishment of temporary housing for residents and evacuees received (total number)				13 (as of October 15, 2013)		42 (as of March 1, 2013)
Approximate number of voluntary evacuees	Inside Fukushima Prefecture (number of people)		1 (as of March 13, 2013)	40 (as of October 15, 2013)		0 (as of March 1, 2013)
	Outside Fukushima Prefecture (number of people/ prefectures where people are evacuated)		58/10 (″)	28/8 (″)		148/27 (″)
3 Whole efforts						
Countermeasures against external exposure	Personal dose measurement		○		○	○
	Refreshment for expectant mothers (relaxation in low-dose areas)					
	Refreshment for young children		○ (*Waiwai Hiroba* program implemented three times a week accompanied by nursery staff)			
	Refreshment for elementary school and junior high school students		○ (ski schools, etc.)			
	Monitoring of air levels		○	○	○	○
	Real-time measurement of radiation dose (Ministry of the Environment)		○	○	○	
	Measurement of air levels in the whole jurisdiction & creation of maps				○	○
	Replacement of the surface soil on the grounds in childcare facilities, child education facilities and schools		○	○	○	○
	Decontamination of houses		○	○		○
	Decontamination of public and medical institutions		○	○		○
Countermeasures against internal exposure	Examination of breast milk					
	Whole Body Counter measurements (conducted by municipalities)		○	○		
	Whole Body Counter measurements (conducted by Fukushima Prefecture, targeting those age 4 to 18)		○	○		○
	Food and water quality inspection		○	○	○	○
	Thyroid gland examination (conducted by Fukushima Prefecture)		○	○		○
	Inspection of school meals		○	○		○
Others	Debriefing sessions for measurement results of exposure dose		○			
	Study sessions on radiation		○	○		○
	Cancer screening		○	○		○
	Replacement of the surface soil in rice paddies					○
	Measurement of radiation dose in soil in the whole jurisdiction & creation of maps		○			○
	Lecture meetings on radiation		○	○		○
	Sampling of respondents for a basic survey in the Fukushima Health Management Survey		○	○		○
	Publication of disaster information magazines					
	Issuance of citizen health cards (containing a column for recording radiation exposure levels)		"*Kokoro to Karada no Sukoyaka File*" created independently by the village (distributed to those age 18 or younger)			○
	Other measures					

421

Name of municipality				Hanawa Town	Bandai Town	Hinoemata Village	Hirata Village
1 Situation of the municipality							
Population (persons) (upper part: as of January 1, 2011; lower part: as of January 1, 2013)				10,081 9,727	3,874 3,792	612 600	6,899 6,673
Ratio of the elderly aged 65 or older (%) (upper part: as of January 1, 2011; lower part: as of January 1, 2013)				29.8 30.2	29.99 30.22	34.4 34.3	25.3 26.1
Total area (km²)				211.60	59.69	390.50	93.53
Distance from Fukushima Daiichi Nuclear Power Station of the Tokyo Electric Power Company (km)				70	93.6	152	46.78
2 Situation of damage by the earthquake, tsunami and the nuclear power station accident							
Property damage	House		Completely destroyed	0 (as of October 31, 2013)	0 (as of November 13, 2013)		1 (as of October 15, 2013)
			Half destroyed	0 (″)	0 (″)		15 (″)
			Partially destroyed	247 (″)	405 (″)		418 (″)
	Public institution		Completely destroyed	0 (″)	0 (″)		0 (″)
			Half destroyed	0 (″)	0 (″)		0 (″)
			Partially destroyed	74 (″)	0 (″)		0 (″)
	Other		Completely destroyed	0 (″)	0 (″)		0 (″)
			Half destroyed	0 (″)	0 (″)		0 (″)
			Partially destroyed	80 (″)	16 (″)		23 (″)
Human damage	Deaths by disaster			0 (as of October 31, 2013)	0 (as of November 13, 2013)		0 (as of October 11, 2013)
	Disaster-related deaths			0 (″)	0 (″)		0 (″)
	Missing persons			0 (″)	0 (″)		0 (″)
	Injured persons			0 (″)	0 (″)		0 (″)
Establishment of evacuation centers (total number)				2 (as of October 31, 2013)	2 (as of November 13, 2013)		2 (as of October 11, 2013)
Evacuees received (total number)				1,624 (as of October 31, 2013)	404 (peak period) (as of May 18, 2011)		376 (as of April 12, 2011)
Establishment of temporary housing for residents and evacuees received (total number)				0 (as of October 31, 2013)	0 (as of November 13, 2013)		0 (as of October 11, 2013)
Approximate number of voluntary evacuees	Inside Fukushima Prefecture (number of people)			7 (as of October 31, 2013)	0 (as of November 13, 2013)		0 (as of October 11, 2013)
	Outside Fukushima Prefecture (number of people/ prefectures where people are evacuated)			9/3 (″)	0 (″)		24/7 (″)
3 Whole efforts							
Countermeasures against external exposure	Personal dose measurement			○		○ (conducted in FY 2011)	○
	Refreshment for expectant mothers (relaxation in low-dose areas)						
	Refreshment for young children			○			
	Refreshment for elementary school and junior high school students			○	○		
	Monitoring of air levels			○	○	○	○
	Real-time measurement of radiation dose (Ministry of the Environment)			○	○	○ (conducted from FY 2011)	○
	Measurement of air levels in the whole jurisdiction & creation of maps			○	○		
	Replacement of the surface soil on the grounds in childcare facilities, child education facilities and schools			○			○
	Decontamination of houses						
	Decontamination of public and medical institutions			Conducted only in kindergartens, elementary schools and junior high schools			○
Countermeasures against internal exposure	Examination of breast milk				○		
	Whole Body Counter measurements (conducted by municipalities)			○			
	Whole Body Counter measurements (conducted by Fukushima Prefecture, targeting those age 4 to 18)			○	○	Conducted in August 2013	○
	Food and water quality inspection			○	○		○
	Thyroid gland examination (conducted by Fukushima Prefecture)			○	○	Planned to be conducted in December 2013	○
	Inspection of school meals			○	○		○
Others	Debriefing sessions for measurement results of exposure dose						
	Study sessions on radiation			○			○
	Cancer screening			○		○ (screenings for breast cancer, uterine cancer, gastric cancer, colorectal cancer, lung cancer and prostate cancer conducted annually)	○
	Replacement of the surface soil in rice paddies						
	Measurement of radiation dose in soil in the whole jurisdiction & creation of maps						
	Lecture meetings on radiation			○	○		○
	Sampling of respondents for a basic survey in the Fukushima Health Management Survey				○	○	
	Publication of disaster information magazines						
	Issuance of citizen health cards (containing a column for recording radiation exposure levels)						
	Other measures						

		Name of municipality		Furudono Town	Mishima Town	Miharu Town	Minamiaizu Town
1 Situation of the municipality							
Population (persons) (upper part: as of January 1, 2011; lower part: as of January 1, 2013)				6,349 6,088	2,020 1,907	18,144 17,662	18,577 17,975
Ratio of the elderly aged 65 or older (%) (upper part: as of January 1, 2011; lower part: as of January 1, 2013)				30.1 30.7	46.24 47.51	26.2 27.7	34.7 34.9
Total area (km²)				163.47	90.83	72.76	886.52
Distance from Fukushima Daiichi Nuclear Power Station of the Tokyo Electric Power Company (km)				57	122	Approximately 45	114.3
2 Situation of damage by the earthquake, tsunami and the nuclear power station accident							
Property damage	House		Completely destroyed	0 (as of February 1, 2013)	0 (as of October 1, 2013)	32 (as of March 31, 2012)	0 (as of January 1, 2012)
			Half destroyed	28 (″)	0 (″)	236 (″)	0 (″)
			Partially destroyed	706 (″)	0 (″)	1,550 (″)	0 (″)
	Public institution		Completely destroyed	0 (″)	0 (″)	0 (″)	0 (″)
			Half destroyed	0 (″)	0 (″)	1 (″)	0 (″)
			Partially destroyed	8 (″)	0 (″)	22 (″)	0 (″)
	Other		Completely destroyed	0 (″)	0 (″)	84 (″)	0 (″)
			Half destroyed		0 (″)	251 (″)	0 (″)
			Partially destroyed		0 (″)	182 (″)	0 (″)
Human damage	Deaths by disaster			0 (as of February 1, 2013)	0 (as of October 1, 2013)	0 (as of January 18, 2012)	0 (as of January 1, 2012)
	Disaster-related deaths			0 (″)	0 (″)	1 (″)	0 (″)
	Missing persons			0 (″)	0 (″)	0 (″)	0 (″)
	Injured persons			0 (″)	0 (″)	2 (″)	0 (″)
Establishment of evacuation centers (total number)				2 (as of February 1, 2013)	1 (as of October 1, 2013)	16 (as of November 15, 2013)	36 (as of March 23, 2011)
Evacuees received (total number)				3,279 (as of February 1, 2013)	4 (as of October 1, 2013)	38,135 (as of September 1, 2011)	181 (as of January 1, 2012)
Establishment of temporary housing for residents and evacuees received (total number)				2 (as of February 1, 2013)	0 (as of October 1, 2013)	770 (as of November 15, 2013)	0 (as of January 1, 2012)
Approximate number of voluntary evacuees	Inside Fukushima Prefecture (number of people)			0 (as of February 1, 2013)	0 (as of October 1, 2013)	14 (as of November 15, 2013)	0 (as of January 1, 2012)
	Outside Fukushima Prefecture (number of people/ prefectures where people are evacuated)			11/4 (″)	0 (″)	103/Unknown (″)	0 (″)
3 Whole efforts							
Countermeasures against external exposure	Personal dose measurement			○	○	○	○
	Refreshment for expectant mothers (relaxation in low-dose areas)						
	Refreshment for young children						
	Refreshment for elementary school and junior high school students						
	Monitoring of air levels			○	○	○	
	Real-time measurement of radiation dose (Ministry of the Environment)			○	○	○	
	Measurement of air levels in the whole jurisdiction & creation of maps			○	○	○	
	Replacement of the surface soil on the grounds in childcare facilities, child education facilities and schools			○	○	○	
	Decontamination of houses					○	
	Decontamination of public and medical institutions			○		○	
Countermeasures against internal exposure	Examination of breast milk					○	
	Whole Body Counter measurements (conducted by municipalities)			○		○	
	Whole Body Counter measurements (conducted by Fukushima Prefecture, targeting those age 4 to 18)			○	○	○	○
	Food and water quality inspection			○	○	○	
	Thyroid gland examination (conducted by Fukushima Prefecture)					○	Planned to be conducted in FY 2013
	Inspection of school meals			○		○	○
Others	Debriefing sessions for measurement results of exposure dose					○	
	Study sessions on radiation				○	○	
	Cancer screening			○	○	○	
	Replacement of the surface soil in rice paddies						
	Measurement of radiation dose in soil in the whole jurisdiction & creation of maps				○	○	
	Lecture meetings on radiation			○	○	○	
	Sampling of respondents for a basic survey in the Fukushima Health Management Survey			○	○	○	
	Publication of disaster information magazines						
	Issuance of citizen health cards (containing a column for recording radiation exposure levels)						
	Other measures					*Misho* project conducted; measures for inhibiting absorption taken by spraying potassium fertilizers in paddy fields	

Name of municipality				Motomiya City	Yanaizu Town	Yabuki Town	Yamatsuri Town
1 Situation of the municipality							
Population (persons) (upper part: as of January 1, 2011; lower part: as of January 1, 2013)				31,761 / 31,166	4,135 / 3,927	18,167 / 18,036	6,570 / 6,403
Ratio of the elderly aged 65 or older (%) (upper part: as of January 1, 2011; lower part: as of January 1, 2013)				22.26 / 23.2	36.6 / 37.8	23.1 / 24.2	31.92 / 31.97
Total area (km²)				87.94	176.07	60.37	118.22
Distance from Fukushima Daiichi Nuclear Power Station of the Tokyo Electric Power Company (km)				57.4	116.5	66	80
2 Situation of damage by the earthquake, tsunami and the nuclear power station accident							
Property damage	House		Completely destroyed	16 (as of February 25, 2013)	0 (as of October 1, 2013)	294 (as of October 1, 2012)	0 (as of October 1, 2013)
			Half destroyed	220 (″)	0 (″)	1,586 (″)	73 (″)
			Partially destroyed	3,225 (″)	4 (″)	1,723 (″)	112 (″)
	Public institution		Completely destroyed	1 (″)	0 (″)	940 (″)	0 (″)
			Half destroyed	1 (″)	0 (″)		0 (″)
			Partially destroyed	11 (″)	0 (″)		0 (″)
	Other		Completely destroyed	79 (″)	0 (″)	269 (″)	0 (″)
			Half destroyed	145 (″)	0 (″)	432 (″)	0 (″)
			Partially destroyed	745 (″)	9 (″)	429 (″)	0 (″)
Human damage	Deaths by disaster			0 (as of March 6, 2013)	0 (as of October 1, 2013)		0 (as of October 1, 2013)
	Disaster-related deaths			0 (″)	0 (″)	1 (as of May 31, 2011)	0 (″)
	Missing persons			0 (″)	0 (″)		0 (″)
	Injured persons			0 (″)	0 (″)	7 (″)	0 (″)
Establishment of evacuation centers (total number)				18 (as of March 6, 2013)	2 (as of October 1, 2013)	10 (as of May 20, 2011)	1 (as of October 1, 2013)
Evacuees received (total number)				1,146 (as of January 29, 2013)	5,090 (as of October 1, 2013)	675 (as of May 20, 2011)	872 (as of October 1, 2013)
Establishment of temporary housing for residents and evacuees received (total number)				421 (as of February 14, 2013)	0 (as of October 1, 2013)	84 (as of January 18, 2012)	0 (as of October 1, 2013)
Approximate number of voluntary evacuees	Inside Fukushima Prefecture (number of people)			2 (as of March 6, 2013)	0 (as of October 1, 2013)		0 (as of October 1, 2013)
	Outside Fukushima Prefecture (number of people/ prefectures where people are evacuated)			116/14 (″)	0 (″)	Approximately 150/ throughout Japan (as of October 1, 2013)	0 (″)
3 Whole efforts							
Countermeasures against external exposure	Personal dose measurement			○	○	○	
	Refreshment for expectant mothers (relaxation in low-dose areas)						
	Refreshment for young children			○		○	
	Refreshment for elementary school and junior high school students			○			
	Monitoring of air levels				○	○	○
	Real-time measurement of radiation dose (Ministry of the Environment)			○	○	○	19 units
	Measurement of air levels in the whole jurisdiction & creation of maps			○	○ (only measurement)	○	
	Replacement of the surface soil on the grounds in childcare facilities, child education facilities and schools			○		○	
	Decontamination of houses			○		○	
	Decontamination of public and medical institutions			○	○ (partially conducted)	○	
Countermeasures against internal exposure	Examination of breast milk					Conducted by the prefecture	○
	Whole Body Counter measurements (conducted by municipalities)			○	Conducted in FY 2013	○	
	Whole Body Counter measurements (conducted by Fukushima Prefecture, targeting those age 4 to 18)			○	Conducted in FY 2013	○	○
	Food and water quality inspection			○	○	○	○
	Thyroid gland examination (conducted by Fukushima Prefecture)			○	Conducted in FY 2013	○	○
	Inspection of school meals			○	○	○	
Others	Debriefing sessions for measurement results of exposure dose						
	Study sessions on radiation			○		○	
	Cancer screening			○	○	○	○
	Replacement of the surface soil in rice paddies			Spraying potassium fertilizers		○	
	Measurement of radiation dose in soil in the whole jurisdiction & creation of maps					△ (partially conducted)	
	Lecture meetings on radiation			○	○	○	
	Sampling of respondents for a basic survey in the Fukushima Health Management Survey			○	○	○	○
	Publication of disaster information magazines			○	○ (town's public relations magazines)	○	
	Issuance of citizen health cards (containing a column for recording radiation exposure levels)					Issued by the prefecture	
	Other measures			Thyroid gland examination (conducted by the city)			

Name of municipality			Yugawa Village
1 Situation of the municipality			
Population (persons) (upper part: as of January 1, 2011; lower part: as of January 1, 2013)			3,548 3,421
Ratio of the elderly aged 65 or older (%) (upper part: as of January 1, 2011; lower part: as of January 1, 2013)			28.04 29.03
Total area (km²)			16.36
Distance from Fukushima Daiichi Nuclear Power Station of the Tokyo Electric Power Company (km)			103
2 Situation of damage by the earthquake, tsunami and the nuclear power station accident			
Property damage	House	Completely destroyed	0 (as of October 16, 2013)
		Half destroyed	3 (″)
		Partially destroyed	38 (″)
	Public institution	Completely destroyed	0 (″)
		Half destroyed	0 (″)
		Partially destroyed	0 (″)
	Other	Completely destroyed	0 (″)
		Half destroyed	0 (″)
		Partially destroyed	125 (″)
Human damage	Deaths by disaster		0 (as of October 16, 2013)
	Disaster-related deaths		0 (″)
	Missing persons		0 (″)
	Injured persons		
Establishment of evacuation centers (total number)			1 (as of October 16, 2013)
Evacuees received (total number)			207 (as of October 16, 2013)
Establishment of temporary housing for residents and evacuees received (total number)			0 (as of October 16, 2013)
Approximate number of voluntary evacuees	Inside Fukushima Prefecture (number of people)		0 (as of October 16, 2013)
	Outside Fukushima Prefecture (number of people/ prefectures where people are evacuated)		0 (″)
3 Whole efforts			
Countermeasures against external exposure	Personal dose measurement		○ (conducted by lending equipment to those who are interested)
	Refreshment for expectant mothers (relaxation in low-dose areas)		
	Refreshment for young children		
	Refreshment for elementary school and junior high school students		
	Monitoring of air levels		○
	Real-time measurement of radiation dose (Ministry of the Environment)		○
	Measurement of air levels in the whole jurisdiction & creation of maps		○ (only measurement)
	Replacement of the surface soil on the grounds in childcare facilities, child education facilities and schools		○
	Decontamination of houses		○
	Decontamination of public and medical institutions		○
Countermeasures against internal exposure	Examination of breast milk		
	Whole Body Counter measurements (conducted by municipalities)		
	Whole Body Counter measurements (conducted by Fukushima Prefecture, targeting those age 4 to 18)		
	Food and water quality inspection		○
	Thyroid gland examination (conducted by Fukushima Prefecture)		
	Inspection of school meals		○
Others	Debriefing sessions for measurement results of exposure dose		
	Study sessions on radiation		
	Cancer screening		○
	Replacement of the surface soil in rice paddies		
	Measurement of radiation dose in soil in the whole jurisdiction & creation of maps		○ (only measurement in the Shuraku Park)
	Lecture meetings on radiation		
	Sampling of respondents for a basic survey in the Fukushima Health Management Survey		
	Publication of disaster information magazines		
	Issuance of citizen health cards (containing a column for recording radiation exposure levels)		
	Other measures		

Index

A

A vague sense of anxiety   346
A vague sense of loss   346
abuse   141, 211
Act on Special Measures Concerning Nuclear Emergency Preparedness   27, 29, 46, 56, 200, 306, 401
activities   4, 16, 32, 34, 35, 36, 37, 38, 39, 40, 41, 42, 59, 60, 62, 63, 65, 67, 69, 70, 71, 72, 75, 76, 77, 78, 80, 82, 83, 84, 85, 87, 89, 92, 94, 96, 97, 98, 99, 100, 101, 102, 103, 105, 106, 107, 118, 119, 120, 123, 138, 142, 143, 144, 151, 154, 162, 163, 166, 171, 178, 179, 189, 190, 203, 204, 205, 206, 211, 214, 216, 226, 227, 228, 236, 238, 245, 247, 249, 251, 256, 257, 258, 259, 271, 272, 274, 275, 280, 281, 289, 291, 295, 298, 299, 303, 304, 306, 308, 310, 312, 314, 316, 318, 320, 322, 326, 328, 330, 334, 338, 340, 342, 344, 346, 350, 354, 356, 358, 360, 362, 364, 366, 368, 370, 372, 374, 376, 378, 382, 384, 386, 391, 394, 401, 403, 409, 410
activities of daily livings   269, 278
activity   138, 152, 154, 156, 189, 193, 196, 235, 269, 275, 279, 282, 298, 334, 336, 346, 360, 378, 397
Acupuncture   358, 360, 362
acupuncturists   116, 358
ADLs   269, 278
adult health study   19
aftershocks   36, 58, 146, 156, 268, 277, 279, 280, 362
Aging   382
AHS   19
aid station   42, 69, 116, 122, 304, 322
air dose rate   12, 15, 16, 30
Aizu-Wakamatsu City   138, 186, 294, 295
alcohol abuse   117, 122, 129, 243
alcohol dependence   117
alcohol dependency   141, 147
allergies   40, 133, 168, 288
ambulance   48, 50, 138, 140, 143
anger   49, 163, 171, 352
Animal Rescue Headquarters   63
apathy   164
artificial dialysis   15, 31, 46, 59, 75, 76, 89, 155, 170, 183, 184, 210, 211, 242, 281
artificial milk   15, 40, 119, 132, 140, 147, 153, 165, 179, 192, 206, 216, 218, 227, 248, 257, 272, 288, 298, 342, 408
Atomic bomb radiation   18
atomic bomb survivors   7, 19, 20, 21, 22, 23, 24
atomic bomb survivors exposed in utero   19, 22, 23, 24
atomic bombing   396, 398
attentively listen   153, 156, 177, 191, 197, 208, 240, 251, 293

B

baby food   140, 145, 147, 153, 154, 165, 166, 180, 192, 272, 273, 274, 288, 298, 342
baby massage programs   193
baby wipes   179, 180, 293
barrier-free   84
base center   41, 42, 65
Basic Resident Registration System   92
basic survey   7, 16, 37, 43, 44, 126, 139, 151, 161, 175, 187, 201, 215, 224, 233, 246, 255, 266, 287, 296, 376, 415, 416, 417, 418, 419, 420, 421, 422, 423, 424, 425
bathing service   123
beam   18, 19
Becquerel   3
bedridden elderly   209, 282, 364
behavior record   7, 16, 19, 30
beta ray burn   392
biological dose assessment system   394
biological effect ratio   19
Blog   141
breast milk   113, 145, 146, 154, 239, 257, 258, 265, 286, 288, 298, 370
breast-feeding   265
bullying   120, 141, 167, 168, 177

C

calumnies   141
care managers   250, 251, 338, 386
care prevention   129, 138, 144, 148, 156, 157, 159, 163, 169, 190, 211, 230, 340
care preventive   136, 182, 183
cause-and-effect relationship   21, 32
CBT   129
certificate   6, 48, 49, 69, 81, 98, 130, 143, 159, 209, 231, 324, 330
certificate of completion of screening   7
certificate of residence   130
certified health and athletic trainers   358
certified nursing-care recipients   279
certify the need for long-term care   97, 100
Chernobyl accident   17
Chernobyl Nuclear Plant accident   12, 15, 16, 23
child abuse   146
child health checkups   368, 370
child obesity   66
childcare workers   167, 181, 193, 194, 348, 350, 352, 354
child-rearing   146, 275, 277, 298
children with special needs   69
chromosomal abnormalities   22, 24
citizens' salons   60
Class Meeting   348, 352, 354
clinical psychotherapists   41, 55, 70, 72, 100, 103
cloud shine   28
clouds   86
clubs for elderly people   269

cognitive behavioral therapy 129
cognitive impairment 123, 164, 197
committed effective dose 3, 29
communication problems 261
communities 17, 94, 216, 220, 226, 251, 261, 279, 280, 308, 348, 354, 356, 358, 370, 384, 386, 396
community medicine 384, 386
community's resilience 271, 281
Compensation 308, 348
complaints 63, 141, 171, 177, 191, 225, 241, 256, 270, 275, 280, 293, 297, 334
complex disaster 3, 4, 12, 13, 58
comprehensive health check 44, 376, 378
comprehensive home visits 63
comprehensive livelihood consultations 281
comprehensive regional care system 87
conservative side 8
constipation 37, 162, 168, 225, 360
consultation 6, 11, 36, 37, 40, 41, 58, 59, 60, 63, 71, 72, 76, 78, 80, 85, 89, 90, 91, 92, 94, 98, 100, 102, 103, 105, 106, 113, 129, 131, 134, 145, 146, 184, 203, 214, 217, 219, 220, 221, 228, 240, 261, 276, 278, 280, 281, 299, 320, 326, 342, 352, 358, 366, 370, 378, 380, 410, 411, 420
contact for consultation 31
contact point for support workers 99
cooking practice 115, 342, 346
cooking program 128, 152, 164
COOP 179
cooperation agreement on disaster management 308, 310, 320
cooperation of the Japanese Consumer Co-operative Union 179
coordinating function 82
core city 58
correct knowledge 10, 121, 145
Council of Developmental Support Center 97, 100, 101
Council on Linkages between Academia and Public Health Practice 372
counseling 116, 117, 120, 134, 138, 141, 142, 144, 145, 146, 151, 152, 153, 154, 155, 156, 157, 164, 165, 167, 169, 170, 172, 177, 194, 203, 204, 224, 228, 234, 236, 237, 241, 248, 256, 257, 260, 265, 266, 268, 270, 271, 272, 273, 275, 280, 281, 292, 297, 299, 318, 338, 352
counts per minute 3
county and city dental associations 308, 312
county and city medical associations 303, 304, 306, 312, 330
crisis communication 82, 86
crisis management staff members 27
CT scan 7
cysts 378

D

daily exercise 340
Date City XXI, 68, 70, 72, 253, 254, 256, 258, 350, 376
day care services 101, 251
day-care programs 136
debriefing 234, 255, 352, 380
Decentralization 382
decision-making system 291
decontamination 6, 10, 13, 15, 32, 48, 49, 61, 64, 86, 92, 93, 98, 112, 113, 138, 150, 151, 154, 161, 174, 187, 200, 201, 204, 206, 207, 214, 215, 221, 224, 233, 245, 248, 249, 254, 258, 260, 261, 262, 265, 274, 285, 286, 289, 295, 296, 308, 322, 324, 326, 328, 368, 374, 391, 393, 403, 406, 408, 415, 416, 417, 418, 419, 420, 421, 422, 423, 424, 425
dedicated social worker 250
deep vein thrombosis/pulmonary embolism 116, 128, 152, 203, 256, 299
dementia 334
Dental and oral health support 60
dental consultation 85, 310, 314
dental health guidance 71, 310, 312
dental hygienists 60, 72, 80, 167, 188, 308, 312, 318, 320
Dental Hygienists' Association 38, 179
dental procedures 310, 312
dental relief activities 308, 310, 312
dentures 184, 188, 189, 195, 196, 310, 312
depression 129, 141, 156, 257, 348, 380
detailed surveys 43, 44, 376
deterministic effect 18, 21
developing human resource 398
development of human resources 298, 398
developmentally disabled children 122, 133, 134
developmentally disabled children/persons 122
DHEAT 82, 86
dietary environment 40, 114, 166, 225, 342, 344
dietary supplements 60, 229
Dietetic Association 38
dietitians 34, 38, 40, 60, 72, 76, 77, 80, 89, 90, 106, 167, 256
digital dose meters 64
Disaster Countermeasures Basic Act 35, 401
disaster damage certificates 92
Disaster Health Care Agreement 306
Disaster Health Emergency Assistance Team 82
disaster information magazines 113, 126, 134, 139, 151, 161, 215, 224, 245, 246, 255, 266, 288, 291, 415, 416, 417, 418, 419, 420, 421, 422, 423, 424, 425
Disaster Medical Assistance Team 13, 27, 42, 60, 80, 191, 304
disaster mitigation measures 87
disaster nursing 318, 320
disaster prevention guide for households 282
Disaster Psychiatric Assistance Team 82

428

Disaster Public health Assistance Team   82, 86
Disaster Relief Act   27, 51, 84, 223, 226, 230, 231, 364
disaster relief nurses   314, 316, 318, 320
disaster response manual   128, 230, 314, 336
Disaster Simulation   56
disaster stress   318
disaster victim certificates   92
disaster volunteer centers   356
disaster-affected animals   80
Disaster-affected pet protection activities   97, 98, 100, 102, 103
disaster-related death   14, 58, 111, 304, 306, 328, 348, 384, 407
discrimination   7, 48, 49, 164, 324
dispatched healthcare teams   34, 38, 39
dispensing information   86
disposable diapers   119, 133, 140, 147, 154, 165, 179, 180, 192, 206, 250, 257, 258, 261, 272, 273, 274, 281, 282, 288, 293, 298
dissatisfaction   163, 171, 241
district centers   42, 65
distrust   259, 264, 271, 272, 293, 370, 410
disuse syndrome   77, 128, 133, 152, 160, 163, 168, 169, 176, 219, 334, 338, 340, 380
DMAT   14, 27, 28, 32, 42, 60, 80, 86, 191, 194, 198, 304, 306
DOE   23
dose-response relationship   19, 20, 21, 24
DPAT   82, 86
drinking   13, 15, 27, 43, 64, 85, 87, 89, 96, 98, 99, 101, 102, 103, 106, 107, 164, 165, 188, 191, 192, 195, 206, 219, 262, 298, 366, 378
drug diary   163, 170, 184
dyslipidemia   216

E

early detection   134, 207, 274, 378
early treatment   378
easy-to-take food   182
economy-class syndrome   116, 128, 152, 155, 203, 256, 269, 277, 278, 279, 299
educational curriculum   86
educational research institutions   374
effective dose   3, 9, 16, 376
effective exposed dose   10
elder people   127
electric beds   282
electric fans   299
electronic integrating dose meters   93
e-mail   316, 336, 380
emergency evacuation-ready zone   14, 49, 53, 99
emergency exposure screening   42, 60, 81, 86
emergency food   121, 122, 168, 178, 180, 182, 186, 202, 235, 272, 273, 277, 288
emergency medical system   90, 306
emergency medical transport vehicles   330
emergency medical treatment   4, 5, 7, 13, 251, 295,

392
emergency monitoring   43, 306
Emergency night clinics   281
Emergency Response Headquarters   4, 13, 36, 40, 45, 46, 50, 51, 52, 53, 57, 68, 74, 79, 82, 85, 88, 89, 95, 96, 104
Emergency Room   392
EMIS   87
empowering   350
environmental behavior   16
environmental health officers   80
Environmental Radiation   394
epidemiological surveys   7, 23
equivalent dose   3, 15, 16, 306
ER   392
Estimated external exposure levels   376
evacuation order   XX, 12, 28, 34, 36, 46, 69, 75, 111, 112, 118, 124, 137, 138, 140, 149, 150, 158, 160, 165, 174, 185, 200, 219, 221, 230, 232, 245, 259, 271, 285, 289, 314, 324, 346, 362, 393, 395, 407
evacuation order zones   14
event volunteers   270
evidence   17, 324, 372, 410
Examination of breast milk   113, 121, 125, 138, 161, 174, 214, 286, 415, 416, 417, 418, 419, 420, 421, 422, 423, 424, 425
exchange salons   37, 102, 103
excrement   183
exercise instructions   169, 190, 239
exercise instructors   90, 247, 249, 251, 257
expectant and nursing mothers   64, 227, 228, 229, 378, 380
external exposed dose   7, 8, 10, 16
external exposure   16, 19, 28, 30, 31, 44, 75, 89, 92, 94, 105, 107, 112, 150, 160, 174, 187, 214, 228, 233, 240, 245, 249, 254, 255, 259, 261, 264, 275, 282, 285, 328, 332, 376, 415, 416, 417, 418, 419, 420, 421, 422, 423, 424, 425
external radiation exposure   7
externally-contaminated evacuated resident   393

F

face-to-face relationship   382
facilitators   350
FETP   90
Field Epidemiology Training Program   90
firefighters   162, 394
flavoring agents   332
follow-up study   19, 22, 23
food allergy friendly foods   342
food chain   16
food poisoning   78, 81, 101, 155, 202, 235, 342
Food Sanitation Act   29
food sanitation inspectors   80
food stocks   122, 168, 176, 188, 189, 192, 235
free comments   380

Fukushima Acupuncture and Moxibustion Association 358

Fukushima Association of Medical Social Workers 362, 364

Fukushima Association of Occupational Therapists 100, 336, 338, 340, 364

Fukushima Center for Disaster Mental Health 41, 65, 72, 103, 107, 117, 120, 220, 270, 276, 378

Fukushima City XXI, 12, 43, 55, 68, 180, 186, 196, 217, 263, 264, 265, 268, 271, 272, 273, 276, 277, 278, 281, 282, 283, 304, 306, 322, 336, 350, 356, 368, 372

Fukushima Dental Association 308, 314

Fukushima Dietetic Association 38, 40, 90, 342

Fukushima Disaster Medical Support Network 96

Fukushima Disaster Volunteer Center 356

Fukushima Disaster Volunteer Liaison Council 356

Fukushima Emergency Exposure Medical Activities Manual 98

Fukushima health management survey XXI, 16, 30, 31, 37, 43, 44, 87, 94, 99, 113, 126, 139, 143, 151, 161, 175, 187, 201, 215, 224, 233, 234, 246, 255, 266, 287, 296, 372, 374, 376, 380, 394, 403, 415, 416, 417, 418, 419, 420, 421, 422, 423, 424, 425

Fukushima Medical Association 54, 303, 308

Fukushima Medical University XX, XXI, 13, 15, 16, 30, 36, 38, 41, 51, 54, 60, 97, 116, 143, 144, 164, 167, 183, 184, 204, 231, 306, 330, 332, 368, 370, 374, 376, 380, 392, 393, 401, 409, 411

Fukushima Mental Health and Welfare Centre 54, 354

Fukushima Nursing Association 38, 40, 314, 316, 318, 320

Fukushima Nutrition Support Team 342

Fukushima office of the Japan Health Insurance Association 36, 38

Fukushima Pharmacists Association 134, 328, 332

Fukushima Physical Therapy Association 100, 334, 336, 338, 340, 364

Fukushima Prefecture Council for Promotion of Diet Improvement 40

Fukushima Preservative Service Association of Health 36, 38, 116

Fukushima Professional Team for Counseling and Support 336, 362, 364, 366

Fukushima resident health management file 44

Fukushima Society of Certified Clinical Psychologists 346, 352, 354

Fukushima University XXI, 374, 397, 398

Fukushima Ward Council on Social Welfare 356, 366

Fukushimaken Association of Radiological Technologist 96, 322, 324, 326

Futaba Town XXI, 7, 45, 54, 71, 85, 124, 127, 128, 129, 130, 131, 132, 133, 134, 136, 328, 350, 376, 404, 406

G

gambling 366

gatekeepers 226

genetic effects 18, 22, 23, 24

genetic influence 7, 370

germanium semiconductor detector 43, 64

glass badge 16, 44, 64, 121, 138, 146, 154, 160, 167, 174, 187, 208, 228, 240, 249, 250, 254, 259, 262, 264, 282, 285, 289, 291, 298, 368, 380

governor of Fukushima Prefecture 51, 303, 304, 394

governor of Nagasaki Prefecture 51

gray 3, 19

Great Hanshin-Awaji Earthquake 271, 334, 338, 364, 370

grief care 346

ground shine 28

group activities 72, 225

group and individual nutritional guidance 342, 346

group home 170

group medical examinations 116, 144

Gy 3, 19, 20, 21, 22, 322

H

half-life 4, 6, 16, 31, 43

Headquarters for Emergency Disaster Control of the government 27

health 3, 5, 6, 7, 10, 13, 16, 17, 18, 19, 20, 21, 22, 23, 27, 29, 30, 31, 32, 34, 35, 36, 37, 38, 39, 40, 42, 43, 44, 56, 59, 60, 62, 63, 64, 65, 66, 67, 71, 72, 75, 77, 78, 80, 82, 83, 85, 86, 87, 89, 90, 91, 92, 93, 94, 96, 97, 98, 100, 102, 103, 105, 106, 107, 112, 113, 116, 117, 122, 123, 126, 127, 129, 131, 132, 133, 134, 135, 136, 138, 141, 142, 144, 146, 154, 157, 158, 159, 160, 161, 162, 163, 164, 168, 169, 171, 172, 173, 175, 177, 178, 180, 181, 183, 186, 189, 191, 194, 195, 196, 197, 198, 204, 205, 207, 208, 210, 211, 212, 214, 215, 216, 217, 218, 219, 220, 221, 224, 225, 226, 227, 228, 230, 231, 234, 236, 237, 238, 239, 240, 241, 242, 246, 247, 248, 250, 251, 254, 256, 257, 261, 262, 264, 266, 267, 268, 269, 270, 271, 272, 273, 275, 276, 277, 278, 279, 280, 281, 282, 287, 289, 292, 297, 299, 303, 304, 306, 308, 310, 312, 314, 318, 320, 322, 324, 328, 330, 332, 334, 336, 338, 340, 342, 344, 346, 348, 350, 352, 354, 358, 362, 366, 368, 370, 372, 374, 376, 378, 380, 382, 384, 386, 393, 394, 396, 401, 402, 403, 404, 405, 407, 408, 409, 411, 415, 416, 417, 418, 419, 420, 421, 422, 423, 424, 425

health care 38, 39, 47, 48, 100, 116, 117, 122, 129, 130, 131, 132, 133, 134, 136, 142, 143, 146, 148, 153, 154, 156, 165, 167, 169, 170, 172, 177, 178, 181, 182, 191, 194, 198, 203, 204, 217, 220, 234, 236, 241, 250, 260, 262,

264, 276, 277, 291, 292, 293, 296, 297, 298, 299, 316, 318, 332, 348, 352, 354, 358, 360, 376, 378, 380, 393, 397, 407
health center 36, 227, 237, 241, 249, 323, 350
health checkups for the elderly (age 75 years or older) 378
health consultation Yorozu 380, 382, 384, 386
health consultations 6, 16, 39, 60, 69, 70, 76, 77, 82, 100, 102, 276, 320
health counseling 237
health festival 268
Health Fund for Childeren and Adults Affected by the Nuclear Incident 31
Health insurance pharmacies 332, 334
health management advisers 157
health management information of affected people 82, 86
health promotion plans 272
health risk management 48, 396
health salon 37, 77, 78
Health Support Program for Affected People 40
health support project 37, 38, 77
health support teams 76, 82, 86
health survey 39, 77, 129, 138, 141, 142, 230, 234
healthcare teams 34, 35, 37, 38, 39, 41, 54, 80, 81, 82, 85, 90
helplessness 141, 142, 153
Higashi Nippon International University 374
high density liquid diet 40
high risk 115, 116, 142, 177, 203, 211, 320, 334, 384
high-dose-rate exposure 18
Hirono Town 7, 45, 54, 75, 199, 202, 203, 204, 205, 206, 207, 208, 210, 211, 212, 306, 328, 376, 406
Hiroshima University 48, 374, 391, 392, 393, 394, 398
home oxygen therapy 242
homebound 78, 128, 196, 197, 229, 236, 257, 276, 340
home-care helpers 386
human dignity 366
human rights 362
hydrated lime 63
hydrogen explosions 4, 50, 59
hyperactive children 120
hypothesis 18

I

IAEA 6, 10, 398
ICRP 11, 15, 23, 398
ICT 374
identification 133, 200, 234, 316
identity 308, 348, 403
Iitate Village XX, XXI, 8, 29, 30, 37, 45, 71, 72, 213, 214, 215, 216, 304, 328, 376, 378, 380, 382, 384, 386, 393
incidence 15, 24, 332, 334

Inclusive and Comprehensive Research Cooperation Agreement 393
individual consultation 106, 228, 368
individual medical examination 116
indoor evacuation order XX, 15, 28, 69, 189, 193, 196, 241, 304
indoor playing spaces 206, 249, 258, 259, 265, 274, 275
inequality 164, 202
INES 12, 46
infection observation room 316
infection prevention measures 76
Infectious Disease Surveillance Center of the National Institute of Infectious Diseases 62
infectious disease surveillance system in shelters 62
infectious gastroenteritis 41, 76, 83, 89, 90, 91, 211
influenza 76, 91, 121, 188, 195, 197
Information and Communication Technology 374
information disclosure 82, 86
initial exposure 66, 175
initial health care 13
insomnia 141, 156, 170, 360
instant experts 62
instant noodles 115, 135, 140, 188
insulin 183, 184
Integrating dose meters 92
integration 54, 87, 91, 136
internal exposed dose 8, 9, 15, 16
Internal exposure 19, 64, 282
International Atomic Energy Agency 6, 398
International Commission on Radiological Protection 11, 15, 23, 398
International Nuclear Event Scale 12, 46
intractable disease 69
iodine preparations 303, 306, 308, 330, 332, 405, 406
island medicine 384
Isodine gargle solution 332
Isodine solution 332
isolation 226, 230, 356, 358, 366
Iwaki City Public Health Center 57, 58, 61, 62, 65, 322
Iwaki Meisei University 374

J

JAEA 8
Japan Agricultural Cooperative 269
Japan Association of Obstetricians and Gynecologists 380
Japan Association of Operational Therapists 340
Japan Association of Radiological Technologists 322, 324, 326, 328, 406
Japan Atomic Energy Agency 8
Japan Committee for UNICEF 350, 354
Japan Dietetic Association 229, 342
Japan Health Insurance Association 90
Japan Medical Association 303, 304, 306, 308, 372
Japan Medical Association Team 41, 59, 80, 282,

303

Japan Society of Obstetrics and Gynecology 380

Japanese Nursing Association 38, 130, 131, 143, 314, 316, 401

Japanese Psychiatric Nurses Association 38

Japanese Red Cross Society 69, 96, 178, 256, 306

Japanese traditional massage 360

JCO criticality incident 306

JMAT 41, 59, 60, 62, 80, 282, 303, 304, 306, 308

JOC criticality accident at Tokai-mura 61

judo healing therapists 358

Judo therapists 72

K

Katsurao Village 8, 37, 45, 77, 96, 99, 185, 188, 189, 190, 192, 193, 194, 195, 196, 197, 328, 350, 376, 406

Kawamata Town XXI, 30, 68, 70, 127, 131, 134, 135, 244, 249, 284, 304, 322, 332, 376

Kawauchi Village XXI, 7, 45, 75, 92, 112, 114, 115, 116, 117, 118, 119, 122, 149, 150, 153, 156, 190, 328, 354, 356, 376, 406

Kazo City 42, 127, 129, 131, 132, 133, 134, 135, 136

Koriyama City Public Health Center 88, 324

L

late health effects 19

lavatories 62, 76, 86

leaflet 40, 266, 368, 370

learning centers 269, 270, 279, 280

Lecture meetings 126, 152, 153, 154, 155, 156, 157, 161, 201, 204, 215, 223, 246, 255, 259, 266, 273, 278, 286, 415, 416, 417, 418, 419, 420, 421, 422, 423, 424, 425

leukemia 20, 21, 22, 23, 24

liaison 97, 98, 99, 116, 128, 165, 171, 172, 356, 380, 384, 403

Liaison Conference 72, 83, 85

liaison meetings 72, 102, 103

life function 39, 77

life inactive diseases 77

life recovery volunteer centers 356

life span study 19

life support counselors 78

lifestyle-related diseases 23, 39, 40, 66, 216, 256, 264, 272, 283, 378, 381, 384

linear non-threshold 18

liquid foods 168, 182, 260

list of indoor play spaces 93

list of residents requiring special health care 131

livelihood reconstruction 107

livelihood support counselors 131, 143, 144, 164, 165, 171, 172, 220, 248

living alone 52, 122, 123, 127, 136, 147, 164, 219, 229, 243, 251, 252, 348, 382, 407

living support counselors 102, 103

LNT 18

local disaster management plan 87

local firefighting team 118

local Nuclear Emergency Response Headquarters of the government 43

local wireless radio 118, 122, 159, 186, 237, 240

logistics 330

loneliness 236, 243, 270, 280, 356, 358

long-term care facilities 13, 14

low dose exposure 16, 18, 30, 66

low dose radiation 64, 394

low-dose-rate exposure 18

LSS 19

M

makeshift beds 105, 169, 408

manuals 31, 312, 318, 322, 346, 402

mass media 53, 86, 132, 160, 223, 264, 290, 299, 410

mass outbreaks 83

massagers 116

maternal and child health handbook 93, 380

maternal and child health system 372

matter implicitly agreed upon 53

MCA radio systems 86

meaningful life 17

medical associations 90, 231, 242, 299, 303, 304, 320, 370

medical care team 36, 39, 41, 42, 51, 75, 205

medical coordinator 312

medical records 86

Medical relief activities 96, 98, 99, 101

medical support registration form 96, 98

medical support teams 76, 85, 360

medicine notebook 51, 54

medium- to long- term dispatch 35

meltdown 328, 410

mental disabilities 122, 133, 170, 183, 184, 261

mental health and lifestyle survey 44, 376, 378

mental health checklist 129

Mental health support 100

mental healthcare team 39, 41, 60, 76, 80, 81, 97, 102, 103, 105, 106

mental retardation 22, 170

MEXT 391, 394, 397

midwives 120, 239, 276, 314, 318, 348, 354, 380

Midwives' Association 90

Minamisoma City XXI, 7, 42, 45, 48, 49, 50, 51, 52, 53, 54, 70, 222, 224, 230, 303, 304, 306, 316, 322, 326, 340, 356, 376, 382, 386, 395, 397, 406

Ministry of Education, Culture, Sports, Science and Technology 30, 42, 150, 240, 264, 289, 290, 326, 374, 391, 397, 415

Ministry of Health, Labour and Welfare 6, 11, 23, 27, 28, 29, 34, 35, 36, 38, 39, 40, 42, 50, 66, 81, 97, 296, 324, 334, 403

Ministry of Health, Labour and Welfare's Support Cen-

ter to Secure Health Workers   54, 56
mischief   141
Monitoring   43, 65, 85, 96, 98, 99, 101, 102, 103,
    112, 113, 125, 138, 150, 160, 174, 187, 200,
    201, 214, 223, 224, 233, 240, 245, 254, 264,
    265, 285, 295, 296, 394, 415, 416, 417, 418,
    419, 420, 421, 422, 423, 424, 425
monitoring mechanism   32
monitoring posts   112, 154, 189, 193, 196, 204,
    240, 259, 264, 289, 290
motor ability   334, 336
motor system diseases   334
moxibustion   358, 360, 362
moxibustionists   358
Municipal Councils on Social Welfare   356
music therapy   153, 156
mutation   22
mutual aid agreement   86
mutual cooperation agreement on disaster prevention
    and disaster relief   159, 176, 190, 193, 197

N

Nagasaki University   51, 223, 230, 268, 308, 374,
    394, 398
Nagasakiken Medical Association   51, 230
Nagomi   55
Namie Town   XXI, 8, 30, 45, 70, 71, 72, 83, 84,
    173, 174, 175, 180, 183, 284, 285, 304, 326,
    328, 350, 356, 376, 406
Naraha Town   7, 45, 96, 99, 101, 158, 159, 163,
    164, 167, 171, 172, 328, 376, 406
National Health Insurance Fujisawa Municipal Hospi-
    tal   386
National Hospital Organization Disaster Medical Cen-
    ter   380, 386
National Institute of Infectious Diseases   41, 81, 90
National Institute of Radiological Sciences   XX, 5, 11,
    30, 44, 47, 217, 241, 332, 374, 376, 393, 398
nationally registered dietitians   40
neighborhood associations   216, 269, 281
Neighborhood community   78
new born infants   69
newsletter   258, 261, 266, 268, 271, 278
newspaper magazine   221
night school courses   386
Nihon University   374
Nihonmatsu City   XXI, 68, 69, 174, 180, 181, 284,
    285, 287, 288, 289, 290, 291, 292, 304, 322,
    350, 356
Niigata Prefecture Chuetsu Earthquake   271
NIRS   5, 7, 8, 11, 17, 30, 31, 47, 48, 393
NMAT   86
nodules   378
non-profit corporations   374
nonprofit organizations   176, 182
norovirus   89, 90, 91, 138, 140, 145, 188, 190,
    193, 195, 196, 211, 316
NPO corporations   374

NPOs   176, 182
nuclear disaster drills   205, 285, 306, 332
Nuclear Disaster Medical Assistance Team   86
nuclear emergency response advisors   92
nuclear emergency response drills   47
Nuclear Emergency Response Headquarters   4, 13,
    27, 28, 29, 30, 43, 47, 87, 214, 324
nuclear emergency situation   46, 56, 200, 401
nuclear emergency situation declaration   12, 27
nurse bank   318, 320
nurse-teachers   119, 120, 354
nutrition assessment   40
nutritional and dietary support   342, 346
nutritional assessment   342

O

obesity   114, 119, 128, 216, 249, 272, 346
object-loss reaction   346
obstetrics and perinatal medicine   380
OFC   4, 5, 12, 42, 43, 47, 48, 205, 306, 322
official register   123, 157, 178, 179
off-site center   4, 12, 42, 47
Ohu University   308, 374
Okidozen Hospital   384
Okuma Town   4, 5, 7, 12, 45, 54, 75, 76, 96, 99,
    137, 138, 141, 142, 143, 144, 146, 147, 205,
    328, 356, 376, 405
on-site learning experience   397
oral care   310, 312
Original Indoor Evacuation Zone   49
outbreak   41, 60, 62, 76, 89, 90, 91, 235, 342
outreach project   55
overestimation   10
overwork   171, 240, 360

P

paper-based patient information   364
Parent and child exchange meetings   102
Parent Meeting   348, 350, 354
Parent-and-child Play   348, 350, 354
Parenting   372
partnership   179, 372
pediatric thyroid cancer   378
peer meetings   350
people who need support   31, 84
people who needed support   13, 28, 36, 37, 72, 78,
    80, 83
personal dose meter   16, 44, 64
Personal dosimeters   146, 154, 187
personal health care services   130
personal information   82, 86, 262, 362
personal services   143
Persons requiring assistance during a disaster   147
Pet Protection Center   63
pets   63, 64, 97, 98, 99, 100, 107, 163, 324
PFA   346
pharmaceutical associations   90

Pharmaceutical product supply activities   97, 98
Pharmacists   66, 98, 157, 330, 332
Phoenix Leader Education Program (Hiroshima Initiative) for Renaissance from Radiation Disaster   391, 396, 397
physical fitness tests   163
physical inactivity diseases   128, 152, 163, 168, 176
physical therapists   72, 128, 182, 190, 304, 336, 354
planned evacuation zone   14, 28, 37, 44, 70, 99, 185
play outdoors   66, 119, 120, 121, 145, 154, 166, 180, 193, 194, 206, 249, 274, 289, 354
pneumococcal vaccinations   197
pneumonia   21, 162, 168
population aging rate   45, 57, 68, 74, 79, 88, 95, 104, 382
postmortem examination   13, 326, 374, 408
post-traumatic stress disorder   129
power milk   40
Prefectural Radiation Health Risk Management Advisor   394
pregnancy and birth survey   44, 376, 378
prejudice   49
prescription records   330, 332, 334
primary prevention   380, 382, 384, 386
primary shelters   34, 40, 41, 70, 77, 80, 81, 82, 85, 96, 97, 99, 105, 106
Prime Minister   28, 29, 48, 174, 308, 392, 401
priority telephone links in disasters   86
privacy   123, 141, 147, 162, 177, 190, 193, 236
private power generator   46
probabilistic effects   18, 19
professional autonomy   304
projected dose   50
prosthetists   338
protection program institution for residents   322
protective clothing   161, 168
Provision of information   11, 32
provisional regulation values   13, 29
psychiatric social workers   55, 70, 72, 90, 100, 167, 336, 364
Psychological First Aid   346, 354
psychosocial crisis   348
PTSD   129, 178, 346, 352, 354
public employment security offices   318
public health   16, 17, 34, 38, 51, 58, 67, 75, 77, 81, 82, 86, 87, 91, 94, 115, 122, 134, 136, 138, 141, 142, 177, 183, 227, 236, 271, 278, 281, 282, 292, 299, 318, 330, 342, 370, 372, 380, 386, 401, 402, 403, 404, 405, 408, 409, 411
public health center   6, 34, 35, 36, 37, 38, 39, 40, 41, 42, 44, 46, 47, 48, 49, 50, 51, 52, 53, 54, 55, 56, 58, 59, 60, 61, 63, 64, 67, 69, 70, 72, 73, 76, 77, 80, 81, 82, 83, 84, 85, 86, 87, 89, 90, 91, 92, 94, 96, 97, 100, 102, 105, 134, 203, 210, 227, 230, 231, 298, 316, 322, 330, 404, 406, 411
public health nurses   16, 29, 34, 35, 36, 37, 38, 39, 40, 41, 46, 51, 54, 60, 63, 64, 69, 70, 72, 76,
77, 80, 87, 89, 91, 101, 105, 106, 107, 115, 116, 117, 120, 130, 131, 134, 135, 142, 147, 165, 167, 171, 173, 177, 181, 183, 190, 191, 196, 197, 207, 229, 237, 243, 271, 281, 299, 304, 314, 316, 318, 320, 338, 348, 354, 368, 370, 372, 378, 380, 382, 384, 386, 401, 402, 409
public health team   75
public relations magazines   125, 128, 134, 161, 187, 216, 226, 235, 242, 247, 248, 378, 416, 420, 424
pulmonary deep vein thrombosis/thromboembolism   168, 269, 278

R

radiation and health advisory group   44
radiation cataracts   21
Radiation Disaster Recovery Studies   398
Radiation Effects Research Foundation   20, 23, 398
Radiation Emergency Medical Assistance Team   82, 391
radiation emergency medicine   10, 326, 380, 391, 406
Radiation Health Management Center   64, 94
Radiation Medical Science Center for the Fukushima Health Management Survey   374, 376, 409, 411
radiation meters   163, 165, 172
radiation pharmacists   330
radiation protection   13, 18, 326
Radiation Protection Fundamental Information Portal Site   394
radiation workers   376, 416
radio gymnastic exercises   128, 169, 176, 203, 256, 338
radioactive cloud   12, 332
radioactive fallout   18, 19
radioactive plume   12, 274, 275, 332
raw milk   XX, 15, 29
RDRS   398
ready-prepared dishes   162
recommendations   368
reconstruction of lives   366
reconstruction plans   221
recreation   72, 82, 83, 85, 338, 340
regional development   216, 226, 271, 336, 374
regional disaster prevention plan   282
regional mutual assistance center   195
region-wide collaboration   271
register of evacuees   157
registry system   293
regular medicines   178, 189, 196, 197, 198, 242
Rehabilitation   336
rehabilitation facilities for children   101
relationship   21, 23, 30, 91, 129, 134, 136, 140, 160, 164, 177, 179, 180, 205, 208, 210, 226, 236, 251, 260, 261, 273, 276, 281, 282, 292, 350, 358, 362, 370, 372, 382, 384, 391, 409
relaxation   85, 102, 214, 264, 285, 350, 352, 415,

416, 417, 418, 419, 420, 421, 422, 423, 424, 425

REM 391, 392, 394, 396

REMAT 82, 86, 391, 392, 393

rendered radioactive 18

rental houses 37, 38, 39, 40, 62, 63, 66, 67, 71, 72, 77, 78, 82, 83, 85, 101, 102, 103, 106, 107

Research Institute of Radiation Biology and Medicine 396

resentment 143, 163, 171, 240, 241

residents on welfare 219

residents' association 130, 216, 220

residual radiation 18, 19

resilience 281, 350

response rate 376

restoration vision 238

retired public health nurse 90

returnees 150, 152, 160, 233, 236

revised screening level 393

revitalize regions 336

risk communication 82, 86, 215, 221, 394, 410

road maps 384

rumors 59, 132, 140, 141, 143, 146, 147, 254, 257, 264, 316, 328, 342, 346, 374, 394, 401

S

safe side 8

salon 99, 117, 122, 128, 131, 138, 142, 144, 145, 157, 164, 234, 236, 237, 252

Salt intake 346

sanitary management 34, 38, 62, 97

satellite phone systems 86

School bus 120

school counselors 207, 352

school lunch centers 206

school pharmacists 332

Science Council of Japan 374

screening 6, 10, 13, 15, 17, 29, 32, 34, 36, 42, 43, 46, 48, 49, 50, 56, 60, 61, 69, 75, 81, 82, 83, 84, 85, 86, 89, 92, 96, 98, 99, 101, 103, 105, 107, 113, 115, 126, 139, 140, 143, 151, 152, 159, 161, 164, 175, 186, 187, 189, 193, 196, 215, 224, 233, 234, 246, 256, 257, 266, 269, 278, 281, 282, 286, 287, 322, 324, 326, 328, 334, 368, 370, 391, 393, 405, 406, 415, 416, 417, 418, 419, 420, 421, 422, 423, 424, 425

SDQ 378

secondary health care 13

secondary medical care area 58

secondary shelters 34, 37, 39, 70, 77, 81, 82, 85, 96, 97, 99, 100, 101, 105, 106

secondary-level hospital for radiation exposure 374, 380

second-generation survey 7

selective mutism 133, 134

self-care 382, 384

Self-determination 346

Self-reliance Support Council 205

separated families 368, 370

shelter surveillance 81, 83

shelter wall newspapers 41

shelters 6, 13, 14, 27, 29, 34, 35, 36, 37, 38, 40, 41, 42, 45, 48, 51, 54, 57, 59, 60, 62, 63, 64, 68, 69, 74, 75, 76, 77, 79, 80, 81, 82, 83, 85, 86, 87, 88, 89, 90, 91, 92, 95, 96, 97, 98, 99, 100, 101, 104, 105, 107, 134, 148, 280

shopping tour on a bus 204

short-term dispatch 35

short-term fieldwork 397

shuttle bus 161, 172, 200

sickroom 120

simplified thyroid screening 15

simply syrup 332

simulation 15, 56, 177, 241, 271, 281

sleeping pills 164, 178

sleeplessness 37, 54, 164, 178, 190, 194, 203, 236, 299

SNS 59

social capital 370

Social gatherings 157, 318

social network 91

social networking service 59

social solidarity 205

social workers 336, 338, 362, 364, 366

solid tumors 20, 21, 22, 23

Soma-gun Medical Association 51, 53, 304, 306

Soso 7, 8, 9, 10, 38, 40, 45, 46, 48, 49, 51, 53, 54, 56, 69, 90, 134, 260, 262, 314, 318, 322, 340, 404

Soso Public Health Center 231

Soviet Union 23

Special Act on Evacuees from Nuclear Accidents 64

Special Act on Measures concerning Nuclear Evacuees 130, 132, 134, 135, 143, 148, 228

special food service facilities 127

Special meals 209

special nutritive foods 342

specific health checkups 378

specific medical checkup 39

specific spots recommended for evacuation 28, 70, 254

SPEEDI 7, 13, 15, 30, 205, 277, 306

stable iodine tablets 12, 13, 15, 50, 61, 82, 86, 87, 143, 159, 167, 168, 233, 241

sticks 334, 338

stock 42, 46, 61, 80, 82, 121, 128, 132, 133, 134, 140, 147, 180, 182, 206, 239, 250, 273, 330, 408, 409

stockings 116

stockpiles for an emergency 154, 155, 166, 195, 198, 256, 293

stockpiles for emergencies 180, 260, 273

Stoma devices 183

storage depots for drugs 330

straw sandal making 166

Strengths and Difficulties Questionnaire 378

stress 37, 38, 54, 87, 90, 101, 102, 117, 141, 145,

146, 153, 154, 156, 160, 162, 164, 165, 167, 169, 171, 177, 178, 179, 190, 191, 193, 194, 204, 228, 236, 289, 293, 299, 306, 318, 320, 346, 348, 350, 354, 358, 360, 380, 397
stretching exercises 116
strokes 334
study sessions 121, 165, 235, 241, 266, 276, 291, 292, 417
suicide 103, 117, 118, 120, 122, 129, 133, 136, 141, 146, 148, 153, 154, 156, 163, 164, 166, 170, 177, 181, 183, 190, 194, 197, 203, 207, 209, 217, 218, 220, 226, 228, 230, 236, 240, 242, 247, 249, 251, 257, 259, 261, 270, 275, 279, 290, 297, 298, 299, 348
Summer camp programs 261
Support Activities 238, 314, 352, 354
support agreement 35
support center 97, 99, 100, 101, 102, 103, 142, 144, 148, 159, 166, 169, 171, 190, 196, 198, 210, 211, 236, 243, 280, 295, 298, 340, 350
Support for a cooking practice course 100
Support Meeting for Affected Persons with Disabilities 97
support shelters 76
support the support worker 73
surface soil 112, 150, 151, 160, 161, 187, 200, 214, 215, 223, 224, 233, 240, 245, 246, 254, 258, 265, 266, 286, 289, 415, 416, 417, 418, 419, 420, 421, 422, 423, 424, 425
surveillance 41, 48, 62
survey meter 6, 13, 42, 44, 60, 93, 258, 289, 324
survey on the health conditions and lifestyle of residents 268, 271
symptoms 3, 4, 7, 18, 37, 41, 49, 51, 133, 145, 160, 170, 178, 257, 360, 372
System for Prediction of Environmental Emergency Dose Information 7, 13, 30, 205, 276, 306

T

Tamura City XXI, 74, 75, 119, 138, 140, 141, 142, 143, 232, 233, 235, 237, 238, 241, 242, 304, 316, 322, 350, 376, 406
Teamwork 364
telephone consultations 378, 380
temporary houses 27, 37, 38, 39, 40, 45, 57, 62, 63, 68, 70, 71, 72, 74, 77, 78, 79, 82, 83, 85, 87, 88, 92, 95, 96, 99, 100, 101, 102, 103, 104, 106, 107
Temporary housing liaison personnel 164
temporary town 66
Temporary welfare facilities 83
TEPCO 10, 17, 348, 410
tertiary radiation emergency hospital 5
Tertiary Radiation Medical Institution 391, 392
tertiary-level emergency hospital 376
thick liquid diets 342
Three Mile Island accident 370
threshold 18, 20, 21, 22

thyroid cancer 15, 16, 17, 24, 66, 332, 406, 410
thyroid gland examination 144, 157, 167, 187, 218, 293
thyroid monitor 15, 30, 31
thyroid nodule 21, 24
thyroid screening 30
thyroid ultrasound examination 44, 146, 376, 378
Tokyo Electric Power Company XX, 3, 12, 17, 27, 34, 46, 58, 69, 105, 111, 112, 124, 137, 149, 158, 159, 173, 174, 185, 199, 200, 213, 222, 232, 244, 253, 263, 276, 284, 293, 294, 303, 314, 322, 328, 334, 342, 346, 348, 368, 374, 380, 404, 410, 415, 416, 417, 418, 419, 420, 421, 422, 423, 424, 425
Tokyo Electric Power Company Fukushima Daiichi Nuclear Power Station Accident 3, 12
Tokyo Metropolitan Geriatric Hospital and Institute of Gerontology 360
Tokyo Metropolitan Institute of Gerontology 360
Tomioka Town XXI, 7, 45, 75, 92, 111, 112, 113, 114, 115, 116, 117, 118, 119, 120, 121, 150, 304, 328, 356, 376, 406
traditional medicine 362
trauma 146, 346
triage 46, 261, 262, 392
troublesome habits 123
truant 133, 134, 167, 168, 181, 207
trust 32, 154, 177, 191, 194, 205, 208, 240, 271, 274, 290, 299, 350, 370, 372, 384, 391
tube feeding nutrients 229
Tyvek suit 47

U

unbalanced nutrition 346
underestimate 10, 410
underpopulated areas 384, 386
United Nations Scientific Committee on the Effects of Atomic Radiation 15, 23
United States Department of Energy 23
University of Aizu 322, 324, 374
UNSCEAR 15, 23

V

vaccinations 87, 100, 116, 130, 132, 134, 143, 154, 157, 159, 171, 193, 250
vegetable intake 346
ventilator 364
victim-centered recovery 356
Visiting health consultations 70
vulnerable people 13, 31, 36, 80, 84, 121, 122, 135, 147, 155, 168, 182, 183, 195, 209, 219, 223, 229, 231, 242, 250, 251, 260, 277, 281, 407, 408

W

walking aids 334

Wandering   123
warning zones   14
website   93, 125, 247, 264, 265, 278, 291, 316,
     374, 376, 382, 411
weighted absorbed dose   19
Welfare commissioners   122
welfare counselors   356, 358
welfare shelters   84, 105, 148
WHO   8, 9, 10, 11
whole-body counter   8, 9, 15, 30, 31, 37, 44, 64,
     94, 328
Wide-Area Disaster & Emergency Medical Information
     System   87
World Health Organization   8, 9, 11

Y

yoga   338

γ

γ-rays   3, 4, 7, 18, 19

Public Health in a Nuclear Disaster: Message from Fukushima

Edited by Seiji Yasumura and Kenji Kamiya

Originally published in Japan as
Genshiryoku Saigai No Koushu Eisei: Fukushima karano Hasshin
by Nanzando Co., Ltd., Tokyo
© 2014

This edition includes a newly added chapter five: Measures taken
by Hiroshima University.

© 2016   Hiroshima University Press
ISBN 978-4-903068-37-4

Printed in Japan